SAUNDERS REVIEW OF
Family Practice

SAUNDERS REVIEW OF
Family Practice

3rd Edition

Edward T. Bope, MD
Residency Director
Riverside Methodist Family Practice Residency
Riverside Methodist Hospital
Clinical Professor
Department of Family Medicine
The Ohio State University College of Medicine
Columbus, Ohio

Michael D. Hagen, MD
Professor
Department of Family Practice
University of Kentucky College of Medicine
Lexington, Kentucky

SAUNDERS
An Imprint of Elsevier Science
Philadelphia   London   New York   St. Louis   Sydney   Toronto

SAUNDERS
An Imprint of Elsevier Science

The Curtis Center
Independence Square West
Philadelphia, Pennsylvania 19106

Notice

Family Practice is an ever-changing field. Standard safety precautions must be followed, but as new research and clinical experience broaden our knowledge, changes in treatment and drug therapy may become necessary or appropriate. Readers are advised to check the most current product information provided by the manufacturer of each drug to be administered to verify the recommended dose, the method and duration of administration, and the contraindications. It is the responsibility of the treating physician, relying on experience and knowledge of the patient, to determine the dosages and best treatment for each individual patient. Neither the publisher nor the editor assumes any liability for any injury and/or damage to persons or property arising from this publication.

THE PUBLISHER

Library of Congress Cataloging-in-Publication Data

Saunders review of family practice/[edited by] Edward T. Bope, Michael D. Hagen.—3rd ed.
   p. ; cm.
      Companion vol. to: Textbook of family practice/[edited by] Robert E. Rakel. 6th ed. c2002.
      Includes bibliographical references.
      ISBN 0–7216–8821–7
   1. Family medicine—Case studies. 2. Family medicine—Examinations, questions, etc.
   I. Title: Review of family Practice. II. Bope, Edward T. III. Hagan, Michael D. IV.
   Textbook of family practice.
      [DNLM: 1. Family Practice—Examination Questions. 2. Comprehensive Health
   Care—Examination Questions. WB 18.2 S257 2002]
      RC46 .T327 2002 Suppl.   610—dc21

                                                                      2002017681

Editor: Liz Fathman
Editorial Assistant: Paige Mosher Wilke
Designer: Steven Stave

KI/MVY

Printed in the United States of America

Last digit is the print number: 9   8   7   6   5   4   3   2   1

Contributors

Avril Anthony-Wilson, MD
Clinical Assistant Professor, Department of Community
and Preventive Medicine, Mount Sinai School of
Medicine, New York, New York; Associate Director,
Department of Family Practice, Jamaica Hospital
Medical Center, Jamaica, New York
Emergency Medicine

Ann M. Aring, MD
Assistant Program Director, Department of Family
Medicine, Riverside Methodist Hospital; Clinical
Assistant Professor, Department of Family Medicine,
The Ohio State University College of Medicine,
Columbus, Ohio
Care of the Dying Patient; Nicotine Addiction

Syved S. Azhar, MD, MBA
Assistant Professor, Department of Family Medicine,
University of Texas Medical Branch, Galveston, Texas
Ophthalmology

Edward T. Bope, MD
Residency Director, Riverside Methodist Family
Practice Residency, Riverside Methodist Hospital;
Clinical Professor, Department of Family Medicine,
The Ohio State University College of Medicine,
Columbus, Ohio
Infectious Diseases, Endocrinology

Chad M. Braun, MD
Assistant Clinical Professor, Department of Family
Medicine, The Ohio State University College of
Medicine, Columbus, Ohio
The Family Genogram

Robert W. Brenner, MD
Clinical Assistant Professor, Department of Family
Medicine, New Jersey Medical School/University of
Medicine and Dentistry of New Jersey; Residency
Director, Mountainside Family Practice Associates,
Mountainside Hospital/Atlantic Health System,
Newark, New Jersey
Alcohol Abuse

Darrin L. Bright, MD
Assistant Professor, Department of Family Medicine,
Division of Sports Medicine, The Ohio State
University College of Medicine, Columbus, Ohio
Sports Medicine

Alvah R. Cass, MD, SM
Associate Professor, Vice Chair, and Director of
Research, Department of Family Medicine,
University of Texas Medical Branch, Galveston, Texas
Practice-Based Research, Clinical Genetics

Ron Cook, DO
Assistant Professor, Department of Family and
Community Medicine, Texas Tech University Health
Sciences Center, Lubbock, Texas
Psychosocial Influences on Health

Steven A. Crawford, MD
Professor and Chair, Department of Family and
Preventative Medicine, University of Oklahoma
College of Medicine; Chief, Department of Family
Medicine Service, Oklahoma University Medical
Center, Oklahoma City, Oklahoma
Endocrinology

Lanyard K. Dial, MD
Associate Professor, Department of Family Medicine,
UCLA School of Medicine, Los Angeles;
Director, Family Practice Residency, Ventura
County Medical Center, Ventura, California
*Preparing to Take the American Board of Family Practice
Examinations*

Charles Driscoll, MD, MSEd
Clinical Professor, Department of Family Medicine,
Medical College of Virginia,
University of Virginia; Residency Director,
Department of Family Practice, Centra Health of
Lynchburg, Lynchburg, Virginia
Arrhythmias

James B. Dunnan, MD
Clinical Assistant Professor, Department of Family
Medicine, The Ohio State University College of
Medicine; Staff Physician, Department of Family
Medicine, Mount Carmel Medical Center,
Columbus, Ohio
Anxiety Disorders

William Elder, Jr, PhD
Associate Professor, Department of Family Practice,
University of Kentucky College of Medicine,
Lexington, Kentucky
Crisis, Trauma, and Disaster Intervention

Wanda Gonsalves, MD
Residency Director and Assistant Professor,
Department of Family Practice, University of
Kentucky College of Medicine, Lexington, Kentucky
Nutrition and Family Medicine

Peter G. Gosselink, MD
Resident Physician, Department of Family Medicine,
University of Texas Medical Branch, Galveston, Texas
Chilhood and Adolescence

Michael D. Hagen, MD
Professor, Department of Family Practice, University of
Kentucky College of Medicine, Lexington, Kentucky
*Evidence-Based Medicine, Establishing Rapport, Clinical Problem
Solving, Endocrinology, Interpreting Laboratory Tests, Clinical
Guidelines, Clinical Informatics in Office Practice*

Robert G. Hosey, MD
Assistant Professor, Department of Family Practice,
University of Kentucky College of Medicine,
Lexington, Kentucky
Hematology, Neurology

Jamal Islam, MD
Assistant Professor, Department of Family Medicine,
University of Texas Medical Branch, Galveston,
Texas
Cardiovascular Disease

Robert L. Keith, PhD
Department of Family Medicine University of Texas
Medical Branch, Galveston, Texas
*Practicing Biopsychosocial Medicine, Behavioral Problems in
Children and Adolescents*

Daniel Knight, MD
Residency Program Director, Department of Family
and Community Medicine, University of Arkansas for
Medical Sciences, Little Rock, Arkansas
Accounting Systems

Richard P. Kratche, MD
Assistant Clinical Professor, Department of Family
Medicine, Case Western Reserve University School
of Medicine; Staff Physician, Associate Medical
Director, CCF Solon Family Health Center,
Department of Family Medicine, The Cleveland
Clinic Foundation, Cleveland, Ohio
Parasitology

Dennis LaRavia, MD
Professor and Program Director, Department of Family
Medicine, Family Practice Residency of the Brazos
Valley, Texas A & M Health Science Center;

Physician, Saint Joseph Regional Medical Center,
Department of Family Medicine, Bryan, Texas
Risk Management

Thomas G. Maddox, MD
Associate Professor, Department of Community and
Family Medicine; Associate Program Director, Family
Practice Residency, and Chair, Department of Family
Practice, St. Luke's Hospital, Kansas City, Missouri
Infectious Diseases, Care of the Adult HIV-Infected Patient

Stephen Markovich, MD
Assistant Clinical Professor, Department of Family
Medicine, The Ohio State University College of
Medicine; Associate Medical Director, Riverside
Hospital, Columbus, Ohio
Obstetrics

George W. Miller, Jr, MD
Clinical Assistant Professor, Department of Family
Medicine, UMDNJ – Robert Wood Johnson Medical
School; Associate Chairman, Department of Family
Medicine, St. Joseph's Regional Medical Center,
New Brunswick, New Jersey
Abuse of Controlled Substances

William F. Miser, MD
Associate Professor and Residency Director,
Department of Family Medicine, The Ohio State
University College of Medicine, Columbus, Ohio
Problem-Oriented Medical Record

Jada Moore-Ruffin, MD
Associate Director, Family Practice Residency Program,
Grant Medical Center, Columbus, Ohio
Growth and Development

Peter M. Nalin, MD
Associate Professor and Residency Director,
Department of Family Medicine, Indiana University
School of Medicine; Member, Clarian Medical Staff,
Clarian Health Partners, Indianapolis, Indiana
Rheumatology and Musculoskeletal Problems

Lisa R. Nash, DO
Assistant Professor, Department of Family Medicine,
University of Texas Medical Branch, Galveston,
Texas
Contraception

David A. Nelsen, Jr, MD
Assistant Professor, Department of Family and
Community Medicine, University of Arkansas for
Medical Sciences, Little Rock, Arkansas
Travel Medicine

Dana Nottingham, MD
Assistant Residency Director, Riverside Methodist
  Family Practice Residency, Riverside Methodist
  Hospital; Clinical Assistant Professor,
  Department of Family Medicine, The Ohio State
  University College of Medicine, Columbus,
  Ohio
Patient Education

Jeri A. O'Donnell, MA, LPCC
Director of Clinical Behavioral Science, Riverside
  Methodist Family Practice Residency, Riverside
  Methodist Hospital; Assistant Professor, The Ohio
  State University College of Medicine; Columbus,
  Ohio
Domestic Violence

John O'Handley, MD
Clinical Associate Professor, Department of Family
  Medicine, The Ohio State University College of
  Medicine; Program Director, Family Practice
  Residency, Mount Carmel Medical Center,
  Columbus, Ohio
Urinary Tract Disorders

Juan A. Perez, MD
Assistant Professor, Department of Family Medicine,
  New Jersey Medical School/University of Medicine
  and Dentistry of New Jersery, Newark, New Jersey
Care of the Elderly

Richard D. Pham, MD
Assistant Professor, Department of Family Medicine,
  University of Texas Medical Branch, Galveston, Texas
Gynecology

R. Michael Ragain, MD
Vice Chair for Academic Programs, Department of
  Family and Community Medicine, Texas Tech
  University Health Sciences Center; Program
  Director, Family Practice Residency, Texas Tech
  University Medical Center, Lubbock, Texas
Periodic Health Examination

Linda Roethel, MD
Faculty Attending, Department of Family Practice,
  South Nassau Communities Hospital, Oceanside,
  New York
Dementia

Alan R. Roth, DO
Assistant Clinical Professor of Community and Preventive
  Medicine, Department of Community and Preventive
  Medicine, Mount Sinai School of Medicine, New
  York, New York; Chairman and Residency Director,

Department of Family Practice, Jamaica Hospital
  Medical Center, Jamaica, New York
Gastrointestinal Diseases

Michael P. Rowane, DO
Assistant Professor of Family Medicine and Psychiatry,
  Department of Family Medicine, Case Western
  Reserve University/School of Medicine; Residency
  Director, Department of Family Medicine, University
  Hospitals of Cleveland Family Practice Residency
  Program, Cleveland, Ohio
Office Evaluation and Management of Personality Disorders

William A. Rowane, MD
Assistant Clinical Professor, Department of Psychiatry,
  Case Western Reserve University/School of Medicine,
  Cleveland, Ohio
Office Evaluation and Management of Personality Disorders

David R. Rudy, MD, MPH
Professor and Chairman, Acting Medical Director of
  University Clinics, Department of Family Medicine,
  Finch University of Health Science; Attending
  Physician, Department of Family Practice, Highland
  Park Hospital, North Chicago, Illinois
Endocrinology

Dennis Ruppel, MD
Program Director, Family Practice Residency
  Program, Mount Carmel Health System, Columbus,
  Ohio
Allergy

Alison Rutledge, PhD
Institute for Medical Humanities, University of Texas
  Medical Branch, Galveston, Texas
Ethics in Family Practice

Samuel A. Sandowski, MD
Assistant Professor, Department of Family Practice,
  State University of New York, Health Science
  Center at Stony Brook, Stony Brook; Assistant
  Director and Residency Director, South
  Nassau Communities Hospital, Oceanside,
  New York
*Interpretation of the Electrocardiogram, Orthopedics, Sexuality in
  Family Medicine*

Mrunal S. Shah, MD
Assistant Program Director, Riverside Methodist
  Family Practice Residency, Riverside Methodist
  Hospital; Clinical Assistant Professor, College of
  Medicine and Public Health, The Ohio State
  University, Columbus, Ohio
Pulmonary Medicine

Gurjeet S. Shokar, MD
Assistant Professor, Department of Family Medicine,
  University of Texas Medical Branch, Galveston,
  Texas
Depression

Navkiran K. Shokar, MD
Assistant Professor, Department of Family Medicine,
  University of Texas Medical Branch, Galveston,
  Texas
Preventive Health Care, Depression

Victor S. Sierpina, MD
Associate Professor, Department of Family Medicine,
  University of Texas Medical Branch, Galveston,
  Texas
Mind-Body Medicine

Nicole Solomos, DO
Clinical Instructor, Department of Family Practice,
  State University of New York, Health Science Center
  at Stony Brook; South Nassau Communities Hospital,
  Oceanside, New York
Orthopedics

Dorothy B. Trevino, LMSW, PhD
Associate Professor and Director of Behavioral
  Medicine, Department of Family Medicine,
  University of Texas Medical Branch, Galveston,
  Texas
Somatic Patient

Ana Catalina Triana, MD
Family Systems Medicine Fellow, Department of
  Family Medicine, University of Texas Medical
  Branch, Galveston, Texas
The Family's Influence on Health

Bruce Vanderhoff, MD
Chair and Associate Residency Director, Department of
  Family Practice, Grant Medical Center; Clinical
  Assistant Professor, Department of Family Medicine,
  The Ohio State University College of Medicine,
  Columbus, Ohio
Otolaryngology

David Vander Straten, MD
Assistant Professor, Department of Family Medicine,
  University of Texas Medical Branch, Galveston, Texas
Dermatology

William A. Verhoff, RN, BSN
Nurse Manager, Riverside Family Practice Center,
  Riverside Methodist Hospital, Columbus, Ohio
*Interviewing Techniques, Managed Health Care: Practicing
  Effectively in the 21st Century*

Mary Jo Welker, MD
Chair and Professor of Clinical Family Medicine,
  Department of Family Medicine, The Ohio State
  University College of Medicine, Columbus, Ohio
The Family Physician

Alex Wilgus, MD
Director of Patient Care, Lynchburg Family Practice
  Residency Program, University of Virginia School of
  Medicine; Centra Health of Lynchburg, Lynchburg,
  Virginia
Oncology

A. Stevens Wrightson, MD
Assistant Professor and Associate Residency Program
  Director, Department of Family Practice, University of
  Kentucky College of Medicine, Lexington, Kentucky
Care of the Newborn, Office Surgery

Foreword

Curiosity is one of the permanent and certain characteristics of a vigorous intellect.
Samuel Johnson

One essential ingredient to a successful career in medicine is a persistent curiosity and enthusiasm for learning. Inquisitiveness, testing, and retesting are natural to family physicians. We thrive on the varied challenges of medicine and enjoy the varied problems that confront us daily in practice. We can properly manage 90% of the problems we encounter as primary care physicians, and we are more comfortable with the unknown than are physicians in other specialties and more willing to let time heal or define the condition more clearly.

Ours was the first specialty to require recertification every six years, so that testing and retesting is a way of life for us. We realize how much more we learn from these challenges and recognize how testing keeps our knowledge sharper and more up to date. We are eager to learn more and to provide the best care possible for our patients. *Saunders Review of Family Practice* helps us do both. It also challenges us to be knowledgeable and to remain current with medical advances.

Drs. Bope and Hagen captured the essence of the content of *Textbook of Family Practice* and have designed a variety of questions related to that content in a manner that is both a challenge and informative. They provide a critique of each question, explaining why the answer is correct or incorrect. Everyone, whether experienced physician or second-year student, can benefit from this challenging review.

ROBERT E. RAKEL, MD

Preface

Preparing to master a subject or discipline involves learning in a great many settings and styles. The traditional didactic form occurs in large and small groups. Many people prefer to learn in this fashion. Others prefer self-study and most everyone gravitates to that form to acquire additional knowledge. Knowledge about the great specialty of family practice is achieved piece by piece, usually in settings where the knowledge is immediately applied to a clinical setting. For that reason, comprehensive textbooks like *Textbook of Family Practice* are ideal. They provide basic discussions and specific details on most topics important to a family physician.

Saunders Review of Family Practice is designed as a companion book so that you can test your knowledge on each chapter of *Rakel's Textbook of Family Practice*.

Each question is written by a family physician or family-physician educator to emphasize what they think are the important ideas. By using this book, you will test your knowledge in all aspects of family practice.

Many physicians tell us that the Saunders Review is widely used for board preparation. A new addition this year is the introduction on test taking skills: Preparing to Take the American Board of Family Practice Examination. This new section will help you to sharpen your test-taking skills so that your knowledge is fairly measured. Have fun using this book, and our labor of love, to master the greatest specialty, family practice.

We acknowledge Paul Young, MD, and Bob Avant, MD, who have been our mentors and friends.

We fondly remember our work with
Nicholas Pisacano, MD,
former Executive Director of the American
Board of Family Practice.

Contents

Preparing to Take the American Board of Family Practice Examinations

Lanyard K. Dial

The American Board of Family Practice Examination (ABFP) is designed to test the cognitive knowledge base of family physicians. To prepare to take this examination, the family physician should be familiar with the content and structure of the examination, study appropriately, and have skills necessary to answer standardized examination questions. This section focuses on these concepts.

CONTENT AND STRUCTURE OF THE ABFP EXAMINATION

Creating the Questions

Questions for the ABFP examination are written by family physicians who have completed an ABFP workshop on test question writing skills. These family physicians are in active practice or are teachers in family practice residencies. They write 20 questions per year and must include documentation to support each answer from a standard text or journal article. The questions are then edited by an ABFP test development staff member and placed into a computer database of potential test questions. Each year more than 800 questions from this database are pulled for placement on the current year's examinations. These questions are reviewed by groups of physicians, including the members of the Board of Family Practice, a panel of multiple specialty physicians, and a panel of family physicians. These groups ensure that each question is relevant and that the answer is correct before the question is placed on the final examination. The family physician panel also provides an estimate of the percentage of questions that need to be answered correctly for a passing score. The process of test preparation takes about 9 to 10 months. Three types of questions are used by the ABFP for the examination.

Multiple-Choice Questions

The most common format of test questions is multiple choice. In these questions, a written sentence or para-graph sets the stage for the examinee to choose the one best answer from a series of options. The written statement is called the "stem," and the answers are structured into 4 or 5 options typically labeled A, B, C, D, and E. The examinee reads the stem, chooses the one best answer, and marks the correct letter on the answer sheet. Each question has only one right answer. No question should have more than one answer marked. Approximately 60% of the questions are in this format.

True-or-False Questions

In these questions, the stem is followed by a sequential list of individually identified answers, each of which must be answered as either true or false. On the examination, each answer is recorded on the answer sheet as either A (True) or B (False). In this manner, a single stem is responsible for more than one scored answer. Approximately 20% of the questions are in this format.

Clinical Set Problem Questions

A unique format is the clinical set questions, which make up the last 20% of the test questions. In this format, a clinical case is presented as the stem. The stem frequently includes physical examination and laboratory results. These data are followed by a sequence of questions about differential diagnosis, management, and treatment. Answers in the clinical set problems are a list of individually numbered true-or-false statements, which are similar to multiple true-or-false statements, but they are designed to test more clinical patient management knowledge and skills.

Preparing the Test Booklets

The questions that are to be used in this year's examination are then placed into test booklets. There are two booklet types: General Knowledge Test Booklets and Discipline-Specific Content Test Booklets.

General Knowledge Test Booklets

The clinical content of the General Knowledge Test Booklet covers the entire field of family practice. The question distribution approximates that of a typical family physician practice. The disciplines covered and their distribution are as follows:

Discipline	Questions in General Knowledge Test Booklet (%)
Internal medicine	36
Pediatrics	13
Geriatrics	12
Gynecology	10
Community medicine	9
Obstetrics	7
Psychiatry	7
Surgery	6

Two types of General Knowledge Test Booklets are prepared. The first, labeled Book A, includes all three question types discussed earlier and has a total of 350 test questions (220 in the clinical set problem test format and 130 others). The second type of General Knowledge Test Booklet, labeled Book C, includes multiple-choice and multiple true-or-false type questions but no clinical set problem type questions. Book C also includes pictorial items, such as x-rays, dermatology slides, ECG tracings, obstetrical monitor strips, and so forth. Book C has 180 questions.

Discipline-Specific Test Booklets

The individual discipline-specific test booklets contain 60 questions. These booklets, called modules, include only questions related to a specific discipline. The current modules are as follows: Medicine, Surgery, Pediatrics, Obstetrics, Gynecology, Geriatrics, and Emergent/Urgent Care.

The clinical content of each module is related only to its individual discipline. The examinee answers only the questions from that specific content area. The question types in these modules are multiple choice and multiple true-or-false with no clinical set problems.

Who Takes Which Examination

The ABFP examination is given both to first-time examinees (first-time certificants or certifiers) and to individuals who are currently certified and are taking the examination for their recertification (recertificants or recertifiers). The structures for these two groups are different.

First-Time Test Takers (Certificants)

The majority of certificants are recent residency graduates. Other family physicians who are eligible to take the examination and are taking it for the first time are also included in this group, such as Canadian family physicians who share reciprocity rights with the ABFP.

The examination for certificants uses only the General Knowledge Test Booklets. The morning examination period uses Book A, and the afternoon examination period uses Book C. In this manner, the certificants are tested in the full spectrum of family medicine.

Recertification Examination

The recertification examination is given to all family physicians who have been previously certified. The examination is offered in two formats: one for physicians who have an active practice in family medicine and another for family physicians who have limited or no patient care responsibilities. These two groups are called Process A recertifiers and Process B recertifiers, respectively. Process B recertifiers must send a letter with their application for recertification to the ABFP that explains why they cannot take the Process A examination format and be granted approval to take the Process B examination.

Process A

The examination for practicing family physicians consists of a morning session utilizing the General Knowledge Examination Booklet Book A and an afternoon testing session that uses three of the 60-question Discipline-Specific Test Booklet Modules. The three modules are chosen by the recertifying physician before the examination from the list of seven available modules. This format allows recertifying family physicians to focus their afternoon examination on clinical content areas that reflect their individual practices.

Process B

The Process B recertificants' examination is identical to that of the certificants. The morning and afternoon examination periods use the General Knowledge Test Booklets. The morning examination uses Book A and the afternoon, Book C. Thus, Process B recertifiers must answer questions across the field of care of a family physician.

Scoring

The completed examinations are scored by the ABFP in the following manner: Points are given for correct answers, and no points are given for incorrect answers. Incorrect answers are not subtracted from the score of the examinee, thus allowing examinees to improve their score by guessing.

The grading of scores is a complex process that utilizes a predetermined passing score set by the ABFP family physician panel and the roughly bell-shaped distribution of scores for the examination itself. Each year the examination fails between 3% and 15% of examinees.

STUDY AND PREPARATION FOR THE ABFP EXAMINATION

All of us approach a standardized examination with some degree of trepidation that creates anxiety. Being in a mildly high epinephrine state as you begin an examination is actually beneficial in that it helps you to focus and be sharp as you answer questions, but you will find that your energy declines as the day goes on and fatigue sets in.

Being in an overanxious state, however, is detrimental to overall performance. You cannot do your personal best on an examination if you are too nervous or too anxious about your performance or abilities. The goal of your study and preparation is to be able to enter the examination room feeling confident in your ability to do well.

Pre-Test Study Plan

The structure of the ABFP examination is such that no single source of material can be used to study for the examination. In fact, the ABFP itself has said that the best preparation is "keeping up through an active practice, peer interactions, CME, review courses, and journals." The examination questions are selected to reflect standard accepted clinical practice material, and because it is prepared over a nine-month period, most of the factual information should be available in textbooks. Certainly, the newest research published in peer review journals will not be included.

It is difficult to learn and retain material simply by reading textbooks or review articles. My suggested approach to study for the examination is to use a set of practice questions. Questions can be found in many texts, such as this one or others, as well as in some journals. Many companies have made questions available either on CD-ROMs or over the Internet. The ABFP has a web site that includes board practice questions at www.familypractice.com. Most of the CME board review courses provide test questions for practice. It is important that practice questions include answers that discuss the information.

Set aside time to practice one to three times a week with questions for four to six months before the examination. Answer 20 to 30 questions per session, and read the discussion about those questions. Have available a standard family practice text to do further reading in areas in which you determine you need more understanding. It is also helpful to create memory sheets as you do these study sessions. Memory sheets are a collection of blank pages of paper on which you write facts that you have difficulty remembering. Over these months, these sheets will be filled with the information you need to memorize before taking the examination. During the last month of your study, set aside 30 minutes two to three times a week to review these sheets. After the examination, these pages make a handy reference source for later needs.

Week of the Examination

It is important to plan some activities for the week of the examination. First, no study of questions or reading of review materials should occur on Thursday, the day before the examination. The memory sheets are important to review on this day, but no other material. This day should be used to do an activity that will best allow you to rest and be stress free.

Plan for the necessary transportation to the test site to ensure that you arrive in a stress-free state. Think through the clothes you will wear to the examination. Plan to wear clothing that is layered for maximum comfort, and if you have a lucky outfit, shirt, blouse, hat, or shoes, wear them. Whatever gives you a sense of pride and confidence is good for your test day. Plan your food needs. Most people will want to have a good breakfast before the morning examination session.

Tips for the Overall Examination Process

When the examination begins and you first open your booklet, it is best to take a minute for an overall look at the examination questions. Start at the last page and see how many total questions are on the examination. Next, flip through the pages to determine the flow of questions—where are the short questions, where are the long questions, and where are the clinical set problems? Look for the possible pictorial questions—ECGs, x-rays, dermatology slides, and obstetrical monitor strips. By doing this one-minute overview, you will know better how to pace your test time and reduce your anxiety as you turn test pages.

Your answer sheet is the key to your test score. You can and should make marks in your test booklet, but you must make sure that your answer sheet is done correctly. Mark your answer on the answer sheet as you do each question. *Do not plan on transferring answers from your booklet to the answer sheet at the end of the test session.* As you are answering questions, periodically ensure that the number of the question is the number of the answer you are marking on the answer sheet. It is very important to not skip a question and mismark your answer sheet.

Testmanship—Tips for Answering Individual Questions

Test questions are designed to determine a physician's cognitive knowledge about the discipline of family practice. Each question has a set of answers from which the examinee must pick the correct answer. In this section, we look at specific suggestions for answering questions, or how to improve your "testmanship."

Tip 1: Read the questions and answers carefully.

One common error is to be in a hurry or anxious and to misread the question. Key words or phrases in many of the questions must not be missed. "Except," "contraindicated," "what is the first step . . .," "most likely," and "least likely" are common examples.

Answers also have some important words buried in them. Because medicine is not black or white, words such as "always," "at all times," "never," or "exactly" should cause the examinee to eliminate these answers as potential choices. Do not confuse these terms with the frequently used "none of the above" and "all of the above," which can be correct answers.

Tip 2: Look for the principle of the question.

Test questions are written to assess your knowledge about a specific principle. If you can determine the underlying principle of the question, you will be able to more successfully answer it. The principle often is not stated but is implied through a short case scenario. As you read the stem, recognize that the written words in the scenario are purposeful to lead you to the principle.

As an example, the following question was designed to determine whether the examinee knew that a functional assessment is fundamental to the field of geriatrics:

Sample question: An 85-year-old woman is admitted after a fall resulting in the fracture of her right hip. After repair of her hip and in-hospital physical therapy, she is scheduled for discharge. She lives alone in a second-floor apartment and must negotiate three steps to get to her bedroom. She has two daughters who live in the community, and both have jobs that occupy their daytime hours. The first step in planning her discharge is to:

A. Discuss her needs with her daughters
B. Determine the patient's financial abilities
C. Determine the patient's functional status
D. Arrange for necessary home care services
E. Plan to send her to a skilled nursing facility for further rehabilitation

The correct answer is C. All the answers are good ideas, but functional assessment is the underlying principle first step. When reading the stem, do not get lost in some of the details (three steps or daughters work).

Tip 3: Avoid getting angry about questions and avoid using anecdotal or local issue information as you look for answers.

Many questions appear confusing or not to have answers that seem to you to be correct. The test question's author believes there is a right answer and, for the purpose of passing the examination, the examinee must determine which answer to choose. Anger about questions is counterproductive to finding the best solution and will linger into future questions. Do not use anecdotal information or local issues in answering questions; search for the underlying principle.

Sample question: A 42-year-old man is being maintained on ventilatory support because of end stage ALS. He is bedbound and his movement is limited entirely to his eyes. He communicates by eye motions using a letter board. He requests that you, as his physician, disconnect his mechanical ventilator. His family does not agree with this request. Your responsibility is to:

A. Ask for an opinion from legal counsel
B. Begin therapy with an antidepressant
C. Refuse to turn off the mechanical ventilator
D. Work with the family and staff to plan for discontinuing the ventilator
E. Remove yourself from the case

This question presents a difficult and potentially contentious problem. Many examinees are angry that there is not a choice about involving an ethics committee, or an examinee chooses the answer to involve legal counsel because of a case that he or she has had in practice. The standard principle that this question addresses, however, is patient rights to decision making at the end of life.

Tip 4: In questions with long stems, read the answers first.

Many questions, particularly the clinical set problems, have long stems that detail a clinical scenario and are followed by a set of answers. It is best in these instances to read the answers first. Doing so will enable examinees to better focus their reading of the stem and reduce the need to reread it.

Tip 5: Eliminate answers you know are incorrect to improve your guessing odds.

One of the fundamentals of testmanship is to find and eliminate wrong answers. Most multiple-choice questions have five answers, so you have a 20% chance of getting the question correct with a guess. If you can find two or three wrong answers, eliminate them from your guessing options, you significantly improve your chance of guessing correctly.

Tip 6: Do not pick choices that are unfamiliar but sound correct.

As test writers develop questions, they must create incorrect answers. One of the ways to create a good incorrect answer is to make up something that sounds good but is not correct. Do not select answers that are unfamiliar to you.

Sample multiple true-or-false question: Which of the following are commonly used to manage patients with erectile dysfunction:

A. Intraurethral implant of a prostaglandin medication
B. Intracorporal injection of vasoactive medication
C. Oral medication that increases cGMP
D. Transdermal vasoactive medication
E. Surgical insertion of an erectile implant
F. External vacuum assistive device

All of these answers are true except D. That answer sounds correct, but such a transdermal system is not available.

Tip 7: Analyze similar answers carefully.

In some questions, two or three answers look alike but have important variations. These answers should catch the attention of the examinee. One of these answers frequently is the correct one, but simple alterations have been made to change it into an incorrect answer.

Sample question: The most common location for the Christmas tree–like rash of pityriasis rosea is:

A. Lower extremity
B. Dorsal aspect of the forearm
C. Anterior aspect of the trunk
D. Posterior aspect of the trunk
E. Scalp

The correct answer is D, but a good wrong answer is the opposite of this: the anterior aspect of the trunk. In addition, a common way to alter a good answer is to change a correct answer that includes a number to an incorrect answer by changing the number. In this manner, the question writer is trying to find out if the examinee knows the correct number.

Another use of similar answers in test writing is to create two wrong answers. If a test writer creates an incorrect answer that seems to be a reasonable choice, then a simple change in that answer will make a second reasonable incorrect answer.

Sample question: A 65-year-old man is admitted for antibiotic therapy for diverticulitis. On the second day of hospitalization, he complains of acute onset of right lateral chest pain and shortness of breath. On examination, he is found to be tachycardic and tachypneic and has splinting respiratory effort. His chest x-ray is clear, his ECG shows a deep S wave in lead I, and his ABGs show a marked hypoxia and hypercapnia. Which of the following statements is correct:

A. This clinical picture is characteristic of a rupture of diverticuli and should be treated with emergency surgery.
B. This clinical picture is characteristic of a rupture of his diverticuli and should be treated with IV triple antibiotic therapy.
C. This patient needs emergent treatment with an intravenous thrombolytic.
D. This is a classic description of a pulmonary embolus.
E. This is most likely a rib fracture from undiagnosed metastatic colon malignancy.

The correct answer to this question is D. Answers A and B are written similarly but are both incorrect.

Tip 8: For answers with numbers or percentages, pick a midrange answer.

If you are strictly guessing about a question with answers that are numbers, pick a midrange value. Correct number answers are commonly placed in the center of a list with smaller and larger flanking numbers.

Tip 9: For answers containing numbers or percentages, pick those that look like other answers.

Another way to approach a question with numbers or percentages is to pick a choice from answers that appear similar.

Sample question: A positive PPD reading, as read by the induration of the placed test at 48 hours, in a patient with known HIV disease is:

A. 2 mm
B. 5 mm
C. 8 mm
D. 10 mm
E. 5 cm

In this question, the correct answer is B. The answer that is unlike the rest, E, should be eliminated if you are guessing. Answers A through D are similar (i.e., they are all measurements in millimeters), and if you are guessing then this is the group from which to choose.

Tip 10: Look for answers that support family physician tenets and avoid answers that have poor values.

This is an examination written by family physicians for family physicians, and it will expose the values that are considered important for family physicians. If an answer does not support the tenets of our specialty, then it should eliminated from your choices.

Sample question: A 23-year-old female presents with complaints of a year-long history of intermittent chest pain associated with a rapid heart rate and a feeling of doom. Her examination is normal. Which of the following is appropriate management at this time:

A. Refer her to a psychiatrist to treat her anxiety.
B. Order an ECG, chest x-ray, chemistry panel, lipid panel, and CT scan.
C. Discuss with her that these complaints are common in patients with a borderline personality.
D. Obtain an ECG to look for a shortened PR interval.
E. Prescribe an anxiolytic and have her return for re-evaluation in 6 months.

The correct answer is D. The other answers are all exaggerated to show how you could write answers that do not fit with good values for family physicians.

PART I

PRINCIPLES OF FAMILY PRACTICE

The Family Physician

Mary Jo Welker

1: The family physician provides care that includes all of the following, except care that:

    A. Is comprehensive, continuing, and personalized
    B. Is for patients of all ages and their families
    C. Is limited to the presence of disease
    D. Is given regardless of the presenting complaint

Answer: C

Page: 3

Critique: The family physician provides continuing, comprehensive care in a personalized way to patients of all ages and to their families, regardless of the presence of disease or the nature of the presenting complaint. This care encompasses all ages, both sexes, each organ system, and every disease entity.

2: Family practice includes knowledge of:

    A. Other medical specialties
    B. Family dynamics
    C. Interpersonal relationships
    D. Counseling and psychotherapy
    E. All of the above

Answer: E

Page: 3

Critique: In addition to sharing medical content with other medical specialties, family practice includes knowledge of family dynamics, interpersonal relationships, and counseling and psychotherapy.

3: The American Board of Family Practice came into being as the 20th medical specialty in:

    A. 1923
    B. 1966
    C. 1969
    D. 1971

Answer: C

Pages: 3, 4

Critique: The American Board of Family Practice came into being in 1969 as the 20th medical specialty. In 1923, Francis Peabody called for a rapid return of the generalist physician to give comprehensive and personalized care. In 1966, the Millis Commission report and the Willard Committee report were published. In 1971, the American Academy of General Practice was renamed the American Academy of Family Physicians.

4: The American Board of Family Practice (ABFP) distinguished itself by being the first to:

    A. Require residency training
    B. Require continuing medical education
    C. Require recertification
    D. Use computerized testing

Answer: C

Page: 4

Critique: The ABFP distinguished itself by being the first specialty board to require recertification every 7 years to ensure the ongoing competence of its members. A member of the ABFP must also participate in 50 hours of continuing medical education each year to be eligible for recertification. The ABFP requires residency training, but does not have a computerized version of its recertification test at present.

5: (True or False) Generalist physicians, as defined by the Council on Graduate Medical Education and the American Association of Medical Colleges, includes:

    A. Family medicine
    B. General internal medicine
    C. General pediatrics
    D. Obstetrics and gynecology
    E. Emergency medicine

Answers: A - True, B - True, C - True, D - False, E - False

Page: 4

Critique: The Council on Graduate Medical Education (COGME) and the Association of American Medical Colleges define generalist physicians as those who have completed 3-year training programs in family medicine, internal medicine, and pediatrics and who do not subspecialize. They do not include emergency medicine or obstetrics and gynecology in the definition of primary care physicians.

6: Family physicians must:

    A. Be the patient's advocate
    B. Be able to live with uncertainty
    C. Be able to recognize their limitations
    D. Be willing to refer when necessary
    E. All of the above

Answer: E

Page: 4

Critique: The family physician must be the patient's advocate; be competent, caring, and compassionate; be able to live with uncertainty; be willing to recognize limitations; and be willing to refer when necessary.

Match the following specialties with the recommended competencies for primary care that are achieved in their respective training programs:

    A. 42% of the time
    B. 47% of the time
    C. 66% of the time
    D. 91% of the time
    E. 95% of the time

7: Internal medicine

8: Pediatrics

9: Emergency medicine

10: Family medicine

11: Obstetrics and gynecology

Answers: 7 - D, 8 - D, 9 - A, 10 - E, 11 - B

Page: 5

Critique: Rivo and associates identified common conditions and diagnoses that generalist physicians should be competent to manage and compared these with the training programs of various "generalist" specialties. They found that the goal of including 90% of these diagnoses was met by family practice 95% of the time, by general internal medicine 91% of the time, by general pediatrics 91% of the time, by emergency medicine 42% of the time, and by obstetrics and gynecology 47% of the time.

12: In relation to the gross domestic product (GDP), in 1998 the cost of health care in the United States was:

    A. 6%
    B. 10%
    C. 14%
    D. 19%

Answer: C

Page: 9

Critique: The cost of health care in the United States was 14% of the GDP in 1998.

13: The cost of health care in the United States is so expensive because of:

    A. A low concentration of specialists
    B. Capitation payments
    C. Patient self-referral directly to specialists
    D. Low dependency on specialists for primary care

Answer: C

Page: 9

Critique: Schroeder believes that the United States will continue as one of the most expensive health care systems in the world as long as a high concentration of specialists, fee-for-service payments, patient self-referral directly to specialists, and a high dependency on specialists for provision of primary care exist.

14: In 1997, the number of Americans without health care had risen to:

    A. More than 5%
    B. More than 8%
    C. More than 12%
    D. More than 16%

Answer: D

Page: 9

Critique: The number of Americans without health insurance has been rising steadily and in 1997 had risen to more than 16% of the population.

15: Of all patients seen by a family physician, how many will never be assigned a final, definitive diagnosis:

    A. One sixth
    B. One fourth
    C. One third
    D. One half

Answer: B. One fourth

Page: 11

Critique: Approximately one fourth of all patients seen will never be assigned a final, definitive diagnosis, because the resolution of a presenting symptom or complaint will come before a specific diagnosis can be made.

16: A family physician:

    A. Must, above all, be an outstanding diagnostician
    B. Does not focus on history in making a diagnosis
    C. Does not allow time to pass before making a diagnosis
    D. Evaluates cases after they have been preselected by another physician

Answer: A

Page: 11

Critique: The family physician must, above all, be an outstanding diagnostician. The family physician does not evaluate a case after it has been preselected by another physician but must use procedures selected from the entire spectrum of medicine. The belief that an accurate history is the most important factor in arriving at a diagnosis is especially appropriate to family medicine. Time is used as an important diagnostic aid in family medicine. After the family physician is satisfied that a patient's symptoms are not those of a serious problem, follow-up visits are scheduled at appropriate intervals to watch for changes in the symptoms.

17: Personalized care means all of the following, except:

    A. Understanding the patient as a person
    B. Dealing only with the individual
    C. Respecting the person as an individual
    D. Showing compassion for the patient's discomfort.

Answer: B

Page: 5

Critique: Family practice emphasizes consideration of the individual in the full context of his or her life. The personalized approach includes understanding the patient as a person, respecting the person as an individual, and showing compassion for his or her discomfort.

18: Settings for primary care include:

    A. Office practice
    B. Hospital practice
    C. Long-term care facility
    D. Home
    E. All of the above

Answer: E

Page: 5

Critique: Primary care can occur in a variety of settings, including an office, a hospital, a long-term care facility, a critical care unit, a patient's home, and a day care facility.

19: Families receiving continuing, comprehensive care have:

    A. A greater incidence of hospitalization
    B. More operations
    C. Fewer physician visits for illnesses
    D. More expensive care
    E. Lower quality care

Answer: C

Pages: 7, 8

Critique: Families receiving continuing, comprehensive care have a lower incidence of hospitalization, fewer operations, and fewer physician visits for illnesses compared with those who have no regular physician. Care is also less expensive and of higher quality.

20: In a comparison of family physicians and obstetricians in the management of low-risk pregnancies, women cared for by a family physician had:

    A. More cesarean sections
    B. More episiotomies
    C. More epidural anesthesia
    D. No difference with respect to neonatal outcomes

Answer: D

Page: 8

Critique: A comparison of family physicians and obstetricians in the management of low-risk pregnancies showed no difference with respect to neonatal outcomes. However, women cared for by family physicians had fewer episiotomies and fewer cesarean sections and were less likely to receive epidural anesthesia.

21: Recommendations to medical schools from the Edinburgh Declaration:

    A. Limit the settings in which medical education is conducted in hospitals
    B. Focus on retention and recall of information
    C. Choose students based on intellectual ability and academic achievement
    D. Ensure continuity of learning throughout life

Answer: D

Page: 10

Critique: The recommendations include enlarging the range of settings in which educational programs are conducted to include all health resources of the community, and not hospitals alone. Another recommendation is to ensure continuity of learning throughout life by shifting to more active learning, including self-directed learning, independent study, and tutorial programs. Also recommended is the building of both curriculum and examination systems to ensure the achievement of professional competence and social values, and not just retention and recall of information. Finally, selection methods are recommended for medical students that go beyond intellectual ability and academic achievements to include evaluation of personal qualities.

22: (True or False) To relate well to patients, a physician must:

    A. Gather information slowly
    B. Organize information logically
    C. Focus on a limited number of problems
    D. Listen
    E. Establish rapport and communicate effectively

Answers: A - False, B - True, C - False, D - True, E - True

Pages: 10, 11

Critique: To relate well to patients, a physician must develop compassion and courtesy, establish rapport and communicate effectively, gather information rapidly and organize it logically, identify all significant patient problems, manage these problems appropriately, motivate people, and observe and detect nonverbal clues.

Match the following specialties with the percent of physicians in that specialty who make house calls:

    A. 15%
    B. 47%
    C. 63%

23: General internal medicine

24: General pediatrics

25: Family practice

Answers: 23 - B, 24 - A, 25 - C

Page: 15

Critique: In a 1994 survey of primary care physicians, Adelman and associates found that 63% of family physicians, 47% of general internists, and 15% of pediatricians make house calls.

26: Of all office visits made in 1997, how many were to a primary care physician?

    A. One half
    B. One fourth
    C. One third
    D. One tenth

Answer: A

Page: 15

Critique: In 1997, about one half of all office visits were to the patient's primary care physician.

27: Primary care includes:

    A. Health promotion
    B. Health maintenance and disease prevention
    C. Counseling and patient education
    D. Diagnosis and treatment of acute and chronic illness
    E. All of the above

Answer: E

Page: 5

Critique: In addition to diagnosis and treatment of acute and chronic illnesses, primary care includes health promotion, disease prevention, health maintenance, counseling, and patient education.

28: Patients consider a good physician to be one who does all of the following, except:

    A. Shows genuine interest in them
    B. Superficially evaluates their problem
    C. Demonstrates compassion, understanding, and warmth
    D. Provides clear insight into what is wrong and what must be done to correct it

Answer: B

Page: 6

Critique: Tumulty found that patients consider a good physician to be one who shows genuine interest in them; thoroughly evaluates their problem; demonstrates compassion, understanding, and warmth; and provides clear insight into what is wrong and what must be done to correct it.

29: Comprehensive care includes consideration of:

    A. Religious beliefs
    B. Personal expectations
    C. Cultural problems
    D. Social or economic issues
    E. All of the above

Answer: E

Page: 9

Critique: Comprehensive care includes all factors that may aid or hinder a patient's recovery and requires consideration of religious beliefs, personal expecta-

tions, cultural problems, social or economic issues, and heredity.

30: As the coordinator of care, the family physician:

    A. Selects specialists whose skills can be applied most appropriately to a given case
    B. Involves appropriate community resources
    C. Communicates with other providers
    D. Explains the nature of the illness and the implications of treatment to the patient
    E. All of the above

Answer: E

Page: 12

Critique: The family physician is best prepared to select specialists whose skills can be applied most appropriately to a given case and facilitates the patient's access to the system. The family physician communicates with the patient about the system, the procedures to be performed, the nature of the illness, the implications of the treatment, and the effect on the patient's way of life. The family physician helps the patient choose the best of all possible alternatives after communication with the other providers. The family physician also involves other community resources when necessary, including nurses, social agencies, the clergy, and other family members.

Match the following practice styles with the percentage of graduating family practice residents who chose that style in 1999:

    A. 41.9%
    B. 12.4%
    C. 10.2%
    D. 4.0%

31: Solo practice

32: Family practice group practice

33: Multispecialty group practice

34: Partnership

Answers: 31 - D, 32 - A, 33 - B, 34 - C

Page: 16

Critique: In 1999, 41.9% of graduating family practice residents entered family practice group practices, 12.4% joined multispecialty group practices, 10.2% formed partnerships with two-person practices, and only 4.0% entered solo practice.

Chapter 2

The Family Genogram

Chad Braun

1: The components of a genogram include all of the following, except:

    A. All members of both spouses' families
    B. The age or year of birth of all family members
    C. Significant diseases or problems of family members
    D. Two or more generations
    E. Dates of marriages and divorces

Answer: D

Pages: 20, 21

Critique: The standard family genogram includes:

- Three or more generations
- The names of all family members
- Age or year of birth of all family members
- Any deaths, including age at death or date and cause
- Significant diseases or problems of family members
- Indication of members living together in the same household
- Dates of marriages and divorces
- A key for interpretation of symbols

2: Who is the index person in the family genogram?

    A. The patriarch
    B. The matriarch
    C. The oldest living relative, regardless of gender
    D. A family member of great medical significance
    E. A family member who inspires a genogram

Answer: E

Page: 20

Critique: The index person (similar to the proband) is the major reason for developing a genogram. Often this member is significant because of a chronic disease or an overwhelming problem. Age and gender have no bearing.

3: Which of the following is *not* proper identification for an index person?

    A. An arrow
    B. A triangle
    C. A double square
    D. A double circle

Answer: B

Page: 20

Critique: Familiarity with the standard symbols used in a family genogram is essential for rapid retrieval of information. An index person may be denoted by an arrow, a double square, or a double circle.

4: (True or False) Which of the following are commonly recognized uses of a family genogram?

    A. Identifying significant family risk factors
    B. Demonstrating family relationships
    C. Building patient rapport by using appropriate family names
    D. Allowing the family physician to quickly review family dynamics
    E. Recognizing the need for screening of patients at increased risk

Answer: A - True, B - True, C - True, D - True, E - True

Page: 22

Critique: Uses of the genogram include:

- Allowing other medical professionals to understand the family
- Building rapport by using appropriate family names
- Identifying at a glance significant risk factors within a family
- Recognizing the need for screening family members at high risk
- Promoting lifestyle changes and placing emphasis on patient education
- Demonstrating that family relationships are of concern to the family physician

5: Which of the following is *not* an example of functional charting?

    A. Depicting various strengths of emotional attachment
    B. Listing of familial occupations
    C. Representing marital discord
    D. Depicting dominant personalities

Answer: B

Page: 22

Critique: Functional charting allows representation of the social and interpersonal influences that operate within a family. This includes depiction of emotional relationships and gives a dynamic picture of the family. Varying strengths of emotional bonds can be shown, as can marital discord and dominant personalities. Occupation, while an important part of the genogram, is not a part of functional charting.

6: Which one of the following is *not* one of the four basic components of the genogram?

    A. Relationships
    B. Structure
    C. Demographics
    D. Events
    E. Problems

Answer: A

Page: 26

Critique: The four basic components of the genogram are structure, demographics, events, and problems. Analysis of these components helps to give insight into the interpretation of the genogram. Specifically, these components may either increase or decrease the likelihood of a specific hypothesis, the occurrence of a preventable disease, or the success rate of a particular therapy. Relationships are not classified as one of the four basic components of a genogram.

7: In which of the following conditions is level of the patient's education *not* associated with decreased mortality rate?

    A. Diabetes
    B. Tuberculosis
    C. Breast cancer
    D. Colon cancer
    E. Suicide

Answer: C

Page: 27

Critique: Genograms are very useful in the evaluation of variables such as marriage and education level on mortality. Breast cancer is the exception to the trend of lower educational levels associated with higher mortality rates (Syme and Beckman, 1976).

8: Which of the following theories does *not* provide an explanation for the relation of family factors to outcomes of interest or intervention based on family factors?

    A. Epidemiological theory
    B. Life-cycle theory
    C. Stress–social support theory
    D. Genetic theory
    E. Family system theory

Answer: A

Page: 28

Critique: Although an epidemiological approach to interpreting genograms may be useful, it does not provide an explanation as to how or why family factors are related to the outcomes of interest, nor does it provide any guidance for interventions aimed at the family factors themselves. The four theories that may be of assistance in addressing these two issues are the life-cycle theory, the stress–social support theory, the genetic theory, and the family system theory.

9: Which of the following is an example of family demographics?

    A. Single-parent family with one child at home
    B. High school–educated parents, mother employed
    C. Divorce of parents 1 year before visit
    D. Patient's father with emotional and work problems

Answer: B

Page: 29

Critique: Family demographic information includes ethnicity, education, and occupation. Examples of family structure, life events, and problems are also represented here.

10: (True or False) The family genogram can also be referred to as:

    A. The family pedigree
    B. The family tree
    C. The family chart
    D. The genealogic chart

Answer: A - True, B - True, C - False, D - True

Page: 19

Critique: The family genogram is a tool used by physicians to summarize on one page a large amount of information relating to a family. It includes hereditary background and the risk this background places on current family members, along with major medical, social, and interactional influences. The genogram can also be referred to as the family pedigree, family tree, or genealogic chart.

11: What is the greatest barrier to the universal adoption of the genogram?

    A. The difficulty in interpreting the genogram
    B. The time required to develop the genogram
    C. The absence of standardization of symbols in the genogram
    D. The lack of physician familiarity with the genogram

Answer: B

Page: 19

Critique: The greatest barrier to the universal adoption of the genogram by practicing physicians is the time required to develop one. The search for methods that require less of the physician's and the office staff's time continues. It is thought that the time needed to develop a genogram will be significantly shortened with the development of the computerized medical record.

The Family's Influence on Health

Ana Catalina Triana

1: In family-oriented primary care, *family* is defined as any group of people:

- A. Who share the same household
- B. Who are related biologically, emotionally, or legally
- C. Who are related genetically
- D. In which a parental unit is clearly identified

Answer: B

Critique: In family-oriented primary care *family* is defined as any group of people who are related biologically, emotionally, or legally. This broader definition of a family reflects the changing demographics of American society.

Page: 31

2: (True or False) Determine whether the following statements regarding how families affect illness are true or false:

- A. The outcomes associated with individual versus family approaches to prevention are the same.
- B. Stress is widely accepted by patients and physicians as influencing health.
- C. Research has clearly demonstrated that family support can influence overall mortality.
- D. Spousal support has a direct protective effect on health and buffers the impact of stress.

Answers: A - False, B - True, C - True, D - True

Critique: Strong evidence supports an increase in the likelihood of changing a health-related behavior when the family is involved, as opposed to focusing solely on the individual. The World Health Organization described families as the "primary social agent in the promotion of health and well-being." Many studies on families have documented the relationship between social support and health outcomes. Family members, and particularly the spouse, appear to be sources of support and account for most of the association between social support and health.

Pages: 31, 32

3: Mrs. Boyd is 68 years old and has type 2 diabetes mellitus, congestive heart failure, and hypertension. You decide to convene a family conference to plan her future care. Your decision was made knowing that:

- A. Health care providers are the primary caregivers for patients with chronic illnesses.
- B. Most families must face chronic illness of a family member during the life cycle.
- C. Nursing home placement is the best option for an elderly person with multiple medical needs.
- D. Current research is concentrating on how families cause illness.

Answer: B

Critique: Chronic illness is increasing in prevalence and has replaced acute illness as the major cause of morbidity and mortality in the United States. Most families must face the chronic illness of a family member during the life cycle. Families, and not health care providers, are the primary caregivers for patients with chronic illnesses. They are the ones who help with most of the physical demands of the illness. Research on families and chronic illness is gradually moving away from looking at how families "cause" illness (a pathogenic model) to examining ways in which families influence, positively or negatively, the course of chronic illness.

Page: 33

4: Maria is a 16-year-old female who was recently diagnosed with type 1 diabetes mellitus. Her last hemoglobin A1C was 14%. Her parents complain about being tired of telling her to avoid sugars in her diet. A strategy that is likely to improve her compliance is:

- A. To empower the parents to supervise her diet more closely
- B. To hospitalize Maria for close monitoring and readjustment of her insulin
- C. To encourage her parents to promote Maria's autonomy
- D. To enroll the whole family in the next available diabetic teaching class

Answer: C

Critique: High and low family cohesion are both associated with poor diabetic control. Optimal management of diabetes requires the support and supervision of the family along with respect for individuality and age-appropriate autonomy. Empowering the parents to exert more control over Maria or hospitalizing Maria would serve only to undermine her autonomy. Diabetic education is important for everyone; however, it will not address the issue of control described in this vignette.

Pages: 34, 35

5: Helpful ways to aid newly formed stepfamilies in anticipating problems include all of the following except:

    A. Discouraging the new couple to take time for themselves without the children
    B. Validating and normalizing conflicting feelings
    C. Letting them know that previous adjustment problems may re-emerge
    D. Encouraging the stepparent to assume a secondary parental role

Answer: A

Critique: Family physicians can provide anticipatory guidance to help stepfamilies. The first 2 years of the remarriage are associated with considerable stress. It is important to give attention to the marriage bond because this is the basis of the new family. Acceptance of ambivalent feelings may help to prevent guilt and anger. Parenting stepchildren is a major task; it is better for the stepparent not to try to take over the parental and disciplinary functions.

Page: 40

6: (True or False) Mr. Greenwood, a 64-year-old male, comes in complaining of chronic back pain that has worsened since his daughter and three children moved back home after a divorce. You suspect that he is experiencing a high level of stress. Appropriate questions to assess his coping mechanisms include:

    A. How have you dealt with stress in the past?
    B. What have you tried so far?
    C. Who do you turn to when you are in trouble?
    D. Is your support system helpful?

Answers: A - True, B - True, C - True, D - True

Critique: The family physician can play an important role in helping individuals and families deal with stress. An open-ended and nonjudgmental approach is imperative. An assessment of coping mechanisms should include previous experiences and availability and usefulness of support systems.

Pages: 34, 35

7: (True or False) Mr. Greenwood tells you that his wife died 2 years ago and his daughter is his main source of support. She is working full-time while Mr. Greenwood takes care of the children at home. He agrees with you about the high level of stress in the house and wants to know how it could affect everyone's health. Research on family stress and health has shown that:

    A. Stressful family events precede the development of a wide range of diseases.
    B. Children are not likely to be affected by stressful family events.

    C. Families undergoing stress tend to avoid medical care.
    D. Stress can decrease immunity and make individuals more susceptible to infections.

Answers: A - True, B - False, C - False, D - True

Critique: Research has shown that 10 of the 15 most stressful life events on the Holmes and Rahe scale are family events. Children are likely to be affected by family events. Research studies have shown an increased rate of streptococcal pharyngitis in children who have recently experienced a significant stressful family event. Family life events have been correlated with increased visits to physicians and an increase in hospital admissions for a wide variety of conditions. Research in psychoimmunology has shown how stress can decrease immunity and may render individuals susceptible to a variety of different diseases.

Page: 35

8: (True or False) Mr. Greenwood is concerned about the impact of divorce on his daughter's health. She has been complaining of frequent headaches. You tell him that:

    A. Divorce is always bad for all family members.
    B. Being married is usually associated with better health outcomes.
    C. Within 2 years after the divorce, most adults have adjusted to the marital breakup.
    D. Separated individuals have 30% more acute illnesses than married counterparts.

Answers: A - False, B - True, C - True, D - True

Critique: Divorce is not necessarily bad for all family members. Ending a very stressful and unhappy relationship may ultimately improve a person's sense of well-being. Children actually adjust better in a stable divorced home than in an unhappy, highly conflictual, intact home. The first year after divorce is highly stressful for adults. Separated and divorced adults have the highest rates of acute medical problems compared with counterparts. Even though divorce is often a positive solution to a destructive family environment, most research indicates that being married is associated with better outcomes and fewer health problems than being divorced or single. Within 2 years after the divorce, most adults have adjusted and have developed a new stability in their lives.

Page: 36

9: (True or False) Mr. Greenwood has noticed that his 9-year-old grandson seems to have a very different reaction to the divorce compared with his 12-year-old granddaughter. He is also concerned about his 6-year-old grandson's regression to bed-wetting. You let him know that:

    A. His 6-year-old grandson needs to have a thorough physical evaluation as soon as possible.
    B. Studies have found that divorce is more difficult for boys than for girls.
    C. School-aged children are likely to respond to a divorce with sadness and upset.

D. Adolescents usually blame themselves for their parents' divorce.

Answers: A - False, B - True, C - True, D - False

Critique: Children's gender and age at the time of divorce influence the type and quality of reactions they have to their parents' divorce. Boys tend to develop more behavior, sex-role adjustment, and academic problems than do girls. Young children tend to regress in their behavior. School-aged children frequently feel responsible for the divorce and tend to blame themselves. Adolescents are usually able to separate themselves from their parents' divorce; however, anger, resentment, and hostility are common adolescent reactions.

Pages: 37, 38

Chapter 4

Psychosocial Influences on Health

Ron Cook

1: Of the items listed, all are important aspects of providing primary care that is sensitive to psychosocial issues, except:

    A. The physician needs to see the patient first, so that symptoms and behaviors are conceptualized in the context of the patient.

    B. The physician needs to evaluate the dynamic nature of multiple biopsychosocial variables.

    C. The physician needs to foster a supportive and empathetic doctor-patient relationship.

    D. The physician needs to evaluate the patient's financial resources before the first visit to ensure that patients can pay for services rendered.

Answer: D

Critique: It is important for the physician to evaluate the context of the patient and the biopsychosocial variables and to foster a supportive and empathetic relationship with the patient. Evaluation of the patient's ability to pay is not appropriate at this visit. Doctors who restrict their attention to purely medical and financial considerations are of limited use to their patients.

Page: 43

2: The idea that psychosocial factors influence the etiology and maintenance of disease is best described by which of the following models:

    A. Ethnomedical

    B. Biomedical

    C. Biopsychosocial

    D. Holistic health care

Answer: C

Critique: The biopsychosocial model involves the incorporation of biologic systems that are simultaneously affected by psychological and social factors. To understand an illness in a population requires knowledge of factors such as social and cultural environment, psychological resources of the individual, and biochemistry and genetics of the disorder.

Page: 43

Questions 3–7: Match each lettered item with the numbered entry that best describes it:

    A. Systems approach

    B. Life span perspective

    C. Holistic health care model

    D. Ethnomedical cultural model

    E. Biopsychosocial model

3: Every encounter between a patient and a physician is a cross-cultural transaction.

4: This approach takes into account an individual's previous development, current level of development, and likely development in the future.

5: This model regards environmental stress or intrapsychic conflict as having pathologic potential for the individual.

6: This model rejects linear causality and conceptualizes smaller, simpler systems within larger, more complex ones.

7: This model emphasizes the importance of education, self-care, and health promotion. It also uses an array of alternative therapies.

Answers: 3 - D, 4 - B, 5 - E, 6 - A, 7 - C

Pages: 44, 45

8: Regarding the biopsychosocial model, all of the following statements are true, except:

    A. Clinical care involves not only biomedical aspects of illness but also psychological and social factors.

    B. All states of health are psychosomatic, and each person is a circular interaction of body, mind, and spirit.

    C. Effective treatment requires integration of biopsychosocial factors.

    D. Biological, psychological, and social factors are interrelated.

Answer: B

Critique: Choice B applies to the holistic health care model. All others encompass the biopsychosocial model. As an example, the loss of a job (social) might lead to depression (psychological symptom) and aggravation of a peptic ulcer (biological phenomenon).

Pages: 44, 45

9: The psychological and physiological response to a stressor is called:

- A. Resistance
- B. Strain
- C. An event
- D. A nuisance

Answer: B

Critique: Strains are physiological symptoms (dry mouth, palpitations) and changes in a psychological state (nervousness). These strains are usually a response to a catastrophic event, a major life event, or the result of chronic daily hassles of a medical condition.

Page: 46

Questions 10–14: How a patient deals with the loss of control precipitated by a stressful event can affect health outcomes. Several different personal control types have been described. Match the example to the type of personal control:

- A. The ability to choose an alternative surgical procedure
- B. Focusing on a pleasant thought during a painful procedure
- C. Having someone or something to blame to reduce anxiety
- D. Using a special breathing technique to reduce pain
- E. Handing out patient education materials and encouraging the patient to learn more about a surgical procedure to lessen anxiety

10: Retrospective

11: Informational

12: Cognitive

13: Behavioral

14: Decisional

Answers: 10 - C, 11 - E, 12 - B, 13 - D, 14 - A

Critique: Retrospective control involves beliefs about who or what caused an event. Informational control involves the opportunity to obtain knowledge about a stressful event. Cognitive control involves the ability to use thought processes to modify the impact of an event. Behavioral control involves the ability to take concrete action to reduce the impact of a stressor. Decisional control involves the opportunity to choose between alternative procedures or courses of action.

Page: 47

15: Choose the best answer: Positive health outcomes have been related to:

- A. Developmentally mature defense mechanisms (humor and intellectualization)
- B. Developmentally immature defense mechanisms (denial and avoidance)
- C. Pessimism in early adulthood
- D. A poor sense of control

Answer: A

Critique: People who tend to use more mature defense mechanisms tend to have better adjustment in both work and family arenas. These mechanisms elicit more favorable and socially supportive responses from others. Pessimism in early adulthood has been associated with poor health in middle and late adulthood. A strong sense of control appears to help a person's health and sustains him or her during a serious illness.

Page: 47

16: Hardiness is a personality resource that may help explain who does and who does not get sick under stress. All of the following are characteristics of hardiness except:

- A. Personal control
- B. Financial control
- C. Commitment
- D. Challenge

Answer: B

Critique: A strong sense of personal control, a commitment or sense of purpose, and the ability to see change (challenge) as an opportunity for growth are all characteristics of hardiness. Control and commitment consistently have been associated with health. The presence of all these characteristics in a patient will help him or her remain healthier than less hardy counterparts.

Page: 47

17: (True or False) Determine which of the following statements are true and which are false:

- A. Social support has been demonstrated to have a positive effect on health outcomes.
- B. A person who has many friends but no close friends has adequate support in time of need.
- C. Social support reduces stress and contributes to negative health outcomes.
- D. Life stresses do not affect health outcomes.

Answers: A - True, B - False, C - False, D - False

Critique: Social support refers to the perceived care, comfort, esteem, or help received from individuals or groups. Strong social support has been demonstrated to have a positive effect on health. The lack of close friends may result in inadequate social support in times of need. It is clearly evident that life stressors do have an effect on health outcomes.

Pages: 47, 48

18: During the collection of psychosocial data, all of the following statements are true except:

- A. Information may be gathered using standardized health questionnaires.
- B. Family members are interviewed.
- C. In the family practice setting, the most common and natural approach to data gathering is a single office visit for at least 90 minutes.
- D. Consultation with multidisciplinary colleagues.

Answer: C

Critique: In the family practice setting the most common approach to psychosocial data collection is patient interviewing over time. The use of standardized health questionnaires, interviewing family members, and consultation with other colleagues represent the variety of ways in which psychosocial data may be gathered.

Pages: 48, 49

19: All of the following represent important times when intervention may be needed in psychosocial issues. Which of these is the least significant:

A. A new or significant change in a medical diagnosis (cancer)
B. Natural transitions in the family life cycle (birth of a child)
C. Compliance issues or lifestyles impinging on health
D. A sudden but mild exacerbation in a patient's chronic pain

Answer: D

Critique: A mild, brief exacerbation of chronic pain in a patient may result in a necessary office work-up, but it does not initially require psychosocial intervention. Any new or dramatic changes in an otherwise stable patient may evoke a consideration of psychosocial factors. The birth of a child, death of a spouse, a new diagnosis of cancer, and compliance issues all should elicit evaluation of the psychosocial environment of the patient.

Page: 49

20: (True or False) To successfully integrate psychosocial concerns with treatment options, the sensitive physician will be able to:

A. Acknowledge his or her own limitations
B. Have an understanding of the community and its culture
C. Have familiarity with his or her own practice
D. Have an understanding and knowledge of the patient's demographic, socioeconomic, and cultural dimensions

Answers: A - True, B - True, C - True, D - True

Critique: Self-knowledge entails an honest assessment of one's knowledge base, skills, and attitudes. This knowledge is vital to primary care. Knowledge and understanding of the physician's practice, including patient demographics, culture, and community socioeconomic status, are important in the care of patients.

Pages: 50, 51

Chapter 5

Mind-Body Medicine

Victor S. Sierpina

1: One of the most common presenting symptoms of depression in a primary care setting is:

    A. Suicidal thoughts
    B. Hypersomnia
    C. Pain
    D. Gastrointestinal complaints
    E. Hallucinations

Answer: C

Critique: A growing body of literature is providing dramatic evidence of the mind-body connection. In family practice, mind-body connections are frequently seen in the form of somatic complaints. For example, stress may present as neck pain. One of the more common ways in which depression presents in primary care settings is pain; however, the connection between psyche and soma is still not widely accepted in allopathic medicine.

Page: 52

2: (True or False) Which of the following is involved as a mediator in the psychoneuroimmunologic reaction:

    A. Neuropeptides
    B. Interleukins
    C. Interferon
    D. Tumor necrosis factor

Answers: A - True, B - True, C - True, D - True

Critique: Neuropeptides are secreted by lymphocytes. Lymphocytes also have receptors for neuropeptides on their surfaces. Interleukin-1 and interleukin-2, interferon, and tumor necrosis factor are the most active immunoregulatory cytokines in the hypothalamic-pituitary axis.

Page: 53

3: Immune system activation is associated with increased activity in the:

    A. Inferior olivary nucleus
    B. Amygdala
    C. Temporal lobe
    D. Ventromedian nucleus of the hypothalamus
    E. Subthalamic cortex

Answer: D

Critique: Research has demonstrated a relationship between activation of the immune system and changes in hypothalamic, autonomic, and endocrine processes. Immune system activation in the body increases the firing rate of neurons in the ventromedian nucleus of the hypothalamus coincident with peak antibody production.

Page: 53

4: Relaxation therapy, biofeedback, and keeping a journal are examples of:

    A. Cognitive behavioral training
    B. Self-hypnosis
    C. Mind-body therapy
    D. Psychiatric nihilism
    E. The Alexander technique

Answer: C

Critique: Mind-body therapy techniques are used to influence or interrupt parts of the cycle that cause physical or emotional turmoil.

Page: 54

5: The placebo effect:

    A. May be as much as 70% of a positive effect
    B. Is independent of the patient's belief system
    C. Has never been shown to be useful clinically
    D. Is a form of medical trickery
    E. Has been well documented in animal studies

Answer: A

Critique: When assessing the body's healing potential, placebo response can be viewed as a powerful tool. Depending on the physician's belief in the anticipated outcome and the ailment, the placebo response can climb to 70%. The response is highly dependent on patient and physician beliefs and can prove to be clinically important.

Page: 54

6: Considering the placebo-"nocebo" effect, the physician's attitude in recommending a treatment or modality:

    A. May reduce responses by 90% when the attitude is negative
    B. Is not a significant variable in treatment outcomes
    C. Is best considered neutral as related to the patient's belief system
    D. Increases response rates if the attitude toward the treatment is positive

Answer: D

Critique: Both patient and physician attitudes and beliefs influence the placebo response. The effect must be taken into account when assessing responses to treatments. Physicians and patients sharing their beliefs about treatment and choosing a treatment that both believe in can have a significant impact on the healing process.

Pages: 54, 55

7: (True or False) Journal writing about stressful events has been shown to:

    A. Improve lung functioning in asthmatic patients
    B. Reduce disease severity in patients with rheumatoid arthritis
    C. Improve physical health only when emotional health improves
    D. Increase infections in openly gay patients

Answers: A - True, B - True, C - False, D - False

Critique: In a study of patients with rheumatoid arthritis or asthma, 20% of the asthmatic patients showed improvement in lung functioning and the arthritic patients showed a 28% reduction in disease severity. Concealing homosexuality has been associated with increased incidences of infections and cancer. Journaling may improve physical well-being but at the same time worsen emotional distress.

Page: 56

8: To find therapeutic benefit from the disclosure of prior traumatic events:

    A. Long periods of psychotherapy are required
    B. Writing about them may be sufficient
    C. Hypnosis is generally required
    D. Corroboration of the event is necessary from an independent source

Answer: B

Critique: Many patients may have difficulty disclosing major traumatic events, even to a trusted friend or health care provider. Studies support the notion that simply writing about the experience gives patients the ability to organize their thoughts and possibly come to an understanding about the event. Confidential "journaling" can lead to clinical improvement in the privacy and comfort of the patient's own environment. Disclosure does not require prolonged periods of psychotherapy to achieve a therapeutic benefit. No corroboration is necessary before suggesting that a patient write about past traumatic events.

Page: 56

9: Which of the following statements about relaxation exercises and meditation is true:

    A. Meditation has not been studied scientifically and is not proven in medical settings.
    B. Relaxation therapy has no effect on blood pressure and cardiac ischemia.
    C. Relaxation therapies and meditation increase catecholamine levels and limbic system activity and strengthen immune activity.

    D. Both techniques are proven to be easily applicable and low in cost for a wide variety of clinical conditions in primary care.
    E. Patients require formal religious instruction under the careful mentoring of a trained psychologist or spiritualist.

Answer: D

Critique: Depending on the patient and the condition, different techniques can be used and treatment can be tailored to meet the patient's specific needs.

Page: 57

10: Which of the following statements about social support is true:

    A. Rodents exhibit increased stress in social groups.
    B. Social integration reduces mortality by a similar magnitude as being a nonsmoker or having low cholesterol.
    C. Social support groups uniformly improve health outcomes in patients with chronic diseases.
    D. Social support has been associated with increased survival rates in cancer patients.
    E. The parenting that children receive in early life is not associated with health outcomes in adulthood.

Answer: D

Critique: Social support has been associated with improved survival for patients with breast cancer, melanoma, and lymphoma. Not all social support is beneficial. It is important that patients be involved in social groups with people who are experiencing a similar phase of the disease. Even rodents in isolation show evidence of stress compared with those in groups, despite being caged. Perception of parental caring predicts health status in midlife. Similarly, overly close families, such as the psychosomatic families described by Minuchin, may stifle development and individuation and have been associated with adverse outcomes and illness such as anorexia nervosa.

Page: 57

11: Regarding patients' beliefs and practices of religion and spirituality, controlled studies have indicated that which of the following statements is true:

    A. Those with greater spiritual awareness experience less stress and anxiety.
    B. Patients do not wish their physicians to discuss religious matters with them.
    C. Denominational religion has the most influential effect on health outcomes.
    D. Religious practice has little or no effect on the outcome of heart surgery.
    E. Most patients do not feel that spiritual health is as important as physical health.

Answer: A

Critique: Better health is a result of having belief, faith, and hope. Relief of stress and anxiety may be a result of the comfort provided by the sense of spirit. Patients with no sense of comfort from spiritual beliefs experience higher mortality after heart surgery. Most patients want their physician to discuss spirituality with them; however, health care providers must be respectful that not all spiritual benefit is derived from only the denominational belief systems.

Page: 59

12: Effective hypnosis requires which of the following:

    A. A prior history of artistic talent
    B. Ability to roll the eyes downward and laterally in response to suggestion
    C. The qualities of absorption, dissociation, and suggestibility
    D. An ability to fall asleep during a hypnosis session
    E. A mental health problem, rather than a physical illness

Answer: C

Critique: During hypnosis, these three factors are reflected in effective sessions. First, the patient becomes fully absorbed in the issue at hand through an induction or relaxation technique. This, in turn, results in dissociation from various distractions. An increased state of awareness is created, which allows the patient to be more open to suggestions that can influence physical change. Spiegel developed an "eye roll" test of hypnosis potential. Patients who can focus on the hypnotist's thumb on their forehead while closing their eyes are better candidates.

Page: 60

13: An example of therapeutic guided imagery is:

    A. Recalling a past traumatic event in detail and then trying to forget it
    B. Using biofeedback to relieve a headache
    C. Using the PET scan to activate the eyes and cerebral cortex
    D. Listening to music during surgery
    E. Picturing white blood cells as sharks devouring bacteria or cancer cells

Answer: E

Critique: Therapeutic imagery may be considered an adjunctive treatment and is used by patients to try to combat difficult conditions. It is based on the assumption that images can directly or indirectly influence the physiologic activity of the body. Picturing white blood cells as sharks devouring bacteria or cancer cells is one such example. This process can possibly create false hope and guilt if it is not successful.

Page: 61

14: The process of biofeedback involves which of the following:

    A. Receiving verbal feedback from a therapist while picturing the hands turning warm

    B. Utilizing a monitoring device to provide visual or auditory images of certain body functions
    C. A series of electrical shocks administered at scheduled intervals to desensitize patients to certain phobias
    D. An intra-arterial catheter to monitor blood pressure and catecholamine and cortisol levels during a trance state

Answer: B

Critique: Neal Miller, in the early 1960s, proposed that all responses could be brought under voluntary control through biofeedback. The process requires three things: a patient, a therapist, and a monitoring device capable of measuring physiologic activity. The monitoring device provides information to the patient as the therapist leads the patient through mental exercises to help the patient achieve the desired result.

Page: 61

15: Stress-related conditions should be considered if a medical work-up is otherwise negative. To inform a patient of the presence of a stress-related problem, which of the following is a useful communication:

    A. "This is all in your head, and there is nothing to worry about."
    B. "All the tests are normal; perhaps we need to send you to a specialist."
    C. "Your condition is chronic and incurable except through psychotherapy."
    D. "Perhaps some relation exists between your pain and the stress in your life."
    E. "Changing your life, especially your work, marriage, and hobbies, probably won't help. Medication is required in all such cases."

Answer: D

Critique: An effective way for the physician to determine stressors is to simply ask questions. With a knowledge of the patient and his or her environment, the physician can analyze the situation to recommend appropriate treatment to help the patient toward better health. Asking questions related to events or circumstances in the patient's life may lead to the root of the illness. Communicating your opinion to a patient can be difficult and yet critical to success. A nonjudgmental, suggestive statement, such as "Perhaps some relation exists between your pain and the stress in your life," is usually the preferred approach. Care must be taken not to "medicalize" a problem by overordering tests, by overprescribing medications, or through the indiscriminate use of referrals and consultations.

Page: 61

Chapter 6

Practicing Biopsychosocial Medicine

Robert L Keith

1: (True or False) With the biopsychosocial model's emphasis on the scientific method in medical education and subsequent myriad discoveries about psychology and pathology, attention has been focused at the cellular level and thus contributed to a reduced focus on people, health, and illness.

Answer: True

Critique: In this model, disease is treated as an independent entity that can be categorized and treated. This emphasis often leads to focus on disease rather than on the patient who has the disease.

Page: 65

2: (True or False) In his biopsychosocial model, George Engel supports the notion of mind-body dualism as a useful way to conceptualize health and illness.

Answer: False

Critique: Engel criticizes the reduction of mind-body dualism in the biomedical model. He states that the crippling flaw of biomedicine is that the patient himself/herself is often overlooked.

Page: 65

3: (True or False) Family physicians work at the confluence of biomedical, behavioral, and social sciences and must integrate these aspects to have a more complete understanding of a patient's health and what affects it.

Answer: True

Critique: Family physicians consider the context in which a person functions in order to understand the patient's health. If the physician separates mind and body paradigmatically, vital information may be lost or misinterpreted, resulting in misguided treatment.

Page: 65

4: The type of power that physicians possess in which deference is given to the physician's knowledge base is:

    A. Referent power
    B. Expert power
    C. Legitimate power
    D. Coercive power

Answer: B

Critique: Expert power relates to the power held because of the physician's training in skills and knowledge. Referent power is a means by which patients support their own sense of self by association with their physician. Legitimate power is provided by state-government regulation, which can have a considerable impact on a patient's freedom and well-being. Coercive power involves the physician's power of influence over the behavior of his or her patients.

Page: 66

5: The acronym presented in the classic text *The Fifteen-Minute Hour* is:

    A. BATHE
    B. BETTE
    C. BARKER
    D. BABY

Answer: A

Critique: The BATHE acronym provides a simple and organized means by which physicians can organize their thinking and interviewing. It starts with getting *b*ackground information, seeks to assess *a*ffect, and then focuses on the thing causing the most *t*rouble. It then assesses how the patient is *h*andling or coping with the trouble to provide some assessment of the patient's functioning and urges the physician to demonstrate an *e*mpathetic response to the patient.

Page: 67

6: (True or False) To demonstrate the best empathetic response, physicians must assume responsibility for being sure that the patient manages the troubling situation.

Answer: False

Critique: Rather than assume responsibility for the problem, the physician assesses the patient's circumstances and offers observations and suggestions as to how the patient might manage the problem.

Page: 68

7: (True or False) Patients who are demanding, manipulative, and entitled usually have severe personality disorders and should be barred from the practice if their behavior persists.

Answer: False

Critique: Patients who demonstrate these behaviors are trying to get their needs met by means that are familiar to them and that may have worked with others. Physicians can, at times, contribute to the exacerbation of these behaviors when they have difficulty managing their own feelings about the patient's behavior.

Page: 69

8: (True or False) Hypochondriacal patients should be seen no more than once per year to show them that they are really healthy.

Answer: False

Critique: Patients who are preoccupied with multiple physical complaints tend to dichotomize emotional and physical complaints. They should be seen on a regular basis, as frequently as two times per month. During office visits, both a basic examination and a general discussion about stress and how things are going in their lives are indicated.

Page: 69

9: (True or False) To practice the highest quality of biopsychosocial medicine, the physician must keep in mind that he or she is the doctor and therefore knows what is best for the patient.

Answer: False

Critique: Although physicians are highly skilled and knowledgeable in their fields, it is vitally important to begin with a focus on the patient as a person, and not a disease entity that must be conquered.

Page: 70

Chapter 7

Domestic Violence

Jeri A. O'Donnell

ELDER ABUSE

1: (True or False) According to Hirsch et al., 1999, prevalence information regarding elder abuse differs from state to state because of:

   A. Physicians' current reduction of time due to managed care

   B. Variances in state laws

   C. Physicians not asking pertinent questions regarding potential abuse

   D. An overall reluctance to report abuse in adults

Answer: A - False, B - True, C - False, D - True

Page: 71

Critique: Several different state laws as well as medical definitions of elder abuse can cause confusion. There tends to be reluctance to report (whether by physician, family or friend, or victim), which greatly compromises the accuracy of incidence information. Physician time and history taking do not seem to influence the reporting of information regarding elder abuse.

2: According to a publication issued by the U.S. House of Representatives Select Committee on Aging in 1991, the number of estimated abused elderly individuals in the United States is:

   A. 1 million

   B. 1.5 million

   C. 2 million

   D. 3 million

Answer: C

Page: 71

Critique: Studies estimate that as many as 2 million older Americans each year suffer from some form of elder mistreatment. (United States Congress, 1991).

3: All of the following are considered true regarding acts of elder abuse, except:

   A. Acts of retribution by adult children who were once so mistreated

   B. Accumulated stress between the dependent older adult and the caregiver causes the caregiver to lash out

   C. Another form of aggressive acting out in a violent society

   D. Frustration of a dependent caregiver

Answer: A

Page: 72

Critique: It is possible that elder abuse is simply one additional form of aggressive acting out in a society that is filled with violent actions. It has been erroneously theorized that acts of elder abuse are essentially acts of retribution by adult children who were once so mistreated; research findings do not bear this out. Early research into the etiologies of elder abuse focused on the dependent elder and accumulated caregiver stress; however, more recent findings are pointing to the dependence of the "abuser" on the elder person as the more critical variable.

4: Regarding elder abuse and mistreatment, in the absence of federal law all of the following are false, except:

   A. All states and the District of Columbia have established statutes

   B. All but eight states have established statutes

   C. All but two states have established statutes

   D. Except for eight states and the District of Columbia, all other states have established statutes

Answer: A

Page: 73

Critique: Even though there is an absence of federal law, all states and the District of Columbia have established statutes pertaining to elder abuse and mistreatment. Further, all states except for eight require some form of reporting by professionals. Given this reporting mechanism though, some states still have no adult protective service statutes, which forces the involvement of the criminal justice system.

PARTNER ABUSE

1: Which of the following is not a risk factor for becoming a victim of partner abuse?

A. Being female
B. Being in the "traditional" homemaker role
C. Being pregnant
D. A female being separated from her partner

Answer: B

Page: 74

Critique: Being female is clearly a risk factor for becoming a victim of partner abuse. Pregnancy is also a time of heightened risk for battery. Women who have separated from their spouses are three times more likely to be victimized than are those who are already divorced and 25 times more likely than are married women. Being a traditional homemaker is not noted in studies as a significant factor for becoming a victim of partner abuse.

2: The average age of husbands who murder their wives is:

A. 22
B. 27
C. 31
D. 41
E. None of the above

Answer: D

Page: 76

Critique: Langan and Dawson showed in their study (1995) that the average age of husbands who murder their wives is 41 years, and of the wives who murder their husbands, the average age is 37.

3: (True or False) Because of access to guns, female violence toward their male partners is likely to result in as serious injury as men's violence toward women.

Answer: False

Page: 76

Critique: Even though some women are violent toward their male partner, their violence tends to be more retaliatory in nature, and therefore it is less likely to result in a serious injury (Feldman & Ridley, 1995).

4: Gun access by male perpetrators is associated with higher levels of abuse toward women in which population?

A. Predominantly in the African American community
B. Predominantly in the Hispanic community
C. Across all ethnic groups
D. Predominantly in minority populations in general

Answer: C

Page: 76

Critique: No matter what the ethnic group, it has been found that access to guns by male perpetrators is associated with higher levels of abuse toward women.

5: (True or False) Because the family physician often cares for both the victim and the perpetrator, he or she is the most capable to counsel the couple.

Answer: False

Page: 77

Critique: The family physician should be careful counseling a couple involved in domestic violence, and couple counseling is discouraged. Each party should be seen separately unless specifically given permission by the victim; still, joint counseling is generally inadvisable and should be attempted only if the violence has completely ended.

6: (True or False) Couple's counseling is often:

A. Still provided by some family physicians in their management of partner abuse
B. Doable especially during the batterer's period of contrition
C. Often requested by the victim
D. Encouraged by the AMA

Answer: A - True, B - False, C - True, D - False

Page: 77

Critique: The AMA, in an earlier publication, similarly discouraged couple counseling in cases of domestic violence and underscored the potential harm of advancing couples' work before the cessation of violence (AMA, 1992). Despite these contraindications, research has demonstrated the continued practice of couple counseling by North American primary care physicians in their management of partner abuse (Ferris et al., 1999). The AMA states: "Rather than entirely fault such physicians, it should be recognized that couple's counseling may be *requested by the victim....* When violence is ongoing, partners should be offered individual counseling rather than couple's counseling."

7: (True or False) Concerning children in homes with domestic violence, which of the following is most true?

A. In households where a male partner beats his female partner, the focus is more on the partner than on the children
B. Child abuse is present in half of the households where a male partner beats his female partner
C. Child abuse is always present in households where there is spousal abuse
D. In households where spousal abuse exists, the children are relatively safe from physical abuse

Answer: B

Page: 76

Critique: When children reside in a household where a batterer beats his or her spouse, research has shown that these children have a 50% chance of being physically abused.

CHILD ABUSE

1: The term "battered child syndrome" was coined by:

A. John Caffey
B. Henry Kemp
C. C. T. Wang
D. B. F. Steel

Answer: B

Page: 79

Critique: Child abuse as a syndrome was first formally described by radiologist John Caffey in the early 1940s. In 1962, Henry Kemp coined the term "battered child syndrome" in describing children who were beaten by their parental figures.

2: (True or False) Because there is a downward trend in child sexual abuse, it is not considered a substantial threat to children.

Answer: False

Page: 79

Critique: Although sexual abuse cases have shown a downward trend, the absolute number of sexual abuse cases continues to represent a substantial threat to children in the United States.

3: (True or False) The methods for reporting child abuse are standardized across the United States.

Answer: False

Page: 79

Critique: Although significant strides have been made in reporting child abuse across the nation, estimating the number of substantiated reports of children maltreated in the United States is still met with major obstacles. Part of the problem in estimating cases is that a wide variety of reporting methods are still used by states.

4: The most common form of child abuse is:

    A. Sexual
    B. Physical
    C. Neglect
    D. Emotional

Answer: C

Page: 79

Critique: Most professionals assessing child maltreatment would suspect that physical abuse is the most prevalent, but Wang, in his 50-state survey of 1997, which provided the five categories of physical abuse, sexual abuse, neglect, emotional maltreatment, and others, showed that neglect represented the most common type of reported and substantiated maltreatment.

5: All of the following are true, except:

    A. There is a downward trend in child sexual abuse
    B. Child maltreatment fatalities remain alarmingly frequent
    C. The majority of children suffering from physical abuse are younger than five years of age
    D. About 38% of child fatalities involve children younger than 1 year of age

Answer: B

Page: 79

Critique: Child maltreatment fatalities, although relatively infrequent, are still alarming. Children cannot defend themselves against adult attacks. About 50% of child maltreatment deaths are caused by physical abuse. The majority of maltreated children are younger than 5 years, and 38% are younger than 1 year at the time of their death.

6: A factor that does not contribute to the likelihood of a family engaging in abusive behavior is:

    A. Substance abuse
    B. Poverty
    C. A parent being under 20 years of age
    D. Domestic violence

Answer: C

Page: 80

Critique: In a 1997 study, substance abuse was the top problem exhibited by families who were reported for maltreatment. Other problems include poverty and economic strains, lack of parental capacity skills, and domestic violence.

7: In recent years the media have identified child maltreatment problems in day care centers and foster homes. These problems account for:

    A. 30% of confirmed abuse cases
    B. 11% of confirmed abuse cases
    C. 18% of confirmed abuse cases
    D. 3% of confirmed abuse cases

Answer: D

Page: 80

Critique: Reports of child maltreatment involving day care centers and foster care homes seem to attract media attention, but only 3% of confirmed abuse cases occur in these or other institutional settings. This figure was constant over the 11 years studied before 1997.

8: In assessing for child abuse, which of the following is not true regarding the history and physical assessment of children?

    A. The diagnosis of child sexual abuse is often made on history alone
    B. The physical examination alone is infrequently diagnostic in the absence of good history or specific laboratory findings
    C. A medical history of missed immunizations and follow-up appointments may be a clue to neglect or abuse
    D. Four-year-olds are often able to provide a reliable history

Answer: B

Page: 80

Critique: In the absence of a good medical history, child abuse is often missed. The diagnosis of child abuse or neglect is often made on *history alone.* Physical examination is infrequently diagnostic in the absence of a good history or specific laboratory findings.

9: (True or False) In the case of sexual abuse occurring more than 72 hours before a medical examination, it is best to examine the child in the emergency department for the most complete physical assessment.

Answer: False

Page: 80

Critique: In the case of alleged or suspected sexual abuse that has occurred more than 72 hours before a medical examination, a comfortable, relaxed setting, often outside the emergency department, is preferred.

10: (True or False) In a nonabusive environment, one rarely sees:

    A. Fractures
    B. Bruises
    C. Lacerations and abrasions on areas of the body such as the wrists or ankles
    D. Ankle sprains

Answer: A - True, B - False, C - True, D - False

Page: 80

Critique: It is always important to remember that injuries of abuse are more severe than one could reasonably attribute to the claimed cause. The story reported must match the injury. Physical signs of abuse include injuries to the face, extremities, and trunk that form a regular pattern resembling the shape of the article used to inflict the injury. Burns inflicted by cigarettes or cigars and immersion burns leave characteristic patterns. Fractures, especially of the skull and facial bones, raise the index of suspicion for abuse. Long bone fractures in various stages of healing, as revealed by x-ray, also support abuse. Lacerations and abrasions on wrists and ankles as well as bruises of the genitalia and abdominal wall are generally rare in a nonabusive environment.

11: (True or False) All but two of the 50 states have a reporting mechanism for child maltreatment.

Answer: False

Page: 81

Critique: All 50 states now have a reporting mechanism for child maltreatment; therefore, a Child Protective Service (CPS) agency must be informed of any actual or suspected abuse or neglect.

SEXUAL ASSAULT

1: The ratio of adult women in the United States who have experienced sexual assault in their lifetime is estimated to be:

    A. 1 in 15 adult women
    B. 1 in 8 adult women
    C. 1 in 5 adult women
    D. 1 in 10 adult women

Answer: B

Page: 82

Critique: It is estimated that 12 million American women have been raped, or one in eight adult women in the United States.

2: (True or False) The highest rates of sexual assault are found among which group of women:

    A. Those age 21–25
    B. Those with low income
    C. Those who live in urban areas
    D. Those age 16–19

Answer: A - False, B - True, C - True, D - True

Page: 82

Critique: In studies reviewing sexual assault, the research has found that the rates are highest among women age 16 to 19 years and women with low income or who live in urban areas.

3: (True or False) Which of the following are true about sexual assault:

    A. The majority of attackers use a weapon
    B. About 70% of victims report using some form of self-protection
    C. The highest percentage of rapes is committed by friends or acquaintances of the victim
    D. About 40% of rape victims suffer major physical injuries, such as fractures, lacerations, or internal injuries

Answer: A - False, B - True, C - True, D - False

Page: 82

Critique: Studies consistently show that approximately 75% of rapes and sexual assaults are committed by persons known to the victim. Many attackers threaten that they have a weapon, but most attackers (80%) did not use a weapon. About 70% of victims reported some form of self-protective action, such as struggling, persuading, screaming, or shouting. About 40% of rape victims suffered physical injury, with 5% receiving major injuries such as fractures, lacerations, internal injuries, or unconsciousness.

4: (True or False) The most common reason victims give for reporting the crime of sexual assault is:

    A. To protect future victims
    B. The support of hospital personnel gave them the courage to report
    C. To prevent further crimes by the attacker
    D. To get even with the attacker

Answer: A - True, B - False, C - True, D - False

Page: 82

Critique: Studies have found that the most common reason given for reporting a sexual assault crime is to prevent further crimes by the attacker. Women who have been victimized try to protect other women from going through the same trauma. The support of hospital personnel is important, but it is not one of the most common reasons women give for reporting the crime. And while "getting even" may seem like a natural response for some, it requires knowing the attacker and having a guaranteed prosecution.

5: The most common reason given for not reporting a sexual assault is:

    A. The attacker was a friend
    B. The attack was viewed as a private matter
    C. The attacker was a relative or intimate
    D. The victim feared the attacker would find out and return

Answer: B

Page: 82

Critique: A 1997 study by Greenfeld found that the most common reason given for *not* reporting a sexual assault was that it was viewed as a private matter. Victims are more likely to report sexual assault or rape if the attack is by a friend or acquaintance (rather than by intimates, relatives, or strangers) or if they sustained physical injuries requiring medical attention.

6: (True or False) Which of the following are true regarding the sexual assault of men:

    A. Men are victims in about 5% of all sexual assaults
    B. The majority of male victims are younger than 6 years of age
    C. Men are more likely to sustain physical trauma
    D. Men are the victims in about 10% of all sexual assaults

Answer: A - True, B - False, C - True, D - False

Page: 82

Critique: Limited research has been done on the nature of sexual assault on men, but the studies done to date show that men are victims in about 5% of all sexual assaults, and the majority of male victims are younger than 18 years of age. Also, men are more likely to sustain physical trauma or to be attacked by multiple assailants.

7: (True or False) After a sexual assault, the following behavioral problems are found in victims:

    A. PTSD (post traumatic stress disorder)
    B. Depression develops in all cases of sexual assault
    C. Suicidal thoughts are reported in 75% of victims
    D. 13% of rape victims attempt suicide

Answer: A - True, B - False, C - False D - True

Page: 83

Critique: Understandably, PTSD frequently occurs following a sexual assault. Surprisingly, though, studies tend to show that depression develops in only an estimated 24% of sexual assault/rape victims within the first month after the attack, and in 50% within the first year. According to the Bureau of Justice Statistics, suicidal thoughts are reported in 33% to 50% of victims, and approximately 13% of rape victims actually attempt suicide.

8: (True or False) Regarding evidence collection, documenting objective evidence for prosecution is necessary only when major injuries are inflicted.

Answer: False

Page: 84

Critique: The goal of prosecution is a successful outcome, and objective evidence of even minor injuries increases the chances of obtaining this result.

Care of the Elderly

Juan A. Perez

1: Which of the following best describes frailty:

    A. A reduction in cardiac output and glomerular filtration rate

    B. A condition in which the risk of death is not increased

    C. A condition in which patients can manage minor stressors without difficulty

    D. A condition that results from multisystem reduction in reserve capacity

Answer: D

Critique: Frailty occurs when a number of physiologic systems are close to or past the threshold of symptomatic failure. As a consequence, a frail person is at increased risk of disability and death from minor external stresses.

Page: 89

2: Which organ system is usually affected by aging:

    A. Connective tissue

    B. Respiratory

    C. Gastrointestinal

    D. All of the above

Answer: D

Critique: All of these systems are affected by aging. It is important to learn these changes to differentiate them from pathologic changes. Collagen shows greater stiffness and decreased tissue elasticity in skin, major blood vessels, heart, lungs, and ligaments. The respiratory system shows decreased compliance of the chest wall, decreased number of alveoli, and increased rigidity of the lungs. The gastrointestinal system shows numerous changes that start with the mouth and end with the rectum. Table 8–1outlines these changes.

Page: 93

3: All of the following are important to perform in evaluating an elderly patient for the first time, except:

    A. History and physical examination

    B. Mini mental state examination

    C. Instrumental activities of daily living (IADL)

    D. Pelvic examination

    E. Depression scale, when appropriate

Answer: D

Critique: Although a pelvic examination is important, other issues such as a full history with a caregiver, spouse, or a family member; assessment of cognition; get up and go test; and IADL take precedence during the first visit.

Pages: 94, 95

4: The physical examination of an elderly patient should include:

    A. Get up and go test

    B. Postural vital signs

    C. Pulse

    D. Hearing and sight

    E. All of the above

Answer: E

Critique: All of the above are important in examining an elderly patient. During the examination and history taking, be sure not to shout, but make eye contact and allow time for the patient to process your question. Do not rush, and adapt your pace to the patient's, because they may not be able to function at yours.

Page: 95

5: Which of the following is the most accurate age-related change in pharmacokinetics:

    A. Absorption is decreased in the elderly patient.

    B. Lean body mass decreases.

    C. GFR improves.

    D. Fat tissue decreases.

Answer: B

Critique: Absorption shows no change in the elderly, but lean body mass and GFR decrease. Fat tissue and alpha$_1$-acid glycoprotein increase.

Page: 99; Table 8–6

6: All of the following medications should be avoided in the elderly, except:

    A. Talwin, pentazocine

    B. Valium, diazepam

    C. Methyldopa

    D. Elavil, amitriptyline

    E. Restoril, temazepam, at a low dosage

Answer: E

Critique: Talwin causes severe nervous system side effects. Valium has a long half-life, and when necessary the short-acting benzodiazepines should be used. Methyldopa has CNS side effects, and Elavil has anticholinergic side effects.

Pages: 100, 101

7: Which best describes a stage 3 pressure ulcer:

    A. Partial-thickness skin loss
    B. Full-thickness skin loss when the damage does not extend through the fascia
    C. Full-thickness skin loss associated with extensive damage to muscle
    D. Nonblanchable erythema

Answer: B

Critique: A stage 1 is nonblanchable erythema, stage 2 is partial-thickness skin loss, stage 3 is full-thickness skin loss when the damage does not extend through the fascia, and stage 4 is full-thickness skin loss associated with extensive damage to muscle.

Pages: 102, 103; Table 8–9

8: All are correct statements concerning pressure ulcers, except:

    A. When an ulcer does not heal, one must consider the possibility of infection.
    B. Pressure and friction must be removed when treating pressure ulcers.
    C. Necrotic tissue should be left intact.
    D. Osteomyelitis should be considered in nonhealing pressure ulcers.

Answer: C

Critique: The necrotic tissue should be removed, and the open area should be kept moist while the surrounding tissue is kept dry.

Page: 103

9: Which statement is most accurate regarding exercise in the elderly:

    A. Exercise can shorten active life expectancy.
    B. Exercise does not affect frailty.
    C. Exercise provides adequate physiologic reserve and enhances well-being.
    D. Elderly patients should not exercise.

Answer: C

Critique: Habitual exercise can improve the quality of life, decreases frailty, and prolongs active life expectancy. It is the physician's responsibility to inquire about level of activity in elderly patients and discuss an exercise program that is adequate for the specific patient.

Pages: 103, 104

10: In dealing with health behavior promotion strategies, which is the best approach:

    A. Advice regarding smoking cessation
    B. Advice regarding the use of seatbelts
    C. Retirement counseling
    D. Screening for home safety
    E. All of the above

Answer: E

Critique: In addition to all of these strategies, fire prevention and hearing and vision screening should be included.

Page: 104

11: Recommendations for cancer screening include all of the following, except:

    A. Annual breast examination
    B. Annual fecal occult blood
    C. Annual Pap smears until three or more in sequence are normal
    D. Annual CA-125

Answer: D

Critique: Annual CA-125 is not recommended nicely outlines the cancer screening recommendations. Other tests that are not recommended include chest x-ray, sputum cytology, and pelvic ultrasound.

Page: 105, Table 8–12

12: Reversible causes of dementia include:

    A. Pernicious anemia
    B. Neurosyphilis
    C. Subdural hematoma
    D. Use of sedatives or hypnotics
    E. All of the above

Answer: E

Critique: All of the above are potentially reversible causes of dementia. In practice, depression and drug-induced dementia are seen more frequently.

Page: 106, Table 8–13

13: All of the following statements about benign senescent forgetfulness, are true except:

    A. It does not produce significant functional impairment.
    B. It always produces disorientation.
    C. Language changes are not detected.
    D. If it progresses, it does so very slowly.

Answer: B

Critique: Benign senescent forgetfulness does not produce disorientation, language changes, or visual-spatial defects, which are some of the necessary components of intellectual decline that are seen in dementia.

Page: 106

14: Which scenario best describes stage 3 of Alzheimer's disease (AD):

    A. Loss of train of thought in midsentence and forgetting to pay bills
    B. Short-term memory loss, disorientation to time, place, and possibly person
    C. Loss of the ability to chew and swallow
    D. Slowed reaction and learning

Answer: B

Critique: Alzheimer's disease has five stages. Stage 1 shows a decrease in energy and spontaneity, minor memory loss and mood swings, slowed reaction and learning, and avoidance of new situations. Stage 2 shows slowing of speech and comprehension, loss of train of thought in midsentence, forgetting to pay bills, and getting lost while traveling. Stage 3 shows short-term memory loss; disorientation to time, place, and possibly person; and paraphasic speech. Stage 4 shows behavioral disturbances, increasing need for care, and incontinence. Stage 5 shows loss of ability to chew and swallow and vulnerability to pneumonia and other illnesses. Frailty precedes coma and death.

Page: 108, Table 8–17

15: Treatment of chronic dementia includes all of the following, except:

    A. Nursing home placement
    B. Direct medications for the disease itself
    C. Treatment of associated conditions
    D. Psychosocial support

Answer: A

Critique: The patient should be cared for in his or her environment. Nursing home placement should be reserved for patients who cannot adequately be cared for at home.

Page: 110

16: Which statement is most accurate:

    A. Depressed mood is found in 20% of patients at the onset of memory loss.
    B. Selective serotonin re-uptake inhibitors (SSRIs) should never be used in patients with AD.
    C. Tricyclic antidepressants are recommended for treating depression.
    D. Delusions and psychosis are never present in AD.

Answer: A

Critique: Low dosages of SSRIs are indicated in depressed patients with memory loss. Tricyclic agents should be avoided because of their many side effects, which may exacerbate confusion and impair memory further. Delusions and psychosis are very common. In some cases, delusions are seen as the first manifestation of AD.

Page: 110

17: Treatment of late-life depression can be accomplished by:

    A. Psychotherapy
    B. Pharmacological therapy
    C. Electroconvulsive therapy
    D. All of the above

Answer: D

Critique: All of these treatments are used in treating elderly patients with depression. Elderly patients are less accepting of psychotherapy; nevertheless, it is a very effective therapeutic intervention, that should always be offered.

Page: 114

18: When using psychopharmacology to treat the depressed elderly patient, all of the following are true, except:

    A. Start with tricyclic antidepressants.
    B. "Start low and go slow."
    C. Prozac (fluoxetine) or Paxil (paroxetine) may be used at low dosages.

    D. Celexa may be used in patients with possible associated dementia.

Answer: A

Critique: Do not use tricyclic antidepressants in the elderly; their side effect profile does not outweigh their benefits. SSRIs are very effective in low dosages, for example, Prozac or Paxil at 5 mg. Celexa appears to be effective in patients with associated dementia. When starting treatment give a 6- to 12-week trial before increasing the dosage.

Page: 114

19: What is the most common cause of urinary incontinence in the elderly:

    A. Stress incontinence
    B. Functional incontinence
    C. Urge incontinence
    D. Overflow incontinence

Answer: D

Critique: Detrussor overactivity, also known as urge incontinence, is the most common form of urinary incontinence in the elderly. It is caused by detrussor muscle contractions before the bladder fills, resulting in urgency and frequency. There are two kinds of detrussor overactivity, one with intact bladder contractions and the other with hyperactive bladder contractions. The latter is most commonly seen in the elderly.

Page: 115

20: Which of the following statements is accurate concerning falls in the elderly:

    A. Poor vision rarely contributes to falls.
    B. Polypharmacy is an important risk factor for falls.
    C. Decreased hearing does not increase the incidence of falls.
    D. Environmental factors will never cause falls in the elderly.

Answer: B

Critique: Falls in the elderly are always multifactorial; they involve the specific environment and the activity itself, as well as the particular problems of the specific patient. Poor vision, polypharmacy, decreased hearing, and environmental factors all contribute to falls in the elderly and may account for up to 40% of falls. Other causes are postural hypotension, vertigo, and "drop attacks" (vertebral basilar insufficiency).

Pages: 117–119

21: Who is at highest risk for developing osteoporosis:

    A. An African American female of medium frame who has been a natural body builder most of her life
    B. A thin, elderly white woman who smokes and has a family history of osteoporosis
    C. An olive-skinned Cuban American woman who is large framed and stopped menstruating at the age of 52
    D. A white female of medium frame who is very active running a small farm in Pennsylvania

Answer: B

Critique: The smaller the bone structure, the more likely it is that a person will develop osteopenia and osteoporosis after menopause. This is the case in thin white and Asian women. It is important to point out that low bone mass diagnosed by densiometry is the most accurate predictor of fracture risk.

Page: 121, Table 8–33

22: Which of the following servings has the highest content of calcium:

    A. An 8-ounce serving of plain yogurt
    B. A 3-ounce serving of salmon
    C. One cup of broccoli
    D. An 8-ounce serving of skim milk

Answer: A

Critique: It is important for the physician to know which foods have the highest content of calcium to properly counsel patients. In this list, 8 ounces of plain yogurt has 345 to 415 mg of calcium, 8 ounces of skim milk has 302 mg of calcium, 3 ounces of salmon has 167 mg of calcium, and 1 cup of broccoli has 100 to 136 mg of calcium.

Page: 122, Table 8–34

23: All of the following statements are true regarding polymyalgia rheumatica, except:

    A. It is characterized by stiffness in the shoulder girdle.
    B. The treatment of choice is steroids.

    C. The sedimentation rate is elevated.
    D. It is associated with temporal arteritis in 20% of cases.
    E. It never involves the pelvic girdle.

Answer: E

Critique: Polymyalgia rheumatica is a disease of the elderly characterized by stiffness in the shoulder and pelvic girdles. Neck pain and stiffness are also seen, and the sedimentation rate is always elevated. It is associated with temporal arteritis in 20% of cases, which if left untreated may lead to blindness.

Page: 123

24: What is the most effective way to diagnose sexual dysfunction in women:

    A. Pelvic examination
    B. Medical history
    C. Interviewing her partner
    D. Pelvic sonogram

Answer: B

Critique: The medical history is most important in diagnosing sexual dysfunction in women. One of the most common complaints heard in the office is dyspareunia, particularly as a result of vaginal dryness, a problem that can be resolved by using vaginal estrogen creams for lubrication.

Pages: 124, 125

Chapter 9

Care of the Dying Patient

Ann M. Aring

1: When discussing the prognosis of a terminal illness with the patient, all of the following are true, except:

  A. Patients usually understand the severity of the illness during the family physician's first conversation with them.
  B. The patient gains comfort from nonverbal contact.
  C. Gradual disclosure of the illness likely leads to better patient acceptance.
  D. Denial is a common means of coping with the illness.
  E. Patients will indicate their wish to discuss the prognosis.

Answer: A

Critique: Patients indicate, verbally or often with nonverbal cues, that they need to discuss their prognosis. They may, however, feel unable to accept bad news all at once, and many family physicians reveal the nature of a terminal illness to patients gradually or in stages. This process may need to be repeated many times. It is important to remain alert to nonverbal cues and not to force such a discussion on an unwilling individual. Even when patients are fully aware of their prognosis, they often continue to employ denial as a means of fighting their disease. Eye contact and gentle touch help to reassure the patient that the family physician will support the patient throughout his or her last illness. It is a very powerful way of reinforcing the patient-family physician relationship.

Pages: 132, 133

2: Perception of chronic pain is influenced by:

  A. Past experience
  B. Fear
  C. Frustration and anxiety
  D. Fatigue
  E. All of the above

Answer: E

Critique: All of these factors may worsen pain for the patient. Analgesia alone is less likely to be effective unless the patient's fears about his or her illness are addressed when he or she is tired, anxious, frustrated, or afraid.

Page: 136

3: The greatest fear of a dying patient is:

  A. A painful death
  B. Being alone

  C. Loss of control of his or her body
  D. Loss of control of his or her affairs

Answer: B

Critique: The greatest fear of a dying patient is that of suffering alone and being deserted. There is less fear of a painful death than of the loneliness and alienation that may accompany it. Other factors are also important. A dying patient needs to feel that he or she is in control of personal affairs, even though body control is lost.

Page: 134

4: Which of the following poses a significant problem of opiate use in terminally ill patients?

  A. Nausea
  B. Sedation
  C. Constipation
  D. Respiratory depression
  E. Dependence

Answer: C

Critique: When opiate dose is titrated to the needs of the patient, sedation, hypotension, and respiratory depression are rarely problems. Nausea associated with opiate use usually abates after a few days and may be controlled effectively with an appropriate antiemetic. Constipation, however, may be a persistent problem with ongoing opiate use. Patients should always be encouraged to use a daily dose of laxative.

Page: 137

5: Arrange the following analgesics from least potent to most potent:

  A. Tylenol No. 3
  B. Morphine, 30 mg
  C. Fentanyl patches, 50 micrograms/hr
  D. Percocet
  E. Hydromorphone, 2 mg

Answer: From least to most potent: A, D, E, C, B

Critique: Understanding the relative potency of analgesics allows the physician to best meet the patient's needs for pain control.

Page: 137, Table 9–1

6: In deciding how to care for a dying patient, the family physician's primary responsibility is to:

  A. Himself

B. The spouse
C. The children
D. The patient

Answer: D

Critique: The physician frequently is torn between the patient and the patient's family. Although the wishes and desires of the family must be considered, when deciding how to care for a dying patient the physician's primary responsibility is to the patient.

Page: 134

7: When sharing information regarding a fatal diagnosis with a patient, which of the following is important:

A. Eye contact
B. Touch
C. Personal closeness
D. Sitting near the patient and not standing
E. All of the above

Answer: E

Critique: All of these gestures convey a sense of support, closeness, and compassion. These gestures also reinforce verbal assurance that the patient will not be abandoned during the difficult time remaining. Sitting with the patient, rather than standing, puts the physician at eye level and conveys a willingness to talk and listen.

Page: 133

8: Standards of hospice care include all of the following, except:

A. An interdisciplinary team providing care
B. Inpatient care services only
C. Care and support for the patient and family
D. Palliative care when a cure is not possible
E. The family as a central part of the hospice care team

Answer: B

Critique: In a hospice program, palliative care is the most appropriate form of care when a cure is no longer possible. A hospice program may provide inpatient care, as well as care in the home setting. Hospice philosophy regards the family as a central part of the hospice care team and considers the patient and family together as the unit of care. An interdisciplinary team provides hospice care.

Page: 142

9: (True or False) Which of the following measures are effective in managing the nutritional status of patients with terminal disease:

A. High-calorie food supplements
B. Gastrostomy tubes
C. Total parenteral nutrition
D. Alleviation of guilt in relatives
E. Corticosteroids

Answer: False - A, B, C, True - D, E

Critique: There is little evidence that forced supplementary feeding improves the prognosis. The most important measure may well be to alleviate the guilt of relatives, who may struggle to feed the patient in the belief that it will be helpful. Oral steroids may stimulate the appetite and encourage the patient to eat better.

Page: 141

10: (True or False) Which of the following statements apply to advance directives or "living wills"?

A. More than 50% of Americans have written a living will.
B. Federal law requires that all patients entering a hospice program must be offered the chance to make a living will.
C. A living will should allow for witnesses appointed by the patient to act as guardians of the patient's wishes and the specific circumstances in which the will may be used.
D. A living will provides a substitute for informed discussion with the family physician.

Answer: False - A, D, True - B, C

Critique: Almost 90% of Americans say that they would not want extraordinary steps taken to prolong their lives if they were dying. However, only 20% have made a living will. All patients entering a hospital or hospice program must be offered the opportunity to create advance directives. To cover any possible circumstances, a witness should be appointed to act on the patient's behalf. A living will is not a substitute for the family physician–patient relationship and discussion with the patient and his or her family.

Page: 145

11: All of the following agents may be used as preferred coanalgesics in terminal care patients, except:

A. Nonsteroidal anti-inflammatory drugs (NSAIDs)
B. COX-2 inhibitors
C. Gabapentin (Neurontin)
D. Amitriptyline
E. Steroids

Answer: E

Critique: All of these drugs may be helpful when caring for terminally ill patients, although steroids are not strictly regarded as coanalgesics. Bony lesions or those within the skeletal muscle may benefit from the addition of NSAIDs. Pain caused by nerve damage may respond well to low-dose amitriptyline or gabapentin.

Page: 139

12: All of the following statements apply to the importance of hope, except:

A. The physician should not raise false hopes in the patient.
B. Hope increases when honest information is withheld from the patient.
C. Hope is defined as the patient believing in what is still possible.
D. The physician should not be overaggressive in trying to help the patient maintain hope.
E. Having one's individuality accepted fosters hope.

Answer: B

Critique: Hope increases when honest information is provided, and it is reduced when information is withheld. The physician should not raise false hopes or be overaggressive to help the patient maintain hope, but the physician can help direct a patient toward achievable goals, such as pain relief or making a trip to visit relatives.

Page: 135

13: Which of the following situations best describes a "conspiracy of silence"?

    A. A physician provides a patient with an overoptimistic prognosis.

    B. A physician agrees to give an unrealistic picture of the prognosis either to the patient or to his or her family.

    C. The physician refuses to tell the family the prognosis.

    D. The physician refuses to tell the patient the diagnosis.

Answer: B

Critique: A conspiracy of silence arises when either the patient or his or her relatives are given, at the request of the other party, an unrealistic picture of the patient's illness and prognosis. This almost always creates tension between the two parties and results in isolation of the patient or the relatives. The family physician becomes entangled in the deception, a position that may be extremely uncomfortable.

Page: 134

14: Which one of the following statements about subcutaneous infusions is correct?

    A. Up to 10 mL of medication may be infused daily.

    B. Subcutaneous infusion should be managed only in an inpatient setting.

    C. Different drugs should be given via separate subcutaneous pumps.

    D. The pump may give booster doses of medication when needed.

    E. The butterfly needle used to deliver the medication may be placed anywhere in the body.

Answer: B

Critique: Up to 50 mL of volume may be infused by a subcutaneous pump daily. Although the infusion may be started in the inpatient unit, most families can manage to maintain the pump at home with appropriate supervision. Various medications (e.g., antiemetics, opiates) may be combined within the same syringe, but it is important to check their compatibility first. Most pumps can deliver a booster dose of medication when required. It is important that the infusion site is located in an area that has adequate subcutaneous tissue. The areas that are used most often are the abdomen, chest wall, or thigh.

Page: 140

15: (True or False) Which of the following statements apply to where patients die?

    A. Sixty percent of American patients still die in hospitals.

    B. Death with dignity is easiest to accomplish when the patient dies amid the surroundings that gave meaning to his or her life.

    C. Death with dignity may be accomplished in the company of those whose companionship provided the patient the most rewards in living.

    D. The family physician should always favor aggressively treating the patient, even when the evidence points to its futility.

    E. The family physician should be sensitive to the style of living and the style of dying that seem most appropriate for each individual patient.

Answer: False - A, D, True - B, C, E

Critique: Although 80% of Americans still die in hospitals, most of them say that they would rather die at home. The family physician must have the courage to discontinue aggressive therapy when the evidence points to its futility. The family physician should not arbitrarily decide what is best for all patients and should be sensitive to each individual patient.

Page: 142

Questions 16 to 18: Match the lettered and numbered entries:

    A. Active euthanasia

    B. Passive euthanasia

    C. Both

    D. Neither

16: Withholding treatment and allowing the disease to run its course.

17: Prescribing large quantities of drugs to allow the patient to take his or her own life.

18: The purposeful administration of drugs to end life.

Answers: 16 - B, 17 - D, 18 - A

Critique: The purposeful administration of drugs to end life is known as active euthanasia. Passive euthanasia is the withholding of treatment and allowing the disease to run its course. *Assisted suicide* is the term for prescribing large quantities of drugs to empower the patient to take his or her own life.

Page: 144

19: After causes such as anemia, bronchospasm, or congestive heart failure have been excluded, dyspnea in the terminally ill patient may be managed by using:

    A. Narcotics alone

    B. Oxygen alone

    C. Antibiotics alone

    D. Narcotics and oxygen

    E. All of the above

Answer: A

Critique: Narcotics are the most effective means of relieving dyspnea in the terminally ill patient. Oxygen may give a little extra benefit. The use of antibiotics will not improve control of dyspnea itself, and their use should be considered carefully so that both of the physician and the patient are clear as to whether antibiotics will improve the quality of life or prolong the dying phase.

Page: 140

20: All of the following statements apply to the patient's denial regarding the reality of his or her disease process and impending death, except:

A. Denial is one way of coping with or protecting against overwhelming anxiety.
B. Denial is seen only when the patient first learns of his or her impending death.
C. Denial provides constant emotional protection until the patient is ready to face the truth.
D. A patient who avoids asking about his or her illness or prognosis when the physician offers every opportunity is experiencing denial.
E. Denial is more pronounced when a patient is told abruptly of his or her impending death.

Answer: B

Critique: Denial can appear in different degrees at different times during the illness. The mental burden of impending death is too heavy to carry all the time, and periodic relief is necessary to carry on customary activities and enjoy the limited time left.

Page: 134

Chapter 10

Ethics in Family Practice

Alison Rutledge

1: (True or False) Which of the following are factors that have transformed ethical issues in the practice of medicine in recent years:

    A. Concern for patient rights
    B. Concern for patient autonomy
    C. Decline in the quality of medical education
    D. Demands of third-party payers
    E. Shortage of physicians in certain areas

Answers: A - True, B - True, C - False, D - True, E - False

Critique: Concern for patient rights and autonomy, plus the pervasive demands of third-party payers, has transformed the practice of medicine in recent years.

Page: 148

2: (True or False) The quality of the doctor-patient relationship is currently threatened. According to Holleman and Brody, which of the following problems are at fault:

    A. Time pressure for physicians
    B. Misunderstandings of patient autonomy
    C. Large numbers of uninsured patients
    D. Interference by third-party payers
    E. Team medical practice

Answers: A - False, B - True, C - False, D - True, E - False

Critique: Misunderstandings about patient autonomy include the perception that the patient is a "customer" who has "hired" the doctor to do his bidding; interference by third-party payers likewise includes the potential problem that the doctor is "hired" to do their bidding. However, the physician is a professional whose commitment is to practice within professional standards of care, despite any pressures or competing loyalties.

Page: 148

3: Which of the following is *not* a purpose of an employee preplacement medical examination:

    A. To determine the person's fitness for working at that particular job
    B. To inform the person about health risks relating to that particular job
    C. To address any physical problems detected during the evaluation whether related to the job or not
    D. To inform the employer about any and all physical problems discovered in the examination

    E. To collect baseline data for the future treatment of job-related injuries and illnesses

Answer: D

Critique: The doctor-patient relationship still includes physician respect and observance of confidentiality even when the examination is work related for the patient. Results given to the third party should be relevant to the narrow question at hand. In this case, the employer does not have a right to information about "any and all" physical problems discovered.

Page: 148

4: Mr. Smith is seeing you for ongoing assessment of an on-the-job back injury for workers' compensation benefits. During the examination, he tells you that he has recently developed a bad cough, probably as a result of a cold he caught at home from one of his children. He would like you to investigate and treat his cough. You should:

    A. Inform Mr. Smith that he should see a specialist for this; you are there only to deal with his on-the-job injury.
    B. Go ahead and investigate and treat his cough as part of the workers' compensation examination.
    C. Treat the cough, but do not mention it in Mr. Smith's chart.
    D. Address the cough, but bill Mr. Smith separately for that portion of your time and any tests.
    E. Ask Mr. Smith to come back later for a separate appointment relating to the cough.

Answer: D

Critique: The issuing of separate billings discourages the abuse of benefits programs and makes clear the physician's allegiances.

Page: 149

5: (True or False) Why is confidentiality an important principle in medical treatment?

    A. It protects doctor and patient alike from lawsuits.
    B. It encourages patients to be open in their communications with physicians.
    C. It respects a patient's right to privacy.
    D. It gives the patient necessary control over his or her medical information.
    E. It discourages harmful gossip.

Answers: A - False, B - True, C - True, D - True,
E - False

Critique: The pledge of confidentiality is crucial if patients are to be forthcoming with their true concerns to the physician. The patient has a right to privacy about his or her health status and should have control over the ultimate uses of personal medical information.

Page: 149

6: (True or False) Under which of the following circumstances would the principle of confidentiality be outweighed by circumstances *requiring* the sharing of confidential information:

    A. The physician strongly suspects child abuse.
    B. The physician strongly suspects the patient has committed spousal abuse.
    C. The physician has diagnosed genital herpes.
    D. The physician strongly suspects the patient will commit a murder.
    E. The physician wants to share concerns about a very elderly patient with the family.

Answers: A - True, B - False, C - False, D - True,
E - False

Critique: Laws vary in different jurisdictions, but mandatory reporting of child abuse and the duty to warn or protect a potential murder victim are two circumstances in which the need for information generally outweighs the principle of confidentiality.

Page: 149

7: (True or False) Which of the following conditions are exceptions to the mandate for informed consent for treatment:

    A. If the patient is not competent to give consent, consent need not be sought.
    B. If the patient has a life-threatening emergency but is unconscious and cannot give consent, the treatment may still be performed.
    C. If knowing the full facts of the situation would psychologically harm the patient, informed consent need not be sought.
    D. If the patient agreed to a similar treatment in the past, new consent need not be obtained.
    E. If all the patient's relatives agree, then the patient's consent need not be sought.

Answers: A - False, B - True, C - True, D - False,
E - False

Critique: If a patient is not competent, then the patient's surrogate must give consent. Consent for each new procedure must be sought, and relatives may not decide for the patient if the patient is competent. Only in a life-threatening emergency or in the rare instance in which seeking consent would itself be damaging may exceptions to the imperative of informed consent be made.

Page: 150

8: (True or False) Which of the following are elements of competency for giving informed consent:

    A. The patient can receive relevant information about the treatment.
    B. The patient can remember the information.
    C. The patient can recite the information back to you.
    D. The patient can explain all the pros and cons of the choices.
    E. The patient can use the information to make a decision.

Answers: A - True, B - True, C - False, D - False,
E - True

Critique: There is no requirement that patients recite back the information or explain the pros and cons of their choices; however, in any given instance these may be good techniques to use to ensure that the patient has received, has remembered, and can use the information.

Page: 150

9: (True or False) Most states have passed special laws that allow physicians to treat teenagers without parental consent for which of the following problems:

    A. Venereal disease
    B. Drug-related problems
    C. Need for contraception
    D. Mental health care
    E. Pregnancy

Answers: A - True, B - True, C - True, D - False,
E - True

Critique: Teenagers presenting for mental health care generally must have parental consent to receive treatment.

Page: 151

10: (True or False) Which of the following are causes of many cases of patient noncompliance with treatment:

    A. The patient is depressed or anxious.
    B. The patient is stubborn and oppositional.
    C. The patient does not understand the importance of treatment.
    D. The patient wants to be sick.
    E. The patient does not trust the physician.

Answers: A - True, B - False, C - True, D - False,
E - True

Critique: Although physicians may perceive noncompliant patients as oppositional, the patient's psychological status, lack of understanding, and lack of confidence in the physician are the primary factors in noncompliance. These problems can often be overcome with more and better communication.

Page: 151

11: (True or False) Which of the following are primary reasons that many patients never fill a doctor's prescription:

    A. The patient is afraid of the medication.
    B. The patient dislikes the side effects of the medication.
    C. The medicine is too expensive.

D. The patient's family members urge the patient not to take the medication.

E. The patient does not think the medication is important.

Answers: A - False, B - True, C - True, D - False, E - False

Critique: Problematic side effects and expense are always two of the primary reasons that patients do not fill prescriptions. It is incumbent on the physician to be aware of prescription costs and to educate the patient about side effects in a sensitive manner.

Page: 151

12: (True or False) Why do Holleman and Brody believe that the family practice physician is in an "ideal position" to manage a patient's care throughout a referral process:

A. The physician knows the patient's medical history and personality.

B. The physician knows the outcome of referral alternatives.

C. The physician knows what is best for the patient.

D. The physician is committed to a personal approach to the patient.

E. The physician has a strong knowledge of general medicine.

Answers: A - True, B - False, C - False, D - True, E - True

Critique: A family practice physician is aware of the patient as a person and is a general medicine practitioner. Presumably, he or she also has positive relationships with referral sources.

Pages: 151, 152

13: (True or False) Which of the following are the physician's responsibilities when initiating a referral:

A. Educating the patient as to the reasons for a referral

B. Recommending a particular specialist or treatment center

C. Providing the specialist with all the data needed to help the patient

D. Going with the patient to the appointment with the specialist

E. Explaining everything the specialist says to the patient

Answers: A - True, B - True, C - True, D - False, E - False

Critique: It is not necessary to accompany the patient or to intervene in communication between the specialist and the patient.

Page: 152

14: (True or False) Of the following possible effects of prospective reimbursement systems, which are ethically problematic:

A. Avoiding wasteful procedures and referrals

B. Streamlining the referral process

C. Encouraging the physician to limit interventions

D. Limiting the physician's freedom to practice medicine autonomously

Answers: A - False, B - False, C - True, D - True

Critique: Avoiding waste and streamlining continuity of care are positive benefits of prospective reimbursement systems. Encouraging the physician to limit interventions in the interests of controlling costs and discouraging autonomous practice are both ethically problematic.

Page: 152

15: (True or False) According to Holleman and Brody, the physician has a unique responsibility in dealing with emotions. Which of the following are examples of best practice:

A. Helping the patient become aware of his or her own emotions

B. Helping the patient become aware of the physician's emotions

C. The physician being aware of his or her own emotions

D. Knowing how to skillfully avoid emotional conversations

E. Sharing all the physician's emotions with the patient

Answers: A - True, B - False, C - True, D - False, E - False

Critique: It is never necessary for a patient to be aware of or attentive to a physician's emotions.

Page: 153

16: (True or False) Oregon passed the Death with Dignity Act in 1997. Which of the following are provisions of that act:

A. The patient must submit within 1 week both a written and an oral request to take a lethal dose of medication.

B. The physician must administer the medication himself or herself.

C. The patient must have a terminal diagnosis and prognosis.

D. The patient's depression must be at a mild level only.

E. The physician's assessment must be backed up with that of a consultant.

Answers: A - False, B - False, C - True, D - False, E - True

Critique: The patient has 15 days, not 1 week, to request a lethal dose of medication. The physician is prohibited from administering the medication. If the patient has any level of depression, a counseling referral must be made.

Page: 154

17: (True or False) Which of the following are issues that complicate the resolution of ethical issues in genetic medicine:

A. Ethicists do not know enough about the scientific issues involved.

B. Guilt, shame, and blame often surround perceptions of inherited diseases.
C. Doctors do not understand the ethical implications of the work in the field.
D. There may be problems in family communication and cooperation.
E. Emotional intensity surrounds the issues of eugenics and abortion.

Answers: A - False, B - True, C - False, D - True, E - True

Critique: Although the technology is new, ethicists and physicians can still be aware of each other's work. The intense feelings often evoked in situations of inherited diseases, the political fervor engendered by issues of eugenics and abortion, and the need for family members to communicate openly very much complicate the resolution of ethical issues in genetic medicine.

Page: 155

PART II

FAMILY MEDICINE IN THE COMMUNITY

Periodic Health Examination

Michael Ragain

1: The proven benefits of a periodic health examination include:

    A. Reassurance to the patient that he or she is healthy
    B. Provides cost effective clues to diseases the patient might develop in the future
    C. Has a low false-positive rate
    D. No proven benefit in asymptomatic individuals

Answer: D

Critique: Multiple studies have failed to show any benefit from periodic complete history and physical exams to asymptomatic patients. The use of these physicals is associated with increased cost (both physician time and perhaps unnecessary testing), a false sense of security provided to the patient, and a high false-positive rate.

Page: 159

2: (True or False) The United States Preventive Services Task Force (USPSTF) has produced evidence-based guidelines to guide the use of preventive services. The following statements relate to these guidelines:

    A. A rating of good or strong is based on clear evidence from randomized controlled trials.
    B. A rating of fair is based on inconclusive evidence from randomized controlled trials.
    C. Good evidence exists for all of the common screening and preventive services.
    D. The USPSTF Guide to Clinical Preventive Services makes specific recommendations regarding the usefulness of methods to screen for morbidity and mortality.

Answers: A - True, B - False, C - False, D - True

Critique: The USPSTF Guide to Clinical Preventive Services is based on the best evidence available to guide the selection of screening services. A rating of good or strong is based on clear evidence from randomized controlled trials. A rating of fair is based on less rigorous studies. For some interventions good evidence does not exist. For these screening and preventive services our decisions must be based on other criteria.

Page: 159

3: (True or False) When assessing development in your office in children age birth to 10 years the following should be considered:

    A. Three percent of the United States' population is mentally retarded.

    B. Up to 5% of children beginning school may have speech delay.
    C. There are no good tools to use to assess development.
    D. The American Academy of Pediatrics (AAP) recommends against screening all infants and children for developmental disabilities.

Answers: A - True, B - True, C - False, D - False

Critique: It is true that 3% of the population is mentally retarded and up to 5% of children entering school have speech delay due to developmental disability. Screening for these problems during each preventative visit with a good tool such as the Denver Developmental Screening Test is recommended by the AAP. This instrument assesses gross and fine motor function, and social and language development. It has a test-retest reliability of 97%.

Page: 160

4: The physical examination of the newborn can screen for the following conditions:

    A. Retinal blastoma
    B. Cleft palate
    C. Undescended testicle
    D. Congenital hip dysplasia
    E. All of the above

Answer: E

Critique: As discussed previously the usefulness of the physical examination for screening is debatable, but it may be helpful in certain conditions common in the newborn period. Absence of the red reflex may indicate retinal blastoma or congenital cataracts. Cleft palate should be recognized early in life because it is often associated with other abnormalities. Male genitals should be examined for descent of the testicles since undescended testicles are a risk factor for testicular cancer and infertility. Use of Ortolani's and Barlow's maneuvers can detect hip instability, which can indicate congenital hip dysplasia, which occurs in 1 out of 80 hips at birth.

Page: 160

5: (True or False) The USPSTF, American Academy of Family Physicians (AAFP), and AAP recommend the following screens at each visit in children older than 2 years of age:

    A. Head circumference
    B. Waist-hip ratio

C. Arm span to height ratio
D. Height and weight

Answers: A - False, B - False, C - False, D - True

Critique: Head circumference measurement is useful in children under the age of two. Waist-hip ratio and arm span to height ratio are not recommended for general screening at each visit. Height and weight measurements are recommended at each visit. Height and weight are useful in younger children to detect failure to thrive because of medical or psychosocial problems and in older children as a screen for obesity.

Page: 160

6: (True or False) When addressing hypertension in children age birth to ten years of age, the following statements are important to consider:

A. There are measurement inaccuracies that limit the usefulness of blood pressures in children younger than three years old.
B. Elevated blood pressure in children is less commonly a result of secondary hypertension than in adults.
C. The USPSTF cites fair evidence in support of blood pressure screening in children older than three years of age.
D. The normal values for blood pressure do not vary with age.

Answers: A - True, B - False, C - True, D - False

Critique: Blood pressure measurement can be very useful and there are age-matched normal values. The main problem with assessing the blood pressure in children less than three years of age is measurement inaccuracies. Secondary hypertension is more common in children (28%) than in adults (5%). The causes of secondary hypertension in children include coarctation of the aorta, renal disease, and hyperthyroidism. The USPSTF (1996) cites fair evidence in support of blood pressure screening in children older than 3 years.

Page: 160

7: Which of the following statements are true regarding vision problems in children:

A. Up to 20% of preschoolers are affected by strabismus and amblyopia.
B. The false-positive rate for visual acuity testing in children is less than 10%.
C. The USPSTF cites strong evidence for screening of visual acuity in children.
D. The USPSTF cites fair evidence for screening for amblyopia and strabismus with the cover-uncover test at 3 to 4 years of age.
E. All the above

Answer: D

Critique: Up to 5% of preschoolers are affected by strabismus and amblyopia. Screening of these conditions is important because they lead to educational difficulties and even blindness. The USPSTF cites fair evidence for screening for amblyopia and strabismus with the cover-

uncover test at 3 to 4 years of age. The false-positive rate for visual acuity testing in children is 30% or more. Screening is especially non-specific in children who do not have visual complaints. The USPSTF cites insufficient evidence for or against screening of visual acuity in children.

Pages: 160, 162

8: Which of the following statements is true regarding hearing problems in children:

A. Moderate hearing loss is not associated with delayed language development.
B. There is no way to check for hearing loss in newborns.
C. Routine hearing screening in asymptomatic children older than 3 years old is associated with a low false-positive rate.
D. In school-aged children the most common hearing impairment is recurrent otitis media.

Answer: D

Critique: Moderate to severe hearing loss is associated with delayed language development. Auditory brain stem response testing is the standard screening tool for the newborn. It is limited in utility due to cost and the need for appropriate user training. Routine hearing screening in asymptomatic children younger than 3 years old is associated with a high false-positive rate. The USPSTF cites fair evidence against routine hearing screening in children older than 3 years. In school-aged children the most common cause of hearing loss is recurrent otitis media and is most often self-limited.

Page: 162

9: (True or False) The USPSTF cites good evidence for routine blood screening during the newborn period for the following disorders.

A. Maple urine disease
B. Hemoglobinopathies
C. Phenylketonuria
D. Congenital hypothyroidism
E. Down syndrome

Answers: A - False, B - True, C - True, D - True, E - False

Critique: The USPSTF cites good evidence for routine blood screening for hemoglobinopathies, phenylketonuria, and congenital hypothyroidism during the newborn period. Infants tested for phenylketonuria in the first 24 hours of life should have the test repeated again at 2 weeks of life. Downs syndrome and maple urine disease are not part of the recommended newborn screening blood testing.

Page: 162

10: Which of the following is true of childhood iron deficiency anemia in the United States:

A. The USPSTF cites insufficient evidence for or against universal screening of infants not in high-risk groups.

B. It is more common in Caucasians.
C. Consuming cow's milk starting at age 6 months lowers the risk of developing it.
D. The prevalence is 15%.

Answer: A

Critique: The prevalence of childhood iron deficiency anemia in the United States is less than 3%. It is more common in African Americans, Native Americans, immigrants from developing countries, preterm infants, lower socioeconomic groups, and infants who consume cow's milk before 12 months of age. The USPSTF cites insufficient evidence to recommend for or against universal screening of infants not in high-risk groups. Infants from high-risk groups should be screened. The Bright Futures, AAP, and AAFP guidelines do recommend universal screening once during infancy.

Page: 162

11: (True or False) A 15-month-old child presents to your clinic and the mother requests lead screening. Important considerations that have a bearing on lead screening in this child include:

A. Lead exposure in children can cause decreased intelligence quotient and attention.
B. Children who live in homes built after 1950 are at increased risk.
C. Venous lead testing is more appropriate than erythrocyte protoporphyrin testing.
D. The CDC recommends universal screening in areas where more than 12% of the children screened have elevated blood lead levels.

Answers: A - True, B - False, C - True, D - True

Critique: The percentage of children with elevated lead levels has declined dramatically from 1981 to 1991 due to the removal of lead from gasoline, paint, and food cans. Lead exposure in children can cause decreased intelligence quotient and attention, and can lead to behavioral and neurodevelopmental disorders. Children who live in homes built before 1950, areas with high lead water levels, or areas with high lead levels from industry are at increased risk. Venous lead testing is more appropriate than erythrocyte protoporphyrin testing. The USPSTF cites fair evidence for recommending lead screening at about 12 months of age. The CDC recommends universal screening in areas where more than 12% of the children screened have elevated blood lead levels or where more than 27% of the houses were built before 1950.

Page: 162

12: (True or False) Which of the following are true regarding screening of children for tuberculosis.

A. Children who have known close contact with a person infected with tuberculosis.
B. Children who have known close contact with a person infected with human immunodeficiency virus (HIV).
C. All children over the age of six years at least once.
D. Children from low-income families.

Answers: A - True, B - True, C - False, D - True

Critique: The AAFP, AAP, and USPSTF all recommend screening children from high-risk groups. A child is considered high risk if he or she has been in close contact with a person infected with tuberculosis or HIV, lives in underserved areas or is from a low-income population, or is a resident in a long-term care facility. Routine screening of children at normal risk is not recommended.

Page: 163

13: The current recommended test for HIV infection in infants immediately after birth is:

A. Low white blood cell count
B. Polymerase chain reaction (PCR)
C. Enzyme linked immunosorbent antibody (ELISA) testing
D. Electron microscopy

Answer: B

Critique: The AAFP and the USPSTF both recommend that infants who are born to mothers at high risk for HIV or known to have HIV infection should be tested immediately after birth. The tests that are currently recommended in these neonates are either the polymerase chain reaction PCR test or viral culture.

Page: 163

14: The leading cause of death of persons between the ages of 1 and 34 years is:

A. Human immunodeficiency virus (HIV)
B. Drug overdose
C. Unintentional injuries
D. Pneumonia

Answer: C

Critique: The most common cause of injuries in this age group is unintentional injuries including household and motor vehicle accidents. Following simple safety recommendations could have prevented many of these accidents.

Page: 163

15: (True or False) Which of the following statements are true regarding baby walkers:

A. Use is associated with low rates of injury.
B. Use is associated with high rates of injury.
C. Assist in the development of infant's ability to walk.
D. The AAP recommends their use.

Answers: A - False, B - True, C - False, D - False

Critique: The use of baby walkers is associated with high rates of injury with annual rates approaching 8.9 per 1000. Their use does not assist in the development of infants' ability to walk. The AAP recommends a ban on their manufacture and use because of the high rates of injury and lack of proven benefit to children.

Page: 163

16: (True or False) Which of the following measures are helpful in preventing injuries to children:

A. Swimming lessons are more helpful at preventing drowning than parental supervision.

B. Keeping the water heater temperature set for 180 degrees helps prevent scalding burns.
C. Proper use of child restraints has decreased the morbidity and mortality associated with MVA.
D. Warnings stickers such as "Mr. Yuck" are effective at preventing children from ingesting poisons and should be used on all household chemicals

Answers: A - False, B - False, C - True, D - False

Critique: Parental supervision is more helpful in preventing drowning than are swimming lessons. Water heaters should be set at less than 120°F to prevent scalding. Proper use of child restraints has decreased the morbidity and mortality associated with MVA. Warnings stickers such as "Mr. Yuck" are ineffective at preventing children from ingesting poisons and should not be used. These stickers may actually attract children's attention to harmful chemicals.

Page: 163

17: (True or False) When advising a mother about her children's dental health, which of the following recommendations are useful:

A. There is no associated dental decay in allowing a child to fall asleep with a bottle.
B. Children 2 years and older should begin brushing their teeth with small amounts of fluoride-containing toothpaste while being supervised by an adult.
C. Regular dental habits should start at the time that a child begins school.
D. Oral fluoride supplementation should be given to all children who breast-feed.

Answers: A - False, B - True, C - False, D - False

Critique: Infants and small children should not be allowed to fall asleep with a bottle because it can promote significant dental decay known as "milk bottle caries." Children should begin brushing with a small amount of fluoride-containing toothpaste under adult supervision starting at age 3. At age 3, children should also begin regular dental visits. The USPSTF, the AAFP, and the AAP recommend supplementation of fluoride in children older than 6 months living in areas with a less than 0.6 parts per million of fluoride in the water supply.

Page: 164

18: Which of the following is true regarding the prevention of chlamydial and comital ophthalmia neonatorum:

A. Only high-risk newborns should receive ophthalmologic prophylaxis within one hour of birth.
B. Penicillin ointment is the drug of choice.
C. Most states do not require prophylactic treatment.
D. Using the appropriate antimicrobials is effective in preventing 80% to 90% of chlamydial and comital infections.

Answer: D

Critique: All newborns should have ophthalmologic prophylaxis within one hour of birth, typically with Erythromycin ointment. Law in most states requires this treatment. It is effective in preventing up to 90% of chlamydial ophthalmia neonatorum infections according to the Canadian Task Force Periodic Health Examination, 1992.

Page: 164

19: Which of the following statements is true regarding obesity in adolescents in the United States:

A. Obesity is an uncommon problem in the United States.
B. Obesity is not a major risk factor for other diseases such as diabetes, hypertension, stroke, or cardiovascular disease.
C. Treatment of obesity has no impact on the prevalence of diabetes, hypertension, cardiovascular disease, or stroke.
D. Adolescent obesity is a significant risk factor and predictor of adult obesity.

Answer: D

Critique: Obesity is a major problem in the United States. It is an independent risk factor for stroke, cardiovascular disease, certain cancers, arthritis, hypertension, and diabetes mellitus. It has been shown that treatment of obesity reduces the prevalence of these diseases. Adolescent obesity is a significant risk factor and predictor for the development of adult obesity. The body mass index is a good tool to determine proper height and weight. A body mass index of greater than 85th percentile is used to define obesity. There is a direct relationship between body mass index and mortality.

Page: 165

20: (True or False) A 20-year-old female presents to your office for annual examination. She reports using oral contraceptives and is sexually active with one partner. Which of the following are true regarding the risk of sexually transmitted diseases in this woman:

A. Up to 70% of women with chlamydial infections may be asymptomatic.
B. The most common sexually transmitted disease (STD) in the United States is gonorrhea.
C. The USPSTF cites fair evidence for routine screening of all sexually active adolescent females for chlamydial infection and gonorrhea in those who are at high risk.
D. Serologic screening for HIV should be offered to all persons being treated for other STDs

Answers: A - True, B - False, C - True, D - True

Critique: Chlamydia trachomatis is the most common STD in the United States affecting approximately four million people. It is often asymptomatic in up to 70% of women. This makes them an unknown reservoir for further transmission. The USPSTF cites fair evidence for routine screening of all sexually active adolescent females who are at high risk for chlamydia and gonorrhea infections. All persons who are being treated for an STD should have HIV serologic screening.

Pages: 165, 167

21: A 17-year-old white male presents to your office for a periodic health-screening visit. In order to assess his risk of problem drinking, you utilize the CAGE questionnaire as a tool. The following are components of the CAGE questionnaire, except:

    A. Have you ever felt annoyed by someone else asking about your drinking?
    B. Have you ever had an eye-opener in the morning?
    C. Have you ever felt curious about how much you drink?
    D. Have you ever felt guilty about your drinking or anything you did while drinking?

Answer: C

Critique: Alcohol use in adolescents is common. Screening questions for alcohol use can be remembered by using the CAGE mnemonic. The CAGE questionnaire can be useful for adolescents at risk. The questions of the CAGE questionnaire include:

C – Have you ever felt you had to *cut* back on how much you drink?
A – Have you ever felt *annoyed* by someone else asking about your drinking?
G – Have you ever felt *guilty* about your drinking or anything you did while drinking?
E – Have you ever had an *eye*-opener in the morning?

Page: 167

22: (True or False) Warning signs for homicide and suicide in adolescents include the following, which would indicate a need for further investigation:

    A. Declining school grades
    B. Family dysfunction
    C. Chronic melancholy
    D. History of substance abuse

Answers: A - True, B - True, C - True, D - True

Critique: Suicide and homicide are the third and fourth leading cause of death in 11- to 24-year-olds. Often there is a comorbid disorder present in these adolescents. The USPSTF cites insufficient evidence for or against routine screening for homicide and suicide. Some warning signs for homicidal and suicidal ideation include declining grades, family dysfunction, chronic melancholy, and history of physical abuse or substance abuse.

Page: 168

23: When counseling adolescents regarding tobacco cessation, which of the following is true:

    A. Most smokers begin smoking as adults.
    B. Ten percent of 12- to 13-year-olds reported experimenting with tobacco.
    C. Of high school seniors, 10% smoke regularly.
    D. Counseling against tobacco use is recommended for all ages on a regular basis.

Answer: D

Critique: Most smokers begin smoking as teenagers. Up to 25% of 12- to 13-year-olds reported experimenting with tobacco and 19% of high school seniors smoke regularly. The initiation of smoking at an early age is associated with more severe addiction. It is recommended that all ages be counseled against tobacco use on a regular basis.

Page: 170

24: Which of the following statements is true regarding screening for hypertension in adults aged 25 to 64 years:

    A. Increased awareness and treatment of hypertension have resulted in no significant decrease in mortality from stroke and myocardial infarction since 1970.
    B. The Joint National Committee on Prevention, Detection, Evaluation, and Treatment of High Blood Pressure recommends screening every year for patients with normal blood pressure.
    C. Normal blood pressure is defined as systolic blood pressure less than 140 and diastolic blood pressure less than 90.
    D. The Joint National Committee on Prevention, Detection, Evaluation, and Treatment of High Blood Pressure recommends screening annually for those patients with systolic blood pressure between 130 and 139 or diastolic blood pressure between 85 and 95.

Answer: D

Critique: Hypertension is a very important cause of morbidity and mortality. Increased awareness and treatment of hypertension has resulted in a significant decrease in age-specific mortality from cardiovascular disease since 1970. The Joint National Committee on Prevention, Detection, Evaluation, and Treatment of High Blood Pressure recommends screening every two years for patients with normal (<130/<85) blood pressures and annually for those with "high normal" (130–139/85–89) readings.

Page: 170

25: (True or False) Obesity is a common problem that increases the incidence of the following diseases:

    A. Diabetes
    B. Hyperlipidemia
    C. Degenerative joint disease
    D. Rheumatoid arthritis
    E. Cirrhosis

Answers: A - True, B - True, C - True, D - False, E - False

Critique: Obesity is a common problem affecting up to 30% of the adult population in the United States. Excess weight clearly leads to increases in the incidence of the following diseases: diabetes, hypertension, hyperlipidemia, coronary artery disease, degenerative joint disease, and obstructive sleep apnea. There does not appear to be an increased incidence of rheumatoid arthritis and cirrhosis in obese patients. Periodic screening for obesity by measurement of height and weight is recommended by both the AAFP and the USPSTF for all patients.

Page: 170

26: A 52-year-old female presents to your office for her annual examination. She has questions about screening for breast cancer with mammography. Which of the following statements is true regarding mammography:

A. Annual screening is clearly advantageous over biannual screening.
B. Once she has reached the age of 75, there is no evidence that she will benefit from mammographic screening.
C. There is no decrease in cancer mortality when screening women between the ages of fifty and sixty-nine years with mammography.
D. False-positive mammography is likely to have little adverse psychological impact.

Answer: B

Critique: There is strong evidence from numerous studies that breast cancer mortality is decreased by up to 25% in women between 50 and 69 who are screened with mammography, clinical breast exam, or both. Mammographic screening has not been proven to decrease mortality in women between the ages of 40 and 49 years. There is no evidence of benefit for women older than 75 years of age. There is little data on the appropriate periodicity of mammography, but no clear advantage has been demonstrated with annual versus biannual screening.

Page: 172

27: When screening women for cancer of the uterine cervix, which of the following statements should be considered true:

A. Death from cancer of the uterine cervix has almost completely been eliminated in the United States.
B. Five-year survival rates are low for localized disease.
C. Mathematical modeling studies predict a definite mortality benefit from screening every three years compared with every ten.
D. The specificity of the Pap smear is low.

Answer: C

Critique: Cancer of the uterine cervix accounts for approximately 5,000 deaths per year in the United States. Five-year survival rates are high (90%) for localized disease, but much lower (less than 20%) for stage 4 disease. Cervical cancer may be one of the best examples of successful screening with up to 70% reduction in mortality resulting from Pap smear screening. The specificity of the Pap smear is high (probably greater than 90%) but the sensitivity is suboptimal (55% to 80%). This limited sensitivity contributes to the controversy over the appropriate screening interval. Mathematical modeling studies predict a definite mortality benefit from screening every 3 years compared with every 10. However, there is very little additional benefit predicted by annual Pap smear screening.

Page: 172

28: A 62-year-old male presents to your office for annual physical examination. Which of the following state-

ments should guide your recommendation for colorectal cancer screening in this patient:

A. There is good evidence from three randomized controlled trials that fecal occult blood testing reduces colon cancer mortality in patients 50 years and older.
B. There are few false-positive results with fecal occult blood testing.
C. Screening with sigmoidoscopy has been shown to protect against mortality from colon cancer in large randomized controlled trials.
D. The USPSTF recommends flexible sigmoidoscopy for screening and follow-up of patients with a strong family history of early colon cancer, hereditary polyposis, inflammatory bowel disease, or a personal history of colon cancer.

Answer: A

Critique: The digital rectal examination has a very low sensitivity; less than 10% of colon rectal cancers are located in the distal rectum within easy reach of palpation. There is good evidence from three randomized controlled trials that fecal occult blood testing reduces colon cancer mortality in patients fifty years and older. There are many false-positives with fecal occult blood testing, especially with rehydration of samples before testing. It is possible that some of the benefit derived from fecal occult blood testing may actually be secondary to the large number of colonoscopies performed for positive fecal occult blood test. Similar decreases in mortality could be seen if one third of the population were randomly screened with colonoscopy. Screening sigmoidoscopy has been shown to protect against mortality from colon cancer in large case control studies. No randomized control trials for screening sigmoidoscopy have been performed. The USPSTF recommends colonoscopy for screening and a follow-up of high-risk patients such as those with strong family history of early colon cancer, hereditary polyposis, inflammatory bowel disease, personal history of high-risk polyps or colon cancer.

Pages: 172, 173

29: (True or False) Which of the following are true regarding hyperlipidemia screening and treatment in adults aged 25 to 60 years of age:

A. Elevation of low-density lipoprotein (LDL) is a major risk factor for coronary artery disease.
B. Treatment of hyperlipidemia has not been shown to decrease the incidence of myocardial infarction in patients with known coronary artery disease.
C. The National Cholesterol Education Program recommends measurement of total cholesterol and high-density lipoprotein (HDL) in the non-fasting state for all adults older than 20 years.
D. Fasting lipoprotein analysis is recommended for anyone with total cholesterol of 200 or higher.

Answers: A - True, B - False, C - True, D - False

Critique: Hyperlipidemia, especially low-density lipoprotein, is a major risk factor for coronary artery disease. Treatment of hyperlipidemia has been shown to decrease the incidence of myocardial infarction in patients with known coronary disease and to decrease overall mortality in both primary and secondary prevention studies. The National Cholesterol Education Program recommends measurement of total cholesterol and high-density lipoprotein in a nonfasting state for all adults older than twenty years of age. If both are desirable (cholesterol less than 200 and HDL greater than or equal to 35) it recommends rescreening at 5-year intervals. Fasting lipoprotein analysis is recommended for anyone with a total cholesterol level of 240 or higher or an HDL of less than 35 and for patients with coronary risk factors and total cholesterol of 200 to 239.

Page: 173

30: (True or False) According to the USPSTF, the following minerals or vitamins should be supplemented:

A. Folic acid 0.4 to 0.8 mg per day in all women of childbearing age who are sexually active and not trying to avoid pregnancy.
B. One multivitamin per day for all adults age 25 to 64.
C. Calcium 1200 to 1500 mg per day is recommended for all women, teenagers and older, to maximize bone density and prevent osteoporosis.
D. Selenium supplementation 50 mg per day for all adults age 25 to 64 who have a BMI greater than 28.

Answers: A - True, B - False, C - True, D - False

Critique: The USPSTF recommends folic acid supplementation for all women of childbearing age who might potentially become pregnant. Calcium supplementation is recommended for all women teenage years and older to maximize bone density and prevent osteoporosis. There are no other recommendations regarding chemoprophylaxis in adults age 25 to 64 in the USPSTF.

Page: 175

31: A 70-year-old female presents to your office for evaluation of high blood pressure. Which of the following statements is true regarding hypertension in older individuals:

A. Hypertension becomes less common with advancing age.
B. The elevated pulse pressure of isolated systolic hypertension is one of the most important markers for increased cardiovascular risk and treatment is definitely indicated.

C. Systolic blood pressures greater than 160 but less than 180 should be considered normal.
D. Periodic measurement of blood pressure is not recommended in adults over the age of 65.

Answer: B

Critique: Hypertension becomes more common with advancing age, as do coronary disease and cerebrovascular disease. Isolated systolic hypertension is a very common finding in older individuals. The elevated pulse pressure of isolated systolic hypertension is now recognized as one of the most important markers for increased cardiovascular risks and treatment is definitely indicated. Systolic blood pressures greater than 160 but less than 180 are considered abnormal. Both the AAFP and the USPSTF recommend periodic measurement of blood pressure for all patients.

Page: 176

32: A 68-year-old female presents to the office for a routine annual examination. She has never had an abnormal Pap smear and is sexually active only with her husband of 30 years. Which of the following statements is true regarding cervical cancer screening in this woman:

A. She should be screened yearly with Pap smear tests.
B. The AAFP recommends biannual Pap smear screening for all currently or formerly sexually active women who have a cervix.
C. The USPSTF cites strong evidence to recommend against screening for cervical cancer over the age of 65.
D. She will probably derive very little benefit from continued yearly testing.

Answer: D

Critique: Cervical cancer is still a concern for patients 65 years and older. However the risk is variable and highly dependent on factors such as sexual practices. Low-risk patients who have a history of negative screening in the past probably derive very little benefit from continued yearly screening. The ACOG recommends Pap smears every 1 to 3 years for all women in this age group. The AAFP recommends Pap smears at least every 3 years for all currently or formerly sexually active women who have a cervix. The USPSTF recommends periodic Pap smears for all currently or formerly sexually active women who have a cervix. They cite insufficient evidence to recommend for or against an upper age limit for screening.

Page: 176

Chapter 12

Preventive Health Care

Navkarin K. Shokar

1: With regard to prevention strategies, which of the following is true?

    A. According to the Centers for Disease Control and Prevention (CDC), preventive activities have accounted for 5 of the 30 years of increased life expectancy achieved in the last century.

    B. More emphasis is placed on prevention than on cure in the United States.

    C. Primary prevention refers to interventions that occur before the disease is diagnosable.

    D. Secondary prevention refers to interventions that occur after disease has been diagnosed and symptoms are present.

Answer: C

Critique: Preventive activities during the last century are thought to account for 25 of the 30 years of increased life expectancy in this country, according to the CDC. Still, there is less research and medical education emphasis on prevention and more on cure once the illness is established. Primary prevention refers to interventions that prevent the onset of the disease, that is, before the disease is diagnosable and before symptoms are present. Secondary prevention refers to interventions aimed at diagnosing the disease before the onset of symptoms. Tertiary interventions are those aimed at patients in whom the disease is diagnosed and symptoms are already present.

Page: 183

2: The prevalence of a disease:

    A. Refers to the total number of new cases occurring in a given time

    B. Is not influenced by the mortality of a disease

    C. Refers to the proportion of cases existing in the population at a given time

    D. Has no effect on the positive predictive value of a test for that disease

Answer: C

Critique: The prevalence of a disease is the number of existing cases in a population at a given time. Prevalence is influenced by both the incidence and mortality of the disease. It has a profound effect on the positive predictive value of any screening or diagnostic test for the disease. An increased prevalence in the population tested dramatically improves the positive predictive value of the test.

Page: 184

The prevalence of disease x in a population of 1000 is 20 percent. One hundred with the disease tested positive. Fifty one hundred patients without the disease also tested positive.

3: The sensitivity of the test is:

    A. 100/1000

    B. 150/1000

    C. 100/200

    D. 150/200

Answer: C

4: The specificity of the test is:

    A. 50/1000

    B. 50/800

    C. 50/750

    D. 750/800

Answer: D

5: The positive predictive value of the test is:

    A. 150/100

    B. 100/200

    C. 150/1000

    D. 100/150

Answer: D

6: The negative predictive value of the test is:

    A. 50/850

    B. 750/850

    C. 900/1000

    D. 50/1000

Answer: B

Critique: The characteristics of a test for a certain condition can be calculated with the use of a 2×2 table. Thus, using the information above, the following can be constructed as:

	Disease present	Disease absent
Test pos	100 (A)	50 (B)
Test neg	100 (C)	750 (D)
Total	200	800

If the prevalence of the disease is 20% in this population, then 200 people have the disease and 800 people are disease free.

Sensitivity is the proportion of those with the disease who tested positive = 100/200 a / a + c.

Specificity is the proportion of those without the disease (1000–200) who tested negative = 750/800 d/d + b.

Positive predictive value refers to the likelihood of those with a positive test having the disease = 100/150 a/a + b.

Negative predictive value refers to the likelihood of those with a negative test being disease free = 750/850 d/d + c.

Pages: 183, 184

7: Which one of the following diseases does *not* have a primary prevention strategy?

    A. Cervical cancer
    B. Measles
    C. Colorectal cancer
    D. Breast cancer

Answer: D

Critique: Screening strategies for the first three diseases result in primary and sometimes secondary prevention. Pap screening aims to detect premalignant changes of cervical intraepithelial neoplasia. Treatment of premalignant tissue prevents the onset of cervical cancer. Colorectal cancer screening aims to detect and remove precancerous polyps through the use of fecal occult blood testing or sigmoidoscopy, thus preventing the progression of polyps to cancer. These two strategies can also lead to secondary prevention because they may detect early asymptomatic cancers. Immunization prevents measles from occurring; this is a primary prevention strategy. Mammography can detect only cancers that already exist. Its aim is to find them in the early presymptomatic stage, and this is secondary prevention.

8: (True or False) Which of the following are accepted parameters for a disease to qualify for screening in the general population?

    A. The natural history of the disease should be understood.
    B. Early detection should be proven to lead to better outcomes.
    C. If a screening test for a disease is available, it should be used.
    D. Effective and acceptable treatments should be known, accepted, and available.

Answers: A - True, B - True, C - False, D - True

Critique: The existence of an effective screening test alone is not sufficient to warrant its use for screening. In addition, the disease must meet certain criteria. First, it must carry a significant burden, and its natural course must be understood to identify the susceptible population or risk factors. Effective treatments should be proven to have a significant impact on the disease and have acceptable risk, morbidity, and cost.

Page: 183

9: The sensitivity of a test:

    A. Refers to the proportion of positive tests in those who do not have the disease
    B. Refers to the proportion of positive tests in those who have the disease
    C. Refers to the proportion of positive tests obtained

    D. Refers to the proportion of negative tests obtained

Answer: B

Critique: The sensitivity of a test is its ability to correctly identify as positive those individuals who have the disease. Sensitivity is the percentage of positive tests obtained in a group that is known to have the disease. This is a fixed property of subsequent tests when they are conducted in the same manner.

Pages: 183, 184

10: Which one of the following is true regarding specificity of a test?

    A. It refers to the proportion of individuals with the disease who tested positive.
    B. It refers to the proportion with disease who tested negative.
    C. It refers to the proportion without the disease who tested positive.
    D. It refers to the proportion without the disease who tested negative.

Answer: D

Critique: The specificity of a test refers to its ability to accurately detect individuals who do not have the disease. When applied to a population, it is expressed as the proportion of those without the disease who tested negative.

Page: 184

11: Which of the following is not listed as one of the top five causes of death in the United States in 1997?

    A. Malignant neoplasm
    B. Diabetes mellitus
    C. COPD
    D. Coronary heart disease

Answer: B

Critique: Available data reveal that the top five causes of death in the United States are heart diseases, malignant neoplasms, cerebrovascular diseases, COPD and related disorders, and accidents. Diabetes mellitus is listed as the seventh leading cause of death.

Page: 184

12: An asymptomatic 50-year-old man who is a smoker with a strong family history of coronary heart disease comes to your office. He is extremely worried that he has coronary heart disease and wants to know if he has it. What tests should you order?

    A. Twelve-lead ECG
    B. Exercise treadmill test
    C. Exercise stress thallium test
    D. Exercise stress echocardiogram

Answer: None

Critique: None of the above tests has a proven role for screening in asymptomatic individuals because of low sensitivity, and treadmill testing has a high false-positive rate. They should be used for diagnostic and therapeutic purposes in individuals with symptoms. The best advice to give this man is to stop smoking and to screen and treat him for other risk factors for coronary heart disease.

Pages: 186–189

13: Which of the following is *not* a risk factor for coronary heart disease (CHD)?

    A. Males >45 years
    B. Females >55 years
    C. Mother c MI aged 60 years
    D. Female aged 45 years on hormone replacement therapy

Answer: D

Critique: The risk for CHD is age dependent, but onset in females is delayed by 10 years because of the protective influence of hormones. Thus, males >45 years have an increased risk and females >55 have increased risk. Family history of CHD becomes a significant risk factor if it occurred prematurely. This is defined as before age 55 in a male first-degree relative and before age 65 in a female first-degree relative. Hormone replacement therapy in the postmenopausal woman has been shown to reduce the risk of coronary heart disease significantly in those without pre-existing disease. In those with prior disease, however, the risk may be increased in the first year and then declines in the second year.

Pages: 187, 188

14: A 63-year-old man without CHD who is a smoker with hypertension is found to have a fasting cholesterol of 220, with HDL of 36 and LDL of 140. Which one of the following is the correct advice according to the National Cholesterol Education Program (NCEP)?

    A. No action is necessary because he does not have CHD.
    B. No action is necessary because his LDL is lower than 160.
    C. He needs to start on medication because his total cholesterol is over 200.
    D. Dietary intervention is indicated.

Answer: D

Critique: The NCEP criteria for treatment are determined by the LDL level and the characterization of risk by the presence or absence of CHD. In the absence of CHD, the guidelines depend on the number of risk factors. In this case, the patient has three risk factors; therefore, he meets the criteria for dietary therapy. Medication would be indicated if his LDL were >160. He should be advised to cut his fat intake to <30% of his total calories, with <10% saturated fat, up to 10% polyunsaturated fat, and 10% to 15% monounsaturated fat. He should be reviewed again in 3 months. His other risk factors should be addressed as well.

Pages: 186, 187

15: (True or False) With regard to CHD, which of the following are true?

    A. CHD is the most common cause of premature disability in the United States.
    B. Over 50% of people who die suddenly with CHD have no prior symptoms.
    C. The overall case fatality rate is 1 in 10.
    D. The lifetime risk of CHD for a 40-year-old male is 20%.

Answers: A - True, B - True, C - False, D - False

Critique: Although the incidence of CHD is falling in the United States, it still has significant morbidity and mortality. The prevalence is 7.2% in those older than 20 years. The overall case fatality rate is 1 in 3, and CHD is responsible for 1 of every 4.9 deaths. It is also the most common cause of premature disability. The lifetime risk of CHD for a 40-year-old male is 49%; for a woman, it is 30%. No prior symptoms appear in 57 % of men and 64% of women dying suddenly from CHD, and hence the importance of primary prevention.

Pages: 185, 186

16: The most important risk factor to address for stroke prevention is:

    A. Hypercholesterolemia
    B. Hypertension
    C. Smoking
    D. Oral contraceptive use

Answer: B

Critique: The single most important risk factor for stroke is hypertension. The presence of diabetes is also a significant risk factor. Other risk factors for CHD are indicated but are less predictive; among them are the known presence of heart disease, especially atrial fibrillation; oral contraceptive use; elevated hematocrit; sickle cell disease; and hyperhomocysteinemia.

Page: 189

17: With regard to alcohol use and abuse, which one of the following is true?

    A. One of the strategies for treating an alcoholic is to recommend controlled drinking.
    B. Fifty percent of Americans have a first- or second-degree relative with alcoholism.
    C. The best recovery rate with treatment is 33%.
    D. The prevalence of alcoholism in a primary care population is 2%.

Answer: B

Critique: The prevalence of alcoholism in a primary care population is thought to be 10% to 17%. This disease has enormous personal and societal costs. A spontaneous recovery rate is reported to be between 4% and 26%, but treatment programs can achieve a recovery rate of 70%. Recommending controlled drinking is not a useful treatment strategy. There is a tendency for the problem to run in families, even if the biological parents are not involved in upbringing. Useful outpatient screening tests include the CAGE, MAST, and AUDIT questionnaires.

Pages: 190, 191

18: (True or False) Which of the following is true regarding cancer?

A. Physical activity, diet, smoking, and alcohol use account for 30% of cancer mortality.
B. The top cause of cancer mortality in men is prostate cancer.
C. The top cause of cancer mortality in females is breast cancer
D. The death rate from lung cancer in women is rising.

Answers: A - False, B - False, C - False, D - True

Critique: Cancers account for 23% of all deaths in the United States. Modifiable risk factors, such as physical activity, diet, smoking, and alcohol use, are thought to account for over 67% of all cancer mortality. Lifestyle changes alone can have a significant impact on mortality from cancer. Prostate cancer and breast cancer, respectively, have the highest incidence in men and women, but the top cause of cancer-related deaths in the United States in both sexes is lung cancer. The death rate from this disease has risen dramatically since the 1960s; the death rate in men appears to be falling, but it continues to rise in women.

Pages: 191–194

19: Which one of the following cancers has the lowest overall 5-year survival rate when all stages are considered?

A. Testicular
B. Breast
C. Prostate
D. Pancreas
E. Ovarian

Answer: D

Critique: The overall 5-year survival rate for pancreatic cancer is only 4%. Unfortunately, no screening test for asymptomatic individuals has been found to be effective. The 5-year survival rates for the other cancers are: testicular, 95%; breast, 85%; prostate, 93%; and ovarian, 50%.

Page: 195

20: The recommendations for screening mammography for breast cancer according to the United States Preventive Task Force (USPTF) are:

A. Annual mammogram starting at age 40 in all women
B. Mammogram every 1 to 2 years starting at age 40 in all women
C. Mammogram every 1 to 2 years from age 50 to 70 in all women
D. Mammograms, clinical breast exam, and breast self-exam every 1 to 2 years from age 50 to 70

Answer: C

Critique: The USPTF recommendations are made on the basis of an evaluation of the evidence available from clinical trials. These recommendations represent the minimum level of preventive health care expected of family physicians. USPTF recommends mammography every 1 to 2 years in all patients aged 50 to 70. The usefulness of mammography beyond age 69 has not been proved. Mammography before the age of 50 is controversial, and USPTF recommends considering it annually in high-risk women only. The value of clinical breast exam has not been proved, nor has the value of breast self-exam.

Pages: 196, 197

21: (True or False) An asymptomatic 50-year-old man comes to the office concerned about colon cancer. Which of the following screening tests should be recommended according to USPTF?

A. Barium enema
B. Colonoscopy
C. FOBT × 3 annually
D. Sigmoidoscopy every 3 to 5 years

Answers: A - False, B - False, C - True, D - True

Critique: The only two screening modalities found to have improved mortality in asymptomatic individuals at average risk are FOBT and flexible sigmoidoscopy. The USPTF recommends either modality alone or both in combination starting at age 50. Some proponents have suggested barium enema and colonoscopy for screening, but studies assessing their impact for screening are not available. Thus, their use should be limited to diagnostic indications.

Page: 195

22: (True or False) A 40-year-old woman presents to her PCP worried about breast cancer because her cousin has been recently diagnosed with it. She has no other risk factors. Her exam is normal. You should:

A. Advise her that a mammogram is necessary.
B. Inform her that she is at increased risk because of positive family history.
C. Advise that she start taking oral contraceptives as a preventive therapy.
D. Tell her that if she has a positive mammogram, she has a 3% to 4% chance of having cancer.

Answers: A - False, B - False, C - False, D - True

Critique: Risk factors for breast cancer include a family history of cancer in a first-degree relative. Other factors include past history of cancer in situ, early menarche, and late menopause. Oral contraceptives slightly increase the risk. Tamoxifen is being studied for primary prevention in high-risk women. Screening mammography in asymptomatic women not at high risk in this age group is controversial because the low positive predictive value of a positive test is only 3% to 4%, which may lead to unnecessary anxiety and further tests. A mammogram is certainly not necessary but may still be ordered after a discussion of risks and benefits.

Pages: 196–198

23: A 53-year-old smoker with a 30-pack year history comes in for a routine visit. You can tell him that:

A. Fifty percent of lung cancer deaths are attributable to smoking.
B. Ten years after quitting, ex-smokers reduce their risk of lung cancer by 50%.

C. Annual chest x-ray (CXR) is now recommended for screening.

D. Annual CXR and sputum cytology are recommended for screening.

Answer: B

Critique: Of lung cancer deaths, 85% are directly attributable to smoking. The best advice to give this man is to stop smoking and to provide him with the support necessary for him to do it. Simple physician advice to quit leads to a 5% to 10% quit rate. The risk of lung cancer drops to 50% after 10 years of not smoking. Although CXR or sputum cytology may detect lung cancer at a presymptomatic stage, no evidence is available that shows a corresponding reduction in mortality. Screening with these modalities is therefore not recommended.

Page: 198

24: With regard to endometrial cancer, which one of the following is false?

A. The incidence is not increasing.

B. Obesity is a risk factor.

C. Opposed estrogen is a risk factor.

D. Diabetes is associated with risk.

Answer: C

Critique: The incidence of endometrial cancer has been stable for the last 20 years. The main risk factor is use of prolonged unopposed estrogen. Situations in which this may arise include chronic anovulation, tamoxifen therapy, and estrogen replacement therapy without cyclic progesterone. Diabetes, hypertension, and gallbladder disease are also associated with endometrial cancer, largely because of the prevalence of obesity in patients with these conditions.

Page: 200

25: A 53-year-old white male asks about prostate cancer screening. You should advise:

A. Annual prostate-specific antibody (PSA) testing

B. Annual PSA and DRE

C. That 1 in 20 men with histological evidence of cancer will die from the disease

D. That 100% of males over the age of 80 have the disease

Answer: D

Critique: PSA is a sensitive test for detection of prostate cancer. However, no study has demonstrated improved survival as a result of earlier detection. The incidence increases with age, and some estimates suggest that 100% of men over 80 years of age have the disease. Most men with the disease die from other causes, however, and only 1 in 380 with the disease will die from it. Still, prostate cancer is the second most common cause of cancer-related deaths in men. Until we can identify those men at risk of the more aggressive type of cancer, mass screening is not justified because of the morbidity associated with treatment. According to the USPTF, the pros and cons of screening should be discussed with the patient and an individual decision should be made. The risk factors

include a family history of the disease, African American race, a diet high in animal fat, and increasing age.

Page: 200

26: A 48-year-old Asian female is on estrogen replacement therapy (ERT), smokes 20 cigarettes a day, and is concerned about osteoporosis. You should advise her:

A. To drink a moderate amount of alcohol to reduce her risk

B. That addition of cyclic progesterone to her ERT will decrease her risk

C. That she is in a high-risk group because of her race

D. To start swimming to reduce her risk

Answer: C

Critique: Primary risk factors for osteoporosis include increasing age, smoking, alcohol intake, family history, and dietary calcium deficiency. Risk is also related to lack of pigment in the skin, and therefore Caucasian and Asian races are also associated. The best advice to give this patient is to stop smoking, to increase weight-bearing exercise, and to supplement calcium intake to at least 1.5 g a day. The addition of estrogen therapy for perimenopausal or postmenopausal women delays onset of the accelerated bone loss associated with estrogen withdrawal at menopause. Cyclic progesterone is indicated only for endometrial protection in women with an intact uterus, because it has no effect on bone loss.

Page: 201

27: Which of the following medications increases the risk of osteoporosis?

A. Prolonged glucocorticoid use

B. Thiazide diuretics

C. Raloxifene

D. Fosamax

Answer: A

Critique: Certain medications increase the risk of osteoporosis, including steroids, anticonvulsants, and excess thyroxine. Certain medical conditions also predispose individuals to osteoporosis, including chronic obstructive pulmonary disease, hyperthyroidism, and subtotal gastrectomy. Raloxifene, Fosamax, estrogen, and calcitonin have been shown to improve this problem. Thiazide diuretics may also be helpful because they reduce urinary calcium excretion.

Page: 201

28: Which of the following is true concerning sexually transmitted diseases (STDs)?

A. Most STDs are symptomatic.

B. The prevalence of chlamydia is thought to be 1 in 100 in women of reproductive age.

C. STDs account for 30% of infertility cases.

D. The most prevalent STD is gonorrhea.

Answer: C

Critique: Most STDs have a high asymptomatic carrier rate. The prevalence of chlamydia is thought to be 1 in 20 in women of reproductive age. The most prevalent STDs are thought to be herpes simplex and human papilloma virus because of their persistent nature. Consequences of STDs include PID, infertility, ectopic pregnancy, cervical cancer, premature delivery, and fetal death. HIV testing should be recommended for anyone diagnosed with an STD.

Page: 203

29: With regard to HIV, which of the following are true?

A. Cases in minority populations are increasing.
B. Just over half of cases are attributable to homosexual or bisexual men.
C. Prophylaxis after occupational exposure to HIV is not effective.

D. Routine vaccination in patients with HIV is not recommended.

Answers: A and B

Critique: The number of cases of HIV in minority populations in the United States is increasing. Fifty-two percent of cases are attributable to homosexual or bisexual men. Prophylaxis after occupational exposure has been proved to reduce the risk of transmission 10-fold. It is recommended that routine vaccines, other than that for varicella, be updated in patients with HIV, especially early in the disease when antibody response rate is likely to be higher.

Pages: 203, 204

Chapter 13

Practice-Based Research

Alvah R. Cass

1: (True or False) Practice-based research networks are a relatively new phenomenon, which support primary care research. In general, practice-based research networks provide:

  A. An infrastructure that unites practice and research in a unique partnership
  B. An environment in which practicing family physicians can study the evidence underlying primary care practices
  C. A scholarly environment that can change the culture of primary care in the community
  D. A research environment free of the rigor usually associated with tertiary care–based research

Answers: A - True, B -True, C - True, D - False

Critique: Practice-based research is the generation of new knowledge from the study of patient care in the practice setting. Practice-based research networks are the organizations that support this approach to primary care research. They have been shown to be a feasible and functional laboratory for the study of important primary care questions in the context of clinical practice. These networks provide an infrastructure for research that unites practice and inquiry in a unique partnership. They provide a climate of inquiry in which practicing family physicians can study the evidence underlying primary care practices and substantially contribute to improving that evidence. They also promote a scholarly environment, which has the potential to change the culture of primary care in the community. Practice-based research networks link the relevant research questions of practicing physicians with rigorous research methods to produce results that are potentially more easily assimilated into everyday practice than is the majority of existing research that emanates from tertiary care centers.

Page: 211

2: Compared with traditional biomedical research conducted in tertiary care centers, practice-based research is better suited to study:

  A. Biomolecular mechanisms, diagnosis, and treatment of specific diseases
  B. Outcomes of specific diseases that are fully developed in the adult population
  C. Single interventions directed at selected diseases
  D. Outcomes such as preservation and restoration of function

  E. Specific mechanisms of diseases apart from associated comorbidities

Answer: D

Critique: In general, traditional biomedical research conducted in tertiary care centers is restricted or constrained by a variety of factors. The most important of these is the high degree of referral or selection bias that operates in the referral to tertiary care centers. Traditional research tends to focus on the biomolecular mechanisms, diagnosis, and treatment of specific diseases. Much of this research investigates single interventions directed at specific or selected diseases and usually focuses on hard outcomes, such as death or change in measurable physical parameters. Primary care–based research is well suited to the study of undifferentiated illness, as well as various diseases, in the context of comorbidities, family and social environments, and within the powerful effects of the physician-patient relationship. Primary care–based research has a better opportunity to look at outcomes such as health-related quality of life, relief of suffering, or preservation or restoration of function.

Pages: 212, 213

3: (True or False) Characteristics and features of practice-based research networks include:

  A. Governance within the organizational structure of professional organizations
  B. Close collaboration between practicing physicians and a multidisciplinary research team
  C. Adequate access to external funding through managed care organizations
  D. Interest in health care events that reflect a community-based patient population characteristic of primary care settings
  E. Development of key research questions by a central research committee

Answers: A - True, B - True, C - False, D - True, E - False

Critique: Practice-based primary care research networks have evolved in different ways and represent a healthy diversity in several important design features. Most of the networks exist within the organizational structure of professional organizations, although a few exist within academic departments, and others are independent organizations. Most of the networks foster a close collaboration between practicing physicians and a multidisciplinary research team. Obtaining funding presents a major challenge to virtually all practice-based research networks. Most practice-based research networks incorporate at least three central features: (1) networks capture health issues and health care events that reflect the community-based patient populations that characterize primary care settings; (2) they provide access to the generalist approach to care provided by full-time primary-care clinicians; and (3) all networks strive for the systematic involvement of network clinicians in defining the research questions and participating in the study, design, and interpretation of results.

Page: 213

4: Which of the following practice-based research networks is credited with pioneering methods that laid the groundwork for studying the common phenomena of primary care?

    A. Dartmouth Primary Care Co-operative Information Project (COOP)
    B. Wisconsin Research Network (WReN)
    C. Ambulatory Sentinel Practice Network (ASPN)
    D. Pediatric Research in Office Settings (PROS)

Answer: C

Critique: ASPN pioneered methods for conducting low-cost, low-burden studies that collect high-quality data in busy primary care practice settings. This pioneering effort laid the groundwork for studying the common phenomena of primary care. Other practice-based research networks have benefited from the early pioneering work of ASPN.

Page: 214

5: Which of the following issues constitutes the greatest challenge facing practice-based research networks in the future?

    A. Identifying gaps in knowledge
    B. Finding adequate answers to clinical questions
    C. Designing appropriate studies suitable for the primary care setting
    D. Collecting high-quality data from a diversity of practices
    E. Uniting the processes that investigate questions with the processes that create lasting changes in practice patterns

Answer: E

Critique: The major challenge for practice-based research networks over the next decade is to close the loop that unites the processes of asking and answering questions in practice with the processes that create durable improvements in the practice patterns of family physicians. Identifying gaps in knowledge, searching for adequate answers to clinical questions, generating and clarifying study questions, designing appropriate studies, collecting high-quality data, and analyzing and interpreting results are all essential elements of practice-based research. Practice-based research networks, however, have had collective success in all of these areas and time-tested methods to address these issues. Judging the adequacy and relevancy of answers and implementing findings in practice settings is a more difficult task. Once a question has been answered and judged to be relevant, the challenge remains of how to incorporate this new information into the practice patterns of primary care physicians in the community setting.

Pages: 215, 217

Chapter 14

Evidence-Based Medicine

Michael D. Hagen

1: Evidence-based medicine (EBM) is best described as which of the following:

- A. An empirical-based estimation of best medical practice
- B. Reliance on the clinician's clinical experience to determine best medical practice for individual patients
- C. Conscientious, explicit use of current best evidence in making decisions about the care of individual patients
- D. Consultation with conveniently available peers to ascertain current best practices for individual patients

Answer: C

Critique: Evidence-based medicine represents the explicit, conscientious, and judicious use of the best currently available evidence in caring for an individual patient. Reliance solely on one's own clinical experience or that of others exposes the decision maker to potential recall and availability bias.

Page: 220

2: Which of the following concepts represents the most appropriate focus of an evidence-based approach to clinical problem solving:

- A. The average response of blood pressure to a new antihypertensive medication
- B. The drop in blood sugar associated with a dose of a hypoglycemic agent
- C. The change in pulmonary artery resistance associated with a new alpha-adrenergic inhibitor
- D. The change in mortality rates associated with a new hypolipidemic agent

Answer: D

Critique: Evidence-based practice focuses on outcomes that are important to patients. Blood pressure, blood sugar, and pulmonary artery resistance responses to medications represent physiologic parameters that do not necessarily translate to outcomes that matter to patients.

Page: 220

3: Evidence-based practice consists of several steps. Which of the following represents the first step in the process:

- A. Formulating and asking a question

- B. Conferring with a colleague regarding his or her approach to the clinical problem
- C. Consulting a general medical textbook to identify possible approaches to a problem
- D. Use of a general World Wide Web search engine to identify Web sites devoted to the clinical area in question

Answer: A

Critique: The first step in practicing evidence-based medicine is to formulate a specific question. The well-framed question then serves as the focus for searching information resources such as the Internet, textbooks, and the research literature.

Page: 221

4: Assume that you have formulated a question and identified information pertinent to a clinical situation. The next step in formulating an evidence-based approach is which of the following:

- A. Conduct an audit of your practice's patient charts to ascertain the outcomes of patients who have the same diagnosis
- B. Evaluate the information you obtained for relevance to and validity in your own practice's patients
- C. Request additional information from a pharmaceutical sales representative regarding the treatments you are considering
- D. Begin treatment immediately based on the information you retrieved

Answer: B

Critique: Once you have identified information pertinent to the clinical question, the next step in the evidence-based approach is to assess the relevance and validity of the information to your practice and patient. Issues such as study design, research patient population, and cost of possible therapies will impact the applicability of research results to your patient's context. Assessment of patient outcomes occurs after you've implemented your evidence-based treatment plans. Pharmaceutical sales representatives would not be considered an unbiased source of information for an evidence-based treatment approach.

Page: 221

5: In the evidence-based medicine model, the usefulness of information has three fundamental components.

Information must be relevant to everyday practice, and the information must be medically correct. Which of the following represents the third component:

A. The brevity of the information source
B. The work required to obtain the information
C. The reputation of the author(s) of the information
D. The date of publication of the information

Answer: B

Critique: As described by the author, the usefulness of information is defined by three characteristics: the relevance to the clinician's everyday practice, the correctness of the information, and the work required to obtain the information.

Page: 221

6: Much of the information encountered in the literature focuses on disease. The mnemonic POEM, as used in evidence-based medicine, means which of the following:

A. A lyrical approach to defining medical content
B. Problems of empirical medicine
C. Patient-oriented evidence that matters
D. Patient opportunities for empirical medical practice

Answer: C

Critique: The evidence-based medicine mnemonic POEM refers to *patient-oriented evidence that matters*. The medical literature contains a great deal of information that focuses on disease but that doesn't provide insight into how a particular intervention or therapy will affect a patient's quality of life. POEM describes information that provides such insights about the *effectiveness* of these interventions when applied in practice.

Page: 221

7: Which of the following examples represents a POEM, rather than DOE (disease-oriented evidence)?

A. Evidence that angiotensin-converting enzyme inhibitors lower blood pressure
B. Evidence that beta-adrenergic blockers decrease heart rate
C. Evidence that aspirin decreases platelet aggregation
D. Evidence that chlorthalidone decreases the risk of stroke and heart attack in hypertensive patients

Answer: D

Critique: Options A, B, and C represent disease-oriented concepts that describe physiologic effects of interventions but do not provide information that indicates how these interventions might improve patients' lives. Option D describes evidence that an intervention actually has a tangible benefit for patients' quality and quantity of life.

Pages: 221, 222

8: POEM information can be differentiated from DOE information using which of the following processes:

A. Examining the evidence to determine whether "thinking" is required to establish effects of an intervention on patient-centered outcomes
B. Examining the evidence to determine whether "knowing" is required to establish effects of an intervention on patient-centered outcomes
C. Examining the evidence for statistical significance to establish the effects of an intervention on patient-centered outcomes
D. Examining the evidence for confidence intervals to establish the effects of an intervention on patient-centered outcomes

Answer: B

Critique: DOE, or disease-oriented evidence, focuses on pathophysiologic concepts such as blood pressure control or control of an arrhythmia. These represent intermediate outcomes that require the user to "think" that the outcome will in turn lead to an important patient-centered outcome such as improved mortality or quality of life. POEM evidence provides direct evidence of such patient-centered outcomes, enabling the user to "know" that the intervention in question has an important effect on outcomes that matter to patients.

Page: 222

9: When searching for the best evidence, which of the following provides a guide to assessing the usefulness of a particular source of information:

A. The statistical significance of the effects observed in the retrieved resources
B. The number needed to treat (NNT) calculated by the author(s) of the information source
C. The relevance and validity of the information and the amount of work needed to find it
D. The length of the articles identified in the search for information sources

Answer: C

Critique: The "usefulness score" provides a means to assess the practical value of identified information. This tool considers the relevance and validity of retrieved information and the amount of work required to find the information. The three concepts are related reciprocally, as relevance x validity/work. The more work required to identify and retrieve the information, the lower will be its usefulness. Likewise, higher relevance and validity contribute to greater usefulness for identified information sources.

Pages: 221, 222

10: A clinical study of the results of two different therapies for hypertension reports that the mean blood pressure using therapy A was less than that using therapy B. The authors report a p value of <0.05 for the difference between the two therapies. Which of the following represents the proper interpretation of this p value:

A. Therapy A is five times better than therapy B.
B. There is a 5% probability that therapy A lowers blood pressure.
C. The difference between mean blood pressure with therapy A and with therapy B is 5%.
D. There is a less than 5% probability that these results occurred by chance alone.

Answer: D

Critique: The p value represents that probability that the results observed could have occurred by chance alone.

Page: 222

11: A study of two antibiotics for prophylaxis against surgical wound infection reports that the rate of infection is 5% with antibiotic A and 3% with antibiotic B. Which of the following represents the relative risk reduction for infection associated with antibiotic B compared to that for antibiotic A:

    A. 2%
    B. 15%
    C. 40%
    D. 66%

Answer: C

Critique: Authors frequently report the relative risk reduction for one therapy compared to another, rather than the absolute difference between the two. In the example, the *absolute risk reduction* is 5% − 3%, or 2%. The relative risk reduction is (5% − 3%)/5%, or 40%. This larger number appears more impressive and can make the effect size for a therapy appear larger than it really is.

Pages: 222, 223

12: In the example described in question 11, the authors also state that the number needed to treat (NNT) for therapy B versus therapy A was 50. Which of the following statements represents the proper interpretation of this number:

    A. The study required 50 patients in each treatment group.
    B. Fifty patients have to be treated with antibiotic B versus antibiotic A to prevent one additional wound infection.
    C. Antibiotic B is 50 times better than antibiotic A in preventing surgical wound infection.
    D. Antibiotic A must be given at 50 times the dose of antibiotic B to achieve equivalent results.

Answer: B

Critique: The NNT describes how many patients must be treated to achieve the additional benefit associated with one therapy versus another. The NNT is calculated by inverting the absolute percentage difference in the results achieved with two competing therapies. In this example, the absolute difference is 2%, and the NNT 50.

Page: 223

13: A number of potential sources exist for finding information to answer clinical queries. Medical journals represent a major source of such information. Journals can be divided into two major types. *Knowledge creation* is one major type. Which of the following represents the other major type:

    A. Knowledge representation
    B. Knowledge translation
    C. Knowledge restriction

    D. Knowledge amplification

Answer: B

Critique: Medical journals can be divided into two major types: those that report medical knowledge creation, and those that contain knowledge translation articles that represent reviews or summaries of the research published in knowledge creation journals.

Page: 223

14: *American Family Physician*, *Family Practice Recertification*, and *Hospital and Staff Physician* are examples of which of the following types of journals:

    A. Knowledge translation
    B. Knowledge creation
    C. Knowledge representation
    D. Knowledge amplification

Answer: A

Critique: *American Family Physician*, *Family Practice Recertification*, and *Hospital and Staff Physician* are all examples of knowledge translation journals. These publications contain reviews and summaries of research presented in knowledge creation–type journals and other sources.

Page: 223

15: (True or False) Knowledge creation journals frequently contain information that clinicians can incorporate into their practices, but they also contain studies that might not relate to primary care contexts. Which of the following are questions a reader should ask when deciding whether or not a particular article is relevant to his or her clinical practice:

    A. Did the authors investigate an outcome important to my patients?
    B. Did the authors investigate a problem that is seen commonly in my practice?
    C. Did the authors report the brand names of the drug therapies they used in their study?
    D. Did the authors report information that, if valid, will require me to make changes in my practice?

Answers: A - True, B - True, C - False, D - True

Critique: Knowledge creation journals frequently report information that might not relate to the primary care context. By asking several questions about a particular article, a reader can determine quickly whether or not the paper relates to his or her own practice. Did the authors study an outcome that would be important to his or her patients? Did they study a problem seen commonly in his or her practice? Is the described intervention feasible in his or her practice population? Would the information in the article require changing current practice?

Page: 224

16: Review articles in medical journals can take two general forms: papers that summarize a broad topic (summary review) and those that synthesize new information related to a narrow topic. Which of the following represents a potential problem with summary reviews:

A. The authors systematically select supporting references on the basis of predefined criteria.
B. The summary review format is often influenced by unrecognized bias on the part of the authors.
C. The results of various studies are combined using the techniques of meta-analysis.
D. Summary review authors frequently include only randomized controlled trials in their discussions.

Answer: B

Critique: Summary reviews frequently do not utilize a systematic approach to identifying pertinent supporting literature and can thus be subject to potential biases in the conclusions drawn by the author(s). Synthesis reviews utilize systematic procedures for identifying and analyzing research articles for inclusion in the review and frequently utilize meta-analytic procedures to combine results from different studies.

Page: 224

17: "Educational seduction" is a phenomenon associated with continuing medical education (CME) presentations. Which of the following statements represents the best description of this term:

A. The CME attendee leaves a presentation with the feeling that she has learned something important, although research indicates that this learning does not happen.
B. The CME attendee leaves a presentation feeling very positively about the speaker.
C. The CME attendee leaves a presentation feeling well satisfied about the validity of the information the speaker delivered.
D. The CME attendee leaves a presentation satisfied that the speaker presented a wealth of disease-oriented evidence that will relate directly to the attendee's practice.

Answer: A

Critique: Despite research evidence to the contrary, CME attendees often believe that they have learned something important for their practices. This phenomenon is called "educational seduction."

Page: 225

18: You are interested in approaches to screening for colorectal cancer and ask a trusted colleague her opinion. She relates that, according to research she has read that appears valid, fecal occult blood screening has been shown to decrease colorectal cancer death rates. She has also found that she can apply this technique readily in her own practice and that patients accept the procedure well. Which of the following statements best describes her role as an expert in this interaction:

A. The colleague has functioned as a content expert in responding to the query.
B. The colleague has functioned as a clinical scientist in responding to the query.
C. The colleague has responded as an epidemiologist in responding to the query.

D. The colleague has responded as a YODA (your own data appraiser) in responding to the query.

Answer: D

Critique: Experts come in several varieties: "Content experts" demonstrate a great wealth of experience and knowledge but can present only very subjective interpretations of this information. "Clinical scientists" display expertise in the evaluation of the quality of information sources, but don't necessarily possess expert knowledge in the area in question. The YODA represents an individual who has deep knowledge of the subject and has skill in evaluating the quality of information sources. Additionally, this expert can relate the information to the clinical context on the basis of her clinical experience.

Page: 225

19: Pharmaceutical representatives can serve as a source for drug-related information. The information they present should, like any source, be evaluated for validity. The mnemonic STEPS provides a reminder for five characteristics of drug performance that a clinician should consider in assessing information about the agent. Which of the following corresponds to the "T" in STEPS?

A. The price *Tag* associated with use of the drug
B. The *Time* of administration for drug doses
C. The *Texture* of the filler used in the drug formulation
D. The *Tolerability* of the drug

Answer: D

Critique: The mnemonic STEPS provides a useful reminder for important characteristics of drug performance: *Safety, Tolerability, Effectiveness, Price,* and *Simplicity.*

Page: 225

20: (True or False) Which of the following characteristics describe the relationship between outcomes research and clinical experience:

A. Outcomes research generates hypotheses for testing in clinical experience.
B. Clinical experience can augment the application of outcomes research results.
C. Clinical experience and outcomes research represent inseparable components of successful clinical reasoning.
D. Outcomes research tests hypotheses generated from clinical experience.

Answers: A - False, B - True, C - True, D - True

Critique: Optimal clinical reasoning includes the application of both clinical experience and results from outcomes research. Our clinical experiences generate questions or hypotheses. Outcomes research designs provide answers about these hypotheses in controlled, scientifically conducted studies. The results of these studies must, in turn, be interpreted in the light of our clinical circumstances and context.

Page: 226

21: Family physicians typically generate about 15 questions per day in their clinical practices. Of these questions, approximately what percentage go unanswered:

    A. 10%
    B. 33%
    C. 67%
    D. 97%

Answer: C

Critique: Family physicians encounter approximately 15 clinical questions daily. About two thirds of these go unanswered, and half of these would have potential effects on patient care.

Pages: 226, 227

22: Adoption of a new therapeutic method or mode of practice requires several steps on the part of the decision maker. Which of the following represents the first step in the process of adopting change in medical practice:

    A. Open our minds to the idea of change
    B. Pay attention to feedback regarding our performance
    C. Determine the state of evidence for problems encountered in practice
    D. Honest self-appraisal of one's current practices

Answer: D

Critique: Adoption of new practices requires several actions on the part of the decision maker. The physician must first examine his or her own practice to identify possible less-than-optimal practices. The physician must then open his or her mind to the prospect of change and must then seek information and feedback from customers, such as patients and hospital committees. Then physicians must determine the current state of evidence regarding the problems under consideration. If good evidence exists for a current modality, then physicians should use it for most patients. If this evidence does not exist, the physician must rely on patient preferences, clinical experience, and inductive reasoning to arrive at possible clinical approaches. Physicians must also keep up with the literature and should consider participating in guideline development activities and managed care committees as means of managing change.

Pages: 227, 228

23: Many efforts to improve quality of health care actually reduce the value of health care services delivered. Which of the following represents the best description of how this phenomenon occurs:

    A. Many of these efforts decrease the quality of care delivered.
    B. Many of these efforts increase the overall cost of care delivered.
    C. Many of these efforts increase quality and decrease the cost of care delivered.
    D. Many of these efforts decrease the cost of care delivered.

Answer: B

Critique: The value of health care services is proportional to the quality of these services and is inversely related to their cost. If quality increases proportionally more than cost, the value of the service increases, and vice versa. However, adding additional services generally raises overall costs, limiting society's ability to expand access to care. Approximately 20% of the services we provide represent practices that could be eliminated without harming our patients. Evidence-based approaches provide guidance in identifying these potentially extraneous practices.

Page: 229

PART III

COMMUNICA-TION IN FAMILY MEDICINE

Chapter 15

Establishing Rapport

Michael D. Hagen

1: Which of the following actions represents the greatest deterrent to establishing rapport with a patient:

    A. A high charge for the initial visit
    B. An attitude of indifference or lack of interest on the part of the physician
    C. A physician's sincere effort to understand the patient's problems
    D. A physician's display of kindness and respect for the patient

Answer: B

Critique: A perceived lack of interest or an attitude of indifference represents the greatest impediment to developing effective rapport with a patient. On the other hand, display of concern, kindness, respect, and efforts to understand the patient's problems promote rapport.

Page: 233

2: (True or False) Determine which of the following statements regarding patient satisfaction are true and which are false:

    A. Patient satisfaction is strongly associated with the length of the clinical visit.
    B. Patient satisfaction is more strongly related to affective support than to specific physician examinations and tests.
    C. Patient satisfaction is affected by the patient's understanding of the illness.
    D. Patient satisfaction is enhanced by avoiding non-medical topics in the clinical interview.

Answers: A - True, B - True, C - True, D - False

Critique: Patient satisfaction depends on multiple dimensions of the clinical interaction. Although satisfaction is associated with the length of the visit, the physician's demonstrated affective support and the patient's understanding of his or her illness also greatly influence satisfaction. Brief discussion of nonmedical topics has been associated with greater satisfaction.

Page: 234

3: (True or False) Decide which of the following statements regarding rapport in different clinical settings are true and which are false:

    A. Physicians who see patients in ongoing relationships communicate more easily with them than do physicians seeing patients for the first time.
    B. Physicians who see patients in an emergency talk less than their patients do during their clinical interactions.
    C. Physicians who see patients in private offices demonstrate a strong reciprocal affective relationship with their patients.
    D. Physicians who know their patients well spend twice as much time talking as do the patients.

Answers: A - True, B - False, C - True, D - True

Critique: Not surprisingly, physicians who have long-standing doctor-patient relationships communicate more readily with their patients than those who do not have such relationships. Physicians in the emergency department spend twice as much time talking as do the patients. Physicians in a private office setting also tend to spend twice as much time talking, but demonstrate reciprocal affective responses to their patients: an affective statement made by the patient elicits an affective physician response, and vice versa.

Pages: 235, 236

4: Communications between individuals consist of both verbal and nonverbal components. Which of the following represents the respective contributions of verbal and nonverbal communication in most contexts:

    A. 90% verbal and 10% nonverbal
    B. 75% verbal and 25% nonverbal
    C. 67% verbal and 33% nonverbal
    D. 50% verbal and 50% nonverbal
    E. 25% verbal and 75% nonverbal

Answer: C

Critique: Most communications between individuals consist of about one third nonverbal content. Nonverbal cues tend to be under less conscious control than verbal ones and thus can serve as a more genuine indicator of emotion and attitude.

Page: 237

5: All of the following are components of paralanguage, except:

    A. Speech velocity
    B. Speech intonation
    C. Speech volume
    D. Speech inflection
    E. Speech vocabulary

Answer: E

Critique: Paralanguage represents components of speech that convey meaning beyond the words used. Speech velocity, volume, tone, and inflection all represent components of paralanguage. Paralanguage serves to modify the meaning of the actual vocabulary words used.

Page: 237

6: In the United States, which of the following represents the most acceptable form of touching:

    A. A pat on the back
    B. A firm handshake
    C. Placing an arm around the shoulder
    D. Placing a hand on the patient's knee

Answer: B

Critique: In the United States, the most socially acceptable form of touch is a handshake.

Page: 237

7: Body position can communicate degrees of tension or relaxation. Which of the following body positions is most consistent with a moderately relaxed demeanor:

    A. Sitting erect with rigid posture
    B. Sitting with a forward lean of about 20 degrees and a side lean of 10 degrees
    C. Sitting with a backward lean of 20 degrees
    D. Sitting with arms folded in tightly hugging manner

Answer: B

Critique: Subtle changes in body positioning can convey substantial information regarding the patient's sense of tension or relaxation. Sitting erect with rigid posture conveys tension. Sitting with a forward lean of 20 degrees and a side lean of 10 degrees communicates moderate relaxation. Sitting with a backward lean of 20 degrees conveys a sense of extreme relaxation. Sitting with arms folded in tightly hugging manner conveys a sense of insecurity.

Pages: 238, 239, 243

8: Head position can serve to indicate an individual's responses in an interaction. Which of the following head positions best indicates interest in and attention to the speaker:

    A. Head held forward
    B. Head held back
    C. Head erect
    D. Head tilted to one side

Answer: D

Critique: Head position can provide clues to the speaker's affective state. The head is typically held forward in states of anger. The speaker holds her head back in states of anxiety or fear. The head is held down in situations of sadness, shame, or guilt. An erect head signals self-confidence. Tilting the head to one side indicates attention to and interest in the speaker.

Page: 240

9: Facial expressions can be used to disguise true underlying emotional responses. In American culture, which of the following facial expressions is used most commonly in this manner:

    A. Furrowing the brow
    B. Tightening one corner of the mouth
    C. Wrinkling the forehead
    D. Smiling

Answer: D

Critique: In American culture, smiling is used most frequently to disguise underlying emotions. However, eye and forehead features, such as a furrowed brow or wrinkled forehead, can serve to indicate true underlying emotions. Tightening one corner of the mouth is associated with contempt for the speaker.

Pages: 240, 241

10: Micro-expressions occur when the speaker starts to register a facial expression, recognizes the emotion, and attempts to mask the expression. How long do these micro-expressions usually last:

    A. 3 seconds
    B. 2 seconds
    C. One-half to three-quarters second
    D. One twenty-fifth to one-fifth second

Answer: D

Critique: Micro-expressions represent transient responses that indicate true underlying emotion but that the speaker quickly recognizes and masks with alternative facial expressions. Micro-expressions typically last one twenty-fifth to one-fifth second and can be easily missed.

Page: 241

11: The eyes can serve as a window to underlying emotions. Pupillary responses can indicate pleasure with or distaste for viewed material. All of the following represent expected pupillary responses in specific circumstances, except:

    A. Pupillary dilation among married women viewing baby pictures
    B. Pupillary dilation among heterosexual men viewing photographs of nude males
    C. Pupillary dilation among heterosexual women viewing photographs of nude males
    D. Pupillary constriction among single men viewing baby pictures

Answer: B

Critique: Pupillary dilation indicates pleasure with the viewed subject; subjects perceived as unpleasant lead to papillary constriction. Married women viewing baby pictures and heterosexual women viewing photographs of nude males demonstrate papillary dilation. Heterosexual men viewing nude male photographs and single men viewing baby pictures demonstrate papillary constriction.

Pages: 241, 242

12: Of the following options, which represents the best method for expressing sincerity:

    A. Frequent eye contact with the speaker
    B. Looking down and away from the speaker

C. Frequent distant stares
D. Maintaining eye contact for longer than 5 seconds

Answer: A

Critique: In U.S. culture, frequent eye contact conveys a sense of sincerity when listening to a speaker. Looking down and away might indicate rejection of the speaker. Frequent distant stares might be acceptable when formulating ideas or responses but should be interspersed with frequent eye contact. In American culture, prolonged eye contact of longer than 3 seconds could be considered impolite when talking with a stranger.

Page: 242

13: The amount of eye contact during an interaction can provide clues to the patient's affective state. Which of the following best describes the frequency of eye contact seen in depressed patients:

A. Three times as much as with nondepressed patients
B. Twice as much as with nondepressed patients
C. Half as much as with nondepressed patients
D. One fourth as much as with nondepressed patients

Answer: D

Critique: Depressed patients demonstrate only about one fourth the eye contact that nondepressed patients do. Although the frequency of contact may not be reduced, the duration is.

Page: 242

14: Which of the following hand arrangements is most associated with confidence and assurance:

A. Hands held in droopy, flaccid configuration
B. Hands fidgeting and grasping
C. Hands clenched tightly
D. Hands held with fingers extended and fingertips touching

Answer: D

Critique: Holding the hands with fingers extended and fingertips touching represents "steepling" and conveys a sense of assurance and confidence in the speaker. Droopy, flaccid hands convey sadness, and fidgety, grasping hands convey anxiety. Clenched hands indicate anger.

Page: 242

15: (True or False) Which of the following hand arrangements can indicate a desire to interrupt:

A. A slight raising of the hand
B. A slight raising of the index finger
C. Pulling at an ear lobe
D. Raising the index finger to the lips

Answers: A - True, B - True, C - True, D - True

Critique: All of the described hand and finger movements can provide subtle clues about the patient's desire to interrupt to provide new information.

Page: 242

16: A nose rub can serve as a subtle clue to a patient's reaction to the clinical interaction. All of the following indicate rejection of a statement made by the physician, except:

A. The patient vigorously and repeatedly rubs her nose
B. The patient lightly rubs her nose once or twice
C. The patient lightly flicks the side of her nose once or twice
D. The patient rubs her nose and clears her throat

Answer: A

Critique: Vigorous and repeated rubbing of the nose usually indicates itching. The patient who lightly rubs the nose or flicks the nose lightly, along with clearing the throat, is providing subtle clues about rejection of the speaker's comments.

Page: 244

17: North Americans typically maintain a space around themselves when interacting with strangers. Which of the following best describes the extent of this area:

A. A 1-foot diameter circle
B. A 2-foot diameter circle
C. A 3-foot diameter circle
D. A 4-foot diameter circle
E. A 5-foot diameter circle

Answer: B

Critique: People in all cultures have various comfort levels with proximity to strangers. North Americans tend to maintain a comfort space of about 2 feet in diameter around themselves when interacting with strangers.

Page: 245

18: Social space is classified as which of the following separation distances:

A. 2 inches to 18 inches
B. 18 inches to 4 feet
C. 4 feet to 12 feet
D. 12 feet to 30 feet

Answer: C

Critique: Social space is classified as 4 to 12 feet separation. Intimate space includes close physical contact out to 18 inches, and personal space extends for 18 inches to 4 feet. Distances beyond 12 feet are considered public space.

Page: 245

19: The "hand on the doorknob syndrome" describes which of the following phenomena in clinical interactions:

A. The patient charges to the door at the conclusion of the office visit.
B. The patient stops at the door to tell you about his grandchildren at the end of the visit.
C. The patient voices a new concern as you begin to exit the room.

D. The patient comments about the style of the doorknob as you prepare to exit the room.

Answer: C

Critique: Patients often voice a new concern as the physician prepares to exit the examination room at the end of a visit. This can occur as a result of patient fears about what might really be wrong or may represent an issue that is sufficiently threatening that the patient could not voice the concern earlier in the interview. This is referred to as the "hand on the doorknob syndrome."

Page: 246

20: Readiness to listen is best conveyed by which of the following nonverbal techniques:

    A. Writing in the medical record while the patient speaks
    B. Looking down and away from the patient while she speaks
    C. Bending forward and maintaining eye contact
    D. Crossing the legs and turning away from the patient

Answer: C

Critique: Nonverbal cues can communicate the physician's willingness, or lack thereof, to listen. Bending forward and maintaining eye contact communicates attentiveness and willingness to listen. Looking away or looking down to write in the medical record can be perceived as an unreceptive behavior. Crossing the legs and turning away can convey a sense of defensiveness and shutting out the patient's comments.

Pages: 243, 246

21: Interruption can break a patient's train of thought and thus impede the physician's acquisition of important clinical information. In clinical interactions, how long are patients allowed to talk about their chief complaint before interruption by the physician:

    A. 35 seconds
    B. 1 minute
    C. 2 minutes
    D. 18 seconds
    E. 49 seconds

Answer: D

Critique: At least one study has found that patients are interrupted after only 18 seconds when presenting their initial complaint. Male physicians tend to interrupt more frequently than do female physicians.

Page: 247

22: Using a sentence such as, "Let me see if I have understood you correctly," and paraphrasing what the patient has said represents which of the following facilitating interview techniques:

    A. Confrontation
    B. Repetition
    C. Summation
    D. Interruption

Answer: C

Critique: Paraphrasing and repeating back to the patient what he or she has said serves to confirm the information and provide an opportunity for the patient to expand on previous comments or to correct inaccuracies. Repetition consists of reiterating the last word or words the patient said as a means to encourage the patient to proceed. Gentle confrontation, such as, "We don't seem to be communicating very well. What is wrong?" can serve to address communication difficulties forthrightly. Interruption is not a facilitative technique.

Page: 248

Chapter 16

Patient Education

Dana Nottingham

1: Which of the following is a demonstrated benefit of patient education?

    A. Better adherence to treatment regimens
    B. Improved patient satisfaction
    C. Lower medical costs
    D. Improved quality of life
    E. All of the above

Answer: E

Critique: In addition to all of these benefits, patient education has also been demonstrated to reduce morbidity and mortality and increase patient autonomy. The more interventions adhere to sound educational principles, the better they work. Cost-benefit analyses have estimated savings of three to four dollars for every dollar invested in patient education. The U.S. Preventive Services Task Force (USPSTF) supports routine health habit counseling based on its evidence-based review of the literature.

Page: 253

2: (True or False) Some of the effects of patient education that more directly affect physicians may include:

    A. Practice marketing through enhanced patient satisfaction
    B. Increased number of unnecessary office visits and phone calls
    C. Less physician responsibility for informed consent
    D. Fewer malpractice actions

Answers: A - True, B - False, C - False, D - True

Critique: Benefits to the physician include practice marketing through enhanced patient satisfaction. There is also evidence that education reduces unnecessary office visits and phone contacts, which "waste time" in the current environment of increasingly managed and capitated medical care. The current legal standard of informed consent holds the physician accountable for injuries resulting from undisclosed risks. Enhanced patient satisfaction that results from more education, together with more realistic expectations, can greatly contribute to the prevention of malpractice actions.

Page: 253

3: Which of the following is a characteristic of the emerging health care paradigm?

    A. A shift to a more traditional, paternalistic family physician-patient relationship
    B. Increasing emphasis by physicians on the personal health practices of patients
    C. Resistance by patients to accept responsibility for their health behaviors
    D. Implementation of this paradigm not requiring much educating of patients

Answer: B

Critique: Based on the review of the evidence by the USPSTF, the most effective interventions available to clinicians for reducing the incidence and severity of the leading causes of disease and disability in the United States are those that address the personal health practices of patients. This implies a movement by health care providers and patients toward a nontraditional relationship in which encouragement of healthy lifestyles by providers and acceptance of responsibility for health behaviors by patients become the cornerstones of a new preventive care paradigm. Education of patients will be critical to the implementation of this paradigm.

Page: 253

4: (True or False) When considering opportunities to get involved in patient education:

    A. Patient education should be seen as a separate step during the patient encounter.
    B. They may include involvement in a local school's health education curriculum.
    C. Certain in-office programs should be offered even if they duplicate available community resources.
    D. Recruiting the assistance of the entire office staff is a viable option.

Answers: A - False, B - True, C - False, D - True

Critique: When observing excellent family physicians, it is evident that education is incorporated throughout the interaction with the patient, and not segregated as a separate step. When taking a patient's history, one can assess attitudes, knowledge, and skills. When performing an examination, one can instruct the patient about the purpose of the examination and the meaning of any findings. When discussing a diagnosis, one can share its meaning and the process of decision making in layman's terms. When suggesting therapy, one can assess understanding, willingness, and barriers to implementation. Although patient education may occur largely in the context of individual provider-patient interactions, there are many additional opportunities to get involved in health education, such as involvement in school programs, workplace programs, community events, and with the media. Some creative solutions for the busy practice to increase the amount of education that can be provided include expanding services to include group classes for common topics (e.g., smoking cessation, perinatal care, healthy diet), making education the responsibility of the entire practice working as a team, and making use of other health professionals (e.g., dieticians, pharmacists). It is also important not to overlook existing resources in the community that can be used to expand what is offered in the physician's office (e.g., American Diabetes Association; American Heart Association; American Cancer Society; Weight Watchers; Alcoholics Anonymous; local library, YMCA, and church programs). Becoming familiar with these organizations and programs allows the physician to guide patients to appropriate resources. Physicians should be seen as health consultants by patients and view themselves the same way.

Page: 254

5: Research has shown that benefits of patient education are greatest when interventions follow sound educational principles. Which one of the following would *not* be included among such principles?

    A. Feedback
    B. Reinforcement
    C. Use of as few educational channels as possible
    D. Relevance
    E. Individualization

Answer: C

Critique: Examples of sound educational principles are feedback, reinforcement, individualization, facilitation, relevance, and use of multiple educational channels. During feedback, the patient is informed about progress toward goals. Reinforcement refers to encouragement or rewards for progress. Individualization takes into account the needs, desires, and characteristics of the patient and demands that specific goals be negotiated for each patient. Facilitation refers to materials, cues, or training to assist the patient in making changes. Relevance, to the individual patient, means that the content is appropriate for his or her circumstances. The use of multiple channels implies combined learning strategies as well as a team approach to education.

Page: 254

6: (True or False) The main purpose of patient education is to improve the patient's knowledge about his or her health and health care.

Answer: False

Critique: Sometimes the goal of patient education is to influence a patient's knowledge about his or her health and health care. More often, though, the purpose is not simply to inform but rather to change behavior. Typically, the goal is to improve adherence to therapeut-

ic regimens, encourage new lifestyles, or help the patient adopt other behaviors that prevent disease and disability.

Page: 254

7: Which of the following is *not* part of the transtheoretical model of behavior change (six stages of change)?

    A. Precontemplation
    B. Contemplation
    C. Motivation
    D. Action
    E. Termination

Answer: C

Critique: One of the most useful ways to understand the process of behavior change is the transtheoretical model, which proposes six stages of change: precontemplation, contemplation, preparation, action, maintenance, and termination. The first three can be thought of as stages of motivation and readiness for change. In at-risk populations, typically 40% are precontemplators, 40% are contemplators, and 20% are in preparation. Research has shown improvements in process and outcome measures when stage-matched interventions and recruitment methods are used. Although the model is described in a linear fashion, experience has demonstrated that patients naturally move back and forth between stages.

Pages: 254, 255

8: On which of the six stages of change should family physicians focus the majority of their patient education efforts?

    A. Contemplation
    B. Preparation
    C. Action
    D. Maintenance
    E. Termination

Answer: B

Critique: Given the typical constraints on time and resources in a primary care practice, it makes sense to focus the majority of patient education efforts on patients in the stage of preparation. Giving such patients the proper cue or knowledge to make a beneficial change is generally easy, perhaps through an instructional pamphlet, strongly supporting the new behavior, or referral to another professional such as a dietician. On the other hand, encouraging action for patients in the precontemplation or contemplation stage is a waste of the physician's energy. Rather, the goal in that case should be to increase the patient's readiness for change either by increasing the number of perceived pros or by decreasing the number of perceived cons.

Page: 255

9: (True or False) When the unmotivated patient is in the precontemplation stage, it may be important for the family physician to assess and help modify which of the following to move the patient toward action?

    A. The patient's beliefs about his or her condition or risk as well as about the treatment or new behavior

B. How successful the patient thinks he or she will be in accomplishing the desired change
C. The supports of and barriers to change that may affect the patient's success
D. The physician should rarely attempt this because it leads to burnout

Answers: A - True, B - True, C - True, D - False

Critique: When patients are unmotivated to change and are in the stage of precontemplation, the physician should decide whether to invest the time necessary to intervene through an assessment and modification of beliefs (about their condition/risk and the treatment/new behavior), level of confidence (or expectation of success/failure), supports, and barriers. This can be accomplished over time in the context of routine office visits. The physician, at the very least, should convey the message that he or she is willing and ready to help the patient make changes when the patient is motivated to make them. Then stage of change should be reassessed on a regular basis. When assessing supports and barriers, keep in mind that social realities come into play, such as family and cultural concerns, the patient's living arrangements, and his or her employment situation and income. The patient's motivation for change is likely to be in direct proportion to his or her level of confidence in the ability to change. The goal is to change a patient's readiness in small increments over time and to detect any change in motivation that will allow for a meaningful change in behavior. This process can be very frustrating for physicians and can easily lead to burnout if steps are not taken to avoid it. Such steps might include focusing mostly on motivated patients in the preparation stage, learning to feel rewarded for small changes that patients make, and learning to accept that some people will not change despite one's best efforts.

Pages: 255, 256

10: All but which one of the following are important to consider in the educational process?

A. The patient's existing knowledge
B. How to define the needed knowledge in a functional, outcome-driven sense
C. How to construct, with the patient, an agenda for education
D. How to best accomplish this in a 15-minute office visit

Answer: D

Critique: Education is a dynamic process, most akin to a cycle of assessing, planning, instructing, and evaluating. A common mistake in patient education is to forge ahead with the educational message or content without first assessing existing knowledge. Physicians must be careful to define knowledge in a functional, outcome-driven sense. The physician and patient need to jointly prioritize the issues to construct an agenda for education, and these issues can be revisited following the delivery of the education. The trick is not to feel that all this must be accomplished during one 15-minute office visit. Despite what one might think, collecting the data necessary for ration-

al patient education planning is possible in a relatively small amount of time if it is integrated properly into the medical interview. In many instances, much important assessment information is already known to the family physician and can be used without spending more time on data gathering.

Pages: 256, 257

11: (True or False) The problem of low literacy can be limited to which of the following?

A. Low intelligence
B. Low educational level
C. Low socioeconomic status
D. Difficulty attaching meaning to what is read

Answers: A - False, B - False, C - False, D - False

Critique: One quarter of the U.S. population has rudimentary reading skills, and another quarter has limited reading skills. Medical literacy refers to patients' ability to read and understand instructions; to give informed consent; and to comprehend, absorb, and retain information presented. The problem of low literacy is *not* limited to patients with low intelligence, low educational levels, or low socioeconomic status. Patients experience low literacy in a variety of different ways, such as never learning to read, inability to attach meaning to what is read, inability to conceptualize information so that it can be applied, and difficulty with language fluency or vocabulary. Regardless of the cause, if patients are unable to read or understand the material presented, they get little benefit from receiving the health information.

Page: 257

12: All but which of the following can be helpful in overcoming a literacy problem?

A. Ensuring that all educational materials are written at the sixth grade reading level
B. Directly questioning a patient about his or her reading and comprehension abilities
C. Making use of standardized instruments developed to assess medical literacy
D. Taking sufficient time to present the information in a way that best meets the patient's needs

Answer: A

Critique: Patients do not commonly inform physicians of their inability to read or understand information and often attempt to hide their low literacy skills because of the social stigma. Serious consequences can result unless the problem is identified and adequately compensated for by the physician. The best method of assessing the degree of literacy involves observing, being alert to cues, and conducting sensitive and timely direct questioning. Several instruments have been developed to assess medical literacy, such as the Rapid Estimate of Adult Literacy in Medicine, the Wide Range Achievement Test—Revised III (both word recognition tests), and the Test of Functional Health Literacy in Adults (reading and comprehension test). If the problem is identified, patients with low literacy skills are capable of learning and understanding information when sufficient time is taken to present the information in a way that best meets the patient's needs (e.g., visually, giving smaller amounts of information at a time, giving written materials that include only the absolutely essential information, eliminating jargon, using materials also available in languages other than English). The printed materials used should be written at a reading comprehension level appropriate for the patients served.

Pages: 257, 259

13: All but which of the following are true concerning giving verbal instructions to patients?

    A. An atmosphere of acceptance and approval is essential to effective verbal communication.
    B. This modality serves as the foundation for further education.
    C. Medical jargon should be avoided.
    D. Instructions should be specific and clear.
    E. It is important to continually check patients' understanding of what they have been told.

Answer: A

Critique: The most common form of patient education is talking to patients within the context of routine family physician-patient contacts. This interaction serves as the foundation for further education that may be provided in the form of printed materials, video materials, classes, or other instructional modalities. An atmosphere of acceptance (i.e., nonjudgmental and understanding), but not necessarily approval, is the first prerequisite to effective communication. This will facilitate collaboration with the patient toward the achievement of common goals. Medical jargon should be avoided. Keep in mind that physicians often do not realize how much of their vocabulary is highly technical and outside of the average patient's understanding. One approach to helping patients decode the jargon is to embed synonyms in the information provided. Specificity and clarity are equally important principles. For example, don't say to a patient, "Exercise more!" but rather spell out for the patient the type of exercise; how often, how long, and how intensely to do it; how to warm up and cool down; and any warning symptoms to watch for. It is also important to continually check patients' understanding of what they have been told. A helpful strategy is to ask patients, in a way that is not condescending, to summarize their understanding of the information they have been given.

Pages: 258, 259

14: (True or False) When considering the modality of printed materials for patient education:

    A. They are usually effective when used alone.
    B. Physicians are responsible for the accuracy of any materials they distribute.
    C. It is always appropriate to use materials produced by pharmaceutical companies.
    D. The information should be clearly presented.
    E. Whether or not the materials will continue to be produced should not be much of a concern.

Answers: A - False, B - True, C - False, D - True, E - False

Critique: After verbal instruction, printed materials are the most commonly used patient education modality. Unfortunately, they are often used alone or without sufficient verbal instruction beforehand. Volumes of research have shown that printed materials are not effective when used in this way. In contrast, studies have shown that, when used to supplement other instruction, printed materials are desired by patients and lead to improved outcomes. It is important to recognize that physicians are responsible for the accuracy of any materials they distribute. Sources of free materials are primarily pharmaceutical companies and national voluntary associations such as the American Cancer Society. Low-cost materials are offered by other national organizations (e.g., American Heart Association) and medical specialty societies. Several issues are important to consider before using existing materials. First, is the content appropriate? Materials provided by pharmaceutical companies may advertise a product or present information in a biased way, or voluntary organizations' guidelines may not agree with the physician's own judgments about proper screening and treatment. Second, is the material clearly presented and does it have a reading comprehension level appropriate for the patients served by the practice? Unfortunately, the majority of materials have not been produced with lower-literacy patients in mind and are typically written at a twelfth grade or higher comprehension level. A third concern is logistics. Will additional copies of the material continue to be available for replenishing supplies, or might the material go out of print? How will the materials be stored and displayed?

Page: 259

15: All but which of the following are important when designing your own printed patient education material?

    A. Keep it short.
    B. Keep it simple.
    C. Use of fear messages is helpful.
    D. Start with a planning process.

Answer: C

Critique: For best results, practices should begin with a planning process that identifies the most important needs, based on the common educational issues the practice deals with and the existing materials and their quality and usefulness. It is a good idea to do a literature search before starting to write your own materials to broaden your knowledge base and ensure accuracy. A common pitfall is to try to include too much information. Restrict the content to three or four salient teaching points. Avoid jargon, extensive statistics, and fear messages. Be clear about advice and specific with instructions. Using short words and sentences works best to improve readers' comprehension. Simple line drawings with a few labels are usually more effective than complex illustrations, and they are easier to reproduce. Subheadings help readers find information. The text should be written in the active tense, using first person for questions and second person for answers. Avoid using negatives and absolutes such as "never," "must," and "always." When laying out material, leave plenty of white space on the page, avoid long strings of capital letters, limit the use of bold and italic type, and use 10- or 12-point type size and a 2- or 3-column format. Ideally, test material on colleagues and on a few patients before reproducing the material in quantity.

Pages: 259, 260

16: All but which of the following are advantages to using computer-assisted instruction with patients?

    A. Computers have desirable traits for education.
    B. The World Wide Web is typically a reliable source for patient information.
    C. The education process can be individualized to a given patient's needs.
    D. Computer-based patient record systems can be helpful.

Answer: B

Critique: Computer-assisted instruction software represents an emerging technology that offers great promise. Computers can be anonymous, nonjudgmental, and infinitely patient—all desirable traits in an educator. Well-written software can individualize the process of instruction to a given patient's needs. Unfortunately, the growth of the World Wide Web is a double-edged sword: many sites provide opinion, hearsay, and outright falsehoods with the same authoritative style as peer-reviewed evidence from published medical research. Patients are ill equipped to tell the difference. As more and more patients go on-line, providers should keep abreast of some of the more reliable Web resources so that they can make useful recommendations to patients and respond to misinformation that patients may encounter. Computer-based patient record systems are becoming more common, but not all of them address the needs of education very well. Those that do so can be helpful, for example, by prompting providers to give recommended health habit counseling, by allowing easy access to visual aids that can be used in patient teaching in the examination room, and by automatically generating appropriate educational materials that can be printed and handed to the patient.

Page: 260

17: (True or False) In general, it is not necessary to make use of visual aids when instructing patients.

Answer: False

Critique: It is generally helpful to supplement printed materials with models, anatomic charts, audio tapes, videotapes, and other visual aids that can be used during the process of instruction. Such materials can be invaluable in trying to explain what a 3-ounce serving of meat looks like, for example.

Page: 260

18: (True or False) When considering how to make the practice setting more educational for patients:

    A. The waiting room should be viewed as more than an attractive room with comfortable chairs and a magazine rack or television.
    B. The examination rooms should not be cluttered with posters and handouts.
    C. Monthly or quarterly health themes are a good idea.
    D. A separate patient education room is essential.

Answers: A - True, B - False, C - True, D - False

Critique: One way to provide effective patient education is to view the practice setting in its totality as an educational experience for patients. From this perspective, health providers can critically examine each staff member and each physical area for its potential to contribute to patient education. For example, the waiting area can be utilized by providing a rack of educational brochures, playing educational videotapes, or making computer-assisted instruction available and can be decorated with educational posters. Examination rooms can also have posters and racks of printed materials, especially materials that patients might be embarrassed to pick up while others are watching. Some practices use monthly or quarterly health themes and rotate posters and materials that relate to the themes. Practices that use audio tapes or videotapes may find it effective to create a patient education room or a mobile cart with the necessary equipment. The important aspects of any system used to store, retrieve, index, and order materials are that providers (1) know what types of materials are available, (2) agree with their content, (3) know how to find desired materials, (4) periodically review existing materials for applicability and accuracy, and (5) order or produce more materials as stocks run low. Office staff may be quite eager to assist with this responsibility.

Pages: 260, 261

Chapter 17

Interviewing Techniques

William A. Verhoff

1: During the 1950s, which specialty began to focus on the interview as a significant element in its therapeutic process?

    A. Family practice
    B. Surgery
    C. Internal medicine
    D. Psychiatry

Answer: D

Critique: In the early 1950s, some psychiatric residency programs audio taped interviews, which were reviewed by senior physicians with the residents.

Page: 262

2: (True or False) In the 1960s, the Willard Report emphasized the role of behavioral science as part of medical education and as clearly an integral part of family practice and its doctor-patient relationship.

Answer: True

Critique: The Report of the Ad Hoc Committee on Education for Family Practice, popularly referred to as the Willard Report, emphasized the role of behavioral science in medical education and its place in training of family physicians.

Page: 262

3: In January 1993, what new organization appeared for membership to those interested in the development of improved interviewing skills and enhancing the family physician-patient relationship?

    A. AAFP
    B. ABFP
    C. AAMC
    D. AAPP
    E. STFM

Answer: D

Critique: The American Academy on the Physician and Patient (AAPP) began accepting members in January 1993. The Society of Teachers of Family Medicine (STFM) Behavioral Science Task Force, along with work done by the Society of General Internal Medicine, led to the formation of this new organization.

Page: 262

4: The impact of managed care on health care has forced many patients to shift their care between physicians, between specialists, between health care delivery sites, and between hospitals, thus placing an increased emphasis on _____ to maintain patients' medical histories.

    A. The government
    B. The primary care physician
    C. A large computer data repository
    D. The patient

Answer: D

Critique: McRonald (1999, p. 10) suggests that in the current managed care and specialist-oriented environment, the only consistent element in the process is the patient and that the patient is the only entity that can maintain a complete patient history.

Page: 263

5: (True or False) The electronic medical history has come of age, and claims that the computer is capable of collecting complete, accurate, and consistent information have been proved to hold up with the newest software products.

Answer: False

Critique: A study of computerized histories found that only 68% of patients could express all or most of their complaints. Some of their physical complaints could not be entered at all, and only 52% of the female patients and 75% of the male patients found the range of answers from which to choose sufficient.

Page: 264

6: The Association of American Medical Colleges (AAMC) found in a public opinion research survey that the top reasons for choosing a physician are:

    A. Cost of visit, access, office location, and hospital affiliation
    B. Board certification and medical school attended
    C. Ability to explain medical information in a patient-friendly way, ability to listen, providing adequate time for questions, and overall caring attitude

Answer: C

Critique: Ranked at the top of the survey was "how well a doctor communicates with patients and shows a caring attitude," with listening and taking time for questions close behind. It was taken for granted by the patients that doctors have adequate knowledge and technical skills and are competent to practice.

Page: 264

7: The medical interview, often referred to as the medical history, has three main functions. Which of the statements below does not qualify as a principal function of the interview?

    A. To determine and monitor the nature of the problem
    B. To develop, maintain, and conclude the therapeutic relationship
    C. To establish care guidelines and limits that must be maintained
    D. To carry out patient education and implementation of treatment plans

Answer: C

Critique: Care guidelines may be discussed during the interview, but limit setting is not part of history taking.

Pages: 265, 266

8: Organizing the medical interview is essential if the physician wants to maximize the accuracy and comprehensiveness of the patient's history. Put the seven steps of the medical interview in the proper order.

    A. Data gathering
    B. The problem or chief complaint
    C. Treatment alternatives and decisions
    D. Purpose and willingness to consider problems
    E. Actions and evaluations
    F. Analysis and definition of the problem
    G. Greeting and sizing up

Answer : D, G, B, A, F, C, E

Pages: 265–268

9: (True or False) Past experiences and stereotypes, along with nonverbal and verbal messages, are instrumental in establishing a successful contract with the patient.

Answer: True

Critique: In the first 20 seconds of the interview, visual input dominates the awareness of the two participants. The environment of the room, posture, dress, sex, age, physical distance, and body build drive our perceptions of the other person. The way words are spoken becomes as important as what is said as the patient and the physician generate opinions about each other.

Page: 266

Conducting an effective interview depends in part on the ability to avoid common interviewing pitfalls. Match the numbered items below with the correct lettered pitfall.

10: _____ When you speak about your boss, you appear somewhat anxious.

11: _____ When was the last time you smoked a pack of cigarettes in one day?

12: _____ Do you participate in an exercise program three times each week?

13: _____ Why did you forget to take your medications?
    A. Accusation question   B. Yes or no question
    C. Direct question   D. Suggestive question

Answers: 10 - D, 11 - C, 12 - B, 13 - A

Critique: These questions limit the information the interviewer can collect. Some of the questions put the patient on the defensive and can cause much uncertainty for the patient and the provider as to what the question and the answer meant.

Page: 268

14: As the physician begins to gather data, it is vital that he or she knows enough about the patient's _____ before dealing with the onset of illness.

    A. Family history
    B. Present state
    C. Medical history
    D. Social history
    E. Sexual history

Answer: B

Critique: A common mistake in medical interviewing is for the physician to deal with the onset of illness before knowing enough about the patient's present state to have a good idea of the organ of involvement.

Page: 267

15: (True or False) Patients generally wish to be involved in decisions about their care, and physicians do not wish to exclude them. This understanding always creates synergy between perceptions and expectations regarding the treatment plan.

Answer: False

Critique: Patients say that their physicians do not listen to them, explain things clearly, or want to be bothered with questions. Physicians say they wish their patients had more realistic expectations and would take a more active role in their care management. Thus, the medical encounter can be like two ships passing in the night.

Page: 267

16: In dealing with the problem patient, the family physician must realize that patients are usually _____ because of an expected negative outcome if they talk freely about the topic at hand.

    A. Manipulative/demanding
    B. Defensive
    C. Angry
    D. Happy
    E. Stoic

Answer: B

Critique: A defensive posture is taken when the information to be discussed may have a negative outcome. Once the outcome is discussed, and it becomes evident to the patient that nothing bad will happen, and as the topic is dealt with, the defensiveness begins to melt away.

Page: 269

17: In the normal, healthy person, anger is the natural result of _____.

    A. Not getting what one wants
    B. Not winning
    C. Being frustrated
    D. Being afraid

Answer: C

Critique: Anger is the natural result of frustration. To overcome the frustration in a socially acceptable manner, the anger takes the form of aggression. But once the anger changes to hostility, it becomes destructive, not constructive, and is considered maladaptive.

Page: 270

18: (True or False) For the interviewer to develop an excellent technique, he or she must have an open state of mind, be free to hear and see anything, and be dedicated to hearing exactly what is being said, with a complete focus on the patient verbally and nonverbally.

Answer: True

Critique: The interviewer must be honest and open to his or her own feelings and interpretations and be spontaneous in responding to the patient. In this state of mind, the interviewer is listening and watching the patient, words and tone, gestures, and body movements and staying in touch with his or her own body reactions.

Page: 271

PART IV

PRACTICE OF FAMILY MEDICINE

Chapter 18

Clinical Problem Solving

Michael D. Hagen

1: Which of the following is the first step in the clinical reasoning process:

   A. Collection of laboratory data and clinical history from the patient
   B. Development of hypotheses regarding potential causes for the clinician's observations
   C. Calculation of Bayes' theorem to determine the likelihood that the patient has a condition
   D. Determination of the pertinent clinical question indicated by the patient's symptoms and signs

Answer: D

Critique: The clinical reasoning process begins with identifying the pertinent clinical question indicated by the patient's complaints. The second step is collecting data needed to answer the question. The third step consists of formulating a diagnosis or hypothesis to answer or explain the clinical question. Calculating Bayes' theorem might occur as one component of analyzing the collected data but is not the first step in the process.

Page: 276

2: The patient's agenda for a clinical visit usually consists of explicit and implicit components. All except which of the following are components of this agenda, which the physician must address to clearly identify the clinical question:

   A. The patient's spoken agenda (e.g., the chief complaint)
   B. The patient's unspoken agenda
   C. The physician's agenda
   D. The insurer's agenda

Answer: D

Critique: The clinical question might not become apparent until the astute clinician has considered the patient's both spoken and unspoken agendas for the clinical encounter. Additionally, the physician should be aware of his or her own agenda, because this could influence interpretation of the patient's complaints. The insurer's agenda is not included in this process.

Page: 277

3: (True or False) Patients' cultural beliefs influence their perceptions of clinical symptoms and illness. Which of the following questions might a clinician consider asking to better understand a patient's health beliefs:

   A. "What do you think caused the problem?"
   B. "What do you fear most about your disorder?"
   C. "What are the most important results you hope to receive from the treatment?"
   D. "What kind of treatment do you think you should receive?"

Answers: A - True, B - True, C - True, D - True

Critique: The patient's cultural beliefs and milieu affect how he or she interprets the clinical symptoms associated with an illness. All of the listed questions can help the clinician develop insight into these beliefs.

Page: 277

4: (True or False) The believability of a clinical finding is determined by which of the following characteristics:

   A. The accuracy with which the patient presents the symptoms
   B. The skill with which the clinician examines the patient
   C. The accuracy of the laboratory tests and clinical procedures performed
   D. The cost of the laboratory tests performed

Answers: A - True, B - True, C - True, D - False

Critique: The believability of a clinical finding depends on the patient's accuracy in defining symptoms, the clinician's skill in performing the examination, and the accuracy of the laboratory procedures conducted in investigating the illness. The cost of the test is not among the factors that influence test believability.

Page: 278

5: Assume that you have performed a clinical test and that the test result is positive for the disease in question. On the basis of your knowledge of the test's sensitivity and specificity, you determine that the positive predictive value for the disease in this patient is 40%. Which of the following statements represents the most accurate interpretation of this determination:

   A. The test has a sensitivity of 40%.
   B. There is a 40% likelihood that this represents a false-positive result.
   C. There is a 40% likelihood that the patient has the disease.
   D. The test has an accuracy of 40%.

Answer: C

Critique: The positive predictive value indicates the likelihood that a patient has a disorder, given the test result. The sensitivity, on the other hand, defines the likelihood that a patient who has the disease will have a positive test. The false-positive rate is the likelihood that a normal patient will have a positive result. The accuracy represents the likelihood that the test will correctly characterize normal and abnormal patients.

Pages: 278, 279

6: Which of the following statements best describes the effect of a decrease in disease prevalence on the positive predictive value of a clinical test:

    A. The positive predictive value will decrease.
    B. The positive predictive value will increase.
    C. The positive predictive value will stay the same.
    D. The disease prevalence and positive predictive value have no predictable relationship.

Answer: A

Critique: The prevalence of a disorder in the tested population has a tremendous impact on the positive predictive value associated with a positive result. As the prevalence increases, so does the positive predictive value and vice versa.

Pages: 278, 279

7: Referring to the 2 x 2 table, which of the following represents the positive predictive value for the test results summarized in the table:

	Disease +	Disease −
Test +	80	20
Test −	10	90

80/(80+20) = 0.80; 80/(80+10) = 0.89;
90/(90+20) = 0.82; (80+90)/(80+90+20+10) = 0.85

    A. 0.80
    B. 0.82
    C. 0.85
    D. 0.89

Answer: A

Critique: The positive predictive value represents the likelihood that a patient with a positive test actually has the disease in question. In this case, 100 patients have positive tests, but only 80 of these patients actually have the disease, or 80/100 = 0.80. Choice B represents the test specificity. Choice C is the overall accuracy of the test, or the likelihood that diseased or nondiseased patients are correctly characterized by the test. Choice D is the test sensitivity, that is, the percentage of diseased individuals who have a positive test.

Pages: 278, 279, Table 18–1

8: A number of reasoning strategies exist to assist in the problem-solving process. Which of the following definitions best describes reasoning with reductionism:

    A. Limiting the diagnostic considerations to the least important possibility
    B. Reducing the patient's problems to the smallest list possible
    C. Spending the least possible amount of time interviewing the patient
    D. Using the smallest number of laboratory tests possible

Answer: B

Critique: Reasoning with reductionism entails reducing the number of problems considered to the smallest number that still describes the patient's illness.

Page: 280

9: Developing a list of possible explanations for each of the patient's problems represents which of the following reasoning styles:

    A. Reasoning with organ systems
    B. Reasoning with organizational levels
    C. Reasoning with time
    D. Reasoning with problems individually

Answer: D

Critique: Before attempting to develop a diagnostic hypothesis that can explain all or most of a patient's problems, the clinician should first think of possible explanations for each problem individually. Doing so will avoid premature closure on a possibly incorrect diagnosis. The clinician should consider at least three possible explanations for each of the identified problems.

Pages: 280, 281

10: (True or False) In reasoning with causality, which of the following statements represent possible relationships between two variables under consideration:

    A. The variables are unrelated to each other.
    B. The first variable causes the second.
    C. The second variable causes the first.
    D. Both variables are caused by a third variable.

Answers: A - True, B - True, C - True, D - True

Critique: Four possible relationships exist for any two variables. They are unrelated to each other; the first can cause the second; the second can cause the first; or both variables may be caused or influenced by a third variable.

Pages: 282, 283

Chapter 19

Infectious Diseases

Thomas G. Maddox and Edward T. Bope

1: Antibiotic prophylaxis to prevent perioperative infections should:

    A. Be used for all surgical procedures
    B. Be continued for a minimum of 3 days
    C. Be administered at the time of or immediately before surgery
    D. Be started at least 5 half-lives before surgery so that a therapeutic level can be achieved
    E. Include the use of an oral antibiotic for any gastrointestinal surgery

Answer: C

Critique: Antibiotic prophylaxis for some procedures is indicated only when the patient has elevated risk factors that predispose him or her to develop postsurgical infections. Appropriate prophylactic use of antibiotics includes administration of the antibiotic immediately before surgery and continued for no more than 24 hours after surgery. The antibiotic chosen should provide coverage for the most likely organisms to be encountered. Antibiotics given after inoculation of a wound are ineffective in preventing infection.

Page: 338

2: Aminoglycoside antibiotics:

    A. Are well absorbed orally
    B. Have bacteriostatic activity
    C. Require dosage adjustments in patients with renal impairment
    D. Are not effective against aerobic gram-negative bacilli
    E. Work by inhibiting cell wall synthesis

Answer: C

Critique: Aminoglycosides are not absorbed orally and must be given parenterally. They have activity against most gram-negative bacilli and some staphylococci. Aminoglycosides are not metabolized and are excreted by the kidneys, requiring dosage adjustment in patients with renal dysfunction. Monitoring of blood levels during treatment is recommended. Aminoglycosides are bactericidal because they bind to ribosomes irreversibly.

Pages: 294–296

3: Match the following statements with the appropriate cephalosporins. (Each choice may be used more than once.)

    A. First-generation cephalosporins (e.g., cephadroxil, cephalexin)
    B. Second-generation cephalosporins (e.g., cefuroxime, cefaclor)
    C. Third-generation cephalosporins (e.g., cefotaxime, ceftriaxone)

    1. Good penetration into the cerebrospinal fluid (CSF)
    2. Weakest staphylococcus coverage
    3. The most limited spectrum of activity against gram-negative organisms
    4. Provides coverage for *Haemophilus influenzae* but has no antipseudomonal activity

Answers: 1 - C, 2 - C, 3 - A, 4 - B

Critique: Cephalosporins are divided into first-, second-, and third-generation classes by virtue of the timing of their development and spectrum of activity. First- and second-generation cephalosporins are active against most gram-positive organisms. The second-generation agents are also active against *H. influenzae*. Third-generation cephalosporins have the weakest staphylococci coverage but are active against *Pseudomonas* species. Third-generation cephalosporins penetrate the CSF more reliably than do first- or second-generation cephalosporins. The spectrum of activity of oral second-generation cephalosporins makes them particularly useful in the treatment of lower respiratory tract infections when simpler and cheaper forms of therapy cannot be used because of allergy or resistance.

Page: 294

4: (True or False) Patients should be cautioned against taking over-the-counter antacids while taking quinolone antibiotics.

Answer: True

Critique: Absorption of quinolone antibiotics is inhibited by antacids containing divalent cations (calcium, iron, zinc). H_2 receptor antagonists, however, do not inhibit absorption.

Page: 299

5: (True or False) The elbow is the most commonly affected joint in children with septic arthritis.

Answer: False

Critique: The knee, hip, and shoulder are the most common joints involved in both adults and children with septic arthritis. The most commonly affected joints in adults include the knees, hips, and shoulders.

Page: 318

6: Which of the following is not a predisposing risk factor for developing infective endocarditis:

    A. Congestive heart failure
    B. Atrial septal defect
    C. Chronic atrial fibrillation
    D. Atherosclerotic cardiovascular disease
    E. Aortic stenosis

Answer: D

Critique: Intravenous drug use, prosthetic heart valves, rheumatic heart disease, and atherosclerotic valvular disease are important predisposing factors for developing infective endocarditis. Valvular lesions with a high-pressure gradient raise a patient's risk for bacterial seeding of heart valves. Congestive heart failure, atrial septal defects, chronic atrial fibrillation, and stenotic valvular lesions usually have low-pressure gradients, placing patients at low risk for bacterial seeding.

Pages: 336–338

7: When bacterial meningitis is suspected, which of the following studies should be completed as soon as possible:

    A. Computerized tomography (CT) scan of head and sinuses
    B. Lumbar puncture
    C. Serum glucose: protein ratio
    D. Magnetic resonance imaging (MRI) of head

Answer: B

Critique: A lumbar puncture should be performed as soon as possible after the diagnosis of bacterial meningitis. The opening pressure should be recorded and the specimen sent for cell count and differential, Gram's stain, India ink preparation, latex agglutination tests for *H. influenzae* B, meningococci, and pneumococci. Imaging studies, including CT and MRI scans, are indicated only when focal neurologic signs are present indicating increased intracranial pressure or the possibility of a mass lesion.

Page: 340

8: Regarding body temperature:

    A. It is mediated by the direct effect of angiotensin II.
    B. It is controlled by the sympathetic nervous system.
    C. It has a normal diurnal variation.
    D. Results of blood cultures should be obtained before initiating antibiotics in febrile patients with neutropenia.
    E. A febrile illness that lasts for more than 3 days without an identifiable cause and with negative cultures is classified as a fever of unknown origin (FUO).

Answer: C

Critique: Body temperature is maintained at an average of 98.6° by the autonomic nervous system. There is a diurnal peak in body temperature, in the late afternoon and early evening. Interleukin-1, released by monocytes and macrophages, exerts a direct effect on the thermoregulatory center to cause fever. FUO is, by definition, a febrile illness that lasts for more than 3 weeks and has no identifiable cause. A neutropenic patient who is febrile should be started on broad-spectrum antibiotics empirically because of the patient's susceptibility to the development of overwhelming sepsis.

Pages: 288, 290–291

9: (True or False) In the United States, diarrheal diseases are among the five leading causes of death in children.

Answer: True

Critique: Diarrheal diseases are among the five leading causes of death in small children each year. In underdeveloped countries, death owing to diarrheal diseases is the leading cause of death in infants.

Page: 310

10: Treatment of infectious diarrhea includes:

    A. Increasing the intake of dairy products for children
    B. Antiperistaltic drugs (diphenoxylate, loperamide) for diarrhea caused by *Shigella*
    C. Oral antibiotics for uncomplicated *Salmonella*
    D. Oral antibiotics when pseudomembranous colitis is identified
    E. Prophylactic administration of antibiotics to prevent traveler's diarrhea

Answer: D

Critique: The most important aspect of treatment for diarrheal illnesses is adequate hydration. Children with diarrhea due to viral gastroenteritis should avoid milk products because of temporary lactase deficiency. Antiperistaltic drugs are contraindicated in patients with invasive diarrhea caused by organisms such as *Shigella*, *Salmonella*, and *Yersinia*. *Salmonella* infection is a self-limited disease, and supportive care is usually all that is necessary unless bacteremia occurs. Treatment with antibiotics in otherwise healthy individuals prolongs the carrier state of Salmonella and raises the risk of person-to-person transmission. Use of antibiotics changes the normal bacterial flora of the bowel and provides an opportunity for overgrowth of *Clostridium difficile*. *C. difficile* produces a toxin that causes diarrhea, fever, and abdominal pain. This condition, called pseudomembranous colitis, is treated by oral metronidazole or vancomycin. Intravenous antibiotics are of no value in clearing *C. difficile*. The use of bismuth subsalicylate (Pepto-Bismol) has been shown to help to prevent infection with toxigenic strains of *Escherichia coli*. Taking antibiotics prophylactically, however, may predispose the person to infection with resistant organisms and is not recommended.

Pages: 309–311, 322–325

11: The most common organisms that cause otitis media in children younger than 3 years of age are:

A. *Streptococcus pneumoniae, Mycoplasma pneumoniae*, and *Klebsiella*
B. *S. pneumoniae, H. influenzae*, and *Moraxella catarrhalis*
C. *Staphylococcus aureus, H. influenzae*, and *E. coli*
D. *M. pneumoniae, Chlamydia pneumoniae*, and *Nocardia asteroides*
E. *M. catarrhalis, Pseudomonas aeruginosa*, and influenza A

Answer: B

Critique: Otitis media is the most common cause of infection in children younger than 3 years of age. Eustachian tube dysfunction (failure to drain secretions from the middle ear), caused by mucosal swelling and congestion of pharyngeal tissue, produces a favorable environment for bacterial growth within the middle ear. The most common organisms cultured from suppurative middle ear infections are *S. pneumoniae, H. influenzae*, and *M. catarrhalis*. Amoxicillin is the antibiotic of choice in the treatment of otitis media.

Pages: 351–352

12: A 5-year-old girl presents to the emergency department with a fever (102°F orally), difficulty breathing, and difficulty swallowing, causing her to drool. Additional information or studies should include:

A. Questioning the parent or guardian about a familial history of similar problems in the child's relatives
B. Lateral soft tissue radiographs of the neck
C. Complete neurologic examination with attention to a stiff neck and the presence of a gag reflex
D. Cultures of the oropharynx for viruses and bacteria
E. Giving the appropriate dose of an antipyretic and observing the child for further evidence of localized infection

Answer: B

Critique: This child is presenting with symptoms suggestive of epiglottitis. Epiglottitis usually occurs in children between 2 and 7 years of age and is preceded by a sore throat, high fever, hoarseness, and respiratory distress. The child may be unable to handle his or her own secretions because of difficulty swallowing, causing him or her to drool. Difficulty breathing may also be seen in severe cases. Care should be taken when examining children with possible epiglottitis, because stimulation of the oropharynx may precipitate acute airway obstruction. Lateral soft tissue radiographs of the neck will show an enlarged epiglottis. There is no familial tendency for this infectious disease. An antipyretic may be appropriate for the child's fever, but the child needs immediate and aggressive antibiotic therapy for this potentially fatal infection. Use of a third-generation cephalosporin or cefuroxime is indicated as soon as the clinical diagnosis is made.

Pages: 352–354

13: Which of the following is correct concerning lower respiratory tract infections:

A. Many cases may be prevented by annual influenza vaccinations for persons at risk.
B. Blood cultures are not necessary in patients with suspected pneumonia when sputum cultures have been obtained.
C. Prophylactic antibiotics should not be given to patients with a history of chronic bronchitis owing to the possible development of resistant organisms.
D. Klebsiella pneumonia is the most common cause of pneumonia in adults.
E. *Mycoplasma pneumoniae* is the most common cause of lower respiratory tract infections in children younger than 8 years.

Answer: A

Critique: Respiratory tract infections in the adult most frequently are caused by *S. pneumoniae*. Respiratory syncytial virus is the most common pathogen that causes lower respiratory tract infections in children. Persons at high risk for development of respiratory tract infections should receive an annual influenza vaccine. Pneumococcal vaccine is also recommended at least once. The use of prophylactic antibiotics is indicated for patients with chronic bronchitis to prevent recurrences of lower respiratory tract infections.

Pages: 354–356

14: In patients with sexually transmitted diseases:

A. Males or females exposed to sexual partners known to have gonorrhea should be cultured and treated if positive.
B. Penicillin G is the treatment of choice for gonorrhea.
C. Venereal Disease Research Laboratory (VDRL) titers may continue to be positive even after adequate therapy for syphilis.
D. Toxic shock syndrome is seen only during menses.
E. Herpes simplex type 1 affects only the oral mucosa.

Answer: C

Critique: The frequency of most sexually transmitted diseases has continued to increase annually, despite education efforts for prevention. Several strains of *Neisseria gonorrhoeae* have developed resistance to penicillin. For this reason, ceftriaxone, cefixime, or ciprofloxacin is the preferred therapy for uncomplicated gonorrhea. Persons known to have been exposed to a sexual partner with gonorrhea should be treated and have cultures taken at the same visit. Follow-up cultures should be done approximately 1 week after treatment to ensure clearance of infection. Even after adequate therapy for syphilis, the VDRL nontreponemal antibody test may continue to be positive. Toxic shock syndrome, caused by *S. aureus* and some strains of *Streptococcus pyogenes*, was first recognized in association with tampon use. Toxic shock syndrome now, however, is predominantly nonmenstrual and is seen as frequently in men as in women. Herpes simplex type 1 is capable of producing infection in both oral and genital mucosal surfaces and is responsible for up to 15% of all genital herpes infections.

Pages: 341–347

15: (True or False) Acute rheumatic fever is a frequent complication of impetigo caused by group A streptococci.

Answer: False

Critique: Impetigo is most commonly caused by *S. pyogenes* (group A) or *S. aureus*. Acute poststreptococcal glomerulonephritis may occur after impetigo caused by *S. pyogenes*. The strains of group A streptococci that cause impetigo do not typically cause acute rheumatic fever. Acute rheumatic fever may be seen as a sequella of pharyngeal infections owing to group A streptococci.

Pages: 332–333, 336–338

16: Which of the following statements regarding tuberculosis is correct:

    A. Tuberculosis is usually spread via fomites.
    B. Miliary tuberculosis results from direct invasion of the *Mycobacterium tuberculosis* organism to adjacent organs.
    C. A Ghon complex refers to calcified lymph nodes.
    D. Erythema of greater than 10 mm is always a positive reaction to an intradermal purified protein derivative (PPD).
    E. Joint involvement is the most common form of extrapulmonary tuberculosis.

Answer: C

Critique: Tuberculosis is caused by *M. tuberculosis*. It is spread by inhalation of aerosolized droplets. Fomites are not usually responsible for transmission. Miliary tuberculosis refers to dissemination of the tuberculosis organisms throughout the body by hematogenous spread. Ghon complexes are lymph nodes that have been infected by the tubercle bacillus and calcify on resolution of primary infection. Intradermal skin testing with PPD is done to screen for possible tuberculosis infection. Interpretation of PPD reactions is dependent on the patient's risk factors for development of tuberculosis. Reactions of greater than 15 mm are considered to be positive in individuals with no other health-related problems. A reaction of greater than 5 mm may be considered positive in patients with human immunodeficiency virus (HIV) infection, a recent history of exposure to tuberculosis, or an abnormal chest radiograph. Extrapulmonary tuberculosis is often seen in patients with HIV infection. The lymph node is the most common area involved in extrapulmonary tuberculosis.

Pages: 326–328

17: A 32-year-old woman is diagnosed as having an acute urinary tract infection. You would be correct in telling her:

    A. The most common cause is bacteria that enter the bladder by hematogenous spread.
    B. A urinary tract infection is often an overgrowth of the usual normal flora of the bladder.
    C. Urinary tract infections are often related to sexual activity.
    D. Klebsiella and *Proteus mirabilis* are the most common bacteria that cause a majority of urinary tract infections.

    E. There is no need for treatment of asymptomatic bacteriuria in pregnant women.

Answer: C

Critique: *E. coli* is the most common bacterium responsible for urinary tract infections. Most urinary tract infections are caused by bacteria entering the normally sterile bladder via ascent through the urethra. Trauma to the external urethra, such as may occur during sexual intercourse, can increase the possibility of bacteria entering the bladder. Asymptomatic bacteriuria in pregnancy should still be treated because of an increased risk of nephritis in the mother. Neonatal complications of bacteriuria in pregnancy include prematurity, perinatal death, stillbirth, and intrauterine growth retardation.

Pages: 318–321

18: Which of the following is characteristic of congenital rubella syndrome?

    A. Low birth weight
    B. Hydrocephaly
    C. Limb malformations
    D. Renal dysfunction
    E. Dental malformations

Answer: A

Critique: Both temporary and permanent problems are associated with congenital rubella syndrome. Temporary manifestations include low birth weight, thrombocytopenia, and hepatosplenomegaly. Permanent manifestations are deafness, cataracts, and patent ductus arteriosus. Developmental problems, including mental retardation, behavior disorders, and seizures, can also be seen.

Page: 365

19: (True or False) A person who is susceptible may contract chickenpox after exposure to someone with herpes zoster (shingles).

Answer: True

Critique: Varicella-zoster virus causes chickenpox (varicella) as a primary illness. After reactivation, the varicella-zoster virus can migrate along a dermatome to cause shingles (herpes zoster). Lesions that occur with zoster shed the varicella-zoster virus. Persons who are susceptible may contract chickenpox after exposure to these lesions.

Pages: 358–360

20: Influenza vaccination is indicated for which of the following patients:

    A. A 46-year-old man with a history of smoking
    B. A 22-year-old healthy woman
    C. A 29-year-old man with HIV infection
    D. A 14-year-old girl with a seizure disorder
    E. A 5-year-old child attending day care

Answer: C

Critique: Annual vaccination of individuals at risk for the development of influenza is recommended. Individuals considered at highest risk include adults and children with chronic cardiovascular or pulmonary diseases. Residents of nursing homes; all individuals older than 65 years; patients with renal dysfunction, anemia, or immunosuppression; and adults and children with diabetes mellitus are all considered to be at modest risk. Children on long-term aspirin therapy are also considered to be at modest risk. Physicians, nurses, medical care personnel, and family members who have extensive contact with high-risk patients should also be vaccinated to prevent transmission of influenza to patients.

Page: 367

21: Match the item with the appropriate disease. (Each item may be used only once.)

    A. *Pneumocystis carinii* pneumonia (PCP)
    B. Lyme disease
    C. Measles
    D. Traveler's diarrhea
    E. Infective endocarditis

    1: Deer tick
    2: Roth spots
    3: HIV
    4: Koplik's spots
    5: Toxigenic *E. coli*

Answers: 1 - B, 2 - E, 3 - A, 4 - C, 5 - D

Critique: Lyme disease is transmitted by the deer tick (genus *Ixodes*) and is caused by the spirochete *Borrelia burgdorferi*. Retinal infarctions, known as Roth spots, are oval hemorrhages with central pallor seen in patients with infective endocarditis. Patients with HIV infection are at increased risk of PCP. This may be prevented with the prophylactic use of trimethoprim-sulfamethoxazole. Koplik's spots are bluish gray specks on an erythematous base on the buccal mucosa. Koplik's spots are associated with measles. Traveler's diarrhea, which is caused by strains of *E. coli* that produce an enterotoxin, is often associated with travel to tropical or semitropical countries.

Pages: 291–292, 323–324, 336–338, 363, 368

22: A 38-year-old male presents to the office with 48 hours of a painful left testicle and fever to 101.5°. You diagnose epididymitis. Which of the following are true concerning this diagnosis:

    A. It is usually STD related in men over age 35.
    B. A gonococcus/chlamydia swab and culture should be performed.
    C. *E. coli* may be the causative agent.
    D. Prostatitis may be the original site of infection.

Answers: A - False, B - True, C - True, D - True

Critique: In patients younger than 35 years, STDs may be the cause of epididymitis, and the physician would expect chlamydia or gonorrhea. In patients over 35, it is more likely a result of UTI, prostatitis, instrumentation, or surgery. *E. coli* may be the organism if anal intercourse is practiced. In most patients, a chlamydia/GC swab and culture are proper care before antibiotics are started.

Pages: 347–348

Chapter 20

Care of the Adult HIV-Infected Patient

Thomas G. Maddox

1: HIV-related illness was first described in what year?

    A. 1957
    B. 1972
    C. 1981
    D. 1993

Answer: C

Critique: HIV-related illness was initially described in 1981. Those originally affected were identified in the Morbidity/Mortality World Report as a group of young homosexual males who were noted to have *Pneumocystis carinii* pneumonia (PCP) and Kaposi's sarcoma.

Page: 371

2: (True or False) The prognosis of HIV infection is currently a terminal illness with rapidly progressing course.

Answer: False

Critique: The antiretroviral medications that are now available have significantly extended the life expectancy of patients infected with the HIV virus. In the early years after the disease was identified, patients were expected to develop a life history of threatening opportunistic infections within 6 months to a year after diagnosis. Currently, most patients live symptom free for many years. The death rate from HIV/AIDS began to decline for the first time in 1996. This is attributed to the effectiveness of antiretroviral medications, and especially the class of drugs known as protease inhibitors.

Pages: 371, 372

3: The highest rates of new infections are seen in which patient population?

    A. Homosexual men
    B. Intravenous (IV) drug users
    C. Hemophiliacs requiring multiple transfusions
    D. Heterosexual women

Answer: D

Critique: HIV infection rates were initially noted to be highest among homosexual men, IV drug users, patients requiring blood transfusions, and infants born to HIV-positive women. Over the past decade, women of minority populations have become the group with the highest new infection rates. In 1999, heterosexual contact accounted for 75% of new infections in women, and 25% were caused by IV drug use. Approximately 50% of all HIV-positive patients worldwide are female.

Pages: 371, 392

4: Which of the following is true of the HIV virus?

    A. Infection with the HIV virus disrupts normal host cellular activity by inhibiting the cytochrome P450 enzyme.
    B. HIV virus is made of viral RNA that has the ability to synthesize DNA and inject its genetic material into the host cell's DNA.
    C. As a retrovirus, the HIV virus is unable to cross the blood-brain barrier.
    D. The HIV virus belongs to the herpesvirus family.

Answer: B

Critique: The human immunodeficiency virus (HIV) is a retrovirus. RNA is the basic genetic material of these retroviruses. After infecting a host cell, the retrovirus incorporates its genetic material into the DNA of the host cell, causing the host cell to produce more viral particles. HIV has an affinity for cells with CD4 receptors on their surface. The most important of these are the T lymphocytes, which are a vital component of the body's immune system. The HIV virus is able to invade the central nervous system by crossing the blood-brain barrier.

Page: 372

5: Primary HIV infection:

    A. Is associated with a low number of circulating viral particles
    B. Is easily recognizable by its unique symptoms
    C. May mimic a mononucleosis-like illness
    D. Occurs when the patient develops an opportunistic infection such as *Pneumocystis carinii* pneumonia or esophageal candidiasis

Answer: C

Critique: Primary HIV infection, which occurs in over half of all patients infected with the HIV virus, is identified by the appearance of flu-like or mononucleosis-type symptoms, such as fever, generalized malaise, headaches, or a maculopapular rash. These symptoms usually occur about 2 to 4 weeks after infection. Unless the family physician maintains a heightened awareness of the possibility of acute HIV infection, the diagnosis of acute HIV may be missed. Opportunistic infections such as esophageal candidiasis or Pneumocystis carinii pneumonia occur later in the disease process, after the person's immune system has been significantly damaged.

Page: 373

6: True statements regarding early recognition and treatment for HIV infection include all of the following, except:

A. The patient may be eligible to participate in clinical drug trials comparing antiretroviral medication combinations.
B. They may help prevent the spread of HIV infection to other individuals.
C. Laboratory values may provide information regarding the long-term prognosis for the individual.
D. Earlier therapy allows for a simpler drug regimen of a single antiretroviral agent.

Answer: D

Critique: Antiretroviral therapy for HIV infection should follow the guidelines developed by the International AIDS Society—USA Panel, published in January 2000. These guidelines outline the possible combinations of nucleoside reverse transcriptase inhibitors (NRTIs), non-nucleoside reverse transcriptase inhibitors (NNRTIs), and protease inhibitors (PIs). Regardless of the combinations used, the guidelines strongly encourage the use of at least three agents. Initial values of the viral load are indicative of the patient's clinical course. Patients with a higher viral load early in the diagnosis of HIV infection have been shown to have more complications.

Pages: 373, 377

7: Which of the following is true of antiretroviral therapy?

A. If the patient's current drug regimen is failing, the agent that is known to have the weakest antiviral activity should be discontinued and replaced with a different medication.
B. Development of resistance to a particular antiviral combination is rare if the patient maintains strict compliance.
C. Combining two protease inhibitors should not be done because of potential drug interactions.
D. Compliance failure is the most common reason for the development of resistance.

Answer: D

Critique: Before a patient is started on antiretroviral therapy, the physician and patient should discuss in detail the issues of risks, side effects, pill burden, and cost. If not addressed, these issues significantly raise the risk of the patient being noncompliant with his or her medications. Noncompliance is the most common reason for the development of resistance. If a patient's therapy is no longer thought to be effective (because of an increase in

the viral load or development of symptoms), consideration should be given to changing the entire regimen. Rarely should a single drug ever be substituted, because the virus is able to quickly develop additional resistance to the new agent. Even with adequate compliance, the virus may be able to develop mutations that provide resistance. The more the viral load is suppressed, the less likely the virus will be able to generate mutations providing resistance to the antiretroviral medications. Combining two agents from the same class (PIs or NRTIs or NNRTIs) is often done when developing an antiretroviral regimen. The two protease inhibitors ritonavir (Norvir) and saquinavir (Fortovase) are often used together. As a result of inhibition of metabolism by the cytochrome P450 enzyme, a smaller dose of each medication is used. This provides fewer side effects while maintaining an adequate serum level of medication.

Pages: 377, 380, 381

8: Which of the following is true?

A. Screening for HIV infection is done by enzyme-linked immunosorbent assay (ELISA) and Western blot testing for viral antigen.
B. Seroconversion usually occurs within 2 weeks after infection.
C. Primary HIV infection is associated with high levels of viremia.
D. Left untreated, HIV infection will cause a continual rise in CD4 counts.

Answer: C

Critique: Screening patients for HIV infection is done initially with an ELISA test. If this is repeatedly positive, a confirming Western blot test is done. Both tests combined achieve greater than 99% sensitivity and greater than 99.9% specificity. These tests both detect antibodies produced against the HIV virus, and not the virus itself. Detection of viremia or viral load (amount of virus present in the patient's blood) is accomplished with either polymerase chain reaction (PCR) or branched-chain DNA techniques. Viral load testing is not done routinely as a screening measure because of greater costs. Antibodies to the HIV virus (seroconversion) can be detected between 2 and 6 months after exposure. After initial infection, the viral load may be extremely high. Studies have shown a correlation between the level of initial viremia and the course of the patient's illness. CD4 lymphocytes gradually decline over time if no treatment is initiated. The CD4 count is an indirect measure of a person's immune system. The viral load continues to rise if no antiviral treatment is provided.

Pages: 374–377

9: Which of the following is true regarding prophylaxis for opportunistic infections in the HIV-positive patient?

A. Prophylaxis for *Pneumocystis carinii* pneumonia (PCP) should be initiated when the CD4 count is less than 200/uL.
B. The agent of choice to prevent PCP is dapsone.

C. Patients with a reaction to tuberculosis (TB) skin testing by purified protein derivative (PPD) greater than 10 mm should be treated with isoniazid (INH).

D. Prophylaxis for *Mycobacterium avium* complex should be initiated when CD4 cell counts are at 200/uL or lower.

Answer: A

Critique: The incidence of *Pneumocystis carinii* pneumonia (PCP) has decreased significantly since implementation of prophylaxis recommendations. It is recommended that patients with no previous history of PCP take one of the prophylactic regimens when their CD4 count falls below 200/uL. The agent of choice in prevention of primary PCP is trimethoprim-sulfa. Alternatives include dapsone, either alone or combined with pyrimethamine and leucovorin, aerosolized pentamidine or atovaquone. HIV-positive individuals with a reaction to TB skin testing with purified protein derivative (PPD) greater than or equal to 5 mm should be evaluated for active disease. Once active disease is ruled out, chemoprophylaxis should be given with close monitoring for development of TB. *Mycobacterium avium* complex prophylaxis should be initiated when a person's CD4 count falls below 50/uL.

Pages: 387–389

10: According to Centers for Disease Control and Prevention (CDC) classification guidelines, an HIV-positive individual who also has each of the following is classified as category C, except one with:

A. A history of *Pneumocystis carinii* pneumonia (PCP)

B. Weight loss of greater than 10% of baseline and diarrhea for 2 months

C. An initial episode of cytomegalovirus (CMV) retinitis

D. A viral load of 150,000

Answer: D

Critique: The CDC classification system for HIV disease was revised in 1993 to take into account the integrity of a patient's immune system. Criteria for meeting the definition of full-blown AIDS is met when a patient develops an AIDS-defining opportunistic infection or malignancy, wasting syndrome (loss of greater than 10% of body weight plus diarrhea lasting longer than 30 days), or if their CD4 count falls below 200/uL. A patient's viral load has no bearing on the patient's category.

Page: 374

11: The most common mode of transmission of HIV worldwide is:

A. Vertical transmission

B. Sharing IV needles

C. Heterosexual intercourse

D. Homosexual intercourse

Answer: C

Critique: Heterosexual intercourse is the most common means of contracting HIV infection in the world.

In many areas of Africa, an entire generation has been devastated by the HIV epidemic. In the United States, sexual transmission, both heterosexual and homosexual, is responsible for the majority of new infections. Other less common means of transmission include sharing IV drug use paraphernalia (works), transmission from mother to baby (vertical transmission), transfusion of infected blood products, and occupational exposure (needle sticks).

Page: 374

12: As of 1999, which of the following groups had the highest increase in rates of new cases of HIV?

A. Homosexual men

B. Hemophiliacs and recipients of blood products

C. IV drug users

D. Women of color

Answer: D

Critique: The epidemiology of HIV disease has changed over the past 20 years since it was first described. Engaging in behaviors that place the patient at risk should be considered instead of potential risk groups. Unsafe sexual activity (heterosexual or homosexual) and sharing IV drug use equipment are risky behaviors that patients can be counseled to change. Unsafe sexual behavior refers to the exchange of body fluids (semen or vaginal secretions) from one person to another. The risk of contracting HIV from a blood transfusion is extremely low. The Food and Drug Administration began testing donated blood and plasma for the HIV p-24 antigen as of 1995. Statistics published in 1999 by the CDC showed that African-American and Latino females had the highest increase in incidence of new HIV infections.

Page: 392

13: Which of the following is associated with transmission of the HIV virus?

A. Household contacts of HIV-positive individuals

B. Male-female intercourse

C. Blood donation

D. Insect vectors (mosquito or tick bites)

Answer: B

Critique: Of the examples given, only heterosexual intercourse is considered to be a mode of HIV transmission. Casual contact with persons that are HIV positive pose no risk for transmission. The act of blood donation does not expose a person to any risk for contracting HIV disease. Insect bites have shown to carry no risk of transmission of HIV.

Page: 376

14: All of the following are indicated in the initial evaluation of an HIV-positive patient, except:

A. Hepatitis B virus serology

B. Plasma HIV RNA measurement (viral load)

C. Blood culture

D. Cytomegalovirus (CMV) serology

Answer: C

Critique: The initial evaluation of a patient who is found to be HIV positive includes a thorough history and physical examination. Focus should be directed toward any potential HIV complications. An assessment of the patient's psychosocial support system and coping abilities should also be addressed. Laboratory studies should include a complete blood count (CBC), CD4 lymphocyte count, viral load measurement, tests for syphilis and CMV, and hepatitis A and B serologies. Skin testing or chest x-ray to screen for tuberculosis should also be completed.

Page: 376

15: Which of the following statements is true?

    A. The goal of antiviral therapy in HIV is eradication of the virus.

    B. The International AIDS Society—USA has published guidelines for using antiretroviral agents in a specific order for the care of HIV disease.

    C. The majority of patients whose CD4 lymphocyte count is below 200 should be encouraged to begin antiviral therapy.

    D. After starting an antiviral regimen, one would expect a decrease in the viral load after 6 months.

Answer: C

Critique: The International AIDS Society—USA has developed guidelines for antiviral therapy in HIV. However, the guidelines do not specify which agents to use or in what order. Choosing an antiretroviral regimen has proved to be one of the most difficult dilemmas in treating HIV patients. The guidelines do provide suggestions on combinations of antivirals from various classes (i.e., two nucleoside reverse transcriptase inhibitors combined with one or more protease inhibitors). The goal of therapy in HIV is to reduce the viral load to the lowest level possible. In most cases, an undetectable viral level is attainable. A drop in the viral load of at least 50% is expected within 2 to 6 weeks after starting antiviral therapy. If this has not occurred, the antiviral regimen should be reconsidered.

Page: 377

16: Which of the following statements is true?

    A. Genotype testing measures how different drugs inhibit viral replication.

    B. Suppression of the viral load has no impact on the rate of mutations developed by the HIV virus.

    C. Phenotype testing detects changes in the virus nucleotide sequence.

    D. Several mutations are required to render the virus resistant to some antiretroviral medications.

Answer: D

Critique: As viral replication takes place more rapidly, random mutations will occur with greater frequency. During ineffective or less than optimal antiviral therapy, chances are greater that the virus will develop random mutations that provide resistance. This ineffective therapy will then selectively allow replication of this resistant strain. Genotype testing is done to determine the nucleotide sequences in the HIV virus of greatest concentration in the person's blood. This is an indirect measurement of a virus's susceptibility to a particular drug. Phenotype testing is a direct measure of a drug's ability to inhibit growth and replication of the virus in vitro. Both assays provide information regarding the strain that is in the highest concentration in the person's blood. Some strains of the virus are present in a person's system that may have already developed mutations that these assays are not able to detect. Resistance to some medications may occur after only one mutation. Several antivirals require multiple mutations before resistance develops.

Pages: 380, 381

17: A patient's ability to adhere to the medication regimen has been associated with all of the following, except:

    A. Side effects of the medication

    B. Advertisements aimed at consumers by drug companies

    C. Number of pills required to be taken daily

    D. Patient education regarding medications

Answer: B

Critique: A patient's ability to comply with a medication regimen is extremely important in the treatment of HIV. If a person is unable to take medications correctly, there is a much greater likelihood that resistance will develop. Several factors have been associated with compliance with a medication regimen. Patient education about the medications, potential side effects that may occur, and the correct way to take the medication are some of the topics that should be discussed with patients before beginning antiviral therapy. Simpler antiviral regimens are being investigated in an attempt to improve patient compliance.

Page: 380

18: Which of the following statements regarding weight loss in HIV is true?

    A. Patients should be told that weight loss of up to 20% of baseline is expected in HIV disease.

    B. Weight loss associated with HIV is usually related to depression.

    C. Anabolic steroids should not be used in HIV disease because of increased side effects.

    D. Replacement of testosterone may help maintain lean body mass.

Answer: D

Critique: Among the many causes of weight loss in patients with HIV infection are opportunistic infections, diarrhea, and malabsorption. Decreased intake may be due to gastrointestinal side effects caused by the patient's antiviral medications. The physician should consider depression, although not the most common cause of weight loss in HIV, as a contributing factor. Replacement of testosterone in patients who are hypogonadic helps maintain or regain lean body mass.

Page: 381

19: The most common opportunistic infection occurring in HIV disease in the United States is:

    A. Tuberculosis
    B. *Pneumocystis carinii* pneumonia (PCP)
    C. Kaposi's sarcoma
    D. Toxoplasmosis

Answer: B

Critique: PCP remains the most common opportunistic infection encountered in HIV disease. The incidence has decreased significantly since the implementation of prophylaxis with one of several suggested regimens. Prophylaxis for PCP should be instituted when the patient's CD4 count falls below 200/uL. After the first episode of PCP infection, prophylaxis should be provided regardless of the patient's CD4 count. Common symptoms of PCP include a nonproductive cough, shortness of breath, or dyspnea on exertion.

Pages: 387, 388

20: All of the following are AIDS-defining opportunistic infections, except:

    A. Toxoplasmosis
    B. Oral candidiasis
    C. *Pneumocystis carinii* pneumonia (PCP)
    d. Mycobacterium intracellulare

Answer: B

Critique: All of these infections are considered to be opportunistic (affecting only people with weakened immune systems) except oral candidiasis. Development of an opportunistic infection constitutes category C (AIDS defining) for HIV infection. The most commonly encountered opportunistic infection is PCP. Esophageal candidiasis is considered an opportunistic infection, but oropharyngeal candidiasis is not.

Pages: 387–390

21: Toxoplasmosis is associated with which of the following findings?

    A. Organisms noted on Gram stain of CSF
    B. Distinctive infiltrates on chest x-ray
    C. Cotton wool spots on retinal examination
    D. Ring-enhancing lesions on computed tomography (CT) scan

Answer: D

Critique: Toxoplasma gondii is responsible for causing central nervous system disease in advanced HIV infection. Symptoms are usually gradual in onset and include confusion, seizures, and focal neurologic deficits. Typical ring-enhancing lesions may be seen on CT scan of the head. Biopsy may be required to differentiate the lesion from central nervous system lymphoma.

Page: 389

22: Women account for what percentage of all HIV infections worldwide?

    A. 2%
    B. 10%

    C. 40%
    D. 70%

Answer: C

Critique: Worldwide epidemiologic studies show that between 40% and 50% of all HIV infections have occurred in females. In the United States, 64% of all new infections were among African-American women and 18% among Latinas. It is estimated that approximately 15 million women are infected worldwide. A sobering estimate of 20 to 30 million children will be left without parents because of deaths related to HIV/AIDS by the twenty-first century.

Page: 392

23: Which of the following is an approved antiviral regimen for treating HIV infection?

    A. Zidovudine (AZT) as a single agent
    B. Combination of two nucleoside reverse transcriptase inhibitors and a protease inhibitor
    C. Combination of interferon and a non-nucleoside reverse transcriptase inhibitor
    D. Combination of famciclovir (Famvir) and a protease inhibitor

Answer: B

Critique: The Department of Health and Human Services developed consensus guidelines for the use of antiretroviral medications in treating HIV disease. One of the fundamentals in the treatment of HIV disease is to never use any agent as monotherapy. Highly aggressive antiretroviral therapy (HAART) refers to combining a minimum of three medications from at least two of the three groups of antiretrovirals (nucleoside reverse transcriptase inhibitors, non-nucleoside reverse transcriptase inhibitors, and protease inhibitors). Interferon and famciclovir are not used as antiretroviral agents in HIV disease.

Page: 377

24: Which of the following would apply to a patient who could defer treatment rather than initiating therapy?

    A. CD4 count 280 u/L, viral load undetectable
    B. CD4 count 405 u/L, viral load 15,000 copies/mL
    C. CD4 count 680 u/L, viral load 46,000 copies/mL
    D. CD4 count 530 u/L, viral load undetectable

Answer: D

Critique: The decision to initiate antiviral therapy is influenced by the patient's CD4 count and the viral load. Measurement of the patient's viral load should be done on two separate occasions before initiating therapy. The International AIDS Society—USA Panel has published guidelines for initiating antiviral therapy in HIV-positive patients. Therapy is strongly recommended for all patients whose CD4 counts have dropped below 350 u/L, regardless of the viral load. Patients with CD4 counts between 350 and 500 u/L may consider starting therapy if the viral load is undetectable; however, therapy should be instituted if the viral load is greater than 5,000 copies/mL. Patient's who have maintained a CD4 count of greater than 500 may defer therapy if they also have an undetectable viral load, but therapy should be considered if the viral load is 5,000 to 30,000 copies/mL. It is strongly recommended to begin therapy for all patients who have a viral load greater than 30,000 copies/mL.

Before beginning antiviral therapy for any patient, an assessment should be done to evaluate the patient's ability to comply with the medication regimen.

Pages: 377, 380

Chapter 21

Pulmonary Medicine

Mrunal S. Shah

1: Interpretation of pulmonary function testing can be critical for any patient with lung disease. All of the following are true, except:

  A. Diffusion capacity (DLCO) is the most helpful for chronic obstructive pulmonary disease (COPD) prognosis.
  B. FEV_1 is the best indicator of the severity of lung disease.
  C. FEV_1 is the best predictor of perioperative risk for pulmonary complications.
  D. FEV_1 correlates *least* with survival in patients with COPD.

Answer: D

Critique: FEV_1 correlates well with COPD survival, and the DLCO determines prognosis in COPD. The FEV_1 is the best indicator of severity and the best predictor of perioperative risks. This is helpful for preadmission testing for patients with asthma and COPD, among other lung diseases.

Pages: 395, 396

2: All of the following are true about pulse oximetry, except:

  A. It is a noninvasive test that is consistent with co-oximetry.
  B. Variability is +/–4% between 70 and 100%.
  C. It is more accurate as the saturation drops below 70%.
  D. Significant carbon monoxide (CO) poisoning can overestimate the SaO_2.

Answer: C

Critique: The variability of pulse oximetry worsens as the saturation drops below 70%. In a patient who looks sicker than the reading alone might indicate, one must consider CO poisoning and treat it early.

Page: 398

3: The chest radiograph is one of the most commonly ordered tests. All of the following are indications for chest x-rays, except:

  A. Cough
  B. Chest pain
  C. Hemoptysis
  D. Routine physical examination
  E. Dyspnea

Answer: D

Critique: All but routine physical examination are indications for chest radiographs as explained by the American College of Radiology's expert panel reports. These indications are hoarseness, dyspnea, cough, hemoptysis, and chest pain. Chest x-rays are not indicated for admission in asymptomatic individuals or as part of a routine examination.

Page: 398

4: Pleural effusions are a common complication in many conditions. All of the following are consistent with an exudate, except:

  A. Pleural fluid protein to serum protein ratio greater than 0.5
  B. Pleural lymphocytosis greater than 50%
  C. Pleural fluid LDH to serum LDH ratio greater than 0.6
  D. Pleural fluid LDH greater than 67% of the upper limits of normal serum LDH

Answer: B

Critique: The two most helpful indicators for exudates versus transudates are LDH and protein. The rest are all true, but lymphocytosis is more suggestive of malignancy or tuberculosis. Many other helpful tests can point toward one or the other, as discussed in the chapter.

Page: 400

5: Because tuberculosis (TB) is on the rise in the United States, the complications must be better understood. All of the following would suggest a pleural effusion caused by TB, except:

  A. Fluid glucose level less than 60 mg/dL
  B. An alkaline pH of >7.4
  C. Elevated level of adenosine deaminase (>50 u/L)
  D. Elevated level of lysozyme III (>20 mcg/mL)

Answer: B

Critique: The pH should range from 7.0 to 7.29. Elevated levels of adenosine and lysozyme III are suggestive of TB, rheumatoid arthritis, or empyema. These levels are both low in malignancy.

Page: 401

6: Your patient presents to you after seeing your partner just 2 weeks prior, having had 1 week of cough. She continues to have the cough and wants you to treat it. The cough is least likely because of:

A. Interstitial lung disease
B. Asthma
C. Gastroesophageal ruflux disease (GERD)
D. Postnasal drip

Answer: A

Critique: In over 65% to 90% of adult patients referred to a tertiary care center for a chronic cough (>3 weeks), the most common causes were postinfectious bronchial inflammation, postnasal drip, asthma, and GERD. Less likely causes would include cancer, tuberculosis, pneumonia, sarcoidosis, interstitial lung disease, and many others.

Page: 401

7: The history of a patient who presents with hemoptysis is the most helpful test. All of the following historical findings match its likely location, except:

A. Throat pain, tongue or mouth lesions, sinus pain, or hoarseness point to an oropharyngeal bleeding source.
B. Frequent nosebleeds and heightened hemoptysis in a supine position point to a nasopharyngeal source.
C. Cough, wheezing, dypsnea, or previous lung disease suggest a pulmonary cause.
D. Systemic symptoms such as fever, chills, night sweats, and weight loss suggest a nasopharyngeal source.

Answer: D

Critique: Fever, chills, night sweats, and weight loss suggest an inflammatory or infectious cause. All the rest are true. Always elicit history of TB exposure, use of tobacco, and bleeding disorders or use of anticoagulants.

Page: 402

8: Acute respiratory failure can be divided into two general groups. Most are a combination of the two, but the management of each is different. They are:

A. Ventilation and perfusion
B. Ventilatory failure and hypoxemia
C. Air loss and air trapping
D. Over-recruitment and under-recruitment

Answer: B

Critique: Patients with acute respiratory failure should be divided into two general groups: those with failure of oxygenation and those with ventilatory failure. This division is helpful for management choices. Ventilation and perfusion relate to causes of hypoxemia, as are over- and under-recruitment. Air loss and air trapping are potential causes of ventilatory failure.

Page: 403

9: All of the following are potential causes of hypoxemia, except:

A. Alveolar shunting
B. Derecruitment
C. Air trapping (auto-PEEP)
D. Low-pressure environment

Answer: C

Critique: Air trapping and auto-PEEP are not causes of hypoxemia. Hypoxemia is a condition in which there is incomplete alveolar emptying because of high airway flow resistance. This raises the alveolar pressure above atmospheric levels and must be overcome with subsequent respirations. This condition will ultimately lead to ventilatory failure because the lungs cannot overcome the rising airway pressures. Alveolar shunting, derecruitment, and hypobaria are all causes of hypoxemia.

Page: 403

10: All of the following are reversible causes of acute ventilatory failure, except:

A. Congestive heart failure (CHF)
B. Amyotrophic lateral sclerosis (ALS)
C. Asthma
D. Guillain-Barré syndrome (GBS)
E. Lobar pneumonia

Answer: B

Critique: CHF, asthma, GBS, and pneumonia are all reversible causes of ventilatory failure and will pass with aggressive treatment. ALS, unfortunately, is not reversible. This disease is progressive and patients die at a very young age. Lung cancer is also a nonreversible cause of ventilatory failure.

Page: 403

11: Your 54-year-old male patient comes to your office complaining of 3 weeks of cough. He has been with you since you started practice 12 years ago. You begin with your usual lecture on smoking cessation. You also ask about his bowel habits and whether he has noted any hematochezia from his recent resection of colon cancer. During your examination, you hear bilateral lower lobe crackles, but you think they are more prominent on the left. You decide to get a chest x-ray to confirm. Just as you had expected, he has a left lower lobe infiltrate. You also notice a 1.5 cm nodule in the right upper lung field, although you can't recall whether this is new or not. Your next step is to:

A. Get serial chest x-rays every 3 to 4 months and check for change in size or margins
B. Obtain old x-rays for comparison and schedule for CT scan
C. Get a fine-needle aspiration under fluoroscopy
D. Surgical referral
E. B and D only
F. All of the above

Answer: E

Critique: This patient has a very high pretest likelihood of malignancy because of his age, smoking, and previous cancer. This nodule is malignant until proven otherwise. It would be inappropriate to wait 3 to 4 months for serial scans to show a change in size or margins. A fine-needle aspiration will not likely change the final outcome. This patient will require resection by bronchoscopy or open thoracotomy. Therefore, you should find old x-rays for comparison and schedule a CT scan to better delineate disease. You will also need surgical evaluation for possible resection.

Page: 406

12: One of the most common diagnoses in the outpatient setting is bronchitis. Of the following statements, which are true?

    A. Antibiotics have been shown to decrease cough and sputum production.
    B. Albuterol has not been shown to be effective in reducing symptoms of cough.
    C. Although rarely bacterial, the most common bacterial pathogen is *S. pneumoniae*.
    D. Antibiotics have been shown to decrease duration of symptoms.
    E. All of the above

Answer: A and D

Critique: Antibiotics have been shown in several clinical trials to reduce cough and duration of cough with sputum by less than half a day. This benefit arguably would not justify the added cost, even though antibiotics are the most commonly prescribed agent for bronchitis. In contrast, albuterol has been shown to improve cough and shortness of breath. Some theorize that there is a bronchospastic component similar to that of asthma with bronchitis.

Pages: 406, 407

13: Bronchiolitis is a common condition that affects children. Most commonly, it can be managed at home or on an outpatient basis, but sometimes children need to be managed as inpatients. Of the following, which one component has been shown to reduce hypoxemia?

    A. Ribavarin (Virazole)
    B. Nebulized albuterol
    C. Oxygen
    D. Corticosteroids
    E. Anti-RSV immunoglobulin

Answer: C

Critique: Many studies have shown the short-term benefits of the other agents, but none have shown a decrease in hospitalization or morbidity. The only agent found to consistently reduce hypoxemia is supplemental oxygen. Anti-RSV immunoglobulin should be considered only in high-risk infants. The other agents should be used as determined on a case-by-case basis.

Pages: 407, 408

14: All of the following are common symptoms of pneumonia, except:

    A. Shortness of breath
    B. Fever
    C. Myalgia
    D. Diarrhea
    E. All of the above are true.

Answer: E

Critique: All these symptoms are common in pneumonia.

Page: 408

15: A 64-year-old male presents to your emergency department with cough and sputum and fever and rigors. On evaluation, it is found that he has a left lower lobe pneumonia. The decision is made to admit him for surveillance, oxygen, and antibiotics. Which one of the following is an acceptable option for community-acquired pneumonia?

    A. Ampicillin IV
    B. Flagyl IV
    C. Levofloxacin IV
    D. High-dose levoflaxocin PO
    E. Ciprofloxacin IV and clindamycin IV

Answer: C

Critique: A good choice to cover typical and atypical organisms is levofloxacin. The parenteral route is preferred when the patient is sick enough to be in the hospital. Ampicillin or Flagyl alone will not cover atypical and typical organisms, respectively.

Pages: 408, 409

16: Routine evaluation of most health care workers includes a complete physical examination, a thorough history, and a purified protein derivative (PPD) test. Determination of a positive PPD depends on several factors. Which one of the following is *not* a positive PPD?

    A. A 64-year-old diabetic with 13 mm induration
    B. A 3-year-old infant with 11 mm induration
    C. A 26-year-old schoolteacher with 13 mm induration
    D. A 34-year-old factory worker with 17 mm induration
    E. An HIV-positive 29-year-old with 7 mm induration

Answer: C

Critique: The three levels of induration are 5 mm, 10 mm, and 15 mm, depending on the individual's risks and age. Individuals with HIV and those with recent known contact or fibrosis on chest x-ray (CXR) are positive with 5 mm or more of induration. IV drug abusers, comorbidities (e.g., diabetes mellitus, cancer, chronic renal failure), children under 4 years of age, foreign-born individuals from high-prevalence areas, or residents in long-term care facilities are positive with 10 mm or more. Anyone else is positive with 15 mm of induration. The only person not positive is the 26-year-old with <15 mm induration.

Page: 410

17: A 28-year-old female patient with a long-standing history of asthma returns to your office to review her medications. She read an article that prompted her to come and see you. She describes her symptoms as occurring three or four times a week, even some nights. Her peak flows in your office have always been 80% to 90% of expected flow. She requires the use of albuterol frequently but knows that there are newer options. You prescribe all of the following, except:

    A. Inhaled corticosteroid twice daily
    B. Zafirlukast daily
    C. Inhaled ipratropium bromide twice daily

D. Self-monitoring with peak flow meter at home daily or with symptoms

E. Albuterol inhaler as needed

Answer: C

Critique: This patient can be classified as having mild, persistent disease, or step 2. The other choices are all recommended for this group except the ipratropium, which is reserved for step 4, severe, persistent disease.

Pages: 411, 412

18: All of the following are true about bronchiectasis, except:

A. Patients will present with large volumes of muco-purulent sputum.

B. Chest x-ray may show honeycombing in advanced disease.

C. High-resolution CT is the test of choice and is now the gold standard.

D. Prophylactic antibiotics are necessary in all patients with disease.

E. Lung function testing typically shows obstructive disease.

Answer: D

Critique: Prophylactic antibiotic therapy is equivocal at best. However, antibiotics are the mainstay of treatment of bronchiectasis. High-resolution CT has replaced bronchoscopy as the gold standard. The rest of the statements are true.

Pages: 412, 413

19: Patients with chronic obstructive pulmonary disease (COPD) need many measures to prolong health and reduce morbidity and mortality. Of the following measures, which one has proved to reduce morbidity and mortality while reducing symptoms the most?

A. Albuterol

B. Theophylline

C. Oxygen

D. None of the above

E. All of the above

Answer: C

Critique: The only factor shown and proven to reduce morbidity and mortality with COPD is oxygen. None of the other modalities has been proved to improve outcomes. Other mainstays of treatment include albuterol, Atrovent, corticosteroids, theophylline, and occasionally parenteral antibiotics.

Pages: 414, 415

20: Cystic fibrosis (CF) is a common inherited disease that affects secretions and exocrine function. Problems can include respiratory, gastrointestinal, and reproductive symptoms. Each of the following is a treatment option for patients with CF, except:

A. Modalities to increase mucus clearance

B. Low-sodium diet

C. Lung transplantation

D. Multivitamins

E. Nebulized tobramycin

Answer: B

Critique: All of the choices are treatment options for CF except a dietary restriction of sodium. The most important aspect of treatment is mucus clearance. There is also a need for multivitamins because of a failure of fat absorption and therefore a lack of the fat-soluble vitamins A, D, E, and K. CF patients are advised to have more sodium in their diet. Because of chronic pseudomonas infection, they benefit from nebulized tobramycin therapy. Of course, transplant is one temporizing measure.

Pages: 415, 416

21: An elderly patient from your office was recently found on the floor after falling. Examination revealed a fractured hip, and the orthopedic surgeon opted to perform a total hip replacement. He then consults you to help with discharge planning. The question of safety becomes important when evaluating deep venous thrombosis (DVT) prophylaxis. All of the following are options, except:

A. Coumadin (warfarin)

B. High-dose aspirin

C. Lovenox (enoxaparin)

D. Intermittent pneumatic compression stockings

Answer: B

Critique: Risks for bleeding must be evaluated, but high-dose aspirin would be inadequate to reduce the risk of DVT. If a patient is at high risk for falls and home health service or teaching can be arranged, Lovenox can be used. If a patient has the option of nursing care or a nursing home, intermittent pneumatic compression stockings are an option but only when anticoagulation therapy cannot be used.

Page: 418

22: Lung cancer is one of the most common cancers currently detected. Which of the following is least accurate about lung cancer?

A. It is the most common cause of cancer death.

B. Patients who can quit "cold turkey" have the highest rate of success.

C. Eight out of ten smokers who quit will likely return to smoking.

D. Routine screening should be done and has been shown to improve survival.

E. Smoking cessation is the only effective tool to reduce risk of cancer.

Answer: D

Critique: No current evidence shows that routine screening improves survival or alters outcomes. There is current debate about helical CT showing some benefit in higher risk individuals. All of the other statements are true.

Pages: 418, 419

Chapter 22

Otolaryngology

Bruce Vanderhoff

1: Which of the following is not a typical symptom of epiglottitis?

    A. A barking, brassy cough
    B. Rapidly developing sore throat
    C. High fever, restlessness, and lethargy
    D. Drooling

Answer: A

Critique: A barking, brassy, spontaneous cough is a typical symptom of croup but not of epiglottitis. All of the remaining symptoms are typical symptoms of epiglottitis. These symptoms can also occur with tonsillitis.

Page: 424

2: Appropriate management of suspected epiglottitis includes:

    A. The placement of a tongue blade to adequately visualize the posterior oropharynx
    B. Immediate intubation in the office or emergency room to prevent airway compromise
    C. Management without antibiotics, because most cases are of viral origin
    D. Lateral extended neck x-ray

Answer: D

Critique: Epiglottitis represents a true emergency. An otolaryngologist should be consulted whenever the diagnosis is in question. Placement of a tongue blade can precipitate acute airway obstruction and should be avoided. Lateral extended neck x-rays can help in the diagnosis and classically demonstrate a "thumbprint" sign. If epiglottitis is suspected, the patient should be taken to the operating room for intubation in the presence of an otolaryngologist and anesthesiologist. After the airway is secured, cultures should be obtained and appropriate antibiotics initiated. Haemophilus influenzae type B is a common cause of this condition.

Page: 424

3: Typical signs and symptoms of peritonsillar abscess include all of the following, except:

    A. Fever and sore throat for 3 to 5 days
    B. Dysphagia and odynophagia
    C. Swelling of the soft palate without displacement of the uvula away from the midline
    D. "Hot potato" voice

Answer: C

Critique: The typical signs and symptoms of peritonsillar abscess include all of the above, except that the uvula is displaced away from the midline. Trismus is also extremely common. Examination will confirm asymmetric tonsils and peritonsillar edema and erythema.

Page: 425

4: Among patients with epistaxis:

    A. Recurrent episodes are common among adolescents, especially males, and generally do not prompt any concern
    B. Bleeding from the anterior nasal cavity is uncommon but when present usually arises from Kiesselbach's plexus
    C. Posterior epistaxis is invariably mild and generally easily controlled
    D. Predisposing factors for epistaxis include digital trauma, dry weather, and poorly controlled hypertension

Answer: D

Critique: Recurrent epistaxis among adolescents requires special consideration because such episodes can be associated with juvenile nasopharyngeal angiofibroma. Epistaxis is most commonly from the anterior nasal cavity, originating from the rich plexus of vessels at the anterior septum called Kiesselbach's plexus. Posterior epistaxis can be quite severe and difficult to control. In addition to the predisposing factors listed, bleeding dyscrasias and anticoagulation therapy may predispose patients to epistaxis.

Pages: 426, 427

5: The most common cause of dizziness is:

    A. Central vestibular etiologies
    B. Peripheral vestibular etiologies
    C. Psychogenic disorders
    D. Medications
    E. Multiple sensory deficits

Answer: B

Critique: Multiple investigators have concluded that peripheral vestibular disorders are the most common cause of dizziness, closely followed by pyschogenic disorders. In the elderly, the combined effects of multiple sensory deficits, medication, and orthostasis become important contributors. Central vestibular disorders represent less than 10% of all causes.

Page: 432

6: Meniere's disease:

    A. Is usually bilateral

    B. Usually results in mild vertigo without hearing loss or tinnitus

    C. Is usually associated with vertigo lasting seconds to minutes

    D. Is usually self-limited, resolving after 1 year or a few attacks

Answer: D

Critique: Meniere's disease is usually unilateral, but it can be bilateral. It is usually associated with disabling attacks of severe vertigo, a sense of ear fullness, roaring tinnitus, and sensorineural hearing loss, which can be fluctuating. The vertigo usually lasts for several hours. In most cases, Meniere's disease is self-limited and resolves after a few attacks.

Page: 433

7: Patients with Meniere's disease:

    A. Require an audiogram and an MRI to make the diagnosis

    B. Should maintain high sodium intake while avoiding caffeine

    C. Typically require therapy for no more than 3 to 6 months

    D. May benefit from daily diuretic therapy

Answer: D

Critique: No test is diagnostic of Meniere's disease. It is a clinical diagnosis. Nevertheless, an audiogram can show hearing loss. If the diagnosis is uncertain, an MRI of the brain can help to rule out an acoustic neuroma, which can mimic the symptoms of Meniere's disease. Patients with this diagnosis should limit sodium intake to less than 2 g/day and minimize caffeine intake. Daily diuretics, typically triamterene (Dyrenium) or hydrochlorothiazide (Dyazide), can be helpful. The typical duration of therapy is no less than 1 year.

Pages: 433, 434

8: Benign paroxysmal positional vertigo:

    A. Is the most common cause of peripheral vestibular vertigo in adults

    B. Is generally preceded by a recent viral illness

    C. Is usually associated with a negative Dix-Hallpike maneuver

    D. Is usually very responsive to treatment with meclizine

Answer: A

Critique: Benign paroxysmal positional vertigo (BPPV) is indeed the most common cause of peripheral vestibular vertigo in adults. BPPV is caused by displacement of otoconia particles from the utricle or saccule, which lodge in the posterior semicircular canal. Vestibular neuronitis, not BPPV, can be temporally associated with a viral illness. The Dix-Hallpike maneuver reproduces the vertigo in patients with BPPV. Treatment of BPPV consists of repositioning maneuvers. Antivertiginous agents,

such as meclizine, may be of no help and can even cause troubling side effects.

Page: 434

9: Otitis externa:

    A. Is often associated with purulent drainage in the external ear canal

    B. Is rarely associated with pain

    C. Is usually the result of inadequate cerumen removal by patients

    D. Is generally treated with systemic antibiotics

Answer: A

Critique: Otitis externa is the most common cause of pain in the external ear. This pain results from inflammation and edema of the ear canal skin that normally adheres to the bone and cartilage of the auditory canal. An absence of cerumen due to excessive cleaning by the patient can predispose the patient to otitis externa. Purulent drainage in the external ear canal with edema or erythema of the external ear canal is a common diagnostic clue of otitis externa. The condition is usually treated through removal of debris or drainage from the ear canal followed by the instillation of antibiotic drops with or without steroids. When the infection is thought to be fungal, clotrimazole drops or 2% glacial acetic acid drops (VōSol) can be effective. Systemic antibiotics are usually reserved for patients with necrotizing otitis externa.

Pages: 436, 437

10: Which of the following is true regarding cerumen?

    A. It is an ideal growth medium for bacteria and fungi.

    B. It is produced in excess in many patients.

    C. Impaction usually causes a problem only once the ear canal has become completely, or nearly completely, obstructed.

    D. Cerumen should generally be prevented by the regular use of cotton-tipped applicators to clean the ear canals

Answer: C

Critique: Cerumen acts to moisturize the external auditory canal and is both bactericidal and fungicidal. The external auditory canal is self-cleaning, and most people should clean the external meatus only with a finger in a washcloth while bathing. Repeated attempts to clean the ear canals with cotton-tipped applicators commonly result in cerumen impaction. Cerumen impaction usually does not cause a problem unless the canal is nearly or fully occluded.

Page: 438

11: All but which of the following are common risk factors for acute otitis media?

    A. Bottle-feeding

    B. Female gender

    C. Parental smoking

    D. Native American ethnicity

Answer: B

Critique: All of the above, except female gender, are common risk factors for otitis media. Male gender, exposure to upper respiratory infections, genetic factors, craniofacial abnormalities, use of a pacifier, and a history of previous acute otitis media, particularly during the preceding 3 months, are additional common risk factors.

Page: 439

12: Which of the following are true regarding acute otitis media?

A. The standard therapy in most countries is an antimicrobial.
B. Resistance rates to *Streptococcus pneumoniae* are similar in adults and children.
C. It may be appropriate to delay antimicrobial therapy for some children.
D. The duration of therapy should generally be 14 to 21 days.

Answers: A, C

Critique: Meta-analyses have concluded that the early use of antibiotics does reduce symptoms, although it does not result in significant differences in middle ear effusions at 6 weeks or 1 year. Resistance rates to *S. pneumoniae* are higher in children than in adults and are believed to be related to injudicious use of antimicrobial agents. For children older than 2 years whose symptoms of acute otitis media are not severe, who are not in day care, and who have no history of previous antimicrobial use, delaying therapy may be appropriate. There must, however, be follow-up within 48 to 72 hours. The traditional duration of therapy has been 10 days, although this is not based on scientific study.

Pages: 439, 440

13: True statements regarding cholesteatoma include:

A. It is a destructive epithelial cyst that is usually associated with perforation of the tympanic membrane and chronic otitis media
B. Cholesteatomas possess enzymatic properties that can result in bone erosion
C. A cholesteatoma should be suspected in all patients with chronic ear drainage
D. Cholesteatomas are generally managed with aggressive medical therapy, and recurrence is uncommon

Answers: A, B, C

Critique: Although the drainage from a cholesteatoma can be decreased with aggressive medical treatment, surgical treatment is necessary. Close follow-up after surgical treatment is important because recurrence is not uncommon.

Pages: 441, 442

14: Which of the following statements regarding Bell's palsy are true?

A. It is the most common cause of facial paralysis in primary care.

B. It is frequently associated with otalgia.
C. Treatment usually includes a burst of prednisone at 1 mg/kg tapering over 10 to 14 days.
D. Treatment usually includes an oral antiviral with activity against the herpes virus.

Answers: A, B, C, D

Critique: The most common cause of facial paralysis in a primary care practice is Bell's palsy. At one time, Bell's palsy was treated expectantly. Current evidence, however, suggests that the majority of cases are related to reactivation of herpes simplex virus. At this time, therefore, it is recommended that patients be treated with corticosteroids and oral antivirals. In addition, the eye should be protected and moisturized with eyedrops and nightly lubrication. Any signs of eye irritation should prompt ophthalmology evaluation.

Page: 445

15: A CT of the sinuses should be ordered:

A. Before making a diagnosis of sinusitis
B. When medical treatment has failed and surgery is being considered
C. When a complication of sinusitis is suspected
D. In cases in which a sinus mass is suspected

Answers: B, C, D

Critique: A CT is not required in the management of uncomplicated sinusitis. The remaining answers are appropriate reasons to obtain a CT of the sinuses. In addition, it may be appropriate to obtain a CT of the sinuses if the diagnosis of acute or chronic sinusitis is not certain.

Page: 446

16: The diagnosis of seasonal allergic rhinitis:

A. Should never be made primarily by history
B. Is suggested by a pale, boggy nasal mucosa
C. May be associated with "allergic shiners" in children
D. May be associated with the finding of eosinophils on nasal smear

Answers: B, C, D

Critique: The diagnosis of seasonal allergic rhinitis is made primarily by history. Although a pale, boggy nasal mucosa indicates allergic rhinitis, a red mucosa is more suggestive of a viral infection.

Page: 448

17: Appropriate treatment of allergic rhinitis includes:

A. Avoidance of known allergens
B. Systemic or topical antihistamines
C. Systemic or topical corticosteroids
D. Leukotriene receptor antagonists

Answers: A, B, D

Critique: After allergen avoidance, antihistamines are the mainstay of treatment for seasonal allergic rhinitis. The topical antihistamine azelastine has shown efficacy in the treatment of allergic rhinitis. Decongestants can also be helpful, although patients should be counseled about their potential side effects, and these agents should be used cautiously in patients with hypertension. Topical corticosteroids can be safe and effective, but systemic steroids are not usually used to treat this condition. The main side effects of topical steroids are epistaxis and nasal dryness. Although corticosteroids can have hypothalamic-pituitary-adrenal axis effects, mometasone (Nasonex) and fluticasone (Flonase) are less than 2% bioavailable. Other topical steroids have greater bioavailability. Leukotriene receptor antagonists have been shown to inhibit the early phase of antigen response, attenuate the late-phase inflammatory response, reduce nasal congestion, and improve the sense of smell.

Pages: 448, 449

18: True statements regarding sinusitis include:

A. Sinusitis represents one of the most common disorders requiring antibiotic treatment in adults
B. The symptoms of rhinitis and sinusitis are often very similar
C. Sinusitis frequently follows a viral upper respiratory infection or an episode of allergic rhinitis
D. Classic symptoms include thick rhinorrhea, facial pressure, headache, and nasal obstruction
E. Fever and cough are rarely observed in true sinusitis

Answers: A, B, C, D

Critique: In addition to the classic symptoms noted, other symptoms often include low-grade fever, cough, otalgia, and an altered sense of smell.

Pages: 450, 451

19: True statements regarding the medical treatment of sinusitis include:

A. Topical decongestants applied for 7 to 10 days are appropriate
B. Mucolytics, such as guaifenesin, are appropriate
C. Nasal toilet with saline mist or irrigations should be advised
D. Broader spectrum antibiotics, rather than amoxicillin or trimethoprim-sulfamethoxazole, should be prescribed due to the increasing incidence of beta-lactamase—producing strains of *Haemophilus influenzae* and *Moraxella catarrhalis*

Answers: B, C

Critique: In acute cases of sinusitis, mucociliary function can be improved through a combination of decongestants, mucolytics, and nasal toilet. Topical decongestants, however, should be used for less than 3 days because of the risk of rhinitis medicamentosa. Although the incidence of beta-lactamase–producing strains of bacteria is increasing, a 10-day course of amoxicillin or trimethoprim-sulfamethoxazole remains appropriate for uncomplicated, nonrecurrent acute sinusitis. In cases of recurrent or severe sinusitis, broader spectrum agents, such as the newer macrolides, quinolones, augmented penicillins, and cephalosporins, are appropriate.

Pages: 451, 452

20: True statements regarding sinusitis in children include:

A. Sinusitis in children is not observed in primary care offices because the sinuses are not fully developed until adolescence
B. Children with sinusitis rarely complain of facial pain
C. Foul breath and nighttime cough are symptoms that may suggest sinusitis
D. Unlike adult sinusitis, pediatric sinusitis is rarely treated with antibiotics

Answer: C

Critique: Although the sinuses are not fully developed until adolescence, children still get sinusitis. The diagnosis is suggested by upper respiratory infection (URI) symptoms lasting more than 2 weeks, nighttime cough, and foul breath. Other diagnoses to consider in children with prolonged URI symptoms are choanal atresia, nasal foreign bodies, environmental allergies, cystic fibrosis, and immunodeficiency. Adenoiditis, however, is the most common condition that mimics sinusitis in children. Differentiating these conditions can be difficult because the symptoms can be identical and the disorders can coexist. The treatment of pediatric sinusitis is similar to that of adults and includes the use of antibiotics.

Page: 452

21: True statements regarding acute pharyngitis include:

A. It is caused by viral agents in the majority of cases.
B. Pharyngitis caused by GABHS has its peak incidence in late summer and early fall.
C. The incubation period for GABHS is 2 to 5 days.
D. Symptoms of pharyngitis caused by GABHS include the sudden onset of sore throat, fever, and chills.

Answers: A, B, C

Critique: The peak incidence for pharyngitis caused by GABHS is in late winter and early spring. Additional, though less frequent, symptoms of streptococcal pharyngitis include headache, abdominal pain, and nausea.

Pages: 454, 455

22: Family physicians caring for patients with known or suspected streptococcal pharyngitis should be aware that:

A. Rapid antigen detection tests have been shown in clinical trials to have typical specificities of about 98% and sensitivities of 95%
B. Throat culture is unnecessary for patients with negative rapid antigen tests
C. Penicillin remains the usual treatment for GABHS
D. After treatment, 15% of throat cultures remain positive

Answers: C, D

Critique: Although the specificities and sensitivities claimed by manufacturers are higher, clinical trials suggest that rapid antigen tests have specificities of about 90% and sensitivities of about 60% to 80%. Therefore, when GABHS is suspected and the rapid antigen test is negative, confirmation with a throat culture is recommended. Treatment for GABHS is penicillin VK, 250 mg four times daily or 500 mg twice daily for 10 days. Intramuscular benzathine penicillin G, 600,000 units for children less than 60 pounds and 1.2 million units for patients above 60 pounds, is a reasonable option for reasons of compliance, difficulty in swallowing, and so forth. Erythromycin should be considered for patients who are allergic to penicillin.

Pages: 454, 455

23: Pharyngitis associated with Epstein-Barr virus (EBV):

A. Can mimic GABHS infection
B. Can occur concurrently with GABHS infection
C. Can manifest signs and symptoms that include fatigue, lymphadenopathy, and hepatosplenomegaly
D. Is frequently associated with spontaneous splenic rupture

Answers: A, B, C

Critique: Studies have shown that GABHS infection and EBV infection present together in up to 33% of cases. Although contact sports should be avoided for 6 weeks to reduce the risk of splenic rupture, this is an infrequent complication. Other complications of EBV infection include thrombocytopenia, hemolytic anemia, Guillain-Barré syndrome, Bell's palsy, transverse myelitis, and aseptic meningitis. These occur in less than 2% of cases. Hepatitis is fairly common, occurring in up to 50% of cases.

Page: 455

24: True statements regarding hoarseness include:

A. Acute hoarseness is often associated with malignancy.
B. Hoarseness associated with cough can indicate cancer of the larynx or lung.
C. Hemoptysis with hoarseness should be considered secondary to malignancy until proven otherwise.
D. Visualization of the larynx is necessary only for patients with a history of tobacco use.

Answers: B, C

Critique: Acute hoarseness is rarely secondary to malignancy. It usually results from vocal abuse, laryngitis, or smoking. Malignancy should be considered in patients with chronic hoarseness; however, the differential diagnosis includes polyps, nodules, neurologic disorders, papillomas, and functional voice disorders. Visualization of the larynx by indirect or direct laryngoscopy is absolutely necessary for all patients who present with hoarseness.

Pages: 462, 463

25: True statements regarding thyroid imaging include:

A. Most thyroid nodules are "cold" on thyroid scans.
B. "Hot" nodules are usually malignant.
C. Ultrasound can distinguish cystic from solid nodules.
D. Lesions that enlarge on serial ultrasound require further work-up.

Answers: A, C, D

Critique: About 90% to 95% of all nodules are cold on thyroid scans, and the rate of malignancy in these nodules varies. Hot nodules are usually benign, and 20% of cold nodules are malignant. Many cold nodules are actually thyroid cysts. Ultrasound is a more sensitive test and can identify lesions as small as 2 to 3 mm. Ultrasound can aid in fine-needle aspiration localization of small nodules.

Pages: 469, 470

Chapter 23

Allergy

Dennis Ruppel

1: (True or False) Determine whether the following statements about CD-4-positive T helper cells are true or false:

  A. The T1 pathway results in increased cellular immunity.
  B. The T2 pathway results in increased allergic response.
  C. T1 responses are triggered by exposure in early life to certain viruses, bacteria, and toxins.
  D. T2 responses are stimulated by an individual's allergic genetic makeup, early exposure to allergens, and factors inhibiting the T1 response.

Answers: A - True, B - True, C - True, D - False

Critique: CD-4-positive T helper cells can be classified into two groups based on the cytokines they produce and their related functional activities. Uncommitted T helper lymphocytes can be influenced to develop into either of these types. The T2 responses are stimulated by an individual's allergic genetic makeup and early exposure to allergens and are inhibited by factors stimulating the T1 response.

Page: 473

2: According to theory about the increase in allergies in developed countries, all of the following statements are correct, except:

  A. Milk is pasteurized.
  B. Food additives are used.
  C. Immunizations are given.
  D. Antibiotics inhibit full exposure to bacteria.
  E. Mycobacterium is seldom encountered.

Answer: B

Critique: The theory about why we are seeing an increase in allergies in developed countries is that there are more "protective" features for children. In addition, they do not contract the viral and bacterial diseases as frequently as the children in underdeveloped countries. These factors may have a suppressive effect on the T1 pathway, which allows the T2 pathway to respond.

Page: 473

3: Family history has limited prognostic value in all the following, except:

  A. Insect stings
  B. Urticaria
  C. Eczema

  D. Food allergic states
  E. Drug allergies

Answer: C

Critique: When evaluating a patient for allergies, his or her history will give you 70% of the information you need to treat the allergies. A positive family history of allergies, asthma, hay fever, and eczema is strongly suggestive that the patient has a genetic atopic predisposition.

Page: 474

4: Intradermal skin testing is rarely used for which of the following:

  A. Dust mites
  B. Mold spores
  C. Food allergies
  D. Pollen sensitivity

Answer: C

Critique: Skin tests determine the presence of tissue-fixed allergic antibody. They also determine the ability of that antibody, when complexed with the antigen, to release mediators. Intradermal skin testing is rarely used for food sensitivity because it produces too many nonspecific reactions.

Page: 475

5: Seasonal allergic rhinitis is estimated to occur in what percent of the population younger than 20 years of age:

  A. 2% to 4%
  B. 4% to 6%
  C. 6% to 8%
  D. 8% to 10%

Answer: D

Critique: Allergic rhinitis can be either seasonal (hay fever) or perennial. Seasonal allergic rhinitis occurs when a high concentration of pollens is in the air. Perennial allergic rhinitis can be intermittent or continuous without seasonal variation. Seasonal allergic rhinitis has been found to be twice as common as the perennial type.

Pages: 475–476

6: The following are all common symptoms of seasonal allergic rhinitis, except:

  A. Paroxysmal sneezing
  B. Watery nasal discharge
  C. Nasal itching
  D. Lowered sneezing threshold

Answer: D

Critique: Patients with seasonal allergic rhinitis commonly complain of paroxysmal sneezing, a watery nasal discharge, nasal congestion, nasal itching, conjunctiva itching, and nasal itching. A lowered sneezing threshold often occurs with perennial allergic rhinitis. The bouts of sneezing may result from temperature changes, head movement, perfume, alcohol, tobacco smoke, and other irritants.

Page: 476

7: Which of the following treatments should be avoided as the primary treatment of seasonal allergies:

A. Around-the-clock antihistamine use
B. Alpha-adrenergic drugs
C. Intramuscular long-acting steroids
D. Topical intranasal glucocorticoid drugs

Answer: C

Critique: Antihistamines offer effective symptomatic relief in the treatment of both seasonal and perennial allergic rhinitis. They are more effective when used before exposure to known allergens and when taken around the clock. Alpha-adrenergic drugs are useful as single agents and in combination with antihistamines. The International Board for the Treatment of Allergic Rhinitis recommends topical intranasal glucocorticoid drugs as the first line of therapy. The use of intramuscular long-acting steroids should be avoided because of their suppression of the pituitary-adrenal axis and decreased efficacy with repeated use.

Page: 477

8: Which of the following second-generation antihistamines has been shown to have anti-inflammatory properties:

A. Fexofenadine (Allegra)
B. Loratadine (Claritin)
C. Diphenhydramine (Benadryl)
D. Cetirizine (Zyrtec)

Answer: D

Critique: Of the newer second-generation antihistamines, only cetirizine has been shown to have anti-inflammatory properties. As a result, Zyrtec may be effective in patients with allergic rhinitis and reactive airway disease. Diphenhydramine is a first-generation antihistamine.

Page: 477

9: The efficacy of immunotherapy has been shown to be:

A. 50% for molds and house dust symptom control, 70% for pollen symptom control
B. 80% for molds and house dust symptom control, 60% for pollen symptom control
C. 60% for molds and house dust symptom control, 80% for pollen symptom control
D. 70% for molds and house dust symptom control, 90% for pollen symptom control
E. 70% for molds and house dust symptom control, 60% for pollen symptom control

Answer: C

Critique: Immunotherapy is more efficacious for seasonal allergic rhinitis than for perennial allergic rhinitis.

Page: 477

10: Which of the following statements is not correct about nasal polyps:

A. They may be associated with perennial allergic rhinitis but usually only when it is complicated by sinusitis.
B. They normally develop as the result of seasonal allergic rhinitis and sinusitis.
C. They are easily visible in the nasal cavity.
D. They arise from infected ethmoid or maxillary sinuses.
E. Polypectomy may be necessary.

Answer: B

Critique: Nasal polyps are only coincidentally associated with allergies. They typically develop in the absence of allergies. A brief treatment of systemic steroids and daily use of topical glucocorticoid drugs for a longer period can help to reduce the size of the polyp.

Pages: 477–478

11: Which of the following statements is correct concerning sinusitis:

A. Chronic allergic rhinitis predisposes individuals to sinus disease.
B. Frontal sinuses are more commonly infected than are the maxillary sinuses.
C. Sinus x-rays are more sensitive than is limited CT scanning.
D. Transillumination is not helpful.

Answer: A

Critique: Sinusitis most frequently involves the ethmoid and maxillary sinuses. Transillumination is helpful but not always reliable. A limited coronal CT of the sinus is more sensitive in detecting sinus disease than x-rays are. Radiologic changes may be only minimally visible on routine sinus films.

Pages: 477–478

12: Which of the following treatments offers the best symptomatic control of vasomotor rhinitis:

A. Ipratropium bromide (0.03%) spray solution
B. Antihistamine-decongestant combinations
C. Topical glucocorticoid drugs
E. Buffered saline lavage

Answer: A

Critique: Patients with vasomotor rhinitis have rhinorrhea, postnasal drainage, and intermittent or chronic nasal obstruction. Although all the drugs can be effective, ipratropium bromide usually is the most effective.

Page: 478

13: All of the following are common precipitating triggers of asthma, except:

A. Cat antigen
B. Food allergies

C. Smoke
D. Viral infection
E. Exercise

Answer: B

Critique: Asthma is rarely precipitated by food allergies except as part of an anaphylactic reaction. An asthma attack occurs quickly after eating a certain food and normally every time that food is consumed. *Chlamydia pneumoniae* and *Mycoplasma pneumoniae* can trigger asthma, but other bacteria rarely trigger asthma. Exercise-induced bronchospasm and asthma occur in 60% to 80% of asthmatics and in up to 60% of teenagers and children with allergic rhinitis. Many biological and chemical agents used in the workplace can trigger asthma.

Pages: 479–480

14: When treating asthma, all of the following drugs have anti-inflammatory effects, except:

A. Theophyllines
B. Anticholinergics
C. Leukotriene antagonists
D. Cromolyn
E. Glucocorticoid steroids

Answer: B

Critique: Theophyllines have a mild anti-inflammatory effect. Leukotriene antagonists are the newest anti-inflammatory agents used in asthma management. The main use of cromolyn is in younger children when the physician wants to limit the use of glucocorticoid drugs. The most potent anti-inflammatory drugs currently available to treat asthma are glucocorticoid drugs.

Pages: 481–483

15: All of the following statements about drugs used during pregnancy are true, except:

A. During attacks, subcutaneous epinephrine is preferable to terbutaline.
B. Theophyllines seem to be safe.
C. Decongestants have not been established as safe.
D. Antihistamines have never been recognized as dangerous.

Answer: A

Critique: Terbutaline is preferred over epinephrine because, in addition to relieving bronchospasm, it relaxes uterine muscles. It is used to treat premature labor in nonasthmatic patients. Epinephrine can decrease uterine perfusion.

Pages: 484–485

16: Patients with moderate to severe persistent asthma whose peak flows are in the red zone should call their physician. The red zone is defined as what percentage of their personal best:

A. 80%
B. 70%
C. 60%
D. 50%
E. 40%

Answer: D

Critique: The use of a peak flow meter is essential in the management of asthma. These devices are recommended for patients with moderate to severe persistent asthma or for patients with a history of severe exacerbations. The green zone is 80% or better of the individual's personal best and no intervention is needed. The yellow zone is 50% to 80% and indicates that additional treatment is needed, including either an increase in the patient's regular medication or an additional medication. Patients need rescue medication when the peak flow reaches the red zone, and they should seek medical help immediately.

Pages: 485–486

17: Which of the following statements about contact dermatitis is not correct:

A. It is a pruritic condition that progresses from erythema and induration to a vesicobullous state.
B. It develops only after previous exposure.
C. *Rhus* oleoresins (poison oak, ivy, and sumac) affect 10% of the population.
D. Systemic glucocorticoid drugs can be used.

Answer: C

Critique: Contact dermatitis requires previous exposure for an individual to develop an allergic reaction. The forearms, ears, eyelids, lips, groin, and the dorsa of the feet are the most commonly involved. *Rhus* oleoresins cause contact dermatitis in almost everyone. Also, most people are sensitive to dinitrochlorobenzene, which is used to induce sensitivity in patients as a test for cell-mediated immune competence.

Page: 487

18: All of the following statements about urticaria are true, except:

A. Ninety percent of chronic urticaria is idiopathic.
B. Eighty percent of acute urticaria is idiopathic.
C. In 90% of all cases, the lesions will be gone in 3 weeks.
D. Cetirizine (Zyrtec) is the best overall medication.

Answer: C

Critique: Although 80% of acute urticaria and 90% of chronic urticaria are idiopathic, the physician should rule out obvious causes, such as drugs, foods, physical, cholinergic sources, and stress. If the cause is not easily determined, the patient should be treated before doing an extensive work-up. Of all cases, 90% will resolve within 3 months.

Pages: 487–488

19: Which of the following conditions is often the first manifestation of a true IgE-mediated latex sensitivity and usually starts at the area of contact within minutes of exposure:

A. Irritant dermatitis
B. Contact dermatitis

C. Contact urticaria
D. Allergic rhinitis

Answer: C

Critique: Latex allergy has become a serious problem since universal precautions made the use of latex gloves common. At lease ten antigens have been identified. Most are water soluble and capable of penetrating either wet or inflamed skin, and particularly mucous membranes. Latex allergy can present as irritant dermatitis in people with previously inflamed skin. The rash of contact dermatitis takes 1 to 2 days to develop. Contact urticaria develops within minutes and can lead to generalized urticaria. Allergy in a patient whose history suggests a latex allergy can be confirmed by a prick testing, which is 99% sensitive and 97% specific.

Page: 488

20: Anaphylaxis is a systemic reaction caused by the potent vasoactive mediators released after an allergen triggers the mast cells. All of the following can cause anaphylaxis, except:

A. Insect venoms
B. Allergenic extracts used for immunotherapy
C. Shellfish
D. Radiographic contrast media
E. Penicillin

Answer: D

Critique: Radiographic contrast media cause the release of histamine directly from mast cells, in addition to generating vasoactive kinins. This type of reaction is called anaphylactoid, as opposed to anaphylactic, because of the lack of any evidence of IgE allergy.

Pages: 488–489

21: The first symptom of systemic anaphylaxis is:

A. A flushing sensation
B. A tingling of the extremities
C. A feeling of apprehension
D. Itching
E. Urticaria

Answer: C

Critique: The sequence of symptoms of systemic anaphylaxis are a feeling of apprehension, tingling of the extremities, a flushing sensation, itching, palpitations, urticaria, angioedema, nausea, abdominal discomfort, cough, difficulty breathing, vomiting, diarrhea, intestinal and uterine cramping, incontinence, convulsions, coma, and death.

Page: 489

22: The most reliable test for hematologic drug reactions is:

A. RAST
B. Lymphocyte stimulation
C. To readminister the drug
D. Mast cell histamine release
E. Leukocyte cytotoxicity

Answer: C

Critique: Most tests used to confirm hematologic drug reactions are unreliable. The most reliable test is to readminister the drug and see whether the symptoms are reproduced. Because there is great risk in doing the test, it should be reserved only for patients for whom no other drug is available.

Pages: 489–490

23: Drugs that have been associated with hepatic reactions that are primarily cholestatic include all of the following, except:

A. Erythromycins
B. Phenothiazines
C. Nitrofurantoin
D. Imipramine
E. Sulfonamides

Answer: E

Critique: Sulfonamides cause hepatocellular reactions and are potentially fatal. Other drugs that can cause this type of reaction are allopurinol, hydantoins, isoniazid, methyldopa, monoamine inhibitors, rifampin, and valproic acid. Cholestatic reactions are usually relatively benign.

Pages: 490–491

Chapter 24

Parasitology

Richard P. Kratche

1: All of the following can result from infection with *Giardia lamblia*, except:

- A. An asymptomatic carrier state
- B. Acute explosive diarrhea
- C. Chronic diarrhea with malabsorption and weight loss
- D. Chronic liver disease with multiple hepatic cysts

Answer: D

Critique: *G. Lamblia* is a lumen-dwelling intestinal parasite. Symptoms caused by this protozoan range from none (in the carrier state) to severe acute or chronic diarrhea. *G. lamblia* does not affect the liver.

Page: 494

2: Once infected with *Giardia lamblia*, symptoms generally develop:

- A. Immediately
- B. Within 48 hours
- C. In 3 to 20 days
- D. After an incubation period of 1 to 2 months

Answer: C

Critique: Once *G. lamblia* cysts are ingested, they must pass through the gastrointestinal tract to the small intestine, where they form a new generation of trophozoites. These trophozoites then cause damage to the intestinal mucosa, alter intraluminal enzyme function, and absorb bile salts, resulting in the usual diarrheal illness. Symptoms begin from 3 to 20 days after infection, with a mean of 7 days.

Pages: 494, 495

3: The diagnostic test of choice for *Giardia lamblia* is:

- A. Stool culture
- B. Stool microscopy for ova and parasites
- C. Serum antibody titers to *G. Lamblia*
- D. Immunoassay for fecal *G. Lamblia* antigen

Answer: D

Critique: Historically, the only means to diagnose *G. lamblia* was microscopy of stool specimens for the detection of ova and parasites (cysts and trophozoites). This test is notoriously insensitive. Recently developed immunoassays for fecal *G. lamblia* antigen are highly sensitive and have become the gold standard for diagnosis of giardiasis.

Page: 495

4: The definitive hosts of *Toxoplasma gondii* are:

- A. Birds
- B. Cats
- C. Humans
- D. Bats

Answer: B

Critique: Members of the cat family are the definitive hosts of *T. gondii*. This parasite reproduces sexually within the intestinal epithelium of the cat. Oocysts are shed in the cat's feces, contaminating soil, kitty litter, grass, and vegetables. These cysts may then be inhaled or ingested by an intermediate host in whom they will reproduce asexually. Birds and all other animals, including humans, may serve as intermediate hosts for *T. gondii*.

Page: 495

5: The following infection treatment pairs are all correct, except:

- A. Giardiasis—metronidazole (Flagyl)
- B. Toxoplasmosis—pyrimethamine, sulfadiazine, and folinic acid
- C. Scabies—permethrin 5% cream (Elimite)
- D. Pinworm—mebendazole (Vermox)
- E. Anisakidosis—albendazole (Albenza)

Answer: E

Critique: All of the treatments listed are appropriate for the paired infection except for E. No studies of anthelmintic drug therapy have been done for Anisakid infection. Intestinal infection is usually self-limited. Gastric infection is usually confirmed by endoscopy, at which time the worm is removed. Albenza is a standard therapy for ascariasis.

Pages: 494, 495, 497, 498, 500, 501

6: (True or False) All of the following can be spread through fecal-oral transmission, except:

- A. Giardiasis
- B. Toxoplasmosis
- C. Pinworm
- D. Babesiosis
- E. Ascariasis

Answer: D

Critique: Babesia organisms are transmitted to humans by the Ixodes ticks from their animal reservoir in the white-footed deer mouse and other rodents. All of the other infections are transmitted via the fecal-oral route. Toxoplasmosis may also be transmitted by inhalation.

Pages: 494, 495, 497, 498, 500, 501

7: All of the following are effective methods for preventing infestation and infection by the paired infectious agents, except:

    A. Storing clothes and bedding in closed plastic container for 1 week—body lice
    B. Boiling water—*Giardia lamblia*
    C. Cooking meat until it is no longer pink and its juices are clear—*Toxoplasma gondii*
    D. Washing all clothes and bedding in hot water and drying them in a hot dryer (>122°F) for 10 minutes—scabies

Answer: A

Critique: Unlike head lice and pubic lice, which cannot survive more than 2 days away from their host, the body louse can survive for a week or more away from humans. Therefore, to kill body lice, one must store clothes and bedding in a closed plastic container for 2 weeks. Four days would be adequate for head lice and pubic lice. Choices B, C, and D are effective means of killing the paired parasite.

Pages: 495, 496, 498, 499

8: All of the following parasites are correctly paired with their classification, except:

    A. Scabies—mite
    B. *Pediculosis humanus*—louse
    C. *Giardia lamblia*—nematode
    D. Cercariae—larva (schistosomes)
    E. Ascariasis—helminth

Answer: C

Critique: *G. lamblia* is a protozoan that exists in two forms: (1) cysts that are infectious and once ingested excyst to form (2) trophozoites, which are not infectious

Pages: 494, 495, 497, 498, 500, 501

9: In immunocompetent children and adults, most toxoplasmosis infections:

    A. Are asymptomatic
    B. Cause focal tender adenopathy
    C. Cause an infectious mononucleosis–like syndrome
    D. Result in myocarditis or pericarditis

Answer: A

Critique: It is true that all of the symptoms listed in B, C, and D can result from infection by *Toxoplasma gondii*. However, the vast majority of patients are asymptomatic.

Page: 495

10: The average number of mites infesting an immunocompetent person who has scabies is:

    A. 3
    B. 11

    C. 29
    D. Thousands to millions

Answer: B

Critique: The average person with an intact immune system who has scabies will be infested by an average of only 11 mites. This results in a severely pruritic rash consisting of erythematous papules and nodules in a classic distribution. However, immunocompromised individuals may develop Norwegian scabies in which thousands to millions of mites cause crusted plaques with extensive scaling and minimal pruritis.

Page: 498

11: (True or False) Effective treatment options for head and pubic lice are:

    A. 1% or 5% permethrin (Nix and Elimite, respectively)
    B. Pyrethrin/piperonyl butoxide (RID)
    C. Malathion (0.5 or 1%)
    D. Lindane 1%
    E. Petroleum jelly

Answers: A - True, B - True, C - True, D - True, E - True

Critique: All of the options listed are effective therapies. Other treatment options include olive oil, trimethoprim-sulfamethoxasole, agricultural insecticides, and ivermectin.

Page: 499

12: (True or False) Poor hygiene is a risk factor for:

    A. Pinworm (enterobiasis)
    B. Body lice
    C. Scabies
    D. Ascariasis

Answers: A - True, B - True, C - False, D - True

Critique: Scabies effects people of all ages and socioeconomic status. Poor hygiene is not a significant risk factor. By contrast, poor hygiene is a major risk factor for pinworm, body lice, and ascariasis infection.

Pages: 497–500, 505

13: (True or False) For each of the following conditions, it is generally recommended that all family members and close contacts be treated in addition to the index case:

    A. Scabies
    B. Head lice
    C. Pubic lice
    D. Pinworm

Answers: A - True, B - False, C - False, D - True

Critique: Most authorities do recommend treating family members and close contacts of individuals with scabies and pinworm. When head lice are diagnosed, all family members and close contacts should be examined and treated if infested. In cases of pubic lice, all sexual contacts should be treated.

Pages: 497–500

14: (True or False) Definitive hosts for Trichobilharzia (schistosome responsible for cercarial dermatitis) include the following:

    A. Aquatic birds
    B. Aquatic snails
    C. Semiaquatic mammals
    D. Humans

Answer: A - True, B - False, C - True, D - False

Critique: Aquatic birds and semiaquatic mammals are the definitive hosts for Trichobilharzia. Eggs are shed from the definitive host through feces, hatch in water, and enter the intermediate host, aquatic snails. Humans are not hosts at all, and the cercaria die within several hours of entering one.

Page: 500

15: Which of the following is appropriate therapy for cercarial dermatitis (swimmers' itch)?

    A. Flagyl
    B. Permethrin cream 5% (Elimite)
    C. Vermox (mebendazole)
    D. Antihistamines and topical or oral corticosteroids
    E. Petroleum jelly

Answer: D

Critique: Treatment of swimmers' itch is symptomatic. Once the larvae have entered the skin, they die within a matter of hours. The subsequent rash and pruritis are immune mediated and resolve spontaneously in 1 to 3 weeks.

Page: 501

16: Of the following countries, which has the highest incident of anisakidosis?

    A. United States
    B. Japan
    C. France
    D. South Africa
    E. Brazil

Answer: B

Critique: Ingesting raw or poorly prepared affected fish causes anisakidosis. Thus, countries where raw fish is a large part of the diet, such as Japan, have the highest incidence of infestation.

Page: 501

17: Worldwide, the third most common cause of death from a parasitic infection is:

    A. Dengue fever
    B. Malaria
    C. Schistosomiasis
    D. Amebiasis
    E. Cyptospridiosis

Answer: D

Critique: Amebiasis is the third most fatal parasitic infection, following schistosomiasis and malaria. Cyptosporidiosis generally causes a self-limited gastro-enteritis. Dengue fever is caused by an arbovirus, not a parasite.

Page: 503

18: All of the following groups are at increased risk for amebiasis, except:

    A. Potato farmers
    B. Travelers
    C. Recent immigrants
    D. Institutionalized individuals
    E. Sexually active male homosexuals

Answer: A

Critique: There is no known association between potato farming and amebiasis. All of the other groups listed are at higher risk.

Page: 503

19: (True or False) Each of the following is an appropriate therapy for the treatment or prevention of amebiasis:

    A. Flagyl
    B. Iodoquinol (Yodoxin)
    C. Paromomycin (Humatin)
    D. Aspiration and drainage of hepatic cysts
    E. Amebiasis vaccine

Answer: A - True, B - True, C - True, D - True, E - False

Critique: Although active research on a vaccine for the prevention of amebiasis is ongoing, no vaccine is currently available. Flagyl is the most common antibiotic used to treat amebiasis. Most authorities recommend using an intraluminal drug as well (such as Yodoxin or Humatin). Although not usually necessary, aspiration and drainage of amebic hepatic abscesses is sometimes indicated.

Page: 503

20: The most important risk factor for developing clinical disease from babesiosis infection is:

    A. Infant/toddler age group
    B. Immunodeficiency
    C. Advanced age (>60 years old)
    D. Splenectomy history

Answer: C

Critique: Advanced age poses the greatest risk for developing clinical disease, followed by splenectomy and immunodeficiency. Infants and toddlers are not at increased risk, and in fact are at lower risk of infection as they tend to have a lower incidence of tick exposure.

Page: 504

21: The preferred treatment for moderate to serious illness with babesiosis is:

    A. Clindamycin (Cleocin) and quinine
    B. Atovaquone (Mepron) and azithromycin (Zithromax)
    C. Pentamidine (Pentam) and trimethoprim-sulfamethoxazole (Bactrim)
    D. Exchange transfusions

Answer: A

Critique: All of the antibiotic options listed have been reported to be effective in babesiosis, but the preferred treatment is clindamycin and quinine. Exchange transfusions are reserved for patients with hemolysis and high parasite loads.

Page: 504

Chapter 25

Travel Medicine

David A. Nelsen, JR

1: The primary and most current source for virtually all consensus in the area of travel medicine is:

    A. The Traveler's Health Service of the Centers for Disease Control and Prevention

    B. The World Health Organization website at http://www.who.org

    C. The International Travelers Bureau publication, *Sourcebook for Travel Medicine*

    D. There is no primary source for all travel medicine questions. The World Health Organization maintains contact information for all regional and national health organizations. These should be contacted individually depending on the area to be visited.

Answer: A

Critique: The Traveler's Health Service of the Centers for Disease Control and Prevention, which is based in Atlanta, Georgia, maintains the most current travel information available. This is published in its *Health Information for International Travel*, also known as the Yellow Book. The most current information is continuously available from the CDC web site at http://www.cdc.gov/ travel/ travel.htm. Updates are posted at the web site continuously. Hard copies are available free of charge to physicians.

Pages: 508, 516

2: Traveling patients should be asked to attend a principal office visit before their departure. During this visit, approximately 2 weeks before departure, the physician should:

    A. Arrange for yellow fever vaccination as well as immune serum globulin to prevent hepatitis A (if the traveler has not been immunized previously for hepatitis A)

    B. Initiate cholera vaccine if indicated

    C. Prescribe regular and travel-related medications and provide appropriate copies of current medical record to the patient

    D. Perform a chest x-ray if the patient has not had a baseline chest x-ray in the last 5 years

Answer: C

Critique: The principal office visit should be used to prescribe regular and travel-related medications and provide the patient with appropriate materials for travel. Hepatitis A and cholera vaccines should be provided in advance of the principal office visit because they are given serially over a period of months. Immune serum globulin should not be given when the traveler will receive any live attenuated virus vaccination; it should be reserved for last-minute travelers who otherwise fit guidelines for hepatitis A prophylaxis. Routine chest x-ray is not necessary in asymptomatic travelers before travel; however, tuberculosis status should be assessed with a purified protein derivative (PPD). Patients over the age of 55 who have not had regular PPD testing should receive a PPD booster more than 1 week after the initial PPD. A small number of additional PPD-positive patients will be identified with this testing strategy.

Page: 509

3: Which of the following statements about hepatitis B is accurate:

    A. Hepatitis B is common in many parts of the world but the traveler is at risk only if he or she has intimate sexual contact or receives a blood transfusion.

    B. A single dose of hepatitis B vaccine provides immunity in approximately 95% of the patients who receive it.

    C. Health care workers should receive the vaccine routinely unless they are going to countries of low prevalence, such as Australia or New Zealand.

    D. All travelers should routinely receive hepatitis B vaccine.

Answer: D

Critique: Although individuals who will have prolonged and/or intimate contact with persons in high-risk countries (such as the Middle East, Mediterranean countries, former Soviet bloc countries, Southeast Asia, the Pacific, tropical Africa, and South America) are at the greatest risk, all travelers should be routinely vaccinated against hepatitis B.

Page: 510

4: Travelers who exhibit a positive reaction to purified protein derivative (PPD) should:

    A. Receive a chest x-ray to be sure that it is not a false-positive test

    B. Not be treated if they received BCG vaccination in childhood

    C. Receive a full course of isoniazid (INH) after they have completed their travel

    D. Receive routine tuberculosis prophylaxis regardless of their travel plans

Answer: D

Critique: The overwhelming majority of new cases of tuberculosis occur in developing nations. Travelers are potentially susceptible to this. All travelers should receive routine PPD testing before travel. Those who test positive should be treated according to the CDC guidelines with no regard to their traveling status.

Page: 510

5: Only three diseases—cholera, plague, and yellow fever—remain subject to quarantine under the rules of the World Health Organization. Which of the following statements is correct relevant to these diseases:

A. Vaccines for cholera, plague, and yellow fever must be completed and certified before travel into certain high-risk zones of South America or Africa.
B. The vaccine for yellow fever is only moderately effective against the virus.
C. Yellow fever vaccine may be difficult to obtain; however, any physician may certify that the traveler has been appropriately vaccinated.
D. Cholera vaccine is safe to use during pregnancy.

Answer: D

Critique: Both the plague and cholera vaccines are made from killed bacteria and are safe to give during pregnancy. Yellow fever vaccine is highly effective and is made from attenuated virus. Yellow fever vaccine is the only vaccination that can be required for travel into World Health Organization–designated risk areas. Only agencies or physicians designated by individual state health departments are allowed to administer yellow fever vaccine and to validate the immunization certificate. Most family physicians refer patients to travel clinics or to state health departments to receive a yellow fever vaccination.

Pages: 512, 513

6: Which of the following statements about hepatitis A is correct:

A. Hepatitis A vaccination is a live attenuated virus.
B. Hepatitis A vaccination is safe and approved the for infants over 6 months of age.
C. Although a single injection will give adequate antibody levels for travel, a booster should be completed 6 to 12 months after the initial immunization.
D. Immune serum globulin is still the preferred prophylaxis for hepatitis A in travelers.

Answer: C

Critique: A single injection of hepatitis A vaccine, preferably given at least 4 weeks before travel, has replaced immune serum globulin as the preferred protection against hepatitis A. Hepatitis A vaccine is prepared from a killed virus and is safe and approved for children older than 2 years of age.

Page: 512

7: Lyme disease vaccination (Lymerix) is currently recommended for:

A. Travelers to high-risk areas in the forested regions of northern Europe and Asia
B. No international travelers
C. Travelers to southern Australia or New Zealand
D. Travelers only to certain areas when epidemic conditions exist. These areas can be found on the Centers for Disease Control website.

Answer: B

Critique: The currently available Lyme disease vaccination has been prepared against North American subspecies of Borrelia. The subspecies of Borrelia that causes Lyme disease in northern Europe is different from that causing Lyme disease in the United States. Therefore, Lyme disease vaccination should be used only against North American strains.

Page: 513

8: Which of the following statements regarding rabies vaccination is correct:

A. Rabies vaccination is not recommended for pre-travel prophylaxis.
B. Persons who take the three-dose pre-exposure series are not at risk for rabies even with a high-risk bite.
C. Rabies vaccination should be given to anyone who is at significant risk, especially those who might be exposed to dogs and other mammals at the village level.
D. The human diploid cell vaccine formulation of rabies vaccine is formulated for intradermal use and is somewhat less expensive.

Answer: D

Critique: Rabies vaccination is recommended for pre-travel prophylaxis for those who will have potential exposures to dogs and other mammals at the village level. The CDC maintains a list of "rabies-free countries," and rabies vaccination is not recommended for travel into those countries. The three-dose pre-exposure series does not negate the need for postexposure treatment; rather, patients who have had the pre-exposure series do not need rabies immunoglobulin and they need only two postexposure boosters. The human diploid cell vaccine formulation of rabies vaccine is approved for intradermal use. The dose for this vaccine is smaller than that for intramuscular use, so the series is less expensive.

Page: 513

9: The potential for malaria affects virtually every traveler who sets foot into a country where malaria is documented. Which of the following statements best characterizes the current guidelines for preventing exposure to malaria-carrying insect vectors:

A. Insect avoidance measures should include barriers and topical repellents. Clothing should cover the arms and legs as much as possible. Permethrin-impregnated mosquito nets should be used in outlying areas. Insect repellents containing 20% to 35% *N,N,*-diethyl-m-toluamide (DEET) should be applied to exposed areas.

B. Insect avoidance measures should include barriers and topical repellents. Clothing should cover the body as much as possible. Sleeping areas should be protected with screens or netting. Insect repellents containing 80% N, N,-diethyl-m-toluamide (DEET) should be applied to exposed areas.

C. Insect avoidance measures should include barriers and topical repellents. Clothing should cover the body as much as possible. Sleeping areas should be protected with screens or netting. Insect repellents containing N,N,-diethyl-m-toluamide (DEET) are now considered to be too toxic for human use in concentrations high enough to prevent bites. Citronella-based repellents are as effective as DEET and are safer.

D. Insect avoidance measures should include barriers and topical repellents. Clothing should cover the body as much as possible. Sleeping areas should be protected with screens or netting. Insect repellents containing N,N,-diethyl-m-toluamide (DEET) are now considered to be too toxic for human use in concentrations high enough to prevent bites. Permethrin-based repellents are as effective as DEET and are safer.

Answer: A

Critique: Avoidance of mosquitoes, tsetse flies, and reduviid bugs is an essential component of malaria prevention. DEET is still the most effective topical repellent and should be used sparingly on unprotected skin and on clothing. Mosquito netting and screened buildings are also important.

Page: 515

10: Chloroquine-resistant *Plasmodium falciparum* have spread rapidly through the malarious world. Chloroquine-sensitive strains can still be found in which area:

A. Central America/Mexico
B. South Africa
C. Malaysia
D. Indonesia

Answer: A

Critique: Chloroquine-sensitive strains of *P. falciparum* are still found in the Middle East, Central America/Mexico, and the Dominican Republic/Haiti. The remainder of the malarious world is infested with chloroquine-resistant strains.

Page: 513

11: Which of the following treatment regimens is effective in preventing malaria in areas with documented chloroquine resistance:

A. Primaquine, 15 mg orally once a day
B. Mefloquine, 250 mg orally once per week
C. Doxycycline, 200 mg orally once per week
D. Chloroquine phosphate, 500 mg once per week plus proguanil 2 mg once per day

Answer: B

Critique: Once-weekly mefloquine is still the most widely recommended prophylaxis for chloroquine-resistant to malaria. Doxycycline, 100 mg daily, is the best alternative but is contraindicated in children and pregnant or lactating women. Chloroquine plus proguanil is much less effective than mefloquine or doxycycline but is more effective than chloroquine alone. Primaquine is useful only for postexposure treatment after return from a malarious area and is indicated only after long exposure to *Plasmodium vivax* or *ovale*.

Page: 513

12: The most common microbial etiology for traveler's diarrhea is:

A. Enterotoxigenic *Escherichia coli*
B. Giardia
C. Cryptosporidium
D. Salmonella species

Answer: A

Critique: Although Giardia, amoeba, cryptosporidium, and other gram-negative species can cause traveler's diarrhea, enterotoxigenic *E. coli* is the most common.

Page: 514

13: A 10-year-old traveler who develops frequent diarrhea, more than eight blood-tinged stools per day, and a temperature to 101°F should be treated with:

A. Loperamide (Imodium) until the diarrhea subsides
B. Ciprofloxacin, 250 mg twice daily for 3 days
C. Trimethoprim, 160 mg/sulfamethoxazole, 800 mg twice daily for 3 days
D. Erythromycin base, 250 mg, TID, for 3 days

Answer: C

Critique: Ciprofloxacin or sulfamethoxazole/trimethoprim in appropriate doses is the most effective treatment for traveler's diarrhea, especially when the traveler appears toxic. Loperamide is appropriate when diarrhea is the only symptom. Ciprofloxacin is contraindicated in children under age 12.

Page: 514

14: Which of the following statements about risk for HIV in developing countries is correct:

A. With the availability of modern-day serologic testing, the blood supply in developing countries is considered to be safe from the risk of HIV transmission.
B. Persons with unavoidable HIV risk, such as health-care workers, should carry a postexposure preventive course of antiretroviral medications.
C. Mosquitoes have been demonstrated to be a vector for HIV in some countries.
D. Postexposure HIV chemoprophylaxis has not been shown to be effective.

Answer: B

Critique: The availability of antiretroviral medications is irregular in many countries, particularly third world countries. Health care workers or others who could possibly sustain a high-risk exposure should carry a postexposure preventive course of antiretroviral medications. Blood supplies in developing countries should be presumed to be unsafe. Mosquitoes have never been proven to transmit HIV.

Pages: 514, 515

15: What is the appropriate duration for malaria prophylaxis after the traveler has returned to a non-malarious area:

    A. Medications may be stopped as soon as the traveler has left the malarious area.

    B. Antimalarial regimens should be continued for 4 weeks after departure from the malarious area.

    C. Antimalarial regimens should be continued for 2 weeks after departure from the malarious area.

    D. Mefloquine should be continued for 2 weeks after departure from the malarious area; however, doxycycline should be continued for 4 to 6 weeks after the traveler has left the malarious area.

Answer: B

Critique: Antimalarial regimens should be continued for 4 weeks after departure from the malarious area. The "malignant" form of *P. falciparum* has an incubation period of 12 to 14 days. Thus, prophylaxis must extend beyond this period.

Page: 515

Obstetrics

Stephen Markovich

1: Which of the following is true concerning U.S. infant mortality rates:

  A. Birth defects are the leading cause of infant mortality.
  B. The use of electronic fetal monitoring has dramatically improved neonatal mortality rates.
  C. The U.S. infant mortality rate is 2.5 per 1000 live births.
  D. No significant disparity exists between morbidity rates for blacks and for whites.

Answer: A

Critique: Birth defects are the leading cause of infant mortality at a rate of 164/100,000 live births. Although many advances in technology have proven benefits, electronic fetal monitoring is not recommended as beneficial for use in low-risk normal deliveries. Black infants are 1.8 times more likely to be preterm.

Pages: 518, 519

2: Patient instructions during routine prenatal evaluations should include all of the following, except:

  A. Expected weight gain of 25 to 35 lb
  B. Review of recommended laboratory tests
  C. Scheduling of 8 to 10 follow-up visits
  D. Immediate cessation of sexual intercourse
  E. A moderate exercise program

Answer: D

Critique: Sexual activity need not stop during pregnancy unless complicated by placenta previa or preterm labor. Many couples have questions regarding this topic, and it should be addressed openly.

Page: 522

3: Adequate maternal weight gain and fetal growth requires how many extra calories per day?

  A. 300 cal/day
  B. 500 cal/day
  C. 1200 cal/day
  D. 3500 cal/day

Answer: A

Critique: Nutritional guidelines have been developed based on maternal weight and body mass index, but, in general, 300 calories per day extra is sufficient for fetal growth.

Page: 520

4: The daily intake of folic acid recommended for prevention of neural tube defects is:

  A. 4.0 mg in the third trimester for routine pregnancies
  B. 0.4 mg before conception for routine pregnancies
  C. 400 IU before conception for women with a previously affected child
  D. 4 mg in the third trimester for women with a previously affected child

Answer: B

Critique: Folic acid taken in the preconception and first trimester has been shown to prevent neural tube defects. Routine pregnancies require 0.4 mg/day. Women with prior neural tube defects in offspring require 4 mg of folate per day starting 1 month before conception.

Page: 519

5: A patient presents for a first visit with a last menstrual period (LMP) of October 24. The expected date of delivery (EDD) is:

  A. July 17
  B. August 31
  C. July 31
  D. September 17
  E. August 17

Answer: C

Critique: Naegle's rule predicts delivery day by subtracting 3 months and adding seven days to the first day of the last menstrual cycle.

Page: 522

6: Which of the following is true regarding home pregnancy tests:

  A. Their sensitivity approaches 95%, but specificity is low.
  B. Their specificity approaches 95%, but sensitivity is low.
  C. A positive test requires serum HCG confirmation.
  D. Many can detect pregnancy by the fifth menstrual week.

Answer: D

Critique: Home pregnancy kits are at least 95% sensitive *and* 95% specific and are capable of detecting pregnancy at the fifth menstrual week. Confirmatory testing is not needed unless clinically indicated.

Page: 522

7: Serologic tests at the first visit should include:

    A. RPR
    B. VZV
    C. HSV
    D. CMV

Answer: A

Critique: Serologic tests for syphilis, rubella immunity, and hepatitis B are routinely performed. HIV tests are now encouraged but not generally required. Varicella, herpes, and CMV testing is not performed unless needed as part of a fetal evaluation.

Page: 522

8: During follow-up prenatal visits, digital cervical examination:

    A. Is performed weekly after 36 weeks
    B. Is required to document placenta previa
    C. Increases the risk of preterm labor
    D. Is not required until 41 weeks gestation

Answer: D

Critique: Internal cervical examination is used to assess fetal lie and cervical dilation. It is contraindicated in placenta previa. With appropriate technique and frequency, it does not increase the risk of preterm labor. It need not be done until 41 weeks.

Page: 523

9: The most common reason to offer genetic testing (amniocentesis, CVS) is:

    A. Intrauterine growth retardation (IUGR)
    B. Advanced maternal age
    C. Previous first trimester miscarriage
    D. Family history or fetal abnormality

Answer: B

Critique: Women over 35 are at risk for aneuploidy, first-trimester miscarriage, or other chromosomal abnormalities. They require specific counseling and should be offered diagnostic testing.

Page: 524

10: Maternal triple screen is most accurate at what gestational age?

    A. 10 to 12 weeks
    B. 13 to 15 weeks
    C. 16 to 18 weeks
    D. 24 to 26 weeks

Answer: C

Critique: Normal values for triple screen (alpha-fetoprotein, estriols, and hCG-B) vary with gestational age and are valid from 15 to 20 weeks. They are most accurate at 16 to 18 weeks.

Page: 525

11: An elevated AFP is consistent with which of the following conditions:

    A. Down syndrome
    B. Trisomy 18
    C. Spina bifida
    D. Club feet

Answer: C

Critique: Elevations in maternal AFP are caused by open neural defects such as spinal bifida or anencephaly.

Page: 525

12: All of the following drugs are acceptable in pregnancy, except:

    A. Tetracycline
    B. Allergy shots
    C. Pseudoephedrine
    D. Acetaminophen

Answer: A

Critique: Although many drugs are used routinely and are quite safe, specific hazards related to pregnancy should be identified whenever considering prescribing to a pregnant patient. Routine cold preparations, with the exception of aspirin and nonsteroidal medications, have been found to be acceptable in pregnancy. Tetracyclines have been shown to discolor the teeth of the fetus.

Pages: 525, 526

13: All of the following are true regarding vaginal birth after cesarean (VBAC), except:

    A. The strongest predictor of safety is the location of a previous uterine scar.
    B. Oxytocin augmentation of labor is contraindicated during VBAC.
    C. The overall safety of VBAC for the mother is comparable to that of operative delivery.
    D. VBAC should only be attempted with adequate, available surgical consultation.

Answer: B

Critique: VBAC requires careful patient selection, preparation, and management. Patients with previous classic incision have an increased risk of uterine rupture and are not candidates for VBAC. The incidence of rupture with low transverse incision is low. Oxytocin is not contraindicated, although it should be used cautiously and internal pressure monitoring is recommended. Complication of VBAC or failure to deliver vaginally generally results in operative delivery.

Page: 526

14: Match the following infections with the statements or fetal complications listed below:

    1. Toxoplasmosis
    2. Syphilis
    3. Rubella
    4. Cytomegalovirus
    5. Herpes simplex virus

    A. Skin, eye, oral lesions; CNS involvement; seizures
    B. Deafness, eye lesions, mental retardation, cardiac lesions

C. Hydrops fetalis, stillbirth, preterm delivery, IUGR

D. Antecedent flu-like illness, deafness, periventricular calcifications

E. Ingestion of contaminated raw meat

Answers: 1 - E, 2 - C, 3 - B, 4 - D, 5 - A

Critique: Congenital toxoplasmosis occurs 1 in 10,000 births to mothers who experience active infection during pregnancy. It is contracted by ingesting raw meat or cat feces containing parasitic cysts. Syphilis, generally transmitted in the primary or secondary stages, causes miscarriage, stillbirth, hydrops, and fetal infection. Congenital rubella syndrome causes deafness, cataracts, chorioretinitis, CNS, and cardiac disease. Primary CMV infection occurs in 2% of women, who may be asymptomatic or have generalized symptoms. The most common manifestation of fetal infection is hearing loss.

Pages: 527–529

15: Regarding HIV and pregnancy, all of the following are true, except:

A. Zidovudine has been shown to decrease maternal-fetal transmission.

B. Viral load is not associated with risk of transmission.

C. Artificial rupture of membranes (AROM) and fetal scalp electrode placement are contraindicated.

D. Amniocentesis and breast-feeding are contraindicated.

E. HIV infection in women is rising throughout the United States.

Answer: B

Critique: AZT decreases maternal-fetal transmission from 25% to 8%. Viral load is a significant factor in fetal transmission. AROM, scalp electrodes, amniocentesis, and breast-feeding are all contraindicated.

Page: 528

16: Physiologic anemia of pregnancy is a result of:

A. Decreased iron consumption

B. First-trimester bleeding

C. Relative plasma volume increase

D. Ineffective maternal reticulocytosis

E. Splenic sequestration

Answer: C

Critique: Although red cell mass increases in pregnancy, the relative increase in plasma volume is greater and results in an apparent physiologic anemia.

Page: 529

17: Which of the following is true regarding pulmonary changes in pregnancy?

A. Respiratory rate is increased to provide more oxygen to the fetus.

B. Increased minute ventilation results in a mild arterial acidosis.

C. The best measure of pulmonary function is the peak flow.

D. Prostaglandin F_2 (Hemabate) is the prostaglandin of choice during labor and delivery.

E. Moderate to severe asthma may result in fetal intrauterine growth retardation.

Answer: E

Critique: Minute ventilation is increased in pregnancy, not because of respiratory rate but, rather, increased tidal volume. This results in a mild respiratory alkalosis. FEV_1 is the best measure of pulmonary function, but it is often substituted with peak flows in the office. Hemabate causes bronchial smooth muscle constriction.

Pages: 529, 530

18: (True or False) Pre-existing hypertension is a risk factor for pre-eclampsia, IUGR, and abruption.

Answer: True

Critique: Fetal morbidity and mortality rates are higher in women who have hypertension. In addition, women with pre-existing hypertension have a 20% risk of developing pre-eclampsia.

Page: 530

19: All of the following medications are used in pregnancy for blood pressure control, except:

A. Hydralazine

B. Nifedipine

C. Enalapril

D. Alpha-methyl dopa

Answer: C

Critique: Alpha methyldopa is the drug of choice for hypertension. ACE-inhibitors are contraindicated in pregnancy.

Page: 530

20: A 3-hour glucose tolerance test is required if the 1-hour challenge exceeds:

A. 126 mg/dL

B. 135 mg/dL

C. 140 mg/dL

D. 145 mg/dL

Answer: C

Critique: The initial, nonfasting glucose tolerance test is performed with a 50 g glucose load. If the 1-hour result exceeds 140 mg/dL, the more definitive test is required.

Page: 531

21: All of the following are true regarding gestational diabetes, except:

A. It affects 10% to 15% of pregnant women.

B. Screening is recommended at 26 to 28 weeks.

C. Initial therapy is diet modification and, if unsuccessful, insulin.

D. The lifetime risk of follow-up Type II diabetes is 30% to 60%.

Answer: A

Critique: Gestational diabetes affects 3% to 5% of women. All women should be screened at 26 to 28 weeks with 50 g of glucose. Initial therapy is diet modification with frequent blood sugar monitoring, followed by insulin. There is an increased lifetime risk. Postpartum and yearly glucose tolerance testing is recommended.

Page: 531

22: Which of the following is true regarding pyelonephritis?

    A. Asymptomatic bacteriuria generally poses no risk of progression to pyelonephritis.
    B. Urine cultures with fewer than 100,000 CFUs do not require treatment.
    C. Patients with sickle cell trait should routinely be screened with urine cultures.
    D. Asymptomatic bacteriuria is most often due to *Proteus mirabilis*.

Answer: C

Critique: Asymptomatic bacteriuria occurs in 3% to 5% of pregnant women and is more frequent in patients with sickle cell trait. Untreated, it may result in pyelonephritis in 30% of affected women. Pyelonephritis may occur with CFU counts as low as 20,000 to 50,000. *E. coli* is the most commonly implicated pathogen.

Pages: 531, 532

23: All of the following are true regarding the evaluation of ectopic pregnancy, except:

    A. The classic clinical triad of ectopic is amenorrhea, abdominal pain, irregular vaginal bleeding.
    B. Of ectopic gestations, 20% to 30% have no sonographic abnormality.
    C. A serum progesterone level of less than 15 ng/ml warrants further evaluation.
    D. Serum HCG levels should double every 72 hours.

Answer: D

Critique: Ectopic pregnancy is usually related to previous PID and presents with painful vaginal bleeding early in pregnancy, often before pregnancy has even been diagnosed. A serum progesterone level of less than 15 ng/ml is seen in only 11% of normal pregnancies. Serum HCG levels should double approximately every 48 hours.

Page: 532

24: A 10-week G1P0 presents to the office with vaginal bleeding, back pain, and menstrual–like cramps. Pelvis examination demonstrates bleeding from the os, with pooling of blood in the posterior vault. The cervix appears closed. The diagnosis is:

    A. Threatened abortion
    B. Inevitable abortion
    C. Incompetent cervix
    D. Missed abortion

Answer: A

Critique: Not all vaginal bleeding results in miscarriage, but pain, bleeding, and a closed os represent a threatened abortion.

Page: 533

25: Counseling of the patient experiencing early vaginal bleeding should include all of the following, except:

    A. Bleeding does not represent inevitable pregnancy loss.
    B. Bedrest has been shown to be beneficial in preventing miscarriage and should be encouraged.
    C. The majority of miscarriages are due to chromosomal abnormalities.
    D. Fever, foul discharge, and abdominal tenderness warrant further evaluation.

Answer: B

Critique: Of pregnant women, 25% experience some vaginal bleeding and approximately half of those will miscarry. The majority of miscarriages are caused by sporadic chromosomal aneuploidy. Incomplete abortions may result in a septic abortion with fever, pain, discharge, and leukocytosis. With the exception of uterine structural abnormalities, bedrest is not helpful in preventing miscarriage.

Page: 533

26: A 32-week G1P0 presents with low back pain and uterine cramping. Digital examination finds the cervix 3 cm dilated and 80% effaced. Initial management would include all of the following, except:

    A. Subcutaneous terbutaline
    B. Saline wet prep, vaginal cultures, and pH
    C. IV hydration and bedrest
    D. Urinalysis
    E. Evaluation for substance abuse

Answer: A

Critique: The patient is suffering from preterm labor. Initial actions should focus on stabilization, usually with IV fluids, and a search for a causative agent, often infection or drugs.

Pages: 534, 535

27: Which of the following is a contraindication to stopping labor in the preterm patient?

    A. Chorioamnionitis
    B. Maternal tachycardia secondary to beta agonist use (terbutaline)
    C. Loss of reflexes secondary to magnesium sulfate
    D. Multiple gestations

Answer: A

Critique: The goal of management of the preterm patient is to safely carry the pregnancy to term. Tachycardia is frequently encountered with use of beta agonists. Loss of reflexes due to magnesium sulfate requires a dosage adjustment. Multiple gestations frequently require aggressive management. Acute chorioamnionitis is a contraindication to pharmacologic arrest of labor.

Pages: 534, 535

28: All of the following are true concerning magnesium sulfate, except:

    A. Plasma levels should be kept between 10 and 20 mg/dL.

    B. Calcium gluconate can be used to treat magnesium toxicity.

    C. Patients should be warned about flushing, warmth, and poor muscle tone.

    D. Urine output and pulmonary status should be closely monitored.

Answer: A

Critique: Plasma magnesium levels should be kept between 5 and 8 mg/dL. Patients should be warned about possible side effects, including flushing, warmth, diplopia, nausea, and vomiting. The kidney excretes magnesium, and its level is affected by urine output. The lungs should be examined frequently for signs of pulmonary edema.

Page: 535

29: Diagnosis of intrauterine growth retardation (IUGR) requires estimated fetal weight to be less than what percentile for gestational age?

    A. 5%

    B. 10%

    C. 15%

    D. 25%

Answer: B

Critique: A weight, determined by ultrasound, to be less than 10th percentile suggests IUGR.

Pages: 535, 536

30: All of the following are true regarding IUGR, except:

    A. Bedrest is the only effective treatment modality.

    B. Maternal hypertension and diabetes can influence fetal growth.

    C. Ultrasound is 80% to 90% sensitive in diagnosing IUGR.

    D. Femur length is the first measured parameter to fall behind in IUGR.

Answer: D

Critique: IUGR is caused by many factors including nutritional status, placental growth, comorbid diseases, fetal infection, and genetic disorders. Ultrasound is very sensitive for the diagnosis of IUGR. The first routinely measured parameter to fall behind is abdominal circumference. The only effective treatment is bedrest in the left lateral decubitus position.

Pages: 535, 536

31: (True or False) Which of the following are risk factors for pre-eclampsia?

    A. Patients younger than 20 years

    B. Caucasians

    C. Multiparous patients

    D. Comorbid medical conditions, including diabetes and hypertension

    E. Previous history of pre-eclampsia

    F. Twins

Answers: A - True, B - False, C - False, D - True, E - True, F - True

Critique: Risk factors include extremes of maternal age, nulliparity, African-American race, multiple pregnancy, comorbid conditions, and previous history.

Page: 536

32: A 19-year-old, previously healthy G1P0 presents to the emergency department at 38 weeks with blood pressure of 160/100 and mental status changes following a seizure witnessed by the squad. Appropriate initial medical management would be:

    A. Magnesium sulfate

    B. Phenytoin (Dilantin)

    C. Diazepam (Valium)

    D. Carbemazepine (Tegretol)

Answer: A

Critique: The most likely diagnosis is eclampsia. Treatment is magnesium sulfate and delivery. Perinatal mortality is 2% to 8.6%.

Page: 536

33: A 33-year-old G2P1 with uncomplicated pregnancy presents at 39 weeks to labor and delivery with an increase in systolic blood pressure of 20 mmHg and slight right upper quadrant pain. Appropriate screening laboratories include all of the following, except:

    A. CBC

    B. Platelets

    C. Electrolytes

    D. AST/ALT

    E. LDH

Answer: C

Critique: The patient is being evaluated for pre-eclampsia with possible progression to HELLP syndrome. This may result in anemia, thrombocytopenia, and elevations in transaminases and LDH. Treatment is emergent delivery of the baby.

Pages: 536, 537

34: A term patient with single gestation presents with abdominal pain and vaginal bleeding. Review of the record shows a first-trimester drug screen positive for cocaine. The pain is getting progressively worse, her blood pressure is 90/60, and her abdomen is firm and exquisitely tender. Fetal monitoring shows occasional contractions and severe fetal bradycardia. Which of the follow represents the best initial management?

    A. CBC, type, and screen

    B. PT (INR)/PTT

    C. Cesarean section

    D. Abdominal ultrasound

    E. Pitocin-augmented induction

Answer: C

Critique: The patient is suffering from severe fetal distress, most likely secondary to placental abruption. Abruption is a clinical diagnosis. Ultrasonography has a high false-negative rate for this disorder. The level of fetal distress requires cesarean section to prevent fetal death.

Page: 537

35: All of the following regarding placenta previa are true, except:

    A. Previa diagnosed in the second trimester generally does not resolve and results in cesarean section.
    B. Tobacco use is a risk factor.
    C. First bleeding is usually painless and occurs at 27 to 32 weeks.
    D. Digital examination of the cervix should be avoided.

Answer: A

Critique: Most cases of placenta previa diagnosed early in pregnancy resolve, although serial ultrasound is recommended for confirmation. Advanced maternal age, increased parity, uterine abnormalities, previous previa or uterine surgery, and tobacco use are risk factors. First bleeding is usually in the third trimester. Digital examination is contraindicated.

Pages: 537, 538

36: The most common risk factor for placenta accreta is:

    A. Bicornuate uterus
    B. Molar pregnancy
    C. Previous cesarean section
    D. Multiple gestations

Answer: C

Critique: Previous cesarean section and uterine surgery are risk factors for placenta accreta, increta, and percreta.

Page: 538

37: A nonreactive nonstress test (NST) indicates:

    A. A fetal sleep state
    B. A damaged central nervous system
    C. A need for further investigation
    D. Fetal jeopardy requiring immediate intervention

Answer: C

Critique: Although the NST assesses the fetal autonomic nervous system and uteroplacental unit, several other factors may be responsible for a nonreactive test. Fetal sleep, maternal narcotics, prematurity, and cardiac abnormalities may affect the results. Further evaluation is required.

Page: 540

38: All of the following are associated with multiple gestations, except:

    A. Predominance of monozygotic twins
    B. Pregnancy-induced hypertension
    C. Gestational diabetes
    D. Premature delivery

Answer: A

Critique: Of twins, 66% to 75% are dizygotic. Preterm labor and delivery, PIH, gestational diabetes, placenta previa, and pyelonephritis are more common with twin gestations.

Page: 539

39: A reactive or reassuring NST requires which of the following:

    A. Two accelerations in a 15-minute period
    B. No previous classical uterine scar
    C. Ten units of pitocin administered over 15 minutes
    D. Vibroacoustic stimulation

Answer: A

Critique: A reactive NST requires two accelerations of 15 beats/min above baseline for 15 seconds. Pitocin and acoustic stimulation are not required for a reactive test. A previous classical scar is a contraindication for a *contraction* stress test.

Page: 540

40: A postdate G2P1 is referred for biweekly NSTs. Despite more than 1 hour of observation, only one acceleration meets the criteria. Subsequently, an ultrasound demonstrates an AFI of 10, normal fetal breathing, and no significant body movements or extension. The biophysical profile score equals:

    A. 2
    B. 4
    C. 6
    D. 8

Answer: B

Critique: The score of 4 is ominous. The score is based on NST (score = 0), amniotic fluid volume (score = 2), fetal breathing (score = 2), body movement (score = 0), and fetal tone (score = 0).

Page: 540

41: Match the following to the appropriate statements below:

    1. First stage of labor
    2. Second stage of labor
    3. Third stage of labor
    4. Active phase of labor
    5. Latent phase of labor

    A. A period of rapid dilation of the cervix, not affected by anesthesia
    B. Can be managed at home in compliant patients with normal pregnancies
    C. Signaled by cord lengthening, increased bleeding, and fundal changes
    D. Progressive, nonlinear change in cervical dilation and effacement
    E. Generally lasts up to 2 hours in nulliparous women without epidural anesthesia

Answer: 1 - D, 2 - E, 3 - C, 4 - A, 5 - B

Critique: Labor is defined as contractions with progressive cervical dilation. Latent phase is characterized as little change in dilation with increased effacement and anterior positioning of the cervix. Active phase is characterized by rapid cervical dilation. The second phase is generally associated with "pushing" and may last as long as 3 hours. The third phase is associated with separation and passage of the placenta.

Pages: 541–543

42: Which of the following Bishop's scores represents a cervix favorable for induction?

    A. 3
    B. 5
    C. 7
    D. 9

Answer: D

Critique: Bishop's scores are used during elective inductions of labor. A scoring system is based on dilation, effacement, station, consistency, and position. A score of 9 or more is favorable for induction.

Page: 543

43: Caution should be used with oxytocin because of its biochemical similarity to:

    A. Prostaglandin E_2
    B. Adrenalin
    C. Antidiuretic hormone
    D. Aldosterone

Answer: C

Critique: Oxytocin is chemically similar to antidiuretic hormone. Prolonged high doses may result in water intoxication.

Page: 544

44: Which of the following is true regarding shoulder dystocia:

    A. Dystocia rarely occurs in normal weight babies.
    B. Advanced maternal age is a risk factor.
    C. Brachial plexus injuries usually result in lifelong disability.
    D. Dystocia requires the Zavanelli maneuver as the initial management technique.

Answer: B

Critique: Although macrosomia, maternal age, and postdate pregnancy are risk factors for dystocia, half of all dystocias occur in normal weight babies. Brachial plexus injuries occur, but most resolve in 6 months. The Zavanelli maneuver (cephalic replacement) is a maneuver of last resort.

Page: 545

45: Match the following to the appropriate statements below

    1. Early decelerations
    2. Late decelerations
    3. Variable decelerations
    4. Accelerations
    5. Sinusoidal patterns

    A. Cord compression
    B. Uteroplacental insufficiency
    C. Severe fetal anemia or hypoxia
    D. Fetal head compression
    E. Forms the basis of the NST

Answers: 1 - D, 2 - B, 3 - A, 4 - E, 5 - C

Critique: Early decelerations are a vagal response to fetal head compression. Late decelerations are worrisome and associated with uteroplacental insufficiency. Variable decelerations are the most common pattern encountered and are related to cord compression, often a nuchal cord. Accelerations are used to assess the NST as reassuring. Sinusoidal patterns are ominous and related to anemia or severe hypoxia.

Pages: 548, 549

46: Complications of epidural anesthesia include all of the following, except:

    A. Hypertension
    B. Spinal headache
    C. Increased need for oxytocin augmentation
    D. Increased rate of cesarean section

Answer: A

Critique: Epidural anesthesia, although generally safe, is occasionally associated with maternal headache and hypotension. It is also associated with increased need for augmentation and operative delivery.

Page: 551

47: The most common indication for amnioinfusion is:

    A. Severe late decelerations
    B. Severe variable decelerations
    C. Severe early decelerations
    E. Chorioamnionitis

Answer: B

Critique: The two most common indications for amnioinfusion are severe variable decelerations and thick meconium. Chorioamnionitis is a contraindication to amnioinfusion.

Page: 551

48: All of the following apply to vacuum extraction deliveries, except:

    A. Anesthesia, preferably epidural, is required.
    B. The bladder should be empty.
    C. The cup should be placed over the sagittal suture, 3 cm from the posterior fontanelle.
    D. Careful inspection of the vagina and cervix should be performed.

Answer: A

Critique: Although all rules for operative delivery apply, vacuum delivery can be accomplished with little to no anesthesia. The perineum should be inspected for lacerations

Page: 554

Chapter 27

Care of the Newborn

A. Steven Wrightson

1: Which of the following statements regarding infant mortality rates is false:

  A. The United States has the lowest infant mortality rate (IMR) among industrialized nations.
  B. The infant mortality rate has been declining in the United States and in 1997 reached an all-time low of 7.1 deaths per 1000.
  C. The infant mortality rate is greater in African Americans than in whites.
  D. The infant mortality rate is declining faster in African Americans than in whites.

Answer: A

Critique: The United States ranks twenty-third among industrialized nations in infant mortality. Progress has been made in lowering the infant mortality rate, which reached a low mark in 1997 at 7.1 deaths per 1000 births. African Americans still have more than twice the rate of infant deaths compared to white Americans (13.7 compared to 6.0); the decline in the infant mortality rate, however, is greater in African Americans than in whites.

Page: 557

2: Which of the following is the leading cause of infant death in the United States:

  A. Premature delivery
  B. Congenital anomalies
  C. Sudden infant death syndrome (SIDS)
  D. Trauma
  E. Respiratory distress syndrome

Answer: B

Critique: The incidence of congenital anomalies is not decreasing, but the number of infants dying from these conditions is. Still, nearly 22% of infant deaths are attributable to congenital anomalies. Premature deliveries account for 10% of all births in the United States and the second highest rate of infant deaths at 13.5%. SIDS deaths have declined dramatically since 1992 in response to recommendation that newborns sleep on their backs rather than prone. Nonetheless, SIDS continues to cause 10% of infant deaths. Respiratory distress syndrome, which may be related to prematurity or conditions that delay surfactant production (such as maternal diabetes), causes 5% of newborn deaths. Finally, trauma accounts for almost 3% of infant deaths.

Pages: 557, 558

3: Which of the following statements concerning the use of preconception folic acid is correct:

  A. The United States Public Health Service and the American Academy of Pediatrics recommend that all women of childbearing capability consume 400 µg of folic acid per day.
  B. Preconception folic acid reduces the risk of neural tube defects by 25%.
  C. Women with a history of a neural tube defect–affected newborn should take 1000 µg of folic acid per day during the 1 month prior to conception, to reduce the risk of a similar anomaly in a subsequent pregnancy.
  D. Women who require more than 400 µg of folic acid daily, the usual amount in a standard multivitamin, may take several multivitamin tablets a day to make up that dose.
  E. Women in the United States are well informed regarding preconception folic acid use to prevent neural tube defects.

Answer: A

Critique: All women capable of becoming pregnant should supplement their diets with 400 µg of folic acid, the amount found in most over-the-counter multivitamins. Because half the pregnancies in the United States are unplanned, adolescent girls to perimenopausal women, both single and married, should take this dose. Preconception folic acid can reduce by half the number of infants born annually with a neural tube defect. Women with a history of a child born with a neural tube defect should take 4000 µg of folic acid daily to prevent a recurrence. Women should not take more than one multivitamin a day, especially if they are anticipating a pregnancy. Although the extra folic acid reduces some birth defects, other vitamins, and particularly vitamin A, may be teratogenic. If a woman needs to take 4000 µg of folic acid a day, a single-component supplement of folic acid should be taken. Women in the United States are not informed and are even less compliant regarding folic acid supplementation. A recent March of Dimes survey showed that 68% of women knew about folic acid, 13% knew taking it prevented birth defects, but only 7% of women knew to take it preconceptually. Women continue to need to hear of the benefits of folic acid.

Page: 557

4: In which of the following cases would you not expect to find symmetric intrauterine growth restriction (IUGR):

A. Trisomy 18
B. Early cytomegalovirus infection
C. Pre-existing hypertension with superimposed preeclampsia
D. Toxoplasmosis infection
E. Fetal alcohol syndrome

Answer: C

Critique: Pre-existing hypertension, even with superimposed preeclampsia, should not result in uteroplacental insufficiency until the third trimester. This premature aging of the placenta leads to asymmetric IUGR. Both CMV infection and toxoplasmosis can affect the development of the central nervous system, resulting in symmetric IUGR. Chromosomal abnormalities, such as trisomy 18, should be suspected in a fetus with symmetric IUGR when no other cause is found. Maternal use of alcohol can have a profound effect on the developing fetus and should also be considered when symmetric IUGR is discovered.

Page: 559

5: Which of the following statements about children born to diabetic mothers is correct:

A. The rate of congenital anomalies in such infants is the same whether the mother has gestational diabetes or diabetes that precedes conception.
B. Macrosomia puts the mother at increased risk for birth trauma but not cesarean delivery.
C. Infants of diabetic mothers are not at risk for small for gestational age (SGA) growth status.
D. Polycythemia can occur in infants of diabetic mothers and should be treated if the hematocrit is greater than 70% in an asymptomatic child or greater than 60% in a symptomatic child.

Answer: D

Critique: Polycythemia can occur in infants of diabetic mothers and can cause nonspecific signs such as poor suck, hypotonia, and plethora. Untreated in a symptomatic child, polycythemia can lead to respiratory distress and other vascular complications, such as persistent pulmonary hypertension of the newborn or venous thrombosis. Congenital anomalies occur more often in women with diabetes that predates conception, because hyperglycemia at conception and during early embryogenesis is teratogenic. Women with gestational diabetes have normal or near normal glucose control during the early stages of fetal development. Macrosomia, defined as an infant weight greater than 4000 grams or higher than the 90th percentile, puts the mother at risk for both birth trauma and cesarean delivery. Infants of diabetic mothers can be large, but they can also be small owing to vascular abnormalities present, particularly with preexisting diabetes.

Page: 561

6: Which of the following represents the birth weight percentile below which a newborn infant is considered small for gestational age (SGA):

A. 10th percentile

B. 15th percentile
C. 20th percentile
D. 25th percentile

Answer: A

Critique: A newborn infant is considered SGA if birth weight falls below the 10th percentile for his or her gestational age. Growth retardation can be symmetric (weight, length, and head circumference all equally affected) or asymmetric (length and head circumference affected less than weight).

Page: 559

7: In examining a normal newborn infant, which of the following configurations would you expect to see for the baby's extremities:

A. Hips fully extended, knees extended, and arms extended
B. Hips flexed, knees extended, and elbows extended
C. Hips extended, knees flexed, and elbows extended
D. Hips, knees, and elbows flexed

Answer: D

Critique: The normal, undisturbed infant should hold his or her hips, knees, and elbows in a flexed configuration.

Page: 562

8: How much weight can a normal newborn be expected to lose during the first week of life:

A. Up to 10% of birth weight
B. Up to 15% of birth weight
C. Up to 20% of birth weight
D. Up to 25% of birth weight

Answer: A

Critique: The normal newborn can lose up to 10% of his or her birth weight during the first week of life.

Page: 562

9: The Ortolani maneuver checks for which of the following musculoskeletal phenomena:

A. Anterior cruciate ligament instability
B. Lateral meniscus tears
C. Direct inguinal hernia
D. Congenital dislocation of the hip

Answer: D

Critique: The Ortolani maneuver consists of abducting the hips while placing the second and third fingers on the femoral heads, with the palms of the hands pressing the femoral shaft toward the mattress. A "clunk" indicates the ability of the infant's femoral head to be dislocated and requires further investigation.

Page: 566

10: A 3600-gram infant is delivered by cesarean section for cephalopelvic disproportion. The initial examination is normal, but over the next several hours the infant develops nasal flaring and grunting. The chest x-ray shows patchy infiltrates. A septic workup is performed, and the infant is placed on 50% oxygen supplementation. Over the next 24 hours, the grunting and flaring resolve and the oxygen is discontinued. Which of the following is the most likely cause of this infant's condition:

A. Respiratory distress syndrome (hyaline membrane disease)
B. Pneumonia owing to chlamydial infection
C. Meconium aspiration syndrome
D. Transient tachypnea of the newborn

Answer: D

Critique: Transient tachypnea of the newborn appears shortly after birth and represents delayed clearance of fluid from the lungs. The transient nature and response to oxygen over 24 hours militate toward this diagnosis rather than toward pneumonia. Chlamydial pneumonia typically occurs at 1 to 3 months of age instead of during the newborn period. The scenario makes no mention of meconium, making meconium aspiration unlikely. The infant's term status makes hyaline membrane disease unlikely.

Pages: 568–570

11: The Apgar score continues to be a useful technique for assessing newborn status. For a newborn with a heart rate of 90, irregular respirations, "glove and booty" cyanosis, weak muscle tone, and a grimace response to irritating stimuli, which of the following Apgar scores would you assign:

A. 3
B. 5
C. 7
D. 9
E. 10

Answer: B

Critique: For an infant who displays a heart rate of 90 and the other described findings, an Apgar score of 5 is appropriate. The Apgar score at 1 and 5 minutes continues to serve as a very important guide to infant resuscitation and should be performed in all newborn infants.

Pages: 571, 573

12: Hyperbilirubinemia is a common newborn metabolic abnormality. A rough clinical correlation exists between the level of hyperbilirubinemia and the infant's level of jaundice. For an infant with facial jaundice but no abdominal or extremity jaundice, which of the following represents a likely bilirubin level:

A. 25 mg/dL
B. 20 mg/dL
C. 15 mg/dL
D. 10 mg/dL
E. 5 mg/dL

Answer: E

Critique: An infant's degree of jaundice bears a rough correlation with the serum bilirubin level. Jaundice visible mainly on the face correlates with a level of 5 mg/dL. Midabdominal jaundice correlates with a bilirubin of 15 mg/dL, and foot sole jaundice correlates with a level of

20 mg/dL. These guidelines are only estimates, and visible jaundice should be investigated with measured bilirubin levels.

Pages: 573–575

13: A healthy appropriate for gestational age infant is delivered with vacuum extraction assistance. The 1 and 5 minute Apgar scores are normal. During your examination in the newborn nursery, you note a fractured left clavicle. Which of the following management strategies should you recommend to the parents:

A. Surgical consultation for anticipated operative repair
B. Placement of a left arm sling
C. Placement of a "figure of 8" clavicle bandage to immobilize the fracture site
D. Advise the parents of the problem and reassure them this will heal with expectant observation

Answer: D

Critique: Fractured clavicles are the most frequently observed birth-related fractures. They usually heal well without specific therapy. The parents should be advised of the injury but reassured that the fracture should heal without active manipulation.

Pages: 575, 576

14: While following the development of a premature infant, which of the following should be used as the point of reference in plotting growth and development:

A. The infant's birth date
B. The infant's due date
C. The infant's birth date minus 2 weeks
D. The infant's due date plus 2 weeks

Answer: B

Critique: In plotting growth and developmental parameters for a premature infant, the clinician should use the infant's due date as the point of reference in charting. Growth charts for premature infants are available and should be used instead of standard growth charts.

Pages: 577, 579

15: Premature infants may require feeding every 2 to 3 hours. How many wet diapers per 24 hours indicates sufficient fluid intake:

A. One to two
B. Two to four
C. Three to five
D. Four to six
E. Six to eight

Answer: E

Critique: The daily frequency of wet diapers can be used to assess the adequacy of infant fluid intake. Six to eight wet diapers per day indicates adequate fluid intake.

Page: 578

16: Which of the following amounts represents the energy requirement for normal growth in newborn infants:

A. 120 kcal/kg/day
B. 100 kcal/kg/day
C. 80 kcal/kg/day
D. 60 kcal/kg/day

Answer: A

Critique: Normal newborn growth requires approximately 120 kcal/kg/day energy intake.

Page: 579

17: A normal newborn infant is being breastfed. The mother gives the child occasional water supplements, but the water supply has no fluoride content. At what age should fluoride supplementation for the infant begin:

A. At birth
B. At 2 weeks of age
C. At 2 months of age
D. At 4 months of age

Answer: B

Critique: Breast milk does not contain significant fluoride. Although this infant also receives occasional tap water, the lack of fluoride content indicates the need for supplementation. The infant should receive 0.25 mg fluoride per day beginning at age 2 weeks.

Page: 581

Chapter 28

Growth and Development

Jada Moore-Ruffin

1: Regarding nutrition in infancy, all of the following statements are true, except:

  A. Human milk is the ideal food for full-term infants during the first 12 months of life and should be promoted by all health care providers caring for children.
  B. Commercial cow's milk and soy-based formulas must contain higher levels of protein to compensate for their lower quality.
  C. The basal metabolic requirements and the energy demands of growth and activity are lowest at birth and increase with age.
  D. Whole cow's milk is not suitable for infants because the higher intake of sodium, potassium, and protein may adversely affect renal clearance.
  E. Whole cow's milk may be a source of blood loss anemia in infants less than 12 months of age.

Answer: C

Critique: It has been well established that human breast milk is the ideal food for infants younger than 1 year of age. Breast milk is well tolerated by virtually all infants, and because it is highly immunopotent with beneficial antibodies and breast-feeding promotes parental bonding, it should be promoted by all who provide health care to children. Commercial cow's milk and soy-based formulas are quite acceptable for mothers who are unable to or choose not to nurse; however, they do contain higher levels of protein to compensate for their lower quality. Whole cow's milk is not suitable for children under 1 year of age because it (a) is too high in sodium, potassium, and proteins for optimal renal clearance; (b) can cause occult gastrointestinal blood loss; and (c) has lower concentrations of iron, zinc, essential fatty acids, and vitamin E and therefore results in deficiencies. Infants require 80 to 120 kcal/kg/day for adequate growth and development during the first months of life; this decreases to 100 kcal/kg/day by 1 year and decreases further to 100 kcal/kg/day for each subsequent 3-year period.

Pages: 591, 592

2: A 27-year-old new mother brings her 2-month-old son in for a well-child routine examination. She reports that he is breast-feeding well, every 2 to 4 hours. The infant's examination is normal, he seems to be well hydrated, and growth and development are appropriate. The mother has some concerns about diet supplementation. Regarding supplementation in infancy, all of the following are true, except:

  A. Breast-fed, full-term infants seldom need iron supplementation before 4 to 6 months of age because of the superior absorption of the iron present in breast milk.
  B. By 3 months of age all infants should have iron-fortified rice cereal or infant formula introduced into their diets because breast milk does not provide enough calories for adequate growth and development.
  C. Breast-fed infants should receive early vitamin D supplementation because breast milk contains only small amounts of vitamin D.
  D. After 6 months of age, fluoride supplementation may be necessary for exclusively breast-fed babies.
  E. Vitamin B_{12} supplementation should be given to breast-fed infants whose mothers are strict vegetarians.

Answer: B

Critique: Human breast milk is actually higher in calories (22 kcal/oz) than most standard infant formulas (20 kcal/oz) and is very adequate caloric intake alone for infants at least up to 6 months of age. Furthermore, solid foods are generally not introduced into the diet until 4 to 6 months of age when the extrusion reflex of early infancy has disappeared and the ability to swallow nonliquid food has become established. Breast-fed infants (as do some formula-fed infants) require nutrient supplementation for optimal nutritional status. These infants should receive 400 IU of vitamin D daily. Also, they should get 1 mg/kg/day of elemental iron. Children 6 months to 3 years of age who do not drink fluoridated water may be given 0.25 mg/day of supplemental fluoride.

Page: 593

3: Which of the following statements is true regarding iron deficiency anemia in adolescents?

  A. Girls are more at risk of developing iron-deficiency anemia than are boys.
  B. Boys are more at risk of developing iron-deficiency anemia than are girls.
  C. Girls and boys share the same risk of developing iron-deficiency anemia.
  D. Neither boys nor girls in this age group are at significant risk for iron-deficiency anemia.

Answer: C

Critique: Adolescents in general are at risk for multiple nutritional deficiencies, including iron, calcium, vitamins

A and C, and sometimes even calories, as a result of their poor eating habits. Boys and girls share the same risk of iron-deficiency anemia, in part because of their greater increase in lean body mass and blood volume.

Page: 594

Using the stem below choose the single best answer for the following sequence of questions 4 to 7.

4: A 4-year-old Asian boy is in for a routine examination. Both parents are present and are concerned that "since birth, his height has been low on the growth chart." Although most people on both sides of their families are considered to be of less than average height, they question if something may be wrong. After careful examination, you determine that history, physical examination, and development are all within normal limits except that he has consistently plotted slightly below the 5th percentile for height. Weight has always been at the 25th percentile.

    A. This child most likely has a growth hormone deficiency.
    B. This child most likely is malnourished.
    C. This child most likely has been plotted incorrectly on the chart.
    D. This child most likely is normal considering his family background.

5: What is the most reasonable next step in this child's work-up?

    A. Begin growth hormone injections to stimulate height growth.
    B. Calculate the midparental height and then plot the corrected height percentile, followed by bone age studies.
    C. Order a series of lab tests to rule out malnourishment and endocrinopathy.
    D. Refer child to an endocrinologist for further evaluation.

6: This child's most likely diagnosis is:

    A. Familial short stature
    B. Constitutional growth delay
    C. Malnutrition
    D. Hormonal endocrinopathy

7: A normal bone age confirms your diagnosis. What can you tell the parents about this child's onset of puberty?

    A. Onset of puberty will be late.
    B. Onset of puberty will be early.
    C. Onset of puberty will be at an appropriate time.
    D. Onset of puberty is not expected without treatment.

Answers: 4 - D, 5 - B, 6 - A, 7 - C

Critique: The child most likely has familial short stature as indicated by his family history, growth curve (consistently on a normal curve below the 5th percentile), and bone age studies consistent with his chronological age. Midparental heights can be obtained by taking the average of both parents' heights, after adding 13 cm to the mother's height for boys and subtracting 13 cm from the

father's height for girls. After correction, these children usually will fall closer to the mean height percentile for age. These children will reach puberty at an appropriate time.

Pages: 584, 585

8: Regarding puberty in girls, all of the following statements are true, except:

    A. The first sign of puberty is breast bud development.
    B. Early menstrual cycles may be irregular and anovulatory.
    C. Girls continue to grow in height velocity after menarche.
    D. Girls generally have onset of puberty 2 years sooner than boys.
    E. Until menstrual cycles become regular, girls are presumed to be infertile.

Answer: E

Critique: Girls will almost always have irregular menses within the first year after menarche. This is a normal occurrence as the ovulation pattern becomes regulated. Nevertheless, the adolescent should be cautioned that pregnancy might still occur, despite menstrual irregularities.

Pages: 589, 590

9: Regarding puberty in boys, all of the following statements are true, except:

    A. Head, hands, and feet tend to reach their adult size first, followed by leg and trunk length.
    B. Change in voice is one of the first signs of puberty.
    C. Boys tend to gain greater muscle strength than do girls.
    D. Some boys may have enlargement of one or both breasts.

Answer: B

Critique: In boys, puberty begins with an increase in growth of the testes and scrotum, with reddening and wrinkling of the scrotal skin. Pubic hair growth then occurs within 6 months, followed by phallic enlargement and peak height velocity. Following the attainment of peak height velocity, boys develop mature spermatozoa, full facial hair, and voice change. However, breaking of the voice is a late and often gradual process.

Pages: 589, 590

10: A 3-week-old female who weighs 8 lb 4 oz consumes 3 oz of iron-fortified infant formula every 4 hours on average. You can reliably counsel the mother that this infant:

    A. Has adequate caloric intake for appropriate growth and development
    B. Has inadequate caloric intake for appropriate growth and development
    C. Has excess caloric intake required for appropriate growth and development

D. Based on the information given, you are unable to comment on this child's caloric intake and growth

Answer: A

Critique: This infant has adequate caloric intake for appropriate growth and development. Using the rule of thumb for growth guidelines in children, this infant is expected to gain 1 kg/mo (0.5 to 1 oz/day) during the first 13 months of life. She should do this by taking in 80 to 120 kcal/kg/day in the first months of life. This child, at 3.75 kg/day, takes in approximately six 3 oz bottles per day at 20 kcal/oz of standard formula. Therefore, she is meeting her daily basal metabolic needs by taking in 96 kcal/kg/day.

Pages: 590–593

Questions 11 to 15: Match the following developmental theories with the associated clinical application. Each choice may be used once, more than once, or not at all.

A. Normative approach (development as maturation)
B. Psychosexual/psychoanalytic (development as resolution of conflict)
C. Behaviorism/social learning (development as learning)
D. Constructivist views (development as cognitive change)
E. Ecologic system (development as cultural/ecologic adaptation)

11: A child's needs must be considered in the context of his or her family and environment.

12: Interpersonal relationships, especially with primary caregivers, influence adjustment, functioning, and self-concept.

13: Children possess an innate drive to learn.

14: Children imitate what they see, so environmental models are important to learning.

15: Basis for age norms for developmental milestones commonly used in the clinical setting.

Answers: 11 - E, 12 - B, 13 - D, 14 - C, 15 -A

Critique: A general understanding of the common theories of child development can enrich the clinician's relationship with young patients. A brief summary of the salient features and proponents of each theory follows:

Normative (Gesell) approach: Behavior depends on neurologic and physical maturation; universal progression of developmental sequence; minimal rule of environment/temperament

Psychosexual/psychoanalytic (Freud, Erikson) approach: Emotional life exerts a strong influence on development and behavior; unconscious conflict between biologic drive and social expectations continuously shapes behavior and self-concept

Behaviorism/social learning (Pavlov, Skinner, Bandura) approach: Behavior, but not its underlying influences and motives, can be studied and changed; environmental stimuli are the major forces shaping development and behavior

Constructivist views (Piaget) approach: Cognitive development depends on both nature and nurture; children use their physical and mental abilities to observe and act on their environment

Ecologic system (Bronfenbrenner) approach: A set of interrelated systems; development is determined by interactions of child and family

Pages: 595, Table 28–6

Choosing from the selections below, match the age with the following developmental milestones. Each choice may be used once, more than once, or not at all.

A. 12 months
B. 15 months
C. 18 months
D. 24 months
E. 36 months

16: Speech 75% intelligible to strangers, alternates feet climbing stairs, counts three objects

17: Listens to story with pictures, can form 2- or 3-word sentences, kicks ball, speech 50% intelligible

18: Drinks from a cup, can place pellet in a bottle, makes symbolic gestures

19: Sits on small chair alone, tower of four cubes, feeds self with utensils, points to one body part

20: Follows 1-step commands without gestures, spontaneously stacks two cubes, walks backward

Answers: 16 - E, 17 - D, 18 - A, 19 - C, 20 -B

Criteria: Key times for formal screening include age 15 to 18 months, when limited expressive vocabulary may signal a need for evaluation and intervention of hearing, language, and global delays, and age 3 years, when more sophisticated language and cognitive skills develop.

Pages: 598–599, Table 28–9

Questions 21 to 25: Answer true or false for the following statements.

21: Persons receiving the varicella vaccine should not become pregnant within 1 month following immunization.

22: The child of a mother who is currently pregnant should not receive the MMR vaccine until after the delivery.

23: Children who are currently taking antibiotics should not be immunized with any vaccine until they have completed the antibiotic course.

24: Premature children should receive their immunizations in smaller dosages than normal, full-term infants.

25: An infant with a family history of convulsions should not receive the DTaP vaccine.

Answers: 21 - True, 22 - False, 23 - False, 24 - False, 25 - False

Critique: Immunizations are a critical part of pediatric and adult preventive care. Therefore, it is necessary to be familiar with immunization schedules, indications and contraindications, and side effects. Many myths exist regarding vaccinations; thus, patient education is essential to facilitate appropriate immunity in both children and adults.

Pages: 601–606

Chapter 29

Childhood and Adolescence

Peter G. Gosselink

1: (True or False) Appropriate anticipatory guidance for parents and their children includes:

   A. Encouraging children to get 30 minutes of exercise per day

   B. Encouraging parents to closely monitor their children's television viewing and Internet access

   C. Discouraging parents from using corporal punishment

   D. Encouraging parents to use syrup of ipecac and activated charcoal in any potential poison ingestion

Answers: A - True, B - True, C - True, D - False

Critique: Children, like adults, need exercise. Evidence has shown that if children witness parental involvement in exercise, sustained and adequate amounts of physical activity throughout childhood and adolescence are seen.

As children become increasingly more sophisticated in their ability to access modern technology, it is imperative that parents retain a direct supervisory role. In addition, there is a direct correlation between the amount of video viewing and obesity.

Although much controversy has been generated about the best methods for disciplining children, the preponderance of evidence suggests that corporal punishment is ineffective as a primary means of discipline and is potentially detrimental to childhood development and health. Parents, therefore, should be asked about punishment techniques and offered alternatives to corporal punishment.

Last, the parents of toddlers and young children should carefully examine their house and safety-proof any lower cabinets that contain poisonous cleansers and other substances. Syrup of ipecac and activated charcoal should be available in the home. These substances, however, should be used only in accordance with the recommendations of a poison control center. The number for this agency should be clearly posted next to telephones.

Pages: 615, 616

2: A father brings his 3-year-old son to the office. The father reports a 2-day history of increased irritability, poor sleeping, fever (up to 103°F rectal), and the child pulling at his left ear. Pneumatic otoscopy is performed and reveals a bulging tympanic membrane with obscured bony landmarks on the left. The diagnosis of acute otitis media is made. Which of the following is the most likely pathogen:

   A. *Haemophilus influenzae*

   B. *Streptococcus pyogenes*

   C. *Streptococcus pneumoniae*

   D. *Moraxella catarrhalis*

Answer: C

Critique: All of these organisms are pathogens associated with otitis media; however, *Streptococcus pneumoniae* is the most prevalent organism in children of all ages. *Haemophilus influenzae* and *Moraxella catarrhalis* are also important pathogens. Other bacteria, including group A streptococci, are less often isolated. Although viral infections are thought to predispose children to middle ear infections, viruses are much less important as pathogens in this condition.

Pages: 617, 618

3: The child discussed in question 2 returns to the clinic in 2 weeks. The physician had prescribed an antibiotic and given the father instructions about symptomatic care. The father reports that the child's fever and other symptoms resolved 3 days after the antibiotics were started. The child has been feeling and behaving normally since this time; however, on examination, an effusion is still present in the left ear. Which of the following is the best management strategy in this case:

   A. Assume that the treatment was ineffective, and switch to a more broad-spectrum antibiotic

   B. Repeat a course of the same antibiotic, but extend the treatment time

   C. Repeat a course of the same antibiotic, but increase the dose

   D. Schedule a follow-up visit for 2 months, with the understanding that if the child has recurrence of symptoms, earlier follow-up is needed

Answer: D

Critique: Residual effusions after treatment of otitis media are common, and up to 70% of children still have effusion present at 2 weeks. For this reason, it would be inappropriate to change antibiotics solely on the presence of an effusion. Most experts recommend that follow-up examination in a patient with a satisfactory clinical response to antibiotic therapy be delayed until about 2 months after treatment. Any child who still has symptoms should be seen when they occur. It is inappropriate, therefore, to make antibiotic changes at this stage, making answers A, B, and C incorrect.

125

Page: 618

4: A 7-year-old previously healthy female is brought to the office by her mother. The mother and child report a 3-day history of mild sore throat, fever, headaches, and general malaise, followed 2 days later by increasing mouth and throat discomfort and the appearance of a rash on the child's hands and feet. Physical examination is most notable for ulcerations of the buccal mucosa and papulovesicular lesions on the palms of the hands and the soles of the feet. The most likely cause of these findings is:

    A. Echovirus 16
    B. Coxsackievirus A16
    C. Adenovirus I47
    D. Epstein-Barr virus (EBV)

Answer: B

Critique: All of these pathogens are known to cause oral and pharyngeal lesions; however, the constellation of findings seen in this patient is pathognomonic for Coxsackievirus A16 infections, the virus responsible for hand-foot-and-mouth disease.

It is important to realize that viruses cause more than 80% of all pharyngitis. A sore throat is often one of several symptoms associated with a viral upper respiratory tract infection. Occasionally, the sore throat is the predominant symptom. Vesicles or small ulcers on the tonsillar pillar or soft palate suggest herpangina, which is also due to Coxsackievirus or can be caused by echoviruses. Infectious mononucleosis, caused by EBV, may cause a sore throat and petechial lesions on the soft palate. Adenoviruses may cause an exudative pharyngitis with or without other symptoms of nasal discharge and cough, particularly in younger children. Echoviruses, EBV, and adenoviruses, however, do not have the skin lesions associated with hand-foot-and-mouth disease.

Pages: 618, 619

5: (True or False) A 3-year-old male toddler is brought to the office by his mother who is concerned about her son's appetite and growth. The mother reports that the child was "hungry all the time" for the first 2 years of life but now eats much more sporadically. The mother tries to stick to three well-balanced meals a day, and mealtime seems to always be a period of conflict. She also states that she feels that his rate of growth has slowed. The child's height and weight are recorded and place the child in the 50th percentile for both height and weight, consistent with the child's growth for the first 2 years of life. Appropriate counseling includes:

    A. Advising the mother to continue with the three meals a day, reassuring her that the child will soon become accustomed to this routine
    B. Showing the mother the patient's plotted growth chart
    C. Educating the mother that frequent meals and snacks are often necessary and provide adequate caloric intake
    D. Educating the mother that attention to the overall caloric intake is generally sufficient to meet the daily requirements for all nutrients

Answers: A - False, B - True, C - True, D - False

Critique: Appetite normally decreases in the second year of life coincident with the normal slowing of the growth rate. Children aged 2 to 5 years have great variability in caloric intake from meal to meal. Parents should be forewarned about these changes to prevent mealtime from being a period of conflict.

For children between the ages of 1 and 10, attention to the four basic food groups (not caloric intake) is needed to meet the daily requirements for all nutrients. Children usually prefer finger foods and single food items to combination foods. In addition, frequent meals and snacks are often necessary because of a child's limited gastric capacity.

The height and weight of children should be recorded at least yearly after the age of 2. The height and weight measurements should be plotted on the standard growth curves and reviewed with the parents. As an example, most parents find that visualizing the tracking of height over time helps them understand how their child can be shorter than other children of the same age and still be growing normally.

Pages: 609, 610

6: A small-town physician is called late one night. A concerned parent states that her 4-year-old child has had a "barking" cough for the last 2 days. The child has also had a subjective low-grade fever. The symptoms began 2 nights ago and seem to be worse in the evening hours. The parent states that her child does not appear to have labored breathing, but the persistent cough is worrisome. The physician makes the preliminary diagnosis of croup. Which of the following is reasonable advice at this time:

    A. Place the child in the bathroom with the shower running and call the physician back in 1 hour to report the child's condition
    B. Rush the child to the emergency room, because croup can rapidly progress to respiratory failure
    C. Keep the child inside, because outside air often exacerbates the symptoms
    D. If the family has a home nebulizer, give the child a trial of nebulized albuterol and call the physician back in 1 hour

Answer: A

Critique: Croup (or laryngotracheobronchitis) is a relatively common syndrome in children. The vast majority of cases are mild and do not require hospitalization. Symptoms typically begin at night and recur nightly for several days. Symptoms are often improved by humidified air. It is possible for croup to lead to respiratory failure; however, the history in this case does not suggest that such failure is imminent. Outside air actually improves symptoms in most cases, particularly the crisp, cold air of winter. Nebulized albuterol is generally ineffective in croup.

Page: 619

7: All of the following are true about croup, except:

A. It typically occurs in children aged 1 to 5, with a peak incidence during the second year of life.

B. Children with this condition are typically afebrile.

C. For children with respiratory compromise, inpatient admission for nebulized racemic epinephrine, oxygen, and systemic corticosteroids are indicated.

D. Croup is most commonly caused by influenza virus.

Answer: D

Critique: The most common cause of croup is the parainfluenza virus (not the influenza virus), accounting for up to 80% of the cases. Croup typically affects children aged 1 to 5, with a peak incidence during the second year of life. Children are usually afebrile. Racemic epinephrine, oxygen supplementation, and systemic corticosteroids have been shown to have beneficial effects in treating the more severe cases.

Page: 619

8: Which of the following statements about vision screening in children is true:

A. Objective evaluation of vision should begin at age 2 years.

B. Visual acuity should reach 20/20 by the age of 3 or 4.

C. Squinting during testing is acceptable and represents a normal compensatory technique during vision development.

D. A difference between the right and left eye of more than one line on the chart is significant and should lead to further testing.

Answer: D

Critique: Evaluation of vision in children younger than 3 years is generally based on subjective reports by the parent. More formal testing should begin routinely at age 3, not 2. Visual acuity may normally be in the 20/30 to 20/40 range at age 3 or 4 and should improve to 20/20 by the age of 6 or 7. Squinting during testing, which creates a pinhole aperture, suggests the presence of an uncorrected refractive error. This is not a normal variation and should prompt further investigation.

Allen cards, which have pictures of easily recognized items such as a telephone and a tree, can be used to test the visual acuity of children around 3 and 4 years of age. Once a child can read letters or numbers, acuity can easily be determined with the Snellen chart. A difference between the right and left eye of more than one line on the chart is significant and should lead to further evaluation.

Page: 613

9: A mother, having recently moved to town, brings her 2-year-old son to the local family physician for a well-child examination. Being the thorough physician that he is, the doctor questions the mother about the child's dental history. The mother states that she has never taken her son to the dentist, but wipes the child's mouth with a rag after each meal. All of the following are important education and counseling points, except:

A. Children should be encouraged to brush their own teeth at the age of 2 to 3 years.

B. By the age of 4, most children have the manual dexterity required to brush satisfactorily without supervision.

C. Flossing is difficult for children, and parents should take responsibility for flossing when there is tight contact between adjacent teeth.

D. Routine dental appointments should begin at age 2 to 3 years and are recommended twice yearly.

Answer: B

Critique: Primary dentition is usually complete by the age of 2 years. The permanent teeth generally begin erupting around age 6 to 7 years and are complete through the second molars by age 12 or 13. Most children lack the manual dexterity to brush satisfactorily until the age of 6; for this reason, parental supervision is essential until this level of dexterity is reached. Therefore, children should be encouraged to brush their own teeth starting at the age of 2 or 3, but the parents should take an active role in brushing and flossing for several years. Routine dental appointments should begin at age 2 to 3 and are recommended twice yearly by pediatric dentists.

Page: 613

10: A father brings his 3-year-old daughter to the emergency room. He states that she has had a fever for the last 2 days, has had a decreased appetite, and complains of abdominal discomfort. A thorough evaluation is performed, but no fever source is clearly evident. The results of a bagged urine specimen are ambiguous, and the decision is made to collect a catheterized specimen. This specimen displays 40 to 50 white blood cells per high-power field. The presumptive diagnosis of UTI is made, and the urine is sent for culture. The father states that his daughter has never had a urinary infection before. The most likely organism to grow from this culture is:

A. *E. coli*

B. Klebsiella species

C. Proteus species

D. *Staphylococcus saprophyticus*

Answer: A

Critique: Up to 90% of first infections are caused by *E. coli*. Other bacteria that may cause UTI in children include Klebsiella species, Proteus species, *S. saprophyticus*, and enterococci. The clinical features of UTI in children are dependent on the age of the child. This case is representative of most presentations in toddlers, who have mostly nonspecific symptoms. Preschool children may have discomfort and secondary enuresis in addition to fever and abdominal pain. Older children are more likely to have the "classic" symptoms of UTI, including frequency, urgency, and dysuria. As discussed in this scenario, appropriate collection of a urine specimen in a child is difficult. Bagged urine is generally contaminated and can be considered reliable only if the specimen is sterile.

Pages: 621, 622

11: (True or False) Further investigation of children with UTI is warranted in:

    A. All males with their first UTI
    B. All females with their first UTI
    C. All females with repeat infections
    D. All females with clinical evidence of pyelonephritis, irrespective of the number of infections

Answers: A - True, B - False, C - True, D - True

Critique: The recommended further evaluation of children with UTI is contingent on several factors. All males with a first UTI and females with repeat infections or clinical evidence of pyelonephritis or growth retardation should be further evaluated. The test of first choice is a voiding cystourethrogram (VCUG) obtained 4 to 6 weeks after treatment of the acute infection. The renal structure should also be evaluated with intravenous pyelography or ultrasound. The finding of significant reflux or obstructive uropathy should prompt referral to a urologist.

Pages: 621, 622

12: The most common pathogen in bronchiolitis is:

    A. Coxsackievirus
    B. Respiratory syncytial virus (RSV)
    C. Parainfluenza virus
    D. Influenza virus

Answer: B

Critique: Bronchiolitis is a syndrome that occurs in small children and is unusual after the age of 2. It is generally viral in origin, and RSVs have been implicated in a large proportion of cases. Symptoms typically seen in bronchiolitis include expiratory wheezing (with or without tachypnea), air trapping, and substernal retractions.

Page: 619

13: A 3-year-old female presents for a well-child examination. The child's mother reports no present concerns. Past medical history includes one episode of bronchiolitis at age 8 months that required hospitalization for 2 days, but it is otherwise unremarkable. Family history includes a brother with asthma and a father who suffers from seasonal allergies (allergic rhinitis). Physical examination is unremarkable except for dry, flaking skin involving the flexural surfaces of the antecubital and popliteal fossae, the wrists, and the area around the neck and face. When asked about this, the mother states, "She's always had dry skin." The most likely diagnosis is:

    A. Contact dermatitis
    B. Psoriasis
    C. Atopic dermatitis
    D. Tinea

Answer: C

Critique: Atopic dermatitis is a chronic condition that is characterized by dry, eczematous skin in a typical distribution. It is often found in association with a personal or family history of other atopic disorders, including allergic rhinitis and asthma. Atopic dermatitis typically begins during infancy, but it is occasionally seen in older children. By childhood, the rash most commonly involves the areas seen in this case.

Pages: 620, 621

14: The most common complication of atopic dermatitis is:

    A. Secondary fungal infections
    B. Secondary bacterial infections
    C. Secondary viral infections
    D. Scarring from lesions

Answer: B

Critique: The most common complication of atopic dermatitis is secondary bacterial infection of affected areas. The infections are usually caused by staphylococcal or streptococcal species. Systemic antibiotics may be necessary to clear up inflammatory lesions that have become secondarily infected.

Page: 621

15: Gastroenteritis is a common problem in children. Which of the following statements concerning gastroenteritis is true:

    A. In small children, most infections occur via the respiratory droplet route.
    B. Children attending day care centers are more likely to suffer bouts of gastroenteritis.
    C. Most cases are caused by bacteria, including *Campylobacter*, *Shigella*, and *Salmonella*.
    D. In children older than 2 years, hospitalization is usually required to maintain adequate hydration.

Answer: B

Critique: Most cases of gastroenteritis in small children occur via the fecal-oral route, not via respiratory droplets. Not surprisingly, data have shown an increased likelihood of gastroenteritis in children attending day care centers. When sought, a pathogen can be found in about half of cases, and approximately 80% of the pathogens identified are viral, not bacterial. In particular, rotavirus has been implicated as a major cause of gastroenteritis in children. *Campylobacter*, *Shigella*, and *Salmonella* have been implicated as the causative agents in gastroenteritis in children; however, they do represent the most common causes. Most cases of gastroenteritis in children older than 2 years are not severe and can be managed without medical intervention, often over the telephone. In an otherwise healthy child, putting the bowel at rest with clear liquids for 24 to 48 hours is generally sufficient. Oral rehydration solutions have been used successfully in the United States as well as in Third World nations. These solutions can be recommended for moderately dehydrated children.

Page: 621

16: (True or False) Additional accurate statements concerning gastroenteritis include:

    A. Diarrhea and abdominal pain of nonviral etiology usually require antibiotic therapy.
    B. *Campylobacter* is the most common bacterial cause of childhood diarrhea.

C. *Shigella* is one of the bacteria associated with bloody diarrhea.

D. *Escherichia coli* 0157:H7 infections usually follow a benign course.

E. Giardia is another example of a bacterial cause of gastroenteritis in children.

Answers: A - False, B - True, C - True, D - False, E - False

Critique: Diarrhea and abdominal pain of nonviral etiology generally resolve without antibiotic therapy. *Campylobacter* is now the most common bacterial cause of childhood diarrhea. Most episodes are of short duration, and although the abdominal pain may be substantial, no therapy is indicated. Prolonged courses with a positive culture should be treated with erythromycin. *Shigella* is one of the infections associated with bloody diarrhea. Oral ampicillin or trimethoprim-sulfamethoxazole (Bactrim) shortens the duration of symptoms and lessens the period of infectivity to others and therefore should be used in treatment. Of recent concern are outbreaks of *E. coli* 0157:H7, which can result in fulminant infections, including bloody diarrhea, hypotension, and even death. Contaminated well water and food products have been shown to harbor this pathogen. Careful hand washing and adequate cooking of meat should eliminate the potential for infection. Giardia is a common organism found in children with diarrhea, but it is a protozoan infection, not a bacterial one.

Page: 621

17: A 13-year-old female comes to the office for a routine examination by the physician who has seen her since she was 3 years old. The doctor and the patient have always had a good relationship; however, the girl's mother has always accompanied the child during previous visits and has been present during all history taking and physical examinations. The 13-year-old has not been to the office in 3 to 4 years. Which of the following is *not* true about this patient encounter:

A. The physician must realize that, in some situations, the adolescent patient is distrustful of the physician.

B. It is often helpful to see the patient with the parent(s) for part of the visit and then alone.

C. Explain to the parents that issues discussed with the adolescent in private will be held confidential, no matter what the content.

D. The time alone with the adolescent should be used for more topics, such as sexuality and concerns about growth and development.

Answer: C

Critique: It is true that medical visits by adolescents are frequently more emotionally charged than are visits by younger children. The family physician must be aware of this and adapt his or her care in appropriate ways. Unconditional confidentiality is usually not possible, because certain information revealed to the physician may not be legally withheld from the parents or other authorities. That is, the protection of information discussed does not apply in life-threatening situations, such as for a suicidal adolescent. The other options present valid points and strategies to use when treating adolescent patients.

Pages: 622, 632

18: Which of the following is not true about care of adolescents:

A. By most criteria, adolescents are a healthy group with low morbidity and mortality.

B. Adolescents are more likely to be uninsured than any other age group in the United States.

C. Adolescents generally express little concern about their health.

D. Concerns of adolescents focus not only on medical problems but also on issues regarding interpersonal relationships, sexuality, substance abuse, and anxiety.

Answer: C

Critique: By most criteria, adolescents are a healthy group with low morbidity and mortality; however, adolescents themselves report much greater concern about their health than might be expected. In short, adolescents see themselves as needing more comprehensive professional care than they typically have access to. One of the barriers to adolescents receiving health care is economic. They are more likely to be uninsured than any other age group in the United States. Other barriers include issues of confidentiality (and the physician's previous alignment with the patient's family) as well as legal and ethical issues.

Page: 622

19: A 14-year-old male comes to the office for a routine examination. After seeing them and discussing the patient's past and present medical history with his mother in the room, the physician asks the mother to leave the room. The adolescent's history was unremarkable, and he has no chronic illnesses. Now alone in the examination room, the 14-year-old male begins to express concern about his sexual maturity. He states that he is shorter than most of his friends, that he is very shy in the locker room (particularly because he has noticed mild enlargement of his breasts), and that most of the girls he is interested in are taller and more "mature looking" than he is. Physical examination reveals mild enlargement of testicles; sparse, long, straight hair at the base of the penis; and mild gynecomastia. Appropriate counseling includes all of the following, except:

A. Although the changes of puberty tend to follow a predictable sequence, the onset and rapidity of the changes are extremely variable.

B. In males, the first sign of puberty is testicular enlargement.

C. The growth spurt in males occurs soon after the onset of puberty.

D. Nearly two thirds of boys have gynecomastia at Tanner stage 2.

Answer: C

Critique: The first sign of puberty in males is testicular enlargement, which typically begins between ages 9.5 and 13.5 years. The growth spurt in males occurs late in puberty, at around Tanner stage 4. Therefore, males start puberty after females and their growth spurt occurs later in puberty. It should be noted, however, that more than 95% have resolution of gynecomastia by the end of puberty. Bear in mind that patients who are preoccupied with changes in their bodies and are concerned about being examined generally benefit the most from information provided by physicians regarding normal developmental processes.

Pages: 623, 624

20: A 15-year-old male presents to the office with a complaint of increasing acne. The patient states that he has had mild acne since the age of 13 but that it has recently worsened. Physical examination reveals a well-nourished, well-developed (Tanner stage 4), extremely shy Caucasian male. The patient has multiple papules and pustules on his face, many of which appear inflamed. In addition, he has multiple inflammatory, nodulocystic lesions, particularly on his back and upper chest. The rest of the examination is unremarkable. The patient states that he has used several over-the-counter medications without success. Which of the following statements is true:

- A. Acne affects approximately 50% of teenagers.
- B. This patient's acne is likely the result of poor hygiene.
- C. Acne often poses a serious medical risk.
- D. This patient's demeanor is potentially associated with his acne.
- E. The etiology of acne is poorly understood.

Answer: D

Critique: Acne affects up to 85% of all teenagers. Although acne poses no serious medical risk, the psychological effects of inflammatory lesions can be devastating. It is not uncommon for adolescents to be socially inhibited secondary to acne. This point emphasizes the fact that acne warrants adequate attention. The etiology of acne is well understood. Androgenic hormones stimulate the proliferation of sebaceous glands. Skin bacteria that release lipases and other substances colonize these glands. These enzymes act on the sebum to release free fatty acids, which cause inflammation in the dermis and act with other substances to produce abnormal keratinization of the glandular ducts. Although good hygiene can help to improve acne, it is not the sole etiological factor.

Page: 631

21: All of the following are true concerning acne, except:

- A. *Propionibacterium acnes* commonly colonizes sebaceous glands in cases of acne.
- B. Noninflammatory comedones can be treated with a topical keratolytic agent alone.
- C. Benzoyl peroxide and isotretinoin are both examples of topical keratolytic agents.

- D. When inflammatory lesions are present, topical antibiotics should generally be tried before systemic antibiotics are used.

Answer: C

Critique: Treatment of acne is directed by an understanding of the pathogenesis of this disease. *P. acnes* is one of the organisms most often implicated in colonization of sebaceous glands. Additionally, noninflammatory comedones can be treated with a topical keratolytic agent alone. Examples of topical keratolytic agents are benzoyl peroxide and retinoic acid, but not isotretinoin. Isotretinoin is a systemic medication reserved for severe cystic acne that has the potential for long-term scarring. Substantiated concerns regarding this drug's teratogenicity mitigate against its use in adolescent females. Additionally, regular monitoring of laboratory parameters (including liver and lipid profiles) is required when this drug is prescribed. Last, most physicians treat acne with a topical antibiotic such as tetracycline, erythromycin, or clindamycin and reserve systemic antibiotics for unresponsive cases.

Page: 631

22: Which of the following statements about scoliosis is true?

- A. Scoliosis is typically a result of an underlying medical problem.
- B. Congenital abnormalities of the spine are responsible for a large majority of cases.
- C. Management of scoliosis depends on the sexual maturity rating (Tanner stage) of the adolescent.
- D. Specific exercises have proved to halt the progression of scoliosis.

Answer: C

Critique: Of cases of scoliosis, 70% are idiopathic, particularly in females. Congenital abnormalities of the spine, including occult spina bifida or hemivertebrae, account for less than 10% of cases. Management of scoliosis depends on the degree of the curve, as well as the sexual maturity rating of the adolescent. Teenagers in early Tanner stages may require closer follow-up, because scoliosis tends to progress during the growth spurt. Exercises are of no proven benefit to halt the progression of scoliosis, although lower back exercises may strengthen muscles that easily fatigue.

Pages: 631, 632

23: A 13-year-old male presents to the office complaining of intermittent left knee pain over the past 3 months, which is exacerbated by activity (e.g., repetitive activities such as running in soccer or climbing stairs) and relieved by periods of rest. He states that he thinks he may have had mild trauma to the left knee, but he is uncertain of the timing. Physical examination reveals soft-tissue swelling and tenderness over the tibial tubercle on the left. Bilateral knee joint examinations are within normal limits. Sexual development is estimated at Tanner stage 2. The rest of the physical examination is within normal limits. The most likely diagnoses is:

A. Stress fracture of the left tibia
B. Osgood-Schlatter disease
C. Avulsion of left medial meniscus
D. Legg-Calvé-Perthes disease
E. Overuse syndrome

Answer: B

Critique: Osgood-Schlatter disease is a painful swelling of the tibial tubercle at the insertion of the infrapatellar tendon. It is a common problem, particularly in males in the early pubertal stages. The pain is typically aggravated by activity and relieved by rest. Physical examination reveals soft-tissue swelling and tenderness over the tibial tubercle. The constellation of history and physical examination findings in this patient are typical for this condition.

Page: 632

24: All of the following are true about suicide and depression in adolescents, except:

A. Suicide is the third leading cause of death in adolescents.
B. Male adolescents (compared with female adolescents) are more likely to complete a suicide attempt.
C. Female adolescents (compared with male adolescents) are more likely to make a suicidal gesture.
D. Adolescents typically have depressive symptoms similar to those found in adults.
E. Suicide attempts in adolescents generally occur in the setting of chronic stress.

Answer: D

Critique: It is important to remember that a depressed adolescent may have symptoms different from those of the adult with typical depression. An older adolescent may have the classic vegetative signs of depression and report low self-esteem, whereas depression in a younger adolescent may be marked by acting-out behavior, excessive anger, a decrease in school performance, or new drug use. For developmental reasons, young adolescents are often unable to articulate their troubles.

Page: 632

25: (True or False) Criteria for the diagnosis of anorexia nervosa include:

A. Amenorrhea
B. Refusal to maintain minimum body weight at 85% of that expected
C. Intense fear of gaining weight
D. A ritualistic exercise history
E. Binge eating followed by self-induced vomiting
F. Onset of disease at younger than 25 years

Answers: A - False, B - True, C - True, D - False, E - False, F - True

Critique: Criteria for the diagnosis of anorexia nervosa include a refusal to maintain minimum body weight at 85% of that expected, an intense fear of gaining weight, a disturbance in body image, onset of disease at younger than 25 years, and no other illness that could account for the weight loss. Other commonly associated findings include amenorrhea, a ritualistic exercise history, and excessive preoccupation with food; however, these findings are not diagnostic criteria. This illness is far more common in females than in males and occasionally coexists with bulimia. Bulimia, unlike anorexia nervosa, is characterized by episodic binge eating followed by self-induced vomiting, use of laxatives, and often abdominal pain.

Pages: 632, 633

Chapter 30

Behavioral Problems in Children and Adolescents

Robert L. Keith

1: (True or False) Well-child visits should be limited to thorough, multisystemic examination and immunization updates; behavioral assessment should be dealt with when more time is available.

Answer: False

Critique: Because it is common for parents to bring a child to the family physician for behavioral problems, addressing behavioral issues is important during the well-child visit.

Page: 635

2: (True or False) Rates of childhood depression and suicide are roughly the same as they have been in recent years and are estimated to remain so for the next 10 years.

Answer: False

Critique: The rates of the psychosocial problems have been rising in recent years throughout Western culture, and it is anticipated that the problems will make up an increased proportion of patient care.

Page: 635

3: (True or False) As children get older, the amount of REM sleep gradually decreases and deep non-REM sleep drops off significantly.

Answer: True

Critique: Children have large quantities of very deep sleep that lessens as they get older.

Pages: 635–636

4: From the age of 1 week to 9 years, the typical child's need for sleep:

    A. Increases by about 5%
    B. Increases by about 1%
    C. Decreases by about 10%
    D. Decreases by about 40%

Answer: D

Critique: The total daily sleep requirements decrease from 16.5 hours at 1 week of age to 14 hours by age 1 year, 13 hours by age 2, 12 hours by age 3, 11 hours by age 5, and 10 hours by age 9.

Page: 636

5: (True or False) Transitional objects, such as teddy bears and special blankets, should generally not be allowed because such items foster dependency on inanimate objects in younger children.

Answer: False

Critique: Many children find such special items to be comforting at bedtime, thus helping the child sleep better.

Page: 636

6: (True or False) Determine which of the following statements are true and which are false:

    A. Very few children and adolescents have sleep problems.
    B. Obstructive sleep apnea is most common in the 3- to 8-year-old group.
    C. Sleep problems in early life are associated with behavioral and emotional problems in adulthood.
    D. 20% to 30% of children and adolescents experience problems with sleep.
    E. Delayed sleep-phase syndrome most commonly occurs in toddlers.

Answers: A - False, B - True, C - True, D - True, E - False

Critique: Of children and adolescents, 20% to 30% experience sleep problems that cause serious concerns in the child and/or his or her family. Delayed sleep-phase syndrome is more common in adolescents.

Page: 636

7: (True or False) Parents should always manage sleep refusal in the same way, regardless of its cause. Parents should keep a sleep diary for the child for 2 weeks and ignore the child whenever he or she gets out of bed.

Answer: False

Critique: If a child is fearful, it is harmful to ignore his or her fears. Sleep refusal, which is oppositional or attention seeking, usually stops when parents do not become emotionally engaged by the behavior.

Page: 636

8: (True or False) Determine which of the following statements are true and which are false:

- A. Night terrors usually occur during the first few hours of sleep.
- B. Children with night terrors scream and appear to be awake.
- C. Night terrors usually occur in children age 6 months to 3 years.
- D. A differential diagnosis for night terrors that should include nocturnal seizure if the events occur at sleep onset or if there is a personal family history of seizures.

Answer: A - True, B - True, C - False, D - True

Critique: Night terrors usually occur in children aged 2 to 6 years and are more common during times of illness, stress, or sleep deprivation.

Page: 637

9: (True or False) Sedatives are the treatment of choice for night waking.

Answer: False

Critique: Behavior management techniques designed specifically for the child and family are more appropriate than medication, although no specific treatment guidelines for night terrors exist.

Page: 637

10: (True or False) In providing education for parents of children with night terrors, the family physician should:

- A. Advise the parent to wake the child up as quickly as possible
- B. Provide reassurance and information about how common the disorder is
- C. Advise an increase of total sleep
- D. Advise a consistent sleep-wake cycle

Answers: A - False, B - True, C - True, D - True

Critique: Waking the child could frighten the child or slow his or her return to sleep.

Page: 637

11: (True or False) Obstructive sleep apnea syndrome in children generally does not cause a large decrease in blood oxygen levels.

Answer: True

Critique: The frequent brief awakening of the child's sleep cycle re-establishes the airway and allow oxygen levels to remain within the appropriate range.

Page: 638

12: (True or False) Delayed sleep-phase syndrome is the most common adolescent sleep problem.

Answer: True

Critique: Factors contributing to such delayed sleep are social activities, part-time jobs, television viewing, and schedule shifts.

Page: 638

13: (True or False) Determine which of the following statements are true and which are false:

- A. Assessment of delayed sleep-phase syndrome is by history.
- B. Secondary gain for choosing a late-night schedule is the primary differential diagnosis.
- C. Treatment involves helping the adolescent and his or her family to make a schedule shift and maintain it.
- D. It is harmful to treat delayed sleep-phase syndrome by remaining awake throughout the night.

Answers: A - True, B - True, C - True, D - False

Critique: An adolescent who is having difficulty initiating timely sleep may respond to staying awake through an entire night and then re-establishing a regular sleep schedule.

Page: 638

14: REM sleep occurs after a person has been asleep for:

- A. 20 to 40 minutes
- B. 30 to 60 minutes
- C. 60 to 90 minutes
- D. 70 to 120 minutes

Answer: C

Critique: REM occurs when a person has been asleep for 60 to 90 minutes and follows all four stages of non-REM sleep.

Page: 638

15: In the case of narcolepsy, the diagnosis is made by:

- A. Sleep study
- B. Patient report
- C. Patient history
- D. Family history

Answer: A

Critique: A sleep study is required to make a diagnosis of narcolepsy. Any child or adolescent with a family history of narcolepsy or with unexplained daytime sleepiness that does not subside with good sleep hygiene should be considered for such evaluation.

Page: 638

16: Management of narcolepsy involves:

- A. Stimulant medications and selective serotonin re-uptake inhibitors
- B. REM suppressants for cataplexy
- C. Behavior modification
- D. Behavioral approaches combined with appropriate medications

Answer: D

Critique: Therapeutic naps can enhance daytime alertness and may help lower the dosage of stimulants required. Stimulants are used to decrease daytime sleepiness and antidepressants are used to help cataplexy and hallucinations.

Page: 638

17: Anxiety disorders occur in:

- A. 2% to 5% of school-aged children
- B. 10% to 20% of school-aged children
- C. 8% to 12% of children between 4 and 8 years
- D. 12% to 15% of school-aged children

Answer: B

Critique: Barrett (1998) states that anxiety disorders occur in 10% to 20% of school-aged children but that only a small portion are serious enough to come to the attention of health care providers.

Page: 638

18: (True or False) Specific phobias are best treated using psychoanalytic techniques, which are used to uncover the unconscious meaning of the feared stimulus and thus allow for integration of the phobic personality.

Answer: False

Critique: The literature on treatment of specific phobias clearly indicates that cognitive-behavioral approaches, and desensitization in particular, are the most efficacious treatment method.

Page: 639

19: (True or False) Determine which of the following statements are true and which are false:

- A. The age at which encopresis may be diagnosed is 3 years.
- B. Constipation is associated with encopresis in the majority of cases.
- C. Encopresis is more common in boys than in girls.
- D. Encopresis is nearly always related to organic problems, usually associated with diet transitions.

Answers: A - False, B - True, C - True, D - False

Critique: The diagnostic criterion for encopresis at first onset is age 4 years. Encopresis is commonly associated with fecal retention, but emotional factors can sometimes account for encopretic incidents or may occur concurrently with physiological causes.

Page: 639

20: The cause of enuresis is most likely:

- A. Genetic in origin
- B. Related to inappropriate parenting
- C. Pathophysiologic
- D. Multifactorial

Answer: D

Critique: Enuresis is a complex issue that frequently is related to multiple causes.

Page: 640

21: The likelihood of a significant contextual issue, such as a family dynamics problem, being related to bedwetting should be considered when the diagnosis is:

- A. Uncomplicated
- B. Nocturnal, not diurnal
- C. Complicated
- D. Both A and B

Answer: C

Critique: Uncomplicated enuresis is diagnosed based on initial history, physical examination, and urinalysis and culture. When these examinations are negative, enuresis is considered complicated and greater weight should be given to the contribution of psychosocial factors to episodes. Whether nocturnal enuresis is complicated or medical, the presence of psychosocial factors may be assumed.

Page: 640

22: Exclusively diurnal enuresis may be related to:

- A. Interpersonal interaction difficulties
- B. Changes in the family
- C. Physical factors only
- D. Both A and B

Answer: D

Critique: Both primary and secondary nocturnal enuresis strongly suggests that contextual dynamics problems are affecting the child. These can be problems in relationships, changes in the family configuration, family roles or losses, sexual abuse, or physical abuse.

Page: 640

23: Although most enuresis is usually not caused by emotional factors alone:

- A. Enuresis can have considerable psychosocial effects
- B. Enuresis rarely occurs in children with high self-esteem
- C. Both A and B
- D. Neither A nor B

Answer: A

Critique: Children who experience enuresis often feel embarrassed and incompetent. This can lead to low self-esteem and negative self-concept, which may affect other areas of performance. Although enuresis may have a purely physical cause, parental response to episodes may have a great emotional impact on the child.

Page: 640

24: Enuresis alarms work as a:

- A. Conditioning mechanism to facilitate arousal
- B. Startling mechanism that uses punishment as the primary change agent
- C. Means of alerting parents to onset of an episode
- D. None of the above

Answer: A

Critique: Alarms help by sounding when a very small volume of urine is secreted, thus creating an association between urine flow sensations and arousal from sleep. The child learns to avoid the alarm by retaining urine and continuing to sleep or by awakening and going to the bathroom before the alarm sounds.

Page: 641

25: Attention deficit hyperactivity disorder (ADHD) is a disorder that:

    A. Is limited to childhood and adolescence
    B. Persists from childhood through adulthood with no significant change in hyperactivity in adulthood
    C. Persists from childhood to adulthood with a significant reduction in hyperactivity in adulthood
    D. Persists from childhood to adulthood with significant increases in inattention in adulthood

Answer: C

Critique: ADHD persists throughout life with hyperactivity disappearing in adulthood.

Page: 641

26: Regarding comorbidity, what percentage of children diagnosed with ADHD have more than one psychiatric diagnosis?

    A. 5%
    B. 20%
    C. 50%
    D. 65%

Answer: D

Critique: According to Biederman, about 65% of children diagnosed with ADHD have at least one other psychiatric diagnosis.

Page: 641

27: (True or False) Numerous validated psychological tests definitively diagnose ADHD.

Answer: False

Critique: No single measure or combination of measures results in a definitive diagnosis of ADHD. Diagnosis may be supported by psychological assessment data; however, diagnosis must be determined through the use of several sources, such as diagnostic interviews, behavioral observations, Conner's rating scales, and others.

Page: 641

28: (True or False) Both medication and parent education are important in treating ADHD.

Answer: True

Critique: Medication alone is rarely adequate to help manage the needs of families with a child with ADHD. Behavioral management and self-management for children are usually necessary.

Page: 642

29: Adverse effects for psychostimulant medication can occur in up to:

    A. 10% of children
    B. 20% of children
    C. 30% of children
    D. Psychostimulant medications rarely cause adverse effects.

Answer: B

Critique: As many as 20% of children treated with medications for ADHD will experience weight loss, anorexia, irritability, abdominal pain, insomnia, dysphoria, rebound effects, impaired cognitive performance, tachycardia, and increased tic symptoms.

Page: 643

30: (True or False) Children who take stimulant medication are at higher risk of developing addictions later in life.

Answer: False

Critique: No current evidence supports this notion.

Page: 643

31: Oppositional defiant disorder is often confused with:

    A. Developing personality disorder
    B. Conduct disorders
    C. Depression
    D. Developmentally appropriate oppositional behavior

Answer: D

Critique: It is expected and developmentally appropriate for toddlers and teenagers to behave oppositionally, because these stages are characterized by the need for increased autonomy.

Page: 644

32: (True or False) Children who meet the criteria for conduct disorder respond differently to punishment than do children who do not meet the criteria.

Answer: True

Critique: The frequency of negative behavior increases following punishment in children with this disorder.

Page: 645

33: (True or False) Medications are often sufficient treatment for children with conduct disorder.

Answer: False

Critique: Medication alone is inadequate treatment for conduct disorder. Family therapy, parent training, and social skills training are generally the most effective treatment. Medications, if used, should target concurrent psychiatric disorders and symptoms.

Page: 646

34: The prevalence of major depression in children and adolescents:

A. Decreases from childhood to adolescence
B. Increases from childhood to adolescence
C. Is three times higher for adolescent boys than for adolescent girls
D. Is three times higher for adolescent girls than for adolescent boys

Answer: B

Critique: The prevalence of major depression in children is about 2% and about 4% to 8% in adolescents; adolescent girls are twice as likely to become depressed as adolescent boys.

Page: 646

35: (True or False) Relatively few children are hospitalized for failure to thrive because of psychosocial causes.

Answer: False

Critique: As many as half of the children hospitalized for failure to thrive have a psychosocial etiology.

Page: 648

36: When diagnosis of a feeding disorder is considered, it is important to:

A. Prescribe appropriate nutrition
B. Scrutinize the parents carefully to assess their knowledge of proper feeding
C. Consult with an expert in child abuse
D. Consult with a physician familiar with growth problems in children

Answer: D

Critique: Because of the extensive differential diagnosis for growth problems in children and the psychosocial issues that often accompany feeding problems, it is important to consult with a physician who has expertise in growth and development.

Page: 648

37: (True or False) Excessive exercise is not to be classified as a method of purging as occurs in bulimia.

Answer: False

Critique: Any form of compensation for binge eating, including excessive exercise, may qualify as purging.

Page: 649

38: (True or False) The erythrocyte sedimentation rate (ESR) and serum albumin level tend to remain at normal levels in people with eating disorders.

Answer: True

Critique: Elevated ESR or lower albumin levels suggest an organic cause for weight loss, rather than an eating disorder.

Page: 649

Chapter 31

Office Surgery

A. Stevens Wrightson

1: Which of the following statements is true concerning wound healing:

- A. Diabetics with glucose greater than 250 mg/dL have impaired leukocyte function, which can delay wound healing.
- B. Chronic steroid use does not affect wound healing as long as the dose is not lowered.
- C. Keloids are unlikely to recur as long as aseptic technique is used.
- D. Wound healing, including the maturation phase, is usually complete 3 months after the procedure.

Answer: A

Critique: The hyperglycemia of poorly controlled diabetes can lead to depressed leukocyte function, which in turn interferes with collagen synthesis. Chronic steroids, even at stable doses, also can impair healing. Although aseptic technique is important, a familial predisposition and the location of the wound more likely determine whether a keloid will occur. Some wounds can take up to 2 years for all phases of healing to be complete.

Pages: 651, 656

2: Which of the following statements is correct regarding universal precautions:

- A. The Occupational Safety and Health Administration (OSHA) recommends voluntary compliance with standard infection control procedures.
- B. The risk of developing an infection with hepatitis B (HBV) after exposure to infected blood or body fluids is greater than the risk of developing human immunodeficiency virus (HIV).
- C. Nearly 100% of health care workers are vaccinated against hepatitis B.
- D. HIV infection in a health care worker after exposure to a contaminated needle from an infected patient ranges from 6% to 30%.

Answer: B

Critique: HBV is much more likely to be spread after a work exposure to a hepatitis B surface antigen–positive patient. The rate of infection in a non-immune patient after an exposure such as a needlestick is 6% to 30%. The rate of transmission of HIV to a health care worker is only 0.09% (for a mucous membrane exposure) to 0.3% (for a percutaneous exposure) and is felt to be less if treatment with antiviral agents is begun immediately. Unfortunately, only 42% to 77% of health care workers are immunized against HBV. By law, OSHA mandates compliance with standard infection procedures.

Page: 652

3: Which of the following is true regarding eutectic mixture of local anesthetics (EMLA) cream:

- A. EMLA cream is appropriate for use in a 2-month-old for her or his immunizations.
- B. EMLA cream is contraindicated in children with glucose-6-phosphate dehydrogenase (G6PD) deficiency.
- C. EMLA cream is made primarily of topical lidocaine.
- D. EMLA cream has virtually no drug interactions.
- E. EMLA cream is an ideal anesthetic for laceration repair in children, because it can be applied directly on the open wound.

Answer: B

Critique: EMLA cream is a combination of 2.5% lidocaine and 2.5% prilocaine. Prilocaine, in toxic doses, can cause methemoglobinemia and therefore should be avoided in patients with G6PD and methemoglobin reductase deficiencies. EMLA cream is relatively contraindicated in children younger than 3 months and in children younger than 1 year who are taking methemoglobinemia-inducing drugs such as acetaminophen, sulfonamides, phenobarbital, and antimalarials, although the risk in normal term children is small. EMLA cream should be applied to intact skin only.

Page: 653

4: All of the following statements concerning local infiltration of anesthetics are correct, except:

- A. It is quicker and safer than a field block but more drug may be required to anesthetize a wound.
- B. It can distort tissues, making alignment and suturing more difficult.
- C. The use of epinephrine with the anesthetic can limit bleeding, making it particularly useful in peninsular areas such as fingers, toes, ears, nose, lips, or penis.
- D. Epinephrine can prolong the duration of the anesthetic and limit bleeding secondary to its vasoconstricting effect.

Answer: C

Critique: Infiltration anesthesia involves local injection of the anesthetic into tissue. It is generally quick and safe, but systemic toxicity is possible if large amounts of anesthetic are required such as for large wounds or lesions. Tissue distortion may make suturing a wound more difficult. The addition of epinephrine to the anesthetic causes local vasoconstriction, which can decrease bleeding and prolong the duration of action of the anesthesia. Epinephrine, however, should not be used in areas where blood supply may be compromised and therefore increase the risk of tissue necrosis.

Pages: 653, 654

5: Which of the following statements regarding keloids and hypertrophic scars is true:

    A. Intralesional corticosteroids can be used to shrink the keloids.
    B. There are no known risk factors for the development of keloids.
    C. Topical steroids reduce the size of the keloids as well as the associated itching.
    D. Thin skin, such as on the arms or face, is more likely to develop keloids.
    E. Keloids develop within a few weeks after the wound repair.

Answer: A

Critique: An intralesional corticosteroid, such as triamcinolone 10 mg/mL, can be injected at 4-week intervals to reduce the size of the keloid or hypertrophic scars. Topical steroids may help relieve the itching of keloids but do not appear to reduce their size. Keloids occur 5 to 15 times more often in nonwhites, and they also occur more often in patients with a personal or family history of keloid formation. Keloid formation occurs more often in wounds across tension lines and on thick skin such as shoulders, anterior chest, and upper back. They tend to develop months to years after the skin disruption. Hypertrophic scars can occur anywhere on the body and appear to be the result of excessive or prolonged inflammation. In both cases, collagen deposition far exceeds the collagen degradation that is taking place.

Page: 656

6: All of the following statements concerning nonhealing wounds are true, except:

    A. The tension across a wound decreases with age, making wound dehiscence less likely in patients older than 60.
    B. Steroids, antineoplastic agents, and cytotoxic drugs interfere with protein synthesis and inhibit fibroblast migration.
    C. Arterial and venous insufficiency contributes to poor wound healing.
    D. Smoking can reduce oxygen tension in a wound by 30%, leading to nutritional deficiencies that impair wound healing.
    E. Drawing wound edges together too tightly can reduce the blood supply, resulting in the inhibition of the body's own defenses against infection.

Answer: A

Critique: Wound dehiscence, on average, occurs three times more often in the elderly because immune responsiveness, epithelization, and collagen synthesis are all impaired. Various medications, including corticosteroids, antineoplastic drugs, cytotoxic agents, and even beta blockers, can interfere with wound healing. Poor blood flow to an area as a result of previous irradiation, surgery, or smoking contributes to poor wound healing. Poor repair technique, by drawing wound edges together too tightly, can lead to tissue necrosis and infection.

Page: 657

7: Which of the following statements concerning the diagnosis and treatment of hemorrhoids is true:

    A. The anorectal area is highly vascular, and wounds in this area heal well despite heavy fecal contamination.
    B. Internal hemorrhoids are located below the pectinate line, are covered with anoderm, and are extremely sensitive.
    C. External hemorrhoids usually cause painless rectal bleeding.
    D. Dietary modifications, such as a high-fiber diet and increased oral fluid intake, along with the use of topical steroids can usually heal all internal hemorrhoids.
    E. Alcoholics, because of their fluid intake, have fewer problems with hemorrhoids.

Answer: A

Critique: When treating a thrombosed external hemorrhoid, local infiltration of an anesthetic followed by an elliptical excision along the intact hemorrhoidal vein and overlying skin will relieve the pain and allow healing. The wound heals by secondary intention and has minimal chance to become infected owing to the highly vascular nature of the tissue. Internal hemorrhoids are located above the pectinate line and typically present with painless rectal bleeding. First-degree hemorrhoids bleed but do not prolapse. Second-degree hemorrhoids may prolapse but spontaneously reduce themselves. Third- and fourth-degree hemorrhoids prolapse more severely and may become thrombosed. Dietary modifications and topical steroids usually affect first- and second-degree hemorrhoids only. Alcoholics who have developed cirrhosis and portal hypertension have an increased incidence of hemorrhoids. Patients with increase in intra-abdominal pressure, such as with chronic constipation, prostate enlargement, chronic cough, and pregnancy, are also predisposed to the development of hemorrhoids.

Pages: 663, 664

8: All of the following are indications for cryosurgery, except:

    A. Seborrheic keratosis
    B. Skin tags
    C. Small (<5 mm) squamous cell carcinoma
    D. Actinic keratosis
    E. Verruca

Answer: C

Critique: Benign lesions such as seborrheic keratosis, actinic keratosis, dermatofibromata, warts, skin tags, and even acne can be treated with cryotherapy. Absolute contraindications include suspected malignancy, cold intolerance, cold urticaria, cryoglobulinemia, or cryofibrogenemia.

Page: 660

9: Which of the following findings does not necessitate surgical referral after performing a breast cyst aspiration:

    A. The aspirate is bloody.
    B. A palpable mass remains after the procedure.
    C. The mass is no longer palpable.
    D. The mass recurs.

Answer: C

Critique: Fine-needle aspiration of a breast mass can help determine whether an open surgical biopsy is necessary. Open biopsy after fine-needle aspiration should occur when: (1) the needle aspiration produces no cyst fluid and a solid mass is discovered; (2) the fluid obtained is bloody and thick; (3) fluid is aspirated, but the mass does not go away; or (4) the cyst or mass reappears in the same location. When the cyst fluid is turbid dark green or amber and the cyst disappears entirely with aspiration, open surgical biopsy is not required at that time.

Page: 665

10: Fine-needle aspiration for cytology is contraindicated in all but which of the following circumstances:

    A. A history of a bleeding diathesis
    B. A pulsatile mass
    C. An enlarged, firm lymph node in the anterior cervical chain
    D. An overlying skin infection
    E. A breast cyst that has resolved completely with aspiration of greenish fluid

Answer: C

Critique: Fine-needle aspiration for cytology is safe and simple to perform and is indicated for any unknown palpable subcutaneous mass. Although most commonly performed on breast masses, the technique can be used elsewhere, such as on a thyroid mass or for an enlarged lymph node. Contraindications include a history of a bleeding disorder, a mass that is pulsatile, or a mass with an overlying infection. If a breast mass has resolved with aspiration of greenish fluid, there is nothing to gain by doing random biopsies on the surrounding normal tissue.

Pages: 665, 666

11: Indications for endometrial biopsy include all but which of the following:

    A. Uterine bleeding in a postmenopausal woman
    B. Diagnosing luteal phase defect in a woman with unexplained infertility
    C. Unexplained amenorrhea in a woman whose pregnancy status is unknown
    D. Abnormal uterine bleeding in a perimenopausal woman

Answer: C

Critique: Pregnancy is the primary absolute contraindication for endometrial biopsy and should be ruled out in a patient with unexplained amenorrhea. Endometrial biopsy is more helpful in the diagnosis of abnormal uterine bleeding, such as is seen in perimenopausal and postmenopausal women. The finding of secretory endometrium by endometrial biopsy is indirect evidence of ovulation. The finding of proliferative endometrium suggests anovulation and may aid in the diagnosis of luteal phase defect in women with unexplained infertility.

Page: 665

12: Appropriate initial treatment of a Bartholin's gland abscess includes all of the following, except:

    A. Marsupialization of the abscess
    B. Placement of a Word catheter
    C. Incision and drainage with packing of the wound
    D. Sitz baths and analgesics after the initial procedure

Answer: A

Critique: Bartholin's gland abscesses are usually polymicrobial, although they may be caused by gonococcus 20% to 30% of the time. Incision and drainage of the abscess or the placement of a Word catheter is the appropriate initial treatment for a Bartholin's gland abscess. The incision should be made behind the hymenal ring to prevent vulvar scarring and to allow packing or catheter placement inside the vagina, which makes it far more controllable. After the procedure, sitz baths and analgesics help alleviate the discomfort. Marsupialization of the abscess is reserved for recurrent abscess formation and should not be used as initial treatment.

Page: 664

13: Initial therapy for anal fissures includes all of the following, except:

    A. Sitz baths
    B. Bran
    C. Bulking agents such as psyllium seed products
    D. Nitroglycerin ointment
    E. Topical steroids

Answer: D

Critique: Sitz baths, bran, and bulking agents are appropriate initial therapy for anal fissures and can allow for healing in 50% to 80% of patients. Patients should be reminded of the added benefit for colon and cardiovascular health of adding bran and psyllium-like agents to the diet. Topical steroids are also an appropriate first-line therapy, although evidence does not indicate any additional benefit to healing over the use of bran alone. Some evidence indicates that topical nitroglycerin helps with recalcitrant fissures, but its use should be reserved for those who fail initial conservative therapy, especially because of the side effects associated with its use (headaches). Crohn's disease, cancer, and sexually transmitted diseases all can cause failure of medical and surgical therapy for anal fissures.

Page: 664

14: Appropriate treatment for subungual hematomas includes all of the following options, except:

    A. For large hematomas that involve more than 50% of the nail, removal of the nail to look for and repair any nail bed laceration

    B. Three-view radiographs to look for distal tuft fractures

    C. Splinting of distal tuft fractures after subungual decompression for 2 to 3 weeks

    D. For hematomas involving less than 50% of the nail, observation alone

Answer: D

Critique: Subungual hematomas are caused by a crushing injury to the distal end of the finger. The nail bed is black or dark violet in color and is very tender. Removal of the hematoma relieves the pain. This is accomplished by drilling a hole in the nail to allow the old blood to escape. Radiographs of the finger are recommended because comminuted fractures of the distal phalanx can occur with these injuries. If such an injury is discovered, the finger should be splinted after the decompression is performed. Large hematomas are associated with nail bed lacerations; they should be repaired to prevent the regrowing nail from splitting or becoming nonadherent and thereby producing a nail that is cosmetically unacceptable or painful. Because of the discomfort involved, most subungual hematomas, even small ones, should be decompressed.

Page: 662

15: Which of the following statements is correct concerning incision and drainage of an abscess:

    A. If no fluctuance is present, the incision can be made over an area of induration, because the abscess is usually located just beneath it.

    B. Packing is not necessary because the use of antibiotics prevents early closure of the wound.

    C. Local infiltration with lidocaine as an anesthetic often does not reduce pain, because the pH of infected tissue causes deactivation of the anesthetic.

    D. If only redness and induration are present, the use of antibiotics should be deferred to allow the infection to localize so incision and drainage can be performed.

Answer: C

Critique: Fluctuance, which is the softening of the central area of infection, allows the physician to determine the area that requires drainage. If the area is red, indurated, and warm, but not fluctuant, incision should not be attempted. Rather, treatment with antibiotics and warm compresses should be started until the infection resolves or localizes. EMLA cream or topical ethyl chloride can be used to reduce the discomfort of the incision. Unfortunately, infected tissue is difficult to anesthetize because it can deactivate an infiltrated anesthetic such as lidocaine owing to the pH changes caused by the infection. Packing is recommended to prevent early closure of an abscess that has been drained. Antibiotics are not necessary when the infection is localized solely to the abscess.

Pages: 661, 662

Chapter 32

Gynecology

Richard D. Pham

1: Which of the following statements is true about Papanicolaou smear screening?

   A. The American Cancer Society recommends that Pap smear screening begin at age 16 or at the onset of sexual activity.
   B. After three consecutive normal Pap smears have been documented, patients at low risk for cervical cancer can be screened every 5 years.
   C. After the age of 55, the U.S. Preventive Health Service Task Forces (USPHSTF) recommend that routine screening be discontinued in women who have had regular screening.
   D. The number one risk factor for adenocarcinoma of the cervix is sexual activity.
   E. Use of the Cytobrush followed by the spatula increases the sensitivity of the smear.

Answer: E

Critique: Use of the Cytobrush before the spatula increases the sensitivity of the Pap smear. The American Cancer Society recommends that Pap smear screening begin at age 18 or at the onset of sexual activity. Most patients require annual screening; however, after three consecutive normal Pap smears have been documented, patients at low risk can be screened at 3-year intervals. Low-risk patients include those who have had two or fewer lifetime sexual partners, who did not have intercourse before age 20, who do not smoke, and who have never had an abnormal Pap smear. After the age of 65, the USPHSTF recommends that routine screening be discontinued in women who have had normal regular screening. The risk of adenocarcinoma of the cervix is not related to sexual activity or the risk factors associated with squamous cell carcinoma of the cervix.

Page: 668

2: Which of the following statements about low-grade squamous intraepithelial lesion (LGSIL) is correct?

   A. LGSIL includes smears that were previously reported as human papillomavirus (HPV) or moderate dysplasia or cervical intraepithelial neoplasia (CIN) type II.
   B. LGSIL responds to antibiotic treatment.
   C. LGSIL can spontaneously regress.
   D. LGSIL can rapidly progress to cervical cancer.
   E. LGSIL can mask higher-grade cervical lesions.

Answer: C

Critique: The majority of low-grade squamous intraepithelial lesions (LGSILs) will resolve spontaneously even without treatment. Even high-grade squamous intraepithelial lesions, previously reported as moderate dysplasia or CIN II or severe dysplasia and carcinoma or CIN III, do not rapidly (within 6 months) progress to invasive cervical cancer. All other statements are incorrect.

Page: 668

3: On colposcopy, which of the following findings is considered normal?

   A. Presence of acetowhite epithelium
   B. Punctation after application of acetic acid
   C. A mosaic pattern of neovascularization
   D. Visualization of the entire transformation zone

Answer: D

Critique: For the colposcopy to be adequate and complete the transformation zone must be fully visualized. All other findings listed are abnormal.

Page: 669

4: Which of the following is the most rapid and effective therapy to control heavy dysfunctional uterine bleeding?

   A. Oral contraceptive pills taken in standard doses but skipping placebo pills
   B. Nonsteroidal anti-inflammatory drugs (NSAIDs) taken in higher than standard doses
   C. Medroxyprogesterone 10 mg taken by mouth daily for 10 days per month
   D. Conjugated estrogen 2.5 mg taken by mouth four times daily

Answer: D

Critique: Oral contraceptive agents may be used but are administered four times per day. NSAIDs may ease the pain of dysmenorrhea but may worsen bleeding secondary to platelet inhibition. Progesterone treatment for 10 days will ease the bleeding, but the patient will experience withdrawal bleeding after the completion of therapy. The most effective agent for the control of heavy dysfunctional bleeding is conjugated estrogen. It is noteworthy that the oral form is as effective as intravenous administration, but nausea may be a side effect.

Page: 670

5: A 17-year-old female is concerned that she might be pregnant. She has had no periods for 6 months, and her periods have been very irregular since menarche at age 13. She became sexually active 6 months ago and has been having unprotected sex. She has always been athletic, is an avid runner, and is the star of her track and basketball teams. She takes no medications and reports eating an adequate diet. Review of systems is negative for weight gain or loss, nausea or vomiting, fatigue, headaches, cold or heat intolerance, or abdominal or pelvic pain. Physical examination reveals a thin, athletic, normally developed female with normal secondary sexual characteristics. She is not hirsute, and her thyroid and cardiac examinations are normal. Pelvic examination revealed no abnormalities, and a urine pregnancy test is negative. She is given a progesterone challenge and responds with some spotting. Her TSH is normal. All of the following statements about this patient are true, except:

 A. Her serum prolactin, follicle-stimulating hormone, and luteinizing hormone will be below normal.
 B. Another diagnosis other than anovulation should be sought, because her progesterone challenge did not result in withdrawal bleeding.
 C. A progestin withdrawal challenge every 2 to 3 months would be an appropriate treatment option.
 D. Oral contraceptive agents would be an appropriate treatment option.
 E. She would benefit from exercise limitation and sexual counseling.

Answer: B

Critique: Stress from severe illness, trauma, weight loss, excessive exercise, or anorexia nervosa can cause suppression of the hypothalamic-pituitary axis leading to secondary amenorrhea and anovulation. Withdrawal bleeding from a progesterone challenge is defined as any vaginal bleeding or spotting. This usually occurs between 2 and 7 days after the completion of therapy. In exercise-related amenorrhea, the serum prolactin, FSH, and LH will be below normal. Polycystic ovarian syndrome is a consideration but is unlikely, because she has no hyperandrogenic traits. Treatment with oral contraceptive pills or progestin withdrawal challenges would be appropriate. Limiting exercise may allow for resumption of normal menses, and she would benefit from safe-sex education.

Pages: 671, 672

6: Clue cells are found in the vaginal pool wet-prep in which of the following conditions?

 A. Physiologic discharge
 B. Candidal vaginitis
 C. Trichomonal vaginitis
 D. Bacterial vaginosis

Answer: D

Critique: Clue cells are vaginal epithelial cells peppered with bacteria and are indicative of bacterial vaginosis. Amsel's criteria for diagnosis of bacterial vaginosis rely on the presence of clue cells plus two of the following three markers: vaginal pH greater than 4.5, a homogeneous discharge adherent to the vaginal walls, and a fishy amine odor on application of 10% KOH. Physiologic discharge comprises secretions from the cervix and vagina, along with bacterial products and shedding epithelial cells. Laboratory evaluation of normal discharge will reveal a pH

of 3.8 to 4.5, few white cells, an absence of clue cells, and a predominance of long rod-shaped bacteria. Pseudo hyphae and budding yeast are seen in candidal vaginitis. The diagnosis of trichomonal infection is based on identification of the motile trichomonads on saline microscopy.

Pages: 672, 673

7: In menopausal women, which of Amsel's criteria is the least specific for bacterial vaginosis?

 A. Vaginal pH below 4.5
 B. Presence of clue cells
 C. A homogeneous discharge adherent to the vaginal walls
 D. A fishy amine odor on application of 10% KOH

Answer: A

Critique: Vaginal pH is not a good marker for menopausal women, because pH normally rises in the postmenopausal period. Of these markers, the presence of greater than 20% clue cells or clue cells and an amine odor are highly specific for bacterial vaginosis.

Page: 673

8: All of the following statements about recurrent candidal vaginitis are true, except:

 A. Predisposing conditions include HIV-positive status, antibiotic use, diabetes mellitus, pregnancy, and zinc and iron deficiencies.
 B. Patients with recurrent infection are more likely to be infected with *C. glabrata* or *C. tropicalis*.
 C. Sexual partners should be examined for Candida and treated if infection is present.
 D. Treatment of recurrent candidal vaginitis involves an extended course of medication.
 E. *Lactobacillus*-containing vaginal suppositories show promise in preventing recurrence.

Answer: A

Critique: Women who are diabetic, pregnant, HIV positive, or zinc deficient or who are taking oral contraceptives, long-term steroids or antibiotics, or immunosuppressive medications are predisposed to recurrent candidal vaginitis. Iron deficiency is not a predisposing factor. All other statements are true.

Pages: 673, 675

9: Which of the following patients is most likely to develop atrophic vaginitis?

 A. A patient on danazol
 B. A patient on tamoxifen
 C. A patient who is postpartum and breast-feeding
 D. A patient on Micronor, a progesterone-only contraceptive
 E. All of the above

Answer: E

Critique: Atrophic vaginitis is most commonly considered a concern of postmenopausal women. However, it can occur in postpartum and lactating women or in association with hormonal medications. The use of low-dose oral contraceptive agents, progesterone-only contraceptives, and estrogen blockers such as danazol and tamoxifen can lead to atrophic vaginitis. Common to these medications and states is a relative deficiency of estrogen. As the estrogen effect decreases, the vulvovaginal tissues thin and produce less glycogen.

Page: 676

10: A female patient with acute pelvic pain should be rapidly evaluated for:

    A. Appendicitis and nephrolithiasis
    B. Nephrolithiasis and pelvic inflammatory disease
    C. Pelvic inflammatory disease and ectopic pregnancy
    D. Ectopic pregnancy and appendicitis

Answer: D

Critique: A female patient with acute pelvic pain should be rapidly evaluated for ectopic pregnancy and appendicitis. These two emergency surgical conditions need to be evaluated before considering other, less serious causes. Ruptured ectopic pregnancies carry a high mortality rate. The ectopic pregnancy rate is increasing, now reported to be 2% of all pregnancies in the United States. An ectopic pregnancy is difficult to diagnose, and patients often make two or more visits before a diagnosis is made. Other causes of acute pelvic pain are listed in Table 32-7.

Pages: 676, 677

11: All of the following statements about ectopic pregnancies are true, except:

    A. Progestational agents such as progesterone-only oral contraceptive pills increase the probability of ectopic implantation of pregnancy.
    B. An office urine pregnancy test sensitive to 50 fg or less of human chorionic gonadotropin (HCG) is sufficient to detect a pregnancy capable of causing pelvic pain.
    C. A serum progesterone level greater than 25 is generally indicative of an extrauterine pregnancy.
    D. An ectopic pregnancy must be presumed if an intrauterine gestational sac is not visible by transvaginal ultrasound with a serum HCG level of more than 2000.
    E. Rupture of an ectopic pregnancy usually occurs at 6 to 8 weeks gestation.

Answer: C

Critique: Serum progesterone levels above 25 generally indicate a normal intrauterine pregnancy. Less than 0.2% of patients with progesterone levels lower than 5 are carrying normal pregnancies. Progestational agents such as progesterone-only oral contraceptives or intrauterine devices increase the possibility of ectopic implantation of pregnancy by slowing tubal motility. Other risk factors include a preceding ectopic pregnancy (25% recurrence rate with a subsequent pregnancy), tubal surgery or infection, and infertility.

Page: 677

12: Medical treatment of ectopic pregnancy with methotrexate is contraindicated in:

    A. Patients who are breast-feeding
    B. Patients who are immunodeficient
    C. Patients with peptic ulcer disease
    D. Patients with hematologic, renal, or hepatic dysfunction
    E. All of the above

Answer: E

Critique: Medical treatment with methotrexate is used only under specific circumstances. The patient must be hemodynamically stable and able to return for follow-up care. Preferably, the unruptured adnexal mass should be less than 3.5 cm in size. Treatment is contraindicated in all of the listed patients.

Page: 677

13: According to the Centers for Disease Control and Prevention 1998 guidelines, which of the following antibiotics is not indicated in the treatment of uncomplicated *Neisseria gonorrhoeae* genital infections?

    A. Ofloxacin (Floxin) 400 mg PO single dose
    B. Ciprofloxacin (Cipro) 500 mg PO single dose
    C. Amoxicillin/clavulanate potassium (Augmentin) 850 mg PO twice daily
    D. Cefixime (Suprax) 400 mg PO single dose
    E. Ceftriaxone (Rocephin) 125 mg IM single dose

Answer: C

Critique: Amoxicillin/clavulanate potassium (Augmentin) is not indicated for the treatment of *N. gonorrhoeae*. All others listed are indicated.

Page: 678

14: (True or False) *Chlamydia trachomatis* is the predominant bacteriologic organism responsible for pelvic inflammatory disease.

Answer: F

Critique: Pelvic inflammatory disease (PID) is usually thought of as a sexually transmitted disease caused by *C. trachomatis* or *N. gonorrhoeae*. Actually, PID is almost always a multiorganism infection with gram-negative organisms, anaerobes that are a part of the normal vaginal flora, streptococci, and *N. gonorrhoeae* and *C. trachomatis*. For this reason, treatment of PID must be capable of eliminating anaerobic infection along with the usual sexually transmitted organisms.

Page: 677

15: Which of the following historical features or physical findings confirms the diagnosis of endometriosis?

    A. Infertility
    B. Increasingly severe dysmenorrhea
    C. Cul-de-sac nodularity
    D. Bilaterally enlarged ovaries
    E. None of the above

Answer: E

Critique: Laparoscopy is the gold standard for the diagnosis of endometriosis. In fact, endometriosis is the most common cause of chronic pelvic pain identified on laparoscopy. Although endometriosis may be suspected from these historical features and physical findings, they are nonspecific because other causes may account for them as well.

Page: 679

16: All of the following statements about leiomyomas are true, except:

    A. Fibroid tumors are more common in white women than in African-American women.

    B. Symptoms of leiomyomas include pelvic pain, heavy menses, and possibly back pain and urinary and bowel problems.

    C. Ultrasound imaging helps further define the size and location of the leiomyoma.

    D. Asymptomatic fibroids should be evaluated clinically at regular intervals to ensure slow growth and stable size.

    E. Pharmacologic treatment for fibroids works by reducing the effects of estrogen on the tumor.

Answer: A

Critique: Fibroid tumors are more common in African-American women than in white women. Symptoms include pain and heavy menses and pressure on surrounding structures, which can cause back pain, as well as urinary and bowel problems. Asymptomatic fibroids should be evaluated clinically at regular intervals. For symptomatic patients, medical treatment consists of progesterone (with or without estrogen), danazol, or GnRH agonists. All medical treatments work by reducing the effect of estrogen on the tumor.

Page: 680

17: On a routine annual well-woman exam, an adnexal mass is discovered in a 35-year-old female. She has no complaints or symptoms, and there is no personal or family history of breast or ovarian cancer. She is on no medications and has never used oral contraceptive pills. Her periods have always been regular, and she is due to start her menses next week. She is married, is monogamous, and denies any history of sexually transmitted diseases. She is a G1P1, and her child is 12 months old. Which of the following statements is true regarding this patient's condition?

    A. Because the differentiation between a simple ovarian cyst and ovarian cancer is critical, the initial work-up is a transvaginal ultrasound.

    B. Delayed childbearing is protective against ovarian cancer.

    C. Because her periods are regular, oral contraceptive pills offer no benefit for this patient.

    D. If she has a simple cyst that is <6 cm, she may be monitored clinically for 2 to 3 months.

    E. Large, noncomplex cysts are managed the same as are small simple cysts.

Answer: D

Critique: When an adnexal mass is found on pelvic examination, a pregnancy test should be performed first to rule out pregnancy. A transvaginal ultrasound may be indicated next, depending on the situation (see Fig. 32–5). The risk of ovarian cancer is increased in women with a family history of breast or ovarian cancer, a personal history of breast cancer, and delayed childbearing. Prevention of ovarian cancer currently focuses on the use of oral contraceptive pills, and 5 years of use has been shown to decrease the risk of ovarian cancer. Because ovarian cysts usually resolve spontaneously—70% disappear within a few months—premenopausal women can be monitored clinically for 2 to 3 months. Complex cysts and large cysts (>6 cm) are more likely to harbor malignancy and should be managed more aggressively.

Pages: 680, 681

18: What proportion of all causes of infertility is due to male factors?

    A. 10%

    B. 20%

    C. 30%

    D. 40%

    E. 50%

Answer: D

Critique: Forty percent of all causes of infertility are a result of male factors, including the delivery of inadequate number of functional sperm from abnormal semen, sperm duct dysfunction, or sexual dysfunction. Female factors account for 50%, and 10% of causes are unexplained. See Table 32–11.

Pages: 682, 683

19: A 55-year-old woman comes to the office for treatment of hot flashes and painful intercourse. She has had no menses for 2 years and does not want her periods to return. She has an intact uterus, and a recent mammogram was normal. Her family history is significant for myocardial infarction in her father at age 50. Her mother has vertebral fractures and sustained a hip fracture at age 70. All of the following statements about this patient are true, except:

    A. Most of her bone loss has already occurred.

    B. On pelvic exam, she will have atrophy of the vaginal mucosa.

    C. Menopause should not increase her risk of incontinence or urinary tract infections.

    D. Her lipid profile will show a decrease in high-density lipoproteins.

    E. If she already has coronary artery disease, starting hormone replacement therapy will have no beneficial effect on the progression of coronary atherosclerosis.

Answer: C

Critique: The bladder and urethra are estrogen-sensitive organs. Loss of estrogen production after menopause will cause atrophy and result in loss of sphincter tone, bladder neck hypermobility, decreased bladder capacity, poor detrusor control, and higher susceptibility to urinary tract infections. Most bone loss occurs in the perimenopausal period. Vaginal atrophy occurs after 1 to

2 years of estrogen deficiency, resulting in vaginal dryness and dyspareunia. Estrogen induces the formation of high-density lipoproteins, and the lack of estrogen is associated with decreased production of these cardioprotective lipids. In addition, besides increasing HDL, hormone replacement therapy (HRT) has also been shown to improve lipid profiles by lowering low-density lipoprotein. Previous observational studies of women taking HRT suggested that mortality from ischemic heart disease and stroke was reduced. The Heart and Estrogen/Progesterone Replacement Study (HERS) found no beneficial effect on the progression of coronary atherosclerosis in post-menopausal women with coronary artery disease.

Page: 684

20: Regarding the above patient, which of the following therapies is most appropriate at this time?

   A. Topical vaginal estrogen
   B. Daily oral estrogen
   C. Daily oral estrogen with cyclical oral progesterone
   D. Daily oral estrogen and continuous oral progesterone
   E. Biweekly transdermal estrogen

Answer: D

Critique: Menopausal symptoms are effectively treated with hormone replacement therapy (HRT). There are some disadvantages and side effects to HRT, but the demonstrated improvement in longevity and quality of life by prevention of osteoporotic fractures outweighs any disadvantages. Estrogen therapy given by any route would benefit this patient. However, because the patient has an intact uterus, she requires concomitant progesterone therapy to prevent endometrial hyperplasia. Because she no longer wants to have menstrual periods, continuous daily administration of estrogen and progesterone is the preferred choice.

Pages: 684, 685

Chapter 33

Contraception

Lisa R. Nash

1: (True or False) A pregnancy rate of 5% or less during the first year of "typical" contraceptive use is associated with:

A. Combination oral contraceptives
B. Progesterone-only pill
C. Depo-Provera
D. Male condom
E. Norplant

Answers: A - True, B - True, C - True, D - False, E - True

Critique: Contraception is both poorly utilized and underutilized in the United States, despite its well-established benefits and wide availability. Of women who experienced an unintended pregnancy, 53% were using a contraceptive method. The patient's ability to cope with an unintended pregnancy is one factor to consider when choosing a contraceptive method and may influence the choice made.

Page: 687

2: (True or False) A 17-year-old G0 presents to your office for contraceptive counseling. She states that she has a single male partner and that they have been using condoms intermittently for contraception. She would like to discuss other methods for contraception. Preferred options (in combination with condoms) include:

A. Depo-Provera (DMPA)
B. Norplant
C. Combination oral contraceptives (COCs)
D. Progesterone-only pill
E. IUD

Answers: A - True, B - True, C - True, D - False, E - False

Critique: Important factors in the choice of contraceptive method for this patient include age, fecundity, and potential risk for STIs. Preferred contraceptive options for adolescents include DMPA, Norplant, or COCs *plus* condoms. Condoms are important for the prevention of STIs, for which adolescents are at increased risk. Progesterone-only oral contraceptives are associated with higher rates of breakthrough bleeding and spotting. IUDs are generally not considered appropriate for nulliparous patients and those not involved in a single, committed relationship because of an increased potential risk for STIs.

Page: 687

3: Combination oral contraceptives (COCs) are recommended for patients with the following conditions:

A. Polycystic ovarian syndrome
B. History of stroke or TIA
C. History of thromboembolism
D. Smoker older than 35 years
E. Gallbladder disease

Answer: A

Critique: COCs suppress androgen excess and are useful in the treatment of patients with polycystic ovarian syndrome. COCs are contraindicated in patients with history of stroke, TIA, or thromboembolism because of an increased incidence of thromboembolism associated with estrogen. Progesterone is not implicated. Women older than 35 years of age who smoke are at increased risk for arterial events (myocardial infarction and stroke) when treated with COCs. Gallbladder disease may be accelerated (but not caused) by COC use.

Page: 688

4: (True or False) The potential benefits of combination oral contraceptives include:

A. Decreased menstrual cramping
B. Decreased blood flow
C. Elimination of ovulatory pain
D. Reduced risk of ovarian cancer
E. Reduced formation of functional ovarian cysts

Answers: A - True, B - True, C - True, D - True, E - True

Critique: COCs have many potential benefits, including all of those mentioned. Other benefits may include protection against atherosclerosis, osteoporosis, endometriosis, and rheumatoid arthritis. Acne is often improved with the use of COCs.

Page: 688

5: (True or False) You are seeing a 25-year-old G3P3 diabetic patient who had an uneventful spontaneous vaginal delivery 6 weeks before the examination. She is bottle-feeding her infant. Her diabetes is well controlled. Her blood pressure is 135/90. She is otherwise healthy and is a nonsmoker. For contraception, you may offer her:

A. Male condoms
B. Diaphragm
C. Combination oral contraceptives

149

D. Depo-Provera
E. Norplant

Answers: A - True, B - True, C - False, D - True, E - True

Critique: Condoms are appropriate for most patients unless allergy exists. The diaphragm is acceptable, although if this was the method used before pregnancy, the patient may need to be resized for appropriate fit. COCs are not appropriate here because of the patient's uncontrolled hypertension. Well-controlled diabetes does not prevent selection of COCs. Because this patient is under the age of 35 and is a nonsmoker, she is not disqualified under those conditions for COCs. The estrogen component of COCs, and not progesterone, is associated with a higher risk of arterial events, and thus Depo-Provera or Norplant would be acceptable for this patient.

Page: 689

6: (True or False) Potential effects of combination oral contraceptives include:

A. Breakthrough bleeding
B. Decreased risk of pelvic inflammatory disease
C. Anovulation
D. Thinning of the cervical mucus
E. Decreased incidence of venous thromboembolism

Answers: A - True, B - True, C - True, D - False, E - False

Critique: Anovulation is an expected effect of COC use. Breakthrough bleeding is a potential side effect during the first 3 months of use, and smoking increases the risk of breakthrough bleeding. COCs cause a thickening of the cervical mucus; this may account for the decreased risk of symptomatic pelvic inflammatory disease, but the risk of STIs is unchanged. The estrogen component of COCs is associated with a dose-related increase in venous thromboembolism.

Pages: 688, 689

7: Compared with progesterone-only pills, combination oral contraceptives are:

A. Associated with fewer serious complications
B. Less effective in preventing pregnancy
C. More likely to cause breakthrough bleeding
D. More likely to inhibit ovulation
E. Likely to confer fewer noncontraceptive health benefits

Answer: D

Critique: Approximately 40% of patients taking progesterone-only pills continue to ovulate. Mechanisms of contraceptive action include thickening of cervical mucus and the production of changes in the uterine lining that are not conducive to implantation. The effectiveness of the two methods in preventing pregnancy is similar. Combination oral contraceptives are associated with more serious complications, are less likely to cause breakthrough bleeding, and confer more noncontraceptive benefits than progesterone-only pills.

Pages: 689, 690

8: (True or False) You are seeing a 22-year-old Caucasian female, G2P2, for her 6-week postpartum examination. She is married and monogamous and has no history of sexually transmitted infections. She is breast-feeding her infant and plans to supplement feedings with formula when she returns to work next week. Both mother and baby are healthy and doing well. The patient's lochia has resolved, and she has not experienced any menstrual bleeding. Her options for contraception include:

A. Combination oral contraceptives
B. Progesterone-only pill
C. Lactational amenorrheic method
D. Intrauterine device (IUD)
E. Depo-Provera

Answers: A - False, B - True, C - False, D - True, E - True

Critique: COCs can decrease the quantity and duration of lactation, for which this patient will already be at increased risk owing to separation from her infant during the workweek and planned formula supplementation. Reliable contraceptive effect of the lactational amenorrheic method requires exclusive breast-feeding on demand. Progesterone does not interfere with the production of breast milk, so both the progesterone-only pill and Depo-Provera are reasonable options. This patient is in a long-term monogamous relationship, presumed at low risk for STIs, and parous, and is thus a good candidate for an IUD.

Pages: 688, 689, 691–693, 697

9: Emergency oral contraceptive pills:

A. Must be taken within 24 hours of unprotected intercourse
B. Require only a single dose
C. Act as an abortifacient
D. Do not affect the endometrium
E. May delay ovulation

Answer: E

Critique: Emergency oral contraceptives may delay ovulation, alter the transport of sperm or ova, or alter the endometrium to prevent implantation, depending on when during the menstrual cycle they are taken. Emergency oral contraceptives should be taken within 72 hours of unprotected intercourse, and all require two doses taken 12 hours apart. Emergency oral contraceptives are not abortifacients, because they do not disrupt an already established pregnancy.

Page: 691

10: Potential effects of Depo-Provera include increased risk of the following:

A. Pain in women with endometriosis
B. Reduced bone mineral density
C. Ovarian cancer
D. Pelvic inflammatory disease
E. Sickle cell crisis in women with sickle cell disease

Answer: B

Critique: Depo-Provera produces beneficial effects of decreased pain in women with endometriosis and reduced risk of ovarian cancer, symptomatic pelvic inflammatory disease, endometrial cancer, and sickle cell crisis in women with sickle cell disease. A potential risk exists in the reduced bone mineral density related to the suppression of estrogen caused by Depo-Provera. This effect is similar to that seen with breast-feeding and is presumed to be reversible. HDL levels may also be decreased by the use of Depo-Provera.

Pages: 691, 692

11: A significant difference between levonorgestrel implants (Norplant) and Depo-Provera is:

- A. Rapid return to ovulation
- B. Thickening of cervical mucus
- C. Changes in the uterine lining that are not conducive to implantation
- D. Reduced menstrual flow
- E. Reduced risk of ectopic pregnancy

Answer: A

Critique: Both methods produce thickening of the cervical mucus, changes in the uterine lining that are not conducive to implantation, reduced menstrual flow, and a reduced risk of ectopic pregnancy compared to non-users. Residual amounts of Depo-Provera may be found in the circulation up to 9 months after injection, and amenorrhea may persist for months after discontinuation. In contrast, a return to fertility after removal of the Norplant may be as rapid as 3 days.

Pages: 691, 692

12: A 23-year-old black female, G2P2, presents to your office with complaints of pelvic pain and vaginal discharge for 3 days. Her method of contraception is an IUD, which was placed 3 years ago. She reports having unprotected sexual intercourse with a new partner for the past 2 months, most recently 5 days ago. Physical examination reveals positive cervical motion tenderness, purulent vaginal discharge with foul odor, and tenderness of the uterus on bimanual palpation. The adnexa are without mass and are not tender. Temperature is 38.2°C. White blood count is 15,500. Appropriate actions include all of the following, except:

- A. Rocephin 250 mg IM
- B. Azithromycin 1 g PO
- C. Cultures for gonorrhea and chlamydia
- D. Close follow-up in 24 to 48 hours
- E. Leave IUD intact if symptoms improve within 24 hours

Answer: E

Critique: Administration of antibiotics, appropriate cultures, and close follow-up are all components of a treatment regimen for pelvic inflammatory disease. Removal of the IUD is also a necessary component of therapy.

Pages: 692, 693

13: The copper T 380A IUD may cause:

- A. Long return-to-fertility times
- B. Abortions
- C. A sperm-hostile environment
- D. Infertility
- E. PID

Answer: C

Critique: It is a common misperception, particularly among the lay public, that modern IUDs cause abortions, pelvic inflammatory disease, and infertility. In fact, the mechanism of action is the production of a sterile, inflammatory, sperm-hostile environment in the endometrium. Local prostaglandin and endometrial enzyme production is also increased, which may increase spermicidal effects. Return-to-fertility times are typically short after removal of the device.

Page: 693

14: (True or False) Risk factors associated with a high risk of regret after sterilization and a request for reversal include:

- A. Young age
- B. Unstable marriage or relationship
- C. Recent pregnancy
- D. High socioeconomic status
- E. Caucasian ethnicity

Answers: A - True, B - True, C - True, D - False, E - False

Critique: Factors known to be associated with high risk of regret include young age, unstable marriage, recent pregnancy, low socioeconomic status, and Hispanic origin. Patients with one or more of these factors warrant additional counseling.

Page: 696

15: (True or False) Methods of contraception that reliably inhibit ovulation include:

- A. Combination oral contraceptives (COCs)
- B. Progesterone-only oral contraceptives
- C. Depo-Provera
- D. Norplant
- E. Lactational amenorrheic method at 8 months postpartum

Answers: A - True, B - False, C - True, D - False, E - False

Critique: COCs and Depo-Provera reliably inhibit ovulation. Up to 40% of progesterone-only oral contraceptive users continue to ovulate normally. Norplant does not reliably suppress ovulation but, instead, relies on thickened cervical mucus and changes produced in the endometrial lining that are not conducive to implantation for its contraceptive effect. The lactational amenorrheic method produces reliable suppression of ovulation only up to 6 months postpartum and requires the additional factor of exclusive breast-feeding on demand.

Pages: 688, 689, 691, 692, 697

16: A 22-year-old Hispanic female, G0P0, requests advice regarding initiation of a convenient and reversible method of contraception before her upcoming marriage. Her medical history is remarkable for a seizure disorder that is well controlled on oral medications. The preferred option for this patient is:

    A. Depo-Provera
    B. Combination oral contraceptives
    C. IUD
    D. Progesterone-only oral contraceptives
    E. Norplant

Answer: A

Critique: The efficacy of COCs, progesterone-only oral contraceptives, and Norplant may be reduced as a result of the oral anti-seizure medications. Depo-Provera is the preferred method because of decreased frequency of seizures related to its sedative effect. An IUD is an acceptable alternative for most patients with seizure disorders, although its use is not recommended in this patient because she is nulliparous.

Page: 689

Chapter 34

Interpretation of the Electrocardiogram

Samuel A. Sandowski

1: A standard ECG records activities in how many planes?

    A. 1
    B. 2
    C. 3
    D. 4
    E. 5

Answer: B

Critique: The ECG records electrical activity of the heart. Although it represents a three-dimensional electrical field, it is recorded only on two planes. The horizontal plane is known as the *precordial* or *chest leads* (V1 to V6), and the vertical plane is known as the *limb leads* (leads I, II, III, AVR, AVF, AVL).

Page: 699 (Tracing 34–1, page 704)

2: Which wave represents repolarization of the ventricle:

    A. P wave
    B. QRS complex
    C. T wave
    D. U wave
    E. All of the above

Answer: C

Critique: The P wave represents depolarization of the atria, and the QRS complex represents depolarization of the ventricle. The T wave represents the repolarization of the ventricle. It is important to remember that activity noted on the ECG represents electrical activity, and not contractions. Atrial repolarization often is not seen because it occurs during ventricular depolarization.

Page: 699

3: Which of the following cannot be determined by ECG:

    A. Heart rate
    B. Rhythm
    C. Blocks in electrical pathways of the heart
    D. Myocardial infarction
    E. The ejection fraction

Answer: E

Critique: Pattern analysis, scalar analysis, and vector analysis are all possible based on ECG tracing. Pattern analysis is done by evaluating the shape and amplitude of the ECG complexes. Scalar analysis is the measurement (in milliseconds) of the duration of a wave. The frequency of repetition of a wave is used to determine rate. Vector analysis is the magnitude and direction of a wave. Specific patterns may suggest blocks in electrical pathways of the heart and myocardial infarction. Scalar analysis is used to determine the rate and rhythm. The ejection fraction cannot be determined on the ECG, because it represents blood flow, and not electrical activity.

Page: 700

4: In a sinus rhythm, the normal sequence of events is as follows:

    A. AV nodal pause, atrial depolarization, ventricular depolarization, ventricular repolarization
    B. Atrial depolarization, ventricular depolarization, AV nodal pause, ventricular repolarization
    C. Atrial depolarization, AV nodal pause, ventricular depolarization, ventricular repolarization
    D. AV nodal pause, ventricular depolarization, atrial depolarization, ventricular repolarization
    E. Ventricular depolarization, atrial depolarization, AV nodal pause, ventricular repolarization

Answer: C

Critique: In a normal sinus rhythm, the sinoatrial (SA) node's automaticity starts the cycle with atrial depolarization. When impulses reach the atrioventricular (AV) node, there is a pause of 0.06 to 0.10 second. Then the ventricle is depolarized and finally repolarized. Normal atrial depolarization occurs in a plane of approximately +45 degrees. Normal ventricular depolarization occurs in a plane of about +60 degrees.

Page: 700

5: What is the axis if an ECG shows an isoelectric wave in lead III, a positive QRS wave in leads I and II, and a negative QRS wave in AVR?

    A. +30 degrees
    B. −150 degrees
    C. +120 degrees

D. −30 degrees
E. +150 degrees

Answer: A

Critique: Einthoven's triangle can be used to calculate an axis, where AVL+AVF+AVR=0. However, another approach is to find the isoelectric lead. The axis is 90 degrees to the isoelectric lead (see Figure 34–7). If lead III is isoelectric, the axis must be toward AVR (−150 degrees) or between leads I and II (+30 degrees). The axis is always toward the positive leads. Because the QRS in this example is positive in leads I and II and negative in AVR, the axis direction must be +30 degrees.

Pages: 701–702

6: Which lead always has a positive P wave in normal sinus rhythm:

A. AVR
B. III
C. AVL
D. II
E. All leads should be positive

Answer: D

Critique: A normal sinus rhythm has an axis of about +45 degrees (between +20 and +70). Therefore, the P wave should be positive in leads reflecting this direction. This would be lead II.

Page: 702 (Tracing 34-2, page 704)

7: What is the normal direction of the axis in newborn infants?

A. Between +90 and +180 degrees
B. Between 0 and +90 degrees
C. Between +180 and -90 degrees
D. Between 0 and -90 degrees
E. None of the above

Answer: A

Critique: Newborn infants normally have right axis deviation (RAD). RAD is defined as an axis direction between +90 and +180 degrees. Extreme right axis is between +180 and −90 degrees. Left axis deviation occurs when the axis lies between 0 and −90 degrees. The direction of the QRS axis in adults and children (but not infants) is between 0 and +90 degrees.

Page: 702 (Tracing 34–8, page 710)

8: Which lead is placed in the fifth intercostal space?

A. V1
B. V2
C. V3
D. V4
E. V5

Answer: C

Critique: ECG tracings reflect lead placement, and leads placed in other than standard positions can lead to misinterpretations of the ECG. V1 and V2 are placed in the fourth intercostal space on the right and left sternal borders, respectively. V3 is placed in the fifth intercostal

space in the midaxillary line. V4 to V6 are all in the sixth intercostal space, where V4 is in the anterior axillary line, V6 in the midaxillary line, and V5 is between them.

Page: 703 (Figure 34–11, page 707)

9: Which of the following does *not* occur with left ventricular hypertrophy (LVH)?

A. A strain pattern
B. A delay in the repolarization sequence of the T wave
C. A large S wave in V1
D. Right axis deviation
E. A large R wave in V5

Answer: D

Critique: The ECG of LVH reflects increased muscle mass of the left ventricle. This increased muscle mass often results in left axis deviation and high-magnitude R waves in the lateral leads, with high-magnitude S waves in the septal leads. (If the S wave in V1 + R wave is V5 >35mm , then LVH should be considered.) With systolic overloading, a delay in the repolarization sequence of the ventricle often causes a strain pattern of the T wave.

Page: 708 (Tracing 34–7, page 709)

10: Which of the following is *not* reflective of right ventricular strain (RVH):

A. Tall R wave in V1 (R >0.7 mV)
B. Deep S wave in V6 (S >0.3 mV)
C. R in V1 + S in V5 >1 mV
D. Right ventricular strain
E. Wide QRS (>0.12 sec)

Answer: E

Critique: RVH reflects increased electromagnetic forces because of increased muscle mass of the right ventricle. This results in right axis deviation and right ventricular strain with a QRS complex of normal duration. The vector forces are pulled vertically and to the right, resulting in the presence of an R wave in V1 and an S wave of significant magnitude in V5 and V6.

Page: 708 (Tracing 34–9, page 710)

11: Which is *not* found in left bundle branch block (LBBB):

A. Right axis deviation
B. QRS >0.12 sec
C. Left ventricular strain
D. Normal amplitude of the QRS
E. Slurring of the QRS in several leads

Answer: A

Critique: In LBBB, the depolarization of the left ventricle occurs slowly. This results in a prolonged QRS complex with left ventricular strain. The amplitude of the QRS, however, is unchanged. Forces initially point toward the back, and there is a left axis deviation.

Page: 711 (Tracing 34–10, page 711)

12: Hemiblocks are caused by a conduction defect in which of the following:

A. SA node
B. Bundle of Kent
C. Bundle of His
D. Purkinje fibers
E. Pericardium

Answer: C

Critique: Conduction defects that occur along the bundle of His cause bundle branch blocks or hemiblocks. Defects can occur anywhere along the pathway, including the AV node. A defect in the right bundle causes a right bundle branch block (RBBB). The left bundle divides into an anterior and posterior portion. A block in either of these portions causes a left anterior hemiblock (LAHB) or left posterior hemiblock (LPHB), respectively. Defects in two of the three bundles, or in the AV node and one of the bundles, cause a bifascicular block.

Page: 712 (Figure 34–19, page 712)

13: Which of the following is diagnostic for left anterior hemiblock (LAHB):

A. Left axis deviation of at least -30 degrees
B. QRS complexes of large magnitude
C. QRS complexes of >0.12 second
D. Significant slurring of the QRS
E. ST elevations

Answer: A

Critique: The location of the block causes a posterior axis and a left axis deviation of at least −30 degrees. The QRS complexes are of normal shape, duration, and magnitude. LAHB does not cause ST elevation, although LAHB can occur with myocardial injury.

Page: 713 (Tracing 34–12, page 713)

14: All of the following are true of P pulmonale, except that it:

A. Is also known as right atrial enlargement
B. Is often caused by pulmonary valve or pulmonary artery disease
C. Has a P wave magnitude of >0.25 mV
D. Is often recognized in lead II
E. Has a P wave of increased duration (>0.08 second)

Answer: E

Critique: P pulmonale reflects and is synonymous with right atrial enlargement. It is often caused by increased pulmonary pressures, which may be secondary to pulmonary valve or artery disease. Peaked P waves of normal duration (<0.08 second) are often noted in lead II.

Page: 714 (Tracing 34–16, page 716)

15: An ECG shows a biphasic P wave in V1 and a notched (double-hump) P wave in lead II. This represents all of the following, except:

A. Right atrial enlargement (P pulmonale)
B. Left atrial enlargement
C. Right atrium depolarizing earlier than the left atrium
D. P mitral
E. Left atrial abnormality

Answer: A

Critique: A notched (double-humped) P wave of prolonged duration (>0.08 second) in lead II and a biphasic or negative P wave in V1 represents the left atrium depolarizing later than the right atrium. This may be secondary to increased left ventricular mass, as in left atrial enlargement, or because of damaged myocardium causing delayed depolarization (as seen with coronary artery disease). This latter term is called left abnormality, because there is no left atrial hypertrophy.

Page: 716 (Tracing 34–17, page 717)

16: Which part of the ECG is typically elevated, representing areas lacking myocardial oxygenation, as seen in a transmural myocardial infarction:

A. P wave
B. QRS wave
C. ST segment
D. T wave
E. U wave

Answer: C

Critique: The P and U waves are often not affected by the lack of oxygenation to the myocardium. The QRS wave (Q wave) is downward and represents dead myocardium, whereas the T wave is downward and represents ischemia. Only the ST segment is elevated, representing the injured myocardium.

Page: 719 (Figure 34–23, page 719)

17: A 67-year-old male presents to the emergency room with chest pain. His ECG reveals a sinus bradycardia with an acute inferior myocardial infarction. Which artery is most likely occluded:

A. Circumflex
B. Right coronary artery (dominant)
C. Left main
D. Left anterior descending
E. Left coronary artery (dominant)

Answer: B

Critique: The left anterior descending artery supplies the anteroseptal and apical portions of the heart. The circumflex artery supplies the anterolateral and anterobasal and superior portions of the heart. The right coronary artery supplies the posterior aspect of the heart. The inferior part of the heart may be supplied by either the right coronary artery or the left coronary artery, whichever is dominant. Because the right coronary artery also supplies the SA node and the AV node, bradycardia is most likely the result of occlusion of the right coronary artery.

Page: 719 (Figure 34–24, page 719)

18: Pick the best answer: Which of the following statements is *not* correct?

A. Anteroseptal myocardial infarctions are noted by QRS and T abnormalities in V1 and V2
B. Apical myocardial infarctions are noted by QRS and T abnormalities in lead I
C. Posterior myocardial infarctions are noted by QRS and T abnormalities in V1

D. Inferior myocardial infarctions are noted by QRS and T abnormalities in II, III, and AVF
E. All of the above

Answer: E

Critique: All of these wave abnormalities correspond to the correct areas of the heart.

Page: 720

19: Which of the following is diagnostic for pericarditis:

A. ST elevations of >2 mm across most of the precordium
B. Q waves in leads with ST elevation
C. Persistence of ST elevations for more than 6 weeks
D. Patients are usually elderly
E. Inverted T waves suggestive of ischemia

Answer: A

Critique: Pericarditis is diagnosed with >2 mm ST elevations across the precordium in the proper clinical scenario. Patients are usually younger than the average patient having a myocardial infarction. Symptoms and ST elevations typically resolve within 1 to 2 weeks. No Q waves or ST changes are consistent with ischemia.

Page: 720 (Tracing 34–25, page 724)

20: Which of the following causes ST elevations:

A. Pericarditis
B. Early repolarization in young people
C. Prinzmetal syndrome
D. Ventricular aneurysm
E. All of the above

Answer: E

Critique: All of these choices cause ST elevations. In pericarditis, ST elevations are >2 mm and are usually accompanied by chest pain, which eases when the patient leans forward. Early repolarization is noted by ST elevations in the anterior chest leads in healthy, asymptomatic patients. Patients with Prinzmetal syndrome have pain at rest secondary to spasm of the epicardial arteries. ST elevations are transient and do not occur at rest. ST elevations secondary to a ventricular aneurysm occur in the leads representing the wall of the aneurysm. The elevations persist as long as the aneurysm is present. The ST elevations seen with ventricular aneurysms are caused by repolarization delays and are not secondary to ischemia.

Pages: 723–725 (Tracings 34–25, 34–26, 34–27, 34–28, pages 724–726)

21: ST depression may be caused by all of the following, except:

A. Digitalis
B. Left ventricular hypertrophy (LVH)
C. Left bundle branch block (LBBB)
D. Prinzmetal syndrome
E. Ischemia

Answer: D

Critique: Prinzmetal syndrome causes ST elevation. All the other choices can cause ST segment depression. With ischemia, the ST segment depression is >2mm . ST segment depression seen in LVH may also be >2mm but is most prominent in the frontal plane (V leads). Digitalis may produce a downward-sloping ST segment that is <2mm .

Page: 726

22: Which of the following statements regarding dextrocardia is true?

A. Dextrocardia cannot occur with situs inversus.
B. Patients with dextrocardia have ECG changes mirroring those of a normal ECG.
C. Typical findings with dextrocardia include left axis deviation.
D. The T axis in patients with dextrocardia is usually 180 degrees from the QRS axis.
E. Patients with dextrocardia do not develop ischemia or bundle branch blocks.

Answer: B

Critique: Patients with situs inversus have dextrocardia. Their heart is located in a mirror image position to the normal heart. Therefore, the ECG changes and abnormalities are also mirrored in a similar fashion. Right axis deviation is present. The T wave axis is usually less than 60 degrees from the QRS axis. Patients with dextrocardia should have precordial (chest) leads placed in a mirror image to the normally placed leads. These leads have an *R* after the number of the lead (e.g., V4, normally placed in the sixth intercostal space in the anterior left axillary line, would be V4R and the lead would be in the sixth intercostal space of the right anterior axillary line.

Pages: 726–727 (Tracing 34–30, page 728)

23: All of the following can cause a short P-R interval, except:

A. Wolff-Parkinson-White syndrome (WPW)
B. Wandering pacemaker
C. Digitalis
D. Nodal rhythm
E. Short P-R interval syndrome (Lown-Ganong-Levine syndrome)

Answer: C

Critique: The normal P wave is <0.08 second, and the normal P-R interval is <0.2 second (at 60 beats/minute). The P wave does not change with heart rate, but the P-R interval does. With increased heart rate, the P-R interval shortens. Conversely, increasing vagal tone, causing bradycardia, lengthens the P-R interval. Digitalis and first-degree A-V block also prolong the P-R interval. If the atrial impulse starts close to the bundle of His (as with a wandering pacemaker or nodal rhythm) or if the atrial impulses reach the bundle of His through a quicker accessory pathway (as in WPW or short P-R interval syndrome), the P-R interval will be short.

Pages: 728–739

24: The ECG of a 38-year-old male reveals a normal sinus rhythm with no acute changes (i.e., a normal ECG). Which of the following statements is *not* true?

A. The QRS complex is 0.08 second.
B. The P wave is 0.08 second.
C. The P-R interval is <0.2 second.
D. The QT interval is 0.4 second in men and 0.44 second in women.
E. The R-R interval is 0.45 second.

Answer: E

Critique: All of the above statements are true, except choice E. An R-R interval of 0.45 second equals a rate of 150 beats/minute. This would be sinus tachycardia, because the upper limit of normal is 100 beats/minute (or an R-R interval of 0.6 second).

Page: 729

25: Shortened QT intervals occur in which situation:

A. Hypokalemia
B. Hypocalcemia
C. Treatment with quinidine
D. Treatment with digitalis
E. None of the above

Answer: D

Critique: Medications and electrolyte disturbances may affect the P wave, QRS complex, ST segment, T wave, and/or the QT interval. Hypokalemia, hypocalcemia, and high quinidine levels prolong the QT interval. Elevated digitalis levels actually shorten the QT interval. Other conditions that shorten the QT interval are hyperkalemia and hypercalcemia.

Page: 730 (Figure 34–28, page 730)

26: Which of the following does *not* cause a significant, upright R wave in V1:

A. Right ventricular hypertrophy
B. Posterior myocardial infarction
C. Right bundle branch block
D. Type A Wolff-Parkinson-White syndrome
E. Type B Wolff-Parkinson-White syndrome

Answer: E

Critique: Wolff-Parkinson-White (WPW) syndrome is a pre-excitation syndrome in which impulses bypass the AV node and pass from the atrium to the ventricle via an accessory pathway. This pathway is called the bundle of Kent. In type A WPW, lead V1 has a delta wave slurred into an R wave. In type B WPW, the delta wave in V1 is slurred into a Q wave. All of the other reasons noted produce an R wave in V1.

Pages: 729–730 (Tracings 34–32 and 34–33, page 731)

Chapter 35

Arrhythmias

Charles Driscoll

1: The most common pacemaker of the heart is located at the:

    A. Atrioventricular (AV) node
    B. Bundle of His
    C. Purkinje fibers
    D. Sinoatrial (SA) node

Answer: D

Critique: Automaticity accounts for the capability of heart cells to produce an electrical impulse. All of the cells may act as pacemakers, but the most common one is the SA node.

Page: 733

2: A 54-year-old man is in the coronary care unit with an acute anterior myocardial infarction. His cardiac monitor shows that an episode of ventricular tachycardia followed a period of time when his oxygen saturation levels were observed to be in the 80s. Which of the following best explains the genesis of the ventricular tachycardia?

    A. Re-entry phenomenon
    B. A shortening of the relative refractory period
    C. A functional lesion of the central nervous system
    D. Wolff-Parkinson-White pre-excitation syndrome
    E. Lown-Ganong-Levine syndrome

Answer: A

Critique: Conduction through Purkinje's branches is usually anterograde, but in the face of hypoxia or electrolyte abnormalities it may be slowed or blocked. An impulse may arrive later in a retrograde fashion through a connecting branch. This is called the re-entry mechanism and causes ventricular tachycardia in the setting of myocardial infarction. Wolff-Parkinson-White pre-excitation syndrome and Lown-Ganong-Levine syndrome can be a result of the re-entry phenomenon. A lengthening, and not a shortening, of the relative refractory period would be expected to cause re-entry. A functional lesion of the central nervous system would not be expected in this setting.

Page: 734

3: A 37-year-old woman is undergoing a somewhat difficult flexible fiberoptic bronchoscopy, and a cardiac monitor shows a sudden bradycardia to 35 beats per minute. Which of the following is the most plausible reason for this occurrence?

    A. Perforation of the trachea
    B. Hypoxic myocardial damage
    C. Irritation of tracheobronchial vagal receptors

    D. Anesthetic reaction
    E. Pulmonary embolization

Answer: C

Critique: Irritation of the vagal receptors in the throat or tracheobronchial tree explains the frequent occurrence of arrhythmias during bronchoscopy, gastroscopy, or nasopharyngeal suctioning in persons who are not anesthetized.

Page: 734

4: In review of an electrocardiogram, numerous QRS and T wave complexes are noted to occur earlier than normal in the cardiac cycle, and they are not preceded by a P wave. Their configuration and duration is different from preceding or following beats, and they are occurring randomly. What is the diagnosis?

    A. Atrial premature beats
    B. Nodal escape beats
    C. U waves due to hypokalemia
    D. Re-entry phenomenon
    E. Ventricular premature beats

Answer: E

Critique: The description given matches that of ventricular premature beats (VPBs) or extra systoles. P waves are present in atrial premature beats, in the presence of U waves, or sometimes following nodal escape beats. Re-entry phenomenon may be a cause of the VPBs.

Page: 735

Match the following drugs with their correct use in the treatment of cardiac arrhythmias.
    A. Digitalis
    B. Adenosine
    C. Magnesium sulfate
    D. Atropine

5: Controls the ventricular tachycardia of torsades de pointes

6: Increases vagal tone and decreases sympathetic tone, causing bradycardia

7: Used to re-establish more rapid rhythm in cases of severe bradycardia

8: Terminates re-entrant supraventricular tachycardias

Answers: 5 - C, 6 - A, 7 - D, 8 - B

Critique: Digitalis and other glycosides have important antiarrhythmic properties in that they increase vagal tone and decrease sympathetic tone. As a result, the discharge rate of the SA node is slowed. Adenosine has fast action and terminates many re-entrant SVTs. Magnesium sulfate is used to control the ventricular tachycardia of torsades de pointes. Anticholinergic and sympathomimetic drugs such as atropine and epinephrine re-establish an adequate rate in cases of severe bradycardia, pulseless electrical activity, and asystole.

Pages: 735, 736

Correctly manage the following patients with their rhythm strips by matching them with their correct action and rationale. Answer choices may be used once, more than once, or not at all.

9: A 76-year-old female is brought to the emergency department complaining of dizziness after having an episode of syncope (Figure A).

10: A 57-year-old man being monitored in the coronary care unit to rule out myocardial infarction shows this finding during his sleep (Figure B).

11: A 66-year-old woman is asymptomatic except for complaining of a "soreness" in the left shoulder and an EKG is done showing this rhythm (Figure C).

12: A 48-year-old man en route to the hospital by ambulance following his collapse in the street with the following rhythm (Figure D).

13: A 48-year-old man en route to the hospital by ambulance following his collapse in the street with the following rhythm (Figure E).

A. CPR and defibrillation with direct current (DC) countershocks are needed immediately.
B. No treatment is needed; observe only.
C. Administer 0.5 mg of atropine IV push and prepare for electrical pacing.
D. Administer 1 to 2 g of magnesium sulfate IV in 100 mL D_5W.
E. Administer a beta blocker from class II (e.g., acebutolol, esmolol).
F. Rapid IV administration of 6 mg adenosine; repeat if necessary.

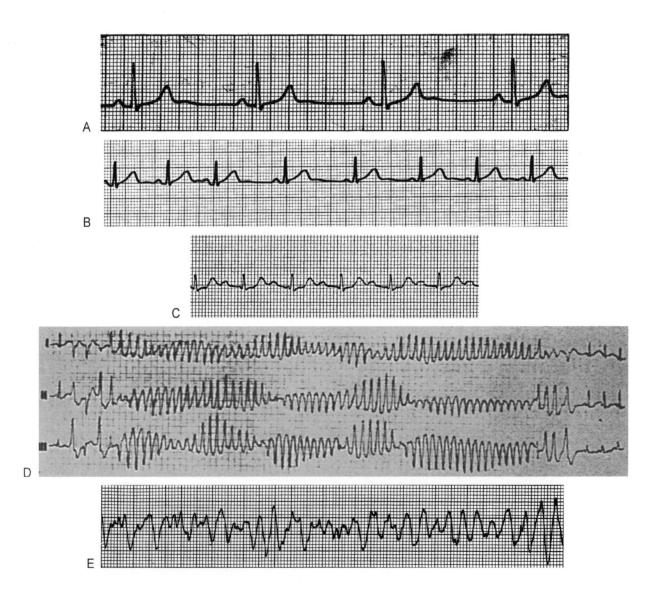

Answers: 9 - C, 10 - B, 11 - B, 12 - D, 13 - A

Critique: The rhythm strip for the patient in question 9 shows sinus bradycardia. The fact that she is symptomatic suggests that treatment of the arrhythmia is indicated. Symptomatic bradycardia may require atropine or pacing. The patient in question 10 is asymptomatic and his rhythm is sinus arrhythmia, which is a common occurrence during sleep. No treatment is indicated. The patient in question 11 shows first-degree AV block on her rhythm strip. No treatment is usually indicated unless the patient is on digitalis, in which case the physician may consider discontinuing the drug. The patient in question 12 has collapsed and shows torsades de pointes on his rhythm strip. This rhythm usually responds only to administration of magnesium or overdrive pacing with isoproterenol. The patient in question 13 has collapsed with cardiac arrest secondary to ventricular fibrillation. The treatment is to initiate CPR and defibrillate immediately.

Pages: (question 9) 736, (10) 736, 737, (11) 748, (12) 747, (13) 747, 748

14: A patient's rhythm strip shows a sustained ventricular tachycardia with a rate of 150 to 160. The patient is stable and does not complain of chest pain. The initial treatment of this arrhythmia is to give an intravenous bolus of:

    A. Lidocaine, 60 to 100 mg
    B. Magnesium sulfate, 1 to 2 g
    C. Atropine, 0.5 to 1.0 mg
    D. Isoproterenol, 2 to 10 μg
    E. Bretylium, 300 to 500 mg

Answer: A

Critique: A stable ventricular tachycardia is treated with an initial bolus of intravenous lidocaine, 60 to 100 mg, followed by a drip of 0.1% to 0.2% lidocaine solution at 100 mL/hr. Thereafter, a beta blocker is indicated for prophylaxis.

Page: 746

15: (True or False) A 25-year-old man experiences recurrent episodes of supraventricular tachycardia. The rate is very rapid, and the etiology is determined to be re-entrant impulses from the bundle of Kent. The ECG after recovery demonstrates a short PR interval and a delta wave of the QRS.

    A. The diagnosis is Lown-Ganong-Levine syndrome
    B. Treatment can be initiated with either verapamil or beta blockers.
    C. Surgical ablation therapy is effective.
    D. In children, digoxin is an effective treatment for this arrhythmia.

Answers: A - False, B - False, C - True, D - True

Critique: The scenario describes the Wolff-Parkinson-White syndrome as a result of an aberrant re-entry pathway. Verapamil, beta blockers, and digoxin should be avoided in this patient because they may make the condition worse by facilitating the re-entry. In young children, however, digoxin may actually be helpful. The treatment of choice is probably electrophysiologic study and ablation of the aberrant pathway.

Page: 750

16: Select the one correct characteristic of second-degree AV block, Mobitz I (Wenckebach's phenomenon).

    A. It occurs only in adults with organic heart disease.
    B. When this block occurs, it can lead to serious consequences.
    C. The PR interval shows progressive lengthening until a QRS is dropped.
    D. The block occurs intermittently, every two or three beats.
    E. There is no relationship of P waves to Q waves.

Answer: C

Critique: Second-degree AV block, Mobitz I (Wenckebach's phenomenon), is the more benign of the two types of second-degree block. The Mobitz I block can occur in adolescents as a result of autonomic lability. Usually not associated with symptoms, this block does not require treatment. If there were no relationship of P waves to QRS waves, the block would be third degree, complete AV dissociation. In Wenckebach phenomenon, the PR interval may start with a normal length, but it progressively lengthens until a normal atrial impulse is completely blocked and not followed by a QRS.

Pages: 747, 748

17: If ventricular fibrillation occurs more than 48 hours after myocardial infarction:

    A. It is easier to treat after magnesium sulfate is administered intravenously.
    B. The prognosis is very poor.
    C. Drug treatment is more efficacious than electrical cardioversion.
    D. It is more likely to be coarse rather than fine fibrillation.
    E. The arrhythmia is invariably resistant to lidocaine therapy.

Answer: B

Critique: If ventricular fibrillation occurs more than 48 hours after myocardial infarction, the prognosis is very poor. Magnesium sulfate is a therapy specific to torsades de pointes and is not helpful in ventricular fibrillation. The only effective course of action is cardiopulmonary resuscitation and immediate electrical defibrillation. A useful sequence of adjunctive drugs is epinephrine, lidocaine, and then bretylium. There is no prediction of whether the fibrillation will appear coarse or fine.

Pages: 746, 747

Match the following drugs with the arrhythmia they commonly cause.

    A. Tricyclic antidepressants
    B. Digitalis
    C. Terfenadine
    D. Atenolol

18: Bradycardia

19: Prolonged QT syndrome

20: First-degree AV block

21: Torsades de pointes

Answers: 18 - D, 19 - A, 20 - B, 21 - C

Critique: The use of beta blockers such as atenolol and acebutolol may produce a symptomatic bradycardia.

Prolonged QT syndrome may be caused by tricyclic anti-depressants, thioridazine, and, rarely, some antihistamines. Digitalis use in older persons can lead to an asymptomatic first-degree AV block. The newer antihistamines (terfenadine and astemizole) have been reported to cause torsades de pointes.

Pages: (question 18) 745, (19) 750, (20) 747, (21) 746

Chapter 36

Cardiovascular Disease

Jamal Islam

1: Which patient mentioned below would require a complete cardiovascular work-up?

 A. A 40-year-old African-American man who complains of shortness of breath, is morbidly obese, and has a short neck, prominent eyeballs, and a protuberant abdomen with striae

 B. A 15-year-old girl, brought in by her mother with complaints that her daughter has not started her menstrual cycle and has no signs of breast development. The girl appears to be short for her age and has multiple pigmented nevi, a shield-shaped chest, and redundant skin in her neck.

 C. A 50-year-old Hispanic female with history of Type II diabetes for 5 years, hyperlipidemia for 5 years, and hypertension for 7 years. She has central obesity, xanthelasma at the elbow, cold skin, poor turgor of mucosa, thinning hair, pallor, and brittle nails.

 D. A 24-year-old white male with no complaints. Has been weight lifting and using anabolic drugs. Salient features on physical examination are muscular build and small testicles.

Answer: B

Critique: Physical examination is an integral part of the cardiovascular examination. Physical appearance provides clues to probable underlying cardiovascular disease and alerts one to consider a more complete cardiovascular work-up. The African-American man will probably need a minimum of ECG but not a full cardiovascular work-up. His obesity is the most likely cause of his breathlessness. The 15-year-old girl has Turner's syndrome. In this population, 20% have congenital heart disease such as aortic stenosis, bicuspid aortic valve, and coarctation of the aorta. Thus, there is a requirement to have a full cardiovascular work-up of this patient. The 50-year-old Hispanic female has several risk factors for cardiovascular disease, but her appearance suggests hypothyroidism and should not require a complete cardiovascular work-up unless she has more specific complaints. Body-builders using anabolic drugs may have cardiovascular manifestation, but without any other symptoms appearance alone does not require a full cardiovascular work-up.

Page: 752

2: During heart failure, all of the following can occur. Which one is the hallmark of heart failure?

 A. Atrial "S4" gallop
 B. Ventricular "S3" gallop
 C. Mitral regurgitation
 D. Tricuspid regurgitation
 E. Increased loudness of the pulmonic component of the second heart sound

Answer: B

Critique: A to E may be found in heart failure. The hallmark of heart failure is the S3 sound. S3 and S4 sound create a cadence similar to the sound of a galloping horse and thus termed occasionally as "gallop" sound or rhythm. Eighty percent of the atrial blood volume fills the ventricle passively and follows the S2 sound. The remaining 20% of the ventricle filling is carried out by virtue of atrial contraction. In volume overload, S3 sound occurs due to rapid expansion and filling of the ventricle. The interval between S2 and S3 is 120 to 170 msec, or the time to say "me too" (ME and TOO representing S2 and S3, respectively). The S4 sound is a result of forceful contraction of the atria into a noncompliant stiff ventricle. It occurs just before S1, approximately equivalent to the time one can say "'middle" (MI and DDLE representing S4 and S1, respectively). Both S3 and S4 are normal in children and young adults. If an S3 or S4 occurs beyond 30 years of age, it usually is pathological. Heart failure with concomitant volume overload can produce both mitral and tricuspid regurgitation. Increased loudness of pulmonic component of second heart sound is found in pulmonary hypertension.

Page: 753

3: Which of the following is not a common finding in aortic stenosis?

 A. Aortic ejection click
 B. S4 and presystolic heave
 C. Pulse small, slow rising, and sometimes prolonged
 D. Second heart sound widely split with inspiration
 E. Blood pressure usually normal

Answer: D

Critique: Ejection clicks are high-pitched sounds. They occur early in systole and are produced by pathological semilunar valve (aortic and pulmonic) opening as soon as blood is ejected from the atria. Because of a hypertrophied and noncompliant left ventricle, an S4 can be heard in patients with a long history of aortic stenosis. Pulse is usually small and slow rising. The second heart sound in aortic stenosis is *paradoxically split*, which means that it widens during expiration, rather than inspiration as found in normal heart. Delay in emptying of the

163

left ventricle is found in aortic stenosis or left bundle branch block. The delay in left ventricle emptying causes a delay in aortic valve closure, and the pulmonic valve thus closes earlier than in normal patients. During inspiration, the pulmonic sound normally moves away from S1, thus causing the pulmonic sound to move closer to the aortic sound in aortic stenosis, which causes narrowing of the split during inspiration. During expiration, pulmonic sound is not shifted, but as the aortic sound is delayed there is a split in the sound. With a normal aortic valve, the aortic and pulmonic split is heard during inspiration and not during expiration as we find in aortic stenosis, and thus the term *paradoxical splitting*. Blood pressure may be normal in patients with aortic stenosis.

Page: 753

4: Which of the following myocardial perfusion imaging agents is not a good choice for patients who are obese or have large breasts?

    A. Thallium-201
    B. Teboroxime (Cardiotec)
    C. Sestamibi (Cardiolite)
    D. Tetrofosmin (Myoview) Tc-9

Answer: A

Critique: Of all the modalities of noninvasive diagnostics for detecting coronary artery disease, myocardial perfusion imaging (MPI) is the most accurate. MPI also helps in the assessment of severity and extent of perfusion defects in patients with coronary stenosis. Until 1990, the tracer used for MPI was thallium-201 (Tl-201). Like Tl-201, technetium 99m (^{99m}Tc) is distributed in the myocardium in proportion to blood flow. Three Tc-99m agents are available: teboroxime (Cardiotec), sestamibi (Cardiolite), and tetrofosmin (Myoview). Two physical features of the ^{99m}Tc label confer advantages over Tl-201: (1) higher photon energy: results in less attenuation and scatter, and (2) shorter half-life allows a higher imaging dose These characteristics of Tc-99m result in superior image quality, with higher count density, improved spatial resolution, and less prominent soft tissue artifacts. This allows good images even in patients who are obese or have large breasts. The high photon flux of ^{99m}Tc also allows the gating of single-photon emission computed tomographic (SPECT) images during multiple intervals of the cardiac cycle, maintaining adequate count density, image contrast, and spatial resolution in each image frame. Running these frames continuously in a cinematic format allows observers to evaluate resting left and right ventricular function in combination with either resting or exercise myocardial perfusion.

Pages: 764, 765

5: High serum cholesterol is found in which of the following conditions?

    A. Hypothyroidism
    B. Amyotrophic lateral sclerosis
    C. Nephritis
    D. Diabetes insipidus
    E. Amyloidosis

Answer: A

Critique: Serum cholesterol has been found to be elevated in several diseases, such as diabetes mellitus, hypothyroidism, and nephrotic syndrome. Treatment of the associated disease has been found to decrease serum cholesterol.

Page: 757

6: Using HMG-CoA reductase inhibitors (statins) in the primary and secondary prevention of coronary artery disease has resulted in:

    A. A 25% to 30% reduction in mortality in both primary and secondary prevention trials
    B. A 25% to 30% reduction in mortality only in secondary prevention trials
    C. A 25% to 30% reduction in mortality only in primary and secondary prevention trials
    D. No reduction in mortality in either primary or secondary trials

Answer: A

Critique: Results of a meta-analysis on randomized, controlled clinical trials of statins in the prevention of both primary and secondary prevention were published recently. It showed a 25% to 30% reduction in mortality from cardiovascular disease in both types of prevention trials.

Pages: 757, 758

7: (True or False) Determine whether each statement below is true or false regarding isolated systolic hypertension (ISH) in patients 60 years and older.

    A. ISH is defined as the systolic pressure above 160 mm Hg with a diastolic reading below 90 mm Hg.
    B. JNV VI guideline recommends lowering blood pressure of patients with ISH to below 150/90.
    C. First-line medication for ISH is a thiazide diuretic.
    D. Using a calcium channel blocker is a contraindication for the treatment of ISH.
    E. Exercise does not help to reduce blood pressure in overweight patients with ISH.

Answers: A - False, B - False, C - True, D - False, E - False

Critique: The Sixth Joint National Committee on Prevention, Detection, and Treatment of high blood pressure defines ISH as the persistent elevation of systolic blood pressure above 139 mm Hg and diastolic pressure below 90 mm Hg. The recommendation is to treat ISH target of BP being below 140/90 mm Hg. First line of treatment is thiazide diuretic. Using calcium channel blockers is not a contraindication in the treatment of ISH. Exercise has been shown to decrease blood pressure in overweight patients.

Page: 759

8: (True or False) A 50-year-old Hispanic man is obese, with a history of diabetes type II for the last 5 years and is on oral hypoglycemic agents with an HgbA1c level below 8. He also has high triglyceride and low HDL levels being treated with a statin. He exercises regularly, has knowledge of how to follow a diabetic diet, has not smoked for the last 10 years and does not have premature deaths due to cardiovascular disease in immediate family members. He has no complaints today. His BP today is 145/95 mm Hg after 15 minutes' rest in a sitting position. Record of previous BP 3 months ago shows 144/90. Determine whether the following statements are true or false.

  A. He does not have hypertension.
  B. He has stage 1 hypertension.
  C. His ideal BP should be below 130/85 mmHg.
  D. He should be advised on nonpharmacologic strategies to decrease his BP and come back after 3 months for recheck of his BP.
  E. He should be started on an ACE inhibitor if serum creatinine level is normal.

Answers: A - False, B - True, C - True, D - False, E - True

Critique: According to JNC, VI hypertension is diagnosed if during two clinical visits after initial screening BP is above 139/89. Mr. Doe is determined to have a category of stage 1 hypertension since this is the second BP that is above 139/89. Since he has diabetes he is in the highest risk group as per stratification by risk. Mr. Doe should be started on an ACE inhibitor as soon as possible once it is determined his creatinine level is stable and below 3 mg/dL

Pages: 759, 760

9: When used for treating hypertension, beta-blocking agents can also improve which of the following comorbid conditions?

  A. Asthma
  B. Diabetes mellitus
  C. Essential tremor
  D. Depression
  E. Peripheral vascular disease

Answer: C

Critique: The two types of beta-adrenoceptors are β_1 and β_2. One has to take into careful consideration the implication of blocking these receptors when choosing a beta-blocking agent. Both β_1 and β_2 receptors are found in the lungs; the β_1 receptors appear in greater numbers. Stimulation of this receptor causes bronchodilatation, and blocking these receptors causes bronchoconstriction. β_2 receptors are found in skeletal muscle and liver, stimulation of which increases glycogenolysis and blocking of which diminishes it. Blocking skeletal β_2 receptors improves essential tremor. Beta-blocking agents have been shown to worsen depression. Blood vessels contain β_2 receptors, which causes vasodilatation. Blocking them causes worsening of the symptoms of peripheral vascular disease.

Page: 766

10: An ideal beta blocker for use as an antihypertensive medication should have all the following effects except

  A. Preferably block β_1 receptors
  B. Hydrophilic
  C. Do not preferably block β_2 receptors
  D. Long acting

Answer: B

Critique: All beta-blocking agents appear to have similar potency to decrease blood pressure in 50% of hypertensive patients. They have different pharmacological properties. Some beta-blocking agents have greater affinity to β_1 receptor rather than β_2, but at higher dose selectivity is lost. Metoprolol, atenolol, and bisoprolol have β_1 selectivity. Beta-blocking agents like labetalol also have blocking action on alpha adrenoreceptors. Some beta-blocking agents have intrinsic sympathomimetic activity such as pindolol, which thus causes less resting bradycardia and lipid changes. Solubility of beta-blocking agents in lipid also varies; carvedilol, metoprolol and propranolol have the highest lipid solubility. Propranolol is the most toxic since it competitively blocks both the β_1 and β_2 adrenoreceptors and also has a direct membrane-depressant and central nervous system effect.

Page: 766

11: The calcium channel blocker that causes the greatest SA and AV node suppression is:

  A. Nifedipine
  B. Verapamil
  C. Diltiazem
  D. Amlodipine
  E. Felodipine

Answer: B

Critique: Calcium channel blockers when used as single-drug therapy reduce BP in approximately 60% of hypertensive patients, irrespective of the stage of hypertension and demographic group. The nondihydropyridines have negative inotropic and chronotropic effects, the most potent being verapamil. Dihydropyridine of the first generation category, nifedipine, has some negative chronotropic and inotropic effect compared with the newer dihydropyridines, which are amlodipine, felodipine, isradipine, and nicardipine.

Pages: 766, 767

12: Which statement is true when comparing the angiotensin converting enzyme (ACE) inhibitors with angiotensin receptor blockers (ARBs)?

  A. ACE inhibitors cause coughing more than do the ARBs.
  B. ARBs increase the level of bradykinin, a vasoactive peptide that causes vasodilatation, more than the ACE inhibitors.
  C. ARBs compared with ACE inhibitors do not have side effects such as hypotension, hyperkalemia, and renal impairment.
  D. ARBs, rather than ACE inhibitors, are indicated first-line therapy for congestive heart failure.
  E. Clinical trials have confirmed the benefits of ARBs as being similar to those of ACE inhibitors for treatment of CHF.

Answer: D

Critique: ACE inhibitors act by blocking the conversion of angiotensin I to angiotensin II, a potent vasoconstrictor and growth factor. The ARBs block the receptors to which the angiotensin II attaches. The ACE inhibitors also inhibit the degradation of bradykinin, which is a vasoactive peptide. The bradykinin promotes vasodilatation by stimulating the endothelium to produce nitric oxide (NO). The NO contributes to maintain vascular structure and function by inhibiting pathological processes such as monocyte adherence, platelet aggregation, and vascular smooth muscle proliferation. Until clinical trials establish the benefit of ARBs to be similar or superior to the ACE inhibitors, the first-line therapy for congestive heart failure continues to be ACE inhibitors. Side effects such as hypotension, hyperkalemia, and renal impairment are seen with the use of either an ACE inhibitor or ARB. Coughing, a bothersome side effect of ACE inhibitors, is not noticed in ARBs.

Page: 762

13: Chest pain is a common challenging complaint. Nature of the chest pain is useful for determining if the pain is cardiac in origin. The descriptions of pain depicted below are all true, except:

    A. Substernal pain that radiates to the jaw
    B. Pain is similar to that of an elephant sitting on the chest
    C. Pain is like a squeezing vice around the chest
    D. Pain is sudden and excruciating in the center of chest
    E. Pain is like an indigestion and produces the urge belch

Answer: D

Critique: All the above descriptions except pain described in statement D have been noticed during episodes of cardiac-related chest pain. One has to keep in mind that acute myocardial infarction may occur with no symptom of chest pain (silent MI). Typical angina is a pressure-like substernal pain radiating to the jaw or arm and back. The above descriptions are typical expressions manifested by patients having angina. The Levine sign, in which the patient forms a squeezing fist in front of the sternum, is strongly correlated to coronary artery disease.

Pages: 767, 768

14: Which statement depicts the truth about the use of transdermal nitroglycerin patches?

    A. They are most effective when placed in the center of the chest.
    B. They lose effectiveness quickly if left in place continuously for 24 hours.
    C. They prevent anginal pain when kept in place continuously for 24 hours.
    D. They have not been proved to be of value for the prevention of angina.
    E. They cause coronary artery vasodilatation.

Answer: B

Critique: Transdermal nitroglycerin patches rapidly lose effectiveness due to tachyphylaxis if they are in place continuously. Increasing the dose does not seem to overcome the ineffectiveness. The effectiveness depends on the absorption through the skin, and they may be placed anywhere that will not hamper absorption. To avoid tachyphylaxis, stop the use of nitroglycerin for at least 8 to 10 hours.

Page: 767

15: A patient presents with symptoms of acute myocardial infarction without any ST segment elevation on ECG. Which of the following findings would provide a strong indication for thrombolysis if no contraindication is found to be documented?

    A. New onset of first-degree heart block
    B. New onset of left bundle branch block
    C. Frequent unifocal ventricular ectopic beats only
    D. New onset of Wenckebach second-degree heart block only
    E. Supraventricular tachycardia

Answer: B

Critique: Left bundle branch block is the only finding that provides a strong indication for thrombolytic therapy when there is absent ST segment elevation of less than 0.1 mV in two or more leads. The other findings mentioned above do not warrant thrombolytic intervention unless cardiac enzymes are increased.

Pages: 770, 771

16: A 75-year-old white female is admitted with shortness of breath, weakness, cough, and difficulty lying flat. She has a history of hypertension for 18 years and treatment with thiazide diuretics. Clinical diagnosis of heart failure is made. An echocardiogram shows no valvular disease and no segmental wall motion abnormalities, left ventricle hypertrophy is noted, and ejection fraction is 55%. The most likely cause of her heart failure is:

    A. Systolic dysfunction
    B. Diastolic dysfunction
    C. Coronary artery disease
    D. High out failure
    E. Cardiomyopathy

Answer: B

Critique: Of all heart failure, at least 20% to 30% is caused by diastolic dysfunction. This occurs as a result of left ventricle hypertrophy produced by the chronic systolic hypertension. This condition causes the left ventricle to be stiff and noncompliant and hampers filling. Of importance is that the ejection fraction is not decreased as found in the systolic type of heart failure.

Page: 774

17: A 51-year-old man comes to your office for a follow-up visit after being discharged from the hospital 4 weeks previously with a diagnosis of inferior myocardial infarction. Cardiac catheterization showed 60% stenosis of the right coronary artery and inferior wall akinesia. His lipid profile showed LDL of 140 mg/dL and HDL of 30 mg/dL He was placed on a beta blocker and aspirin therapy and advised to walk three times a day and reduce his fat intake. Which of the following therapies can be added that would most likely have the greatest effect on secondary prevention of reinfarction?

    A. Coronary artery bypass
    B. Anticoagulation with warfarin to keep the international normalized ratio of 2:3.
    C. Coronary angioplasty with stent placement
    D. Vitamin E 1000 IU/day
    E. Pravastatin 40 mg/day

Answer: E

Critique: The most effective means of preventing secondary infarction is to lower his LDL level below 100 mg/dL as recommended by the National Cholesterol Education Program. Because the stenosis is 60%, angioplasty or CABG at this time will not benefit him the most. Vitamin E would have some additive effect in risk reduction but not as great as lowering LDL. Because the patient is already on aspirin, adding warfarin would not be of much benefit considering the increased risk of bleeding as a side effect.

Pages: 765, 766

18: Atherogenic plaques are likely to fracture:

    A. If patient is not a smoker
    B. If severe stenosis is present
    C. By emotional stress
    D. If there are fewer lipids in the plaque

Answer: C

Critique: Atherosclerotic plaques are formed by lipid-laden foam cells, smooth muscle cells, and calcifications. Factors that increase the likelihood of plaques rupturing are increased lipid content in the plaque, smoking, and emotional stress. There usually is no association of plaque rupture and the degree of coronary artery stenosis.

Page: 765

19: Recommendation of thrombolysis includes all of the following, except:

    A. ST elevation of at least 1 mm or more in two contiguous leads
    B. Onset of typical anginal pain for less than 12 hours
    C. Age below 75 years
    D. New left bundle branch block
    E. Blood pressure of 200/118 mm Hg

Answer: E

Critique: All of these conditions except E are indications of thrombolytic intervention. The risk of intracranial bleeding with uncontrolled hypertension increases; thus, if blood pressure is above 190/110 mm Hg, thrombolysis is contraindicated.

Page: 770, 771

20: Which of the following statements about using cardiac enzymes for diagnosing myocardial infarction is true?

    A. MI can be ruled out if CPK MB fraction is elevated but the total CPK is normal.
    B. Only during MI does CKP MB increase.
    C. Patients with ST segment elevation and an increase in troponin level compared to patients with ST segment elevation and *no* increase in troponin are at greater risk for cardiac deaths within 30 days.
    D. Troponin level needs to be tested even if the ECG shows typical ST segment elevation.
    E. Troponin T is better than troponin I for predicting myocardial injury in patients with renal disease, muscular dystrophy, and polymyositis.

Answer: C

Critique: MI cannot be ruled out if CPK MB is at least 15% of CPK, even if CPK is not elevated. CPK MB can increase with physical exertion, skeletal muscle injury, pericarditis, and renal failure. If new characteristic ST elevation is found in ECG with associated typical clinical presentation of MI, cardiac enzyme has no value in the diagnosis of MI. If the troponin is tested and found to be elevated, however, the prognosis is worse than for those who do not have an increased troponin level. Troponin I is a better indicator of MI in patients with renal disease, muscular dystrophy, and polymyositis.

Page: 769

21: A 68-year-old white male is admitted for the third time in a year for exacerbation of heart failure. IV furosemide and morphine alleviated his dyspnea and he felt better. On discharge, his medication was reviewed and includes digoxin 0.125 mg qid, furosemide 40 mg qid, and lisinopril 40 mg qid, which he was taking for the last year. He is also on a low-salt diet. Which of the following will help prevent future admissions and decrease overall medical costs for the patient during the next year?

    A. Admit the patient to a nursing home.
    B. Start angiotensin receptor blocker (ARB).
    C. Increase the dose of furosemide.
    D. Increase the dose of lisinopril.
    E. Arrange home health care for nurse-directed multidisciplinary services.

Answer: E

Critique: Admitting the patient to a nursing home is not an option because medical cost will increase despite reduction of hospital admissions. Studies have not yet shown that the addition of an ARB will decrease hospital admissions. Increasing the dose of furosemide is not a long-term goal and should be done only when there are signs of volume overload. Increasing lisinopril that is at its maximum dose is not an option. It is has been proved that care by a nurse-directed multidisciplinary intervention team after discharge can reduce rehospitalization, improve quality of life, and reduce the total cost of medical care.

Page: 778

22: In what type of cardiomyopathy can a beta blocker or a calcium channel blocker be of benefit?

    A. Hypertrophic
    B. Restrictive

C. Dilated

D. None of the above

Answer: A

Critique: Half of the patient population with hypertrophic cardiomyopathy obtains relief of their symptoms when a beta blocker is started. Calcium channel blockers have also been used to relieve symptoms. The mechanism of action is probably the improved diastolic function and the vasodilatation effect, overcoming the outflow obstruction. There currently is no effective therapy for restrictive cardiomyopathy. Diuretics can cause some relief, but overdiuresis can aggravate symptoms. The dilated cardiomyopathies also are not amenable to any specific therapy, and the underlying cause has to be eliminated to arrest progression to heart failure. Once heart failure ensues, the standard for treatment is similar.

Page: 774

23: Which of the following statements is true regarding spironolactone and its use in congestive heart failure (CHF)?

A. There is a reduction in mortality when CHF patients use spironolactone.

B. Major side effects in the use of aldosterone are increases in potassium and creatinine.

C. Spironolactone is a short-acting aldosterone receptor inhibitor.

D. Gynecomastia or breast pain occurs in more than 50% of patients taking spironolactone.

E. The hospitalization rate is not decreased when CHF patients take spironolactone.

Answer: A

Critique: A recent study demonstrated that the use of spironolactone in CHF patients decreases the mortality and hospitalization rate. Spironolactone acts as an aldosterone receptor blocker and acts over a long period of time, whereas the angiotensin-converting enzyme (ACE) inhibitors act transiently as an aldactone receptor blocker. Side effects such as elevated creatinine and potassium are minimal and not of clinical significance. Gynecomastia occurs in only 10% of those taking spironolactone.

Pages: 778, 779

24: Which of the following results is the most common found when restoration of coronary artery patency occurs after thrombolysis?

A. Resolution of chest pain

B. ECG resolution of ST-segment elevation

C. Sinus bradycardia

D. Atrial ventricular block

E. Accelerated idioventricular rhythm

Answer: E

Critique: All of these conditions are evident when coronary artery patency is achieved after thrombolysis, but the most common are accelerated idioventricular rhythms.

Pages: 770, 771

25: Which of the following statements regarding treatment of acute myocardial infarction is true?

A. Calcium channel blockers are beneficial in prevention of arrhythmias.

B. Beta-blocking agents reduce the size of infarct and chest pain after acute myocardial infarction.

C. ACE inhibitors cause congestive heart failure.

D. Lidocaine is given routinely after MI to slow down arrhythmias.

Answer: B

Critique: Calcium channel blockers have not shown any benefits after MI. ACE inhibitors prevent congestive heart failure after a myocardial infarction. Beta-blocking agents reduce mortality and reinfarction. Lidocaine is not used routinely after MI.

Page: 770

26: Hypertrophic cardiomyopathy (HCM) is the most common cause of cardiac arrest in young athletes. The following characteristics of murmur, except one, are found in HCM and should alert clinicians to pursue a full cardiovascular work-up, including an echocardiogram. What is the exception?

A. A midsystolic murmur

B. Crescendo–decrescendo murmur

C. Murmur is heard in lower left sternal border or apex

D. Murmur is louder when the patient is supine

E. Murmur is louder during the Valsalva maneuver

Answer: D

Critique: HCM is indicated by harsh, midsystolic, crescendo–decrescendo murmur, heard best in the lower left sternal border or apex. The murmur becomes louder on standing or during the Valsalva maneuver, both of which prompt a decreased blood return to the heart, causing a decrease in diastolic volume and increasing the outlet obstruction. Benign flow murmurs become louder with squatting or lying down, which augment blood flow to the heart and thus increase cardiac output.

Page: 774

27: Which of the following drugs used for peripheral arterial disease (PAD) is contraindicated in patients with heart failure?

A. Cilostazol (Pletal)

B. Clopidogrel (Plavix)

C. Aspirin

D. Dipyridamole (Persantine)

E. Pentoxifylline (Trental)

Answer: A

Critique: The four classes of drugs that have been widely used for PAD diseases are selected antithrombotic agents, lipid-lowering preparations, rheologic drugs, and antioxidants. Antithrombotic drugs are used for the prevention of associated increased incidence of stroke and cardiac infarction. PAD is associated with diffuse atherosclerosis, and it is reasonable to use lipid-lowering drugs to reduce cardiovascular mortality. In patients with PAD, erythrocyte deformability is decreased and platelet activity and blood viscosity increase. Rheologic agents such as cilostazol and pentoxifylline help to increase erythrocyte deformability and decrease platelet activity and viscosity of blood. Cilostazol has been shown to increase patients' maximal walking distance by 38% to 51%, depending on dose. Because cilostazol is a phosphodiesterase inhibitor, the risk for worsening of heart failure increases as a result of a decrease in cardiac muscle contractility.

Page: 784

28: Which of the following statements regarding peripheral arterial disease (PAD) is true?

    A. Pain decreases with elevation of the lower extremities.
    B. The remedy for severe intermittent claudication is surgical intervention.
    C. An arteriogram is required to diagnose PAD.
    D. With PAD, pain at rest occurs in the calf and thigh.
    E. If walking distance varies from one day to the next, pain is experienced.

Answer: A

Critique: Pain from PAD usually worsens when the legs are raised. Severe intermittent claudication can be managed nonsurgically. Diagnosing PAD can be done by measuring the systolic blood pressure at the ankle and brachially and calculating the ankle brachial index (ABI). Pain, if it occurs in PAD, occurs more often in the toes or forefoot. Walking distance must be fixed before pain is experienced. If there is day-to-day variation, causes other than PAD should be considered.

Page: 784

29: Which of the following nonpharmacological interventions would have the most impact in decreasing symptoms of PAD?

    A. Low-fat and low-cholesterol diet
    B. Exercise on a routine basis
    C. Smoking cessation
    D. Weight reduction
    E. Using compression stocking

Answer: C

Critique: Of all the nonpharmacological or surgical interventions, cessation of cigarette smoking has the greatest impact in decreasing symptoms and the progression of the disease. Smoking exacerbates the disease and can lead to severe claudication and ischemia, and ultimately to limb loss. Because there is also increased cardiopulmonary morbidity and mortality associated with smoking, patients with PAD should be aggressively approached to help them stop smoking.

Page: 784

30: (True or False) Determine whether the following statements regarding aortic stenosis are true or false:

    A. There are three major causes of aortic stenosis.
    B. Patients with aortic stenosis may present with syncope or chest pain.
    C. Determination of aortic stenosis requires that all patients undergo cardiac catheterization.

    D. Aortic valve area of less than 0.7 cm^2 is considered to be severe stenosis.
    E. Patients undergoing valvuloplasty usually do not suffer restenosis.

Answers: A - True, B - True, C - False, D - True, E - False

Critique: The three major causes of aortic stenosis are senile calcification, congenital bicuspid valve, and stenosis secondary to rheumatic disease. Presenting symptoms can be chest pain, syncope, or frank heart failure. Chest pain is caused by cardiac muscle anoxia and can occur without any coronary artery stenosis. Syncope occurs on exertion, mostly as a result of peripheral vasodilatation and a fixed cardiac output. It may also occur because of ventricular dysrhythmias. Heart failure occurs at the end stage of left ventricular hypertrophy and has a very poor prognosis. With the advent of advanced echocardiography technology, an echocardiogram will elicit the severity of the stenosis initially. A valvular area below 0.7 cm^2 is considered severe and between 0.7 cm^2 and 1 cm^2 moderate. After undergoing percutaneous valvuloplasty, 50% of patients restenose in 9 months.

Page: 780

31: The Framingham Heart Study demonstrated that 50% of patients with New York Heart Association (NYHA) heart failure class II to IV died within:

    A. 1 year
    B. 2 years
    C. 3 years
    D. 4 years
    E. 5 years

Answer: D

Critique: The Framingham study demonstrated a correlation between congestive heart failure severity, as measured by the NYHA heart failure class, and mortality rate. The correlation is linear and depicts 50% mortality in 4 years in those having NYHA class II to IV.

Page: 776

32: Which one of the following has not been shown to increase survival in patients with congestive heart failure (CHF)?

    A. Captopril
    B. Metoprolol
    C. Digoxin
    D. Carvedilol
    E. Conversion of atrial fibrillation to sinus rhythm

Answer: C

Critique: ACE inhibitors and beta-blocking agents have been shown to increase survival in CHF patients. Conversion of atrial fibrillation to sinus rhythm helps improve the cardiac function and thus survival. Digoxin, though it improves symptoms, has not been found to increase survival.

Page: 779

33: Digitalis is of no benefit, except in:

    A. Hypertrophic cardiomyopathy (HCM)
    B. Right ventricular failure secondary to cor pulmonale
    C. Mitral stenosis and CHF with atrial fibrillation
    D. Wolff-Parkinson-White syndrome with atrial fibrillation

Answer: C

Critique: Digitalis has been used widely for the treatment of CHF. One has to choose patients wisely before starting digitalis therapy. Certain underlying causes of CHF can cause deleterious effects instead of improving cardiac function. Digitalis is contraindicated in HCM and Wolff-Parkinson-White syndrome with atrial fibrillation. Digitalis has no benefit when used in patients with right ventricular failure due to cor pulmonale.

Pages: 778, 779

34: First-line therapy for congestive heart failure is:

    A. Beta-blocking agent
    B. Diuretic
    C. ACE inhibitor
    D. Calcium channel blocker
    E. Digitalis

Answer: C

Critique: Various modalities for treating CHF have been documented. The recent trials with ACE inhibitors not only show an increase in survival but also demonstrate symptom relief. Starting patients on an ACE inhibitor even when no symptoms are apparent helps in prevention of remodeling of the cardiac muscles. The interruption of the renin-angiotensin-aldosterone pathway by ACE inhibitors balances the arterial and venous vasodilatation.

Page: 779

34: (True or False) In regard to abdominal aortic aneurysm:

    A. Risk of rupture is 50% when aneurysm diameter is greater than 6 cm
    B. Risk of rupture is 23% when aneurysm diameter is 4 to 5 cm
    C. Typically arises before the branching of renal arteries
    D. In the majority of cases is caused by atherosclerosis

Answers: A - True, B - True, C - False, D - True

Critique: Diseases of the aorta are usually the result of acquired diseases. Degeneration of the arterial wall is the primary reason for formation of an aneurysm. More than 90% of aneurysms in the abdominal aorta are caused by atherosclerosis. The incidence of rupture is correlated to the size of the aneurysm. A 50% incidence is noted when the diameter of the aneurysm is larger than 6 cm and a 23% incidence when it is 4 to 5 cm. Aneurysms are usually found beyond the branches of the renal arteries.

Page: 783

34: The most common clinical symptom of aortic dissection is:

    A. Syncope
    B. Blurry vision
    C. Shortness of breath
    D. Chest pain
    E. Palpitation

Answer: D

Critique: Chest pain is the most common patient complaint when aortic dissection occurs. Pain is severe and sharp and can mimic symptoms of a myocardial infarction. Associated symptoms may occur, depending on the extent of the dissection.

Page: 784

Chapter 37

Emergency Medicine

Avril Anthony-Wison

1: (True or False) When evaluating life-threatening injuries, a patient in shock who has distended neck veins suggests:

    A. Hemothorax
    B. Extrathoracic injuries
    C. Cardiac tamponade
    D. Tension pneumothorax

Answers: A - False, B - False, C - True, D - True

Critique: Color, chest wall motion, and nature of respiration are vital in assessing for life-threatening injuries. A careful examination of the patient's neck veins is an essential part of a thorough examination. Shock with distended neck veins suggests tension pneumothorax or cardiac tamponade as a cause.

Page: 793

2: (True or False) Tracheobronchial disruptions sustained during a blunt trauma motor vehicle accident present as:

    A. Subcutaneous emphysema
    B. Complete unilateral atelectasis
    C. Tension pneumothorax
    D. Mediastinal crunch

Answers: A - True, B - True, C - True, D - True

Critique: Tracheobronchial disruption may present in several ways, ranging from a mediastinal crunch or subcutaneous emphysema, to pneumothorax with or without tension but with persistent air leak on chest tube drainage or bronchiectasis. Hemoptysis varies from absent to massive, and its presence should be carefully evaluated.

Page: 793

3: After an MVA, a patient is evaluated and found to have pericardial tamponade. Which of the following signs are consistent with this diagnosis?

    A. Narrow pulse pressure
    B. Low-voltage ECG
    C. Electrical alternans
    D. High central venous pressure
    E. Distant heart sounds
    F. All of the above

Answer: F

Critique: If pericardial tamponade is suspected after blunt trauma (narrow pulse pressure, high central venous pressure, distant heart sounds, low voltage on the ECG, electrical alternans of the QRS complex), transthoracic echocardiogram can be used for diagnosis, and pericardiocentesis may be used as a temporizing measure. Transesophageal echocardiogram does not appear to offer any advantages over transthoracic echocardiogram at this time. Open pericardiotomy by a qualified surgeon is the definitive treatment.

Pages: 793, 794

4: The most common injury with blunt chest trauma is:

    A. Pulmonary contusion
    B. Esophageal rupture
    C. Splenic rupture
    D. Compound rib fractures
    E. Simple rib fractures

Answer: E

Critique: Simple rib fractures are probably the most common injury in blunt chest trauma. Rib fractures are managed with analgesia, rest, and careful outpatient follow-up. Fractures of the lower left ribs may be associated with splenic injury, and liver spleen scan, CT scan, focused abdominal ultrasound, or inpatient observation may be indicated.

Page: 794

5: A 40-year-old male is brought to the emergency room and evaluated after sustaining myocardial stab wounds. Tension pneumothorax is ruled out, but cardiac tamponade has been diagnosed. Which procedure is most likely to benefit the patient:

    A. Thoracostomy with pericardicentesis
    B. Thoracostomy without pericardicentesis
    C. Thoracotomy with pericardiocentesis
    D. Thoracotomy without pericardiocentesis

Answer: C

Critique: Generally, emergency thoracotomy is useful only for penetrating thoracic injuries. It is most helpful in myocardial stab wounds with cardiac tamponade in which the tamponade is released readily with pericardial incision and the myocardial lacerations are oversewn with silk sutures. Gunshot wounds of the heart are generally less salvageable.

Page: 796

6: Emergency thoracotomy is required in what percentage of major thoracic traumas?

A. 10%
B. 30%
C. 50%
D. 75%
E. 90%

Answer: A

Critique: Thoracotomy is required in only 10% of major thoracic traumas overall; thus, emergency department thoracotomy is not a common procedure in most centers. Intubation and intravenous access are mandatory before thoracotomy. If possible, it is best that this procedure be performed by a surgeon trained in the technique.

Page: 796

7: In the geriatric population, trauma accounts for what percentage of elderly patient deaths:

A. 40%
B. 20%
C. 10%
D. 5%
E. 2%

Answer: E

Critique: Trauma accounts for 2% of elderly patient deaths but for 28% of all injury fatalities in the United States.

Page: 798

8: A child under the age of 17 is most likely to present to the emergency department with which of the following injuries:

A. Ingestions and poisonings
B. Fractures and dislocations
C. Lacerations and abrasions
D. Bites

Answer: C

Critique: Lacerations and abrasions are the most common injuries in children younger than 17 years, followed by fractures and dislocations, ingestions, and bites.

Page: 798

9: During acute blood loss in children, blood pressure remains unchanged until blood loss exceeds 25% of blood volume. Which physiologic changes in heart rate (HR), stroke volume (SV), and systemic vascular resistance help to maintain blood pressure:

A. ↑ HR, ↑ SV, ↑ SVR
B. ↑ HR, ↑ SV, ↓ SVR
C. ↑ HR, – SV, ↑ SVR
D. ↓ HR, ↓ SV, ↑ SVR
E. ↓ HR, ↓ SV, ↓ SVR

Answer: E

Critique: Acute blood loss responds to increasing heart rate (rather than stroke volume) and systemic vascular resistance, often maintaining blood pressure until blood loss exceeds 25% of blood volume.

Page: 798

10: A 28-year-old G2P101 female at 30 weeks gestation is involved in a motor vehicle accident. She arrives in the emergency department very anxious but in stable condition. The most common obstetric problem you may encounter in this trauma case is:

A. Abruptio placenta
B. Uterine rupture
C. Uterine contractions
D. Fetal tachycardia
E. Placenta previa

Answer: C

Critique: The most common obstetric problem caused by trauma is uterine contractions; 90% stop spontaneously. The patient should be monitored for fetal contraction in all obstetrical trauma cases.

Page: 799

11: Which of the following items listed is most commonly ingested as a foreign body:

A. Food boluses
B. Pull-tabs from aluminum cans
C. Dentures
D. Pins

Answer: A

Critique: Food boluses and coins are the most common foreign bodies ingested. Keep in mind that dentures and pull-tabs from aluminum cans are not radiographically opaque and can easily be missed on x-ray evaluation.

Page: 801

12: Which of the following patient populations is at the highest risk for swallowing foreign bodies:

A. Stroke patients
B. Prisoners
C. Elderly nursing home patients over age 80
D. Children under age 4
E. Psychiatric patients

Answer: D

Critique: More than 50% of cases of foreign-body removal involve children younger than 4 years. Children between the ages of 6 months and 3 years are at the highest risk of swallowing foreign bodies. Other groups include psychiatric patients and prisoners.

Page: 801

13: (True or False) Which of the following statements are true:

A. In third-degree burns, no spontaneous regeneration of tissue is possible.
B. Fourth-degree burns can be pale and include bony involvement.
C. First-degree burns do not blister.
D. Partial-thickness burns involve only partial destruction of the epidermis.
E. Full-thickness burns destroy the skin's natural, spontaneous ability to regenerate.

Answers: A - True, B - True, C - True, D - False, E - True

Critique: Burns are described as superficial (first degree), partial thickness (second degree), or full thickness and deeper (third and fourth degrees). First-degree burns are superficial and involve the epidermis only. They are red, hypersensitive, warm, tender, painful to the touch, and often swollen. There is no blistering. Healing is usually spontaneous within about 1 week; there is often some degree of desquamation of the damaged skin. A classic example of first-degree burn is most sunburn. Partial-thickness or second-degree burns involve destruction of the epidermis and the dermis in varying levels. Partial-thickness burns can be superficial, mid, or deep. Superficial partial-thickness burns involve the epidermis and the superficial (papillary) layer of the dermis. They tend to have a shiny, red, weeping appearance; they heal in 7 to 14 days, producing minimal or no scarring. A mid partial-thickness burn is blistered and ranges in color from pink to red; it heals in 14 to 21 days, often producing pigment changes and scarring. Both superficial and mid partial-thickness burns are exquisitely tender to touch. Deep partial-thickness burns involve the epidermis and most of the dermis, including the deep (reticular) dermis. By definition, there is some dermal sparing, allowing spontaneous re-epithelialization in the future. These burns have a deep cherry-red appearance when fully débrided and may have thick-walled blisters. Skin buds may be seen and can be quite tender or have slightly decreased sensation. Healing tends to occur in 21 to 28 days or longer; there tends to be a significant amount of scarring. Skin grafting is sometimes performed to maximize healing and improve cosmetic outcome. Full-thickness or third-degree burns involve the epidermis and the entire dermis down to the subcutaneous tissue. The dermal structures, including nerves, are destroyed; thus, these burns are usually hard, thick, and anesthetic. The classic appearance of a full-thickness burn is thrombosed blood vessels in a translucent surface with little or no pain. No spontaneous regeneration is possible because the full dermis has been destroyed. Skin grafts are usually needed for eventual repair. Fourth-degree burns involve structures below the subcutaneous tissue, including bone, fascia, and muscle. They appear charred or very pale; these burns usually occur from prolonged thermal contact or electrical burns. They often require extensive débridement, complex reconstructive surgery, flap coverage, or amputation.

Page: 807

14: (True or False) Which of the following are true regarding burn management?

A. The rule of nines is a good method to estimate the evident burn injuries in adults and children.
B. The size of the patient's palm can be used to estimate the extent of burn injuries in adults and children.
C. Generally, first- and second-degree burns can be managed conservatively with office care.
D. Some circumferential burns around an extremity at risk for compartment syndrome do not require hospitalization.
E. Second-degree burns in children involving more than 10% to 20% of the body surface area deserve consultation.

Answers: A - False, B - True, C - True, D - False, E - True

Critique: The rule of nines is a useful way to estimate the surface area of cutaneous burns in adults. In adults, the surface of the body is divided into areas that are a multiple of 9%. This is altered in the child because of the relatively larger size of the head; therefore, the percentages of the extremities, trunk, and other areas are age dependent (Fig. 37–9). Another useful guideline that can be used in adults and children is to note the area of the patient's palm, because this represents approximately 1% of the body surface area (BSA). It can be used as a quick estimate of the extent of irregular burns during initial assessment. Generally, first- and second-degree burns can be managed conservatively with office care. Second-degree burns that involve more than 15% to 25% of the BSA in adults or 10% to 20% in children deserve consultation from a burn center or a colleague with special expertise. Third-degree burns involving more than 2% of the BSA merit consultation.

Page: 808

15: Appropriate management of a first-degree burn should include:

A. Initial first aid should include cold compress to the area for 15 to 20 minutes
B. A cool salve made with petroleum jelly
C. Sterile iodoform gauze wrapping
D. Infiltratation of the area with a local anesthetic
E. High-dose steroids for 3 to 4 weeks until the burn has healed

Answer: A

Critique: Minor burns can be treated effectively on an outpatient basis with analgesics and topical therapy. Most first-degree burns can be treated with cool compresses, antihistamines, and, at times, a rapidly tapering dose of oral steroid for edema and pain (prednisone, 40 mg daily for 3 to 5 days, then 20 mg daily for 3 to 5 days). Initial first aid should include cold compresses for 15 to 20 minutes to stop further destruction of tissue. Generally, retained skin is the body's best dressing. If bullae are present, they should be left intact. If blisters are already ruptured, loose dead tissue or debris should be gently and thoroughly débrided. It is extremely important to handle areas of second-degree burn in a very clean, aseptic manner. Treatment should involve the use of sterile drapes and gloves when cleansing, handling, and dressing the wound, which significantly reduces the chance of infection. After cooling and débridement, a topical antibiotic preparation is applied to second- or third-degree burns but is not necessary for most first-degree burns. Patients often apply many types of home remedies to burns. Butter, petroleum jelly, or other creams are not to be applied to the burn. These agents must be cleaned from the burn wound to assess it and provide proper treatment when the patient arrives in the office or emergency department. Physicians should attempt to educate their patients and local first aid or rescue personnel to avoid this practice.

Pages: 808, 810

16: During the early treatment stage of most minor burn wounds, the family physician should examine the burn wound for proper healing:

    A. Once every 5 to 7 days
    B. Once every 1 to 2 days
    C. Only if pain persists
    D. Only if edema does not resolve in the first 2 to 3 days

Answer: B

Critique: The physician should inspect the burn every 1 to 2 days at the beginning of therapy for evidence of proper healing or signs of infection, even with the most motivated patients. Further débridement or whirlpool treatments may be needed for good wound management and to abort early infection. If signs of infection develop, such as suppuration (pus), increasing redness, and pain, the physician is prudent to implement antibiotic treatment with a penicillinase-resistant penicillin or cephalosporin. Proper analgesia, elevation of the burn to reduce edema, tetanus prophylaxis, and splinting as necessary complete the outpatient management.

Page: 810

17: During fluid resuscitation of the major burn patient, the fluid of choice is:

    A. Crystalloids
    B. Hypertonic saline
    C. Salt-poor albumin
    D. 5% dextrose in water

Answer: A

Critique: Fluid administration, urinary output, and other vital clinical signs should be monitored closely. Prompt fluid resuscitation using the Parkland formula is very popular for adults. Crystalloids (sodium salt solutions) are the essential component of fluid resuscitation; lactated Ringer's solution is the most widely used. Fluid resuscitation formulas using hypertonic saline solutions or the addition of colloid have lost favor over the past few years. This is a result, primarily, of studies indicating that either there is no advantage to these formulas or they are harmful. At least one study reported that the use of hypertonic saline for the treatment of burn shock increased the incidence of renal failure or death. In pediatric patients, maintenance requirements must be added to the resuscitation formula; therefore, the SBH-Galveston Pediatric Formula is recommended. The importance of prompt, early fluid resuscitation in the severely burned patient cannot be overemphasized. In fact, the literature emphasizes that time to intravenous access is a major predictor of mortality in pediatric patients who have burns of greater than 80% of TBSA.

Pages: 810, 811

18: Nonsystemic cold-induced injury that results from repeated cold exposure on the face or extremities without tissue freezing is found in:

    A. Hypothermic cold stroke
    B. Cold tetani
    C. Hypothermia

    D. Frostbite
    E. Chilblains

Answer: E

Critique: Chilblains is a skin reaction or condition that results from repeated exposure to cold weather without actual tissue freezing or frostbite. Chilblains appears as reddish-purple macular lesions on the face or exposed extremities and may progress to include edema and blistering. Protective covering of the skin in extremely cold, humid weather is an important primary prevention. Mild chilblains is managed by rewarming the affected area indoors at room temperature, careful handling (i.e., no massage) of affected tissue, and early treatment of secondary infection. Repeated cold exposure can lead to thick, ulcerated, scarring lesions that require extensive dermatologic treatment.

Page: 815

19: In which disease condition is hypothermia directly related to mortality:

    A. Cancer
    B. Hypopituitarism
    C. Myxedema
    D. Stroke
    E. Vascular diseases

Answer: C

Critique: Diseases such as cancer, severe trauma, vascular disease, cerebrovascular accidents, mental retardation, myxedema, and hypopituitarism all predispose patients to secondary hypothermia. The major determinants of mortality in hypothermia are the presence and severity of associated comorbid disease states and the degree of presenting hypothermia. Reported mortality rates in large series of patients range from 10% to 80%. Only in myxedema coma is the actual depression of core temperature directly related to mortality.

Page: 816

20: Hypothermia can occur at temperatures as high as:

    A. 40°F
    B. 45°F
    C. 50°F
    D. 55°F
    E. 60°F

Answer: C

Critique: A variety of clinical settings predispose individuals to hypothermia (Table 37-11). Primary accidental hypothermia involves accidental direct exposure to a cold environment, with appropriate protection from the cold. Many persons who are active outdoors must be informed that severe hypothermia can occur in temperatures well above freezing if they are not appropriately dressed. The combination of wet clothing, heat loss resulting from wind and evaporation, and inadequate intake of fluid and carbohydrates has led to severe cases of hypothermia in temperatures as warm as the 50s (Fahrenheit).

Page: 816

21: (True or False) ECG changes that are associated with hypothermia include:

    A. J-shaped Osborne waves
    B. T wave inversion
    C. Prolonged QT intervals
    D. Atrial fibrillation
    E. Atrial flutter

Answers: A - True, B - True, C - True, D - True, E - True

Critique: The cardiovascular and neurologic consequences of hypothermia as described are often profound. Progressive bradycardia develops, and all ECG intervals lengthen. Diffuse T wave inversion may occur, and, with distention of the atria, atrial flutter and fibrillation may result. Although gross shivering may begin to disappear below 90°F, fine muscular tremor may be apparent on the ECG. The J-shaped Osborne waves on the ECG (Fig. 37-10) are pathognomonic for hypothermia.

Page: 817

22: Choose the best answer. During evaluation of a patient for drug toxicities, all of the following are true, except:

    A. Obtain a complete toxicologic screen.
    B. Obtain a single urine sample as soon as possible after the episode.
    C. A negative urine sample indicates no need for further urine evaluations.
    D. Urine positive for marijuana often indicates the source of the poisoning.
    E. A complete toxicologic screen should not be routine.

Answer: A

Critique: Obtaining a complete toxicologic screen should not be routine. Rather, obtaining qualitative analysis of urine for street drugs or specific serum levels for certain drugs, especially acetaminophen, aspirin, digoxin, ethanol, iron, lithium, theophylline, and so on, is more useful. Timing of the specimen is important because urine screens may be falsely negative if performed soon after the overdose. Certain drugs, such as marijuana and cocaine metabolites, may create lingering positive urine screens for weeks, thereby leading to a misdiagnosis during an acute ingestion.

Page: 825

23: Changes in vital signs are often a clue to the classification of the drug or poisoning agent causing specific symptoms. Which of the following is correct:

    A. The initial assessment should include a temperature assessment but is not always required.
    B. Tachycardia is associated with *Amanita* muscarinic poisoning.
    C. Bradycardia is often associated with anticholinergic poisoning.
    D. Central nervous system (CNS) depression is often associated with hypothermia induced by narcotics and barbiturates.

    E. Naloxone (Narcan) can be used to reduce barbiturate toxicity.

Answer: D

Critique: Tachycardia is noted in sympathomimetic and anticholinergic poisoning, whereas bradycardia is seen with parasympathomimetics, *Amanita muscaria* poisoning, and cholinesterase inhibitors. The initial assessment must include a temperature measurement, which should represent a core temperature. Hypothermia may be the only indicator for CNS depressants such as narcotics, barbiturates, or ethanol. Hyperthermia is often a complication of cocaine or amphetamine overdose. Pulse oximetry should be included as the fifth vital sign in the patient with altered mental status.

If the patient is obtunded, oxygen, dextrose, and naloxone (2 mg or, in narcotic addiction, a lower dosage of 0.4 mg) should be administered. In the case of alcohol ingestion, 100 mg thiamine should precede dextrose administration for prevention or treatment of Wernicke's encephalopathy.

Page: 823

24: A 65-year-old male presents in your office stating that he sustained a puncture wound with a nail to his foot while doing yard work 1 week ago. He has no complaints and is in your office only at the request of his wife. His only significant medical history is diabetes. What should be done? Choose the best answer.

    A. Inspect the wound and treat it only if there are signs of infection.
    B. Evaluate the patient for signs of tetanus. If they are negative, it is all right to just monitor him periodically over the next 3 to 4 weeks.
    C. Verify tetanus immunization status by history and medical records so that appropriate tetanus prophylaxis can be accomplished.
    D. In the elderly, always give tetanus immune globulin first.
    E. Previous tetanus immunization confers natural immunity.

Answer: C

Critique: Tetanus usually requires 1.5 to 2 weeks of incubation and arrives with the onset of trismus and dysphagia followed by spasms (often over the injured portal site), opisthotonos, respiratory insufficiency, and rhabdomyolysis. Recognition of the clinical features is important because the laboratory evaluation is of limited, and primarily retrospective, value. Once the clinical manifestations are present, specific treatment, including large doses of tetanus immunoglobulin; active immunization with toxoid; antibiotics, usually penicillin; wound débridement; and benzodiazepines are needed. Supportive measures, including neuromuscular blockade, sedation, and analgesia, may be required as well. There is no natural immunity to tetanus, and all injured patients require assessment as to need for immunization. Patients who do not meet the standard for basic immunization may need passive immunization with assurance of completion of active immunization on follow-up.

Pages: 826, 827

25: (True or False) A 7-year-old girl presents in your office with her parents, who report that she was bitten on her left thumb by a skunk earlier in the day. The skunk ran away.

    A. Question the parents and child concerning their use of local wound care, especially washing the site with soap and water

    B. Since a skunk is a high-risk animal for carrying rabies, it is best to provide postexposure treatment.

    C. Postexposure treatment consists only of active immunization.

    D. For passive immunization, always administer the human rabies immunoglobulin (HRIG) vaccine into or around the wound site as much as possible.

    E. Active immunization should be given in the deltoid muscle.

Answers: A - True, B - True, C - False, D - True, E - True

Critique: Rabies is an extremely feared, but increasingly rare, health problem in the United States, with one to two deaths per year. Although, theoretically, any mammal can carry rabies, only a few are of practical concern. High-risk vectors common in the United States are skunks, raccoons, bats, coyotes, and foxes. Rodents (squirrels, gerbils, and hamsters) and lagomorphs (rabbits) are not high-risk vectors. Postexposure prophylaxis should be considered if contact between a high-risk vector and a patient may have occurred, even if a bite, a scratch, or mucous membrane exposure cannot be established (especially if the vector cannot be tested). Immediate care consists of cleansing the wound with soap and water or a povidone-iodine solution or both. Postexposure prophylaxis consists of active and passive immunization. For passive immunization, administer human rabies immunoglobulin (HRIG) 20 IU/kg (all or as much as possible into the wound area and the rest intramuscularly in a more distal site) if necessary. Active immunization uses the inactivated human diploid cell vaccine (HDCV), the rabies vaccine adsorbed (RVA), or purified chick embryo culture (PCEC). Any of these must be given intramuscularly into the deltoid on days 0, 3, 7, 14, and 28 HRIG, and the active vaccine used should be given in different sites using different syringes.

Pages: 827, 828

26: (True or False) A 27-year-old male presents in your office. He explains that his left hand is swollen after he was bitten by a neighbor in a fight. He is unable to extend the hand.

    A. Full evaluation requires both a functional and a neurovascular evaluation.

    B. X-rays are not necessary.

    C. The most likely cause of an infection is *Staphylococcus aureus*.

    D. Open wounds should be sutured and an antibiotic given.

    E. The antibiotic of choice for outpatients is oral pen V-K 500 mg twice daily.

Answers: A - True, B - False, C - False, D - False, E - False

Critique: The hand is the most common location of human bites; the closed or clenched fist injury (CFI) is the typical presentation. When the clenched fist strikes an opponent's face (jaw and teeth) jagged lacerations involving skin, tendons, vessels, nerves, joints, and bones may result. Full evaluation of such a wound requires both functional assessment of neurovascular status and visual inspection of the hand wound through the full range of motion and in the position of contact between fist and jaw to rule out extensor tendon lacerations and foreign bodies (teeth) in the depth of the wound. X-ray evaluation is mandatory. The most frequent aerobic organism is *Streptococcus viridans, followed by S. aureus and Haemophilus;* among the anaerobes, bacteroides, fusobacterium, and peptostreptococcus are commonly represented. *Eikenella corrodens,* a facultatively anaerobic, gram-negative bacterium, is found in one fourth of infected wounds and is associated with an increased risk of osteomyelitis. The initial appropriate antibiotic of choice for outpatients is oral amoxicillin-clavulanate, 500 mg, three times daily or 875 mg twice daily.

Pages: 828, 829

27: (True or False) Determine which of the following statements are correct:

    A. The venom of the brown recluse spider (*Loxosceles reclusa*) may produce a severe systemic syndrome resembling DIC.

    B. Complications from the bite of a black widow spider are mostly rare.

    C. The bite of a tarantula has no systemic toxicity.

    D. The sting of most scorpions in the United States is relatively harmless.

Answers: A - True, B - True, C - True, D - True

Critique: All spiders possess venom designed to immobilize and digest prey.

The clinical presentation from a brown recluse bite is called *loxoscelism* or *necrotic arachnidism.* The recluse is one of the few species whose fangs are able to penetrate human skin. Bites are probably more numerous than were originally suspected, because many bites are not particularly noticeable at the time of the initial event; most bites are probably fairly benign and are not reported. The venom is both cytotoxic and hemotoxic and may cause progressive dermonecrosis as well as a systemic syndrome that resembles DIC. Except in very old, young, immunocompromised, or pregnant patients, complications are rare, and recovery is the rule. Tarantulas produce a painful bite akin to that of a hymenopteran sting, except there is no systemic toxicity. Many species of scorpions exist in the United States, but most are relatively harmless, producing only local reactions to stings. The venom of only one species, *Centruroides exilicauda,* the bark scorpion, produces severe local reactions and systemic neurotoxicity.

Pages: 833, 834

28: A severe hypersensitivity reaction differs from a toxic reaction caused by a bee sting in what way (choose the best answer):

    A. A toxic reaction does not produce bronchospasm.
    B. Urticaria is only seen early in a toxin reaction.
    C. Severe hypersensitivity does not produce bronchospasm.
    D. Toxic reactions are more frequent than are severe hypersensitivity reactions.
    E. A toxic reaction is a more severe form of a severe hypersensitivity response.

Answer: A

Critique: Severe hypersensitivity reactions are thought to be due to immunoglobulin E (IgE) mediators and are seen in a small number of victims, usually within minutes of the sting. The anaphylactic response begins with widespread pruritus and hives; nausea, vomiting, and diarrhea may follow, and bronchospasm, respiratory distress, hypertension, cardiac dysrhythmia, and arrest culminate the attacks in an unfortunate few. A toxic reaction, a rare event, occurs when an abundance of venom has been injected, as opposed to an allergic response. Similar signs and symptoms are seen in both, except urticaria and bronchospasm are absent in the toxic reaction. The amount of venom required is probably that found in dozens to hundreds of bees.

Page: 836

29: In the management of tickborne illnesses, which statement is the best choice:

    A. Transmission of tickborne disease mostly requires attachment and persistent feeding for more than 48 hours.
    B. Weekly evaluation and removal of ticks is adequate for preventive disease management of tickborne illness.
    C. Routine administration of prophylactic antibiotics associated with tick bites is appropriate.
    D. The vaccine against Lyme disease is 90% effective by the second dose.
    E. The best overall disease management strategy is preventive techniques, avoidance, and daily tick checks.

Answer: E

Critique: Except for relapsing fever, disease transmission requires attachment and persistent feeding for more than 24 hours; therefore, daily removal of ticks is adequate for preventive management. Routine administration of prophylactic antibiotics after removal is not advocated. The preferred strategy is avoidance of ticks through the use of appropriate clothing in high-risk environments (closed-toe shoes, long pants tucked into socks, tight-fitting cuffs), along with repellent use (diethyltoluamide for skin and permethrin for clothing). A vaccine is available for Lyme disease; it stimulates the formation of antibodies against *Borrelia burgdorferi*, which are ingested from the patient by the feeding tick and which then kill the spirochetes in the tick. The vaccine is approximately 80% effective after three doses. Candidates may be those who reside in high-prevalence areas (the Mid-Atlantic, Northeast, and North Central United States).

Pages: 837, 838

30: Along the U.S. eastern seaboard, seawater with large algae populations can produce seafood-related toxicities. All of the following toxicities are found in this area, except:

    A. Scombroid toxicity
    B. Paralytic shellfish poisoning
    C. Ciguatera poisoning
    D. Mollusk curariform toxicity

Answer: D

Critique: Scombroid (also known as saurine or pseudoallergic) poisoning is a reaction to ingested histamine-like compounds. Paralytic shellfish poisoning occurs when filter feeders, such as clams, oysters, mussels, or scallops, containing large amounts of dinoflagellate toxin are eaten. The toxins are stable and gastric-acid resistant. Saxitoxin, the best-characterized toxin, has curare-like effects; it blocks sodium conduction and thereby neuromuscular transmission. The toxin is extremely potent, and as few as one mussel or a few clams may be lethal. Ciguatera poisoning may occur when an individual eats a large reef predator fish such as the snapper, jack, sea bass, or grouper (although more than 400 species have been implicated) that has accumulated toxins either directly from dinoflagellates or from the ingestion of smaller fish that have done so. The toxin has anticholinesterase and cholinergic properties; however, the major toxic effect may be the result of the interference of calcium receptor sites that regulate sodium channel function. No known food-processing techniques are protective. Represented in United States waters by *Conus californicum*, a low-toxicity envenomater, cones inject curious people who pick up their shells with a venom-filled dart. The venom is rapid acting and produces pain, swelling, redness, and paresthesias. Hot-water treatment (45°C) is appropriate. Symptoms generally abate within 1 hour.

Pages: 842, 843

Chapter 38

Sports Medicine

Darrin L. Bright

1: A high school football player sustains a forced flexion injury to the neck and collapses on the field. When evaluating this unresponsive player, what should be done first?

A. Immediately remove the helmet and assess the airway.
B. Maintain cervical immobilization with the head tilt–chin lift maneuver.
C. Remove the helmet and shoulder pads together.
D. Assess the airway and carefully remove the facemask while maintaining cervical immobilization to obtain airway access.

Answer: D

Critique: Life-threatening athletic injuries require a stepwise emergency plan. Anyone who is found unresponsive should be treated as having a serious neck injury. Inline cervical immobilization must be maintained. The ABCDE (airway, breathing, circulation, disability, exposure) approach requires the examiner to first ensure that there is an adequate airway and that the patient is breathing spontaneously. The facemask should be carefully loosened and tilted out of the way for airway access. The helmet and shoulder pads should be left on if possible. The head tilt–chin lift maneuver should not be used in an individual suspected of having a neck injury. The jaw-thrust maneuver should be implemented if the victim does not have an adequate airway.

Pages: 847, 848

2: Benefits of regular exercise include:

A. An increase in VO_{2max} by as much as 10% to 30%
B. Strength gains of 25% to 100% in 3 to 6 months
C. Improved joint range of motion and function
D. All of the above

Answer: D

Critique: Numerous health benefits have been documented through aerobic conditioning, strength training, and flexibility training. The benefits of exercise follow a dose-response curve.

Pages: 849–851

Match the following clinical descriptions with the correct heat-related condition:

A. Prickly heat
B. Heat edema
C. Heat cramps
D. Heat exhaustion
E. Heat stroke

3: A 17-year-old football player complains of a maculopapular erythematous rash on his trunk and proximal extremities after the first week of summer conditioning drills. He describes the rash as uncomfortable like "pins and needles" sticking into his skin.

4: An ambulance brings a 76-year-old delirious female to the emergency department during a summer heat wave. She was found wearing a sweater in her apartment without air conditioning. Her core body temperature is 41.6°C.

5: A 22-year-old college football player from North Dakota complains of swelling in his hands and feet following the third day of conditioning at his college in Alabama.

6: A 16-year-old high school cross-country runner collapses at the finish line of the district meet. The wet bulb globe temperature index is 32°C. She reportedly drank no water before or during the race. She is sweating profusely and complains of a headache, dizziness, and nausea.

Answers: 3 - A, 4 - E, 5 - B, 6 - D

Critique: Prickly heat, also known as miliaria rubra, is a maculopapular erythematous rash that occurs with heat exposure. It typically occurs in areas of the body covered by clothing. The rash results from keratin plugs blocking the sweat glands. Patients complain of a sensation of pins and needles sticking into their skin. Treatment is aimed at prevention and includes proper hygiene and loose-fitting clothes. Classical heat stroke occurs in the elderly and results from impaired dissipation of environmental heat. As the core body temperature approaches 42°C multi-organ failure can result from failure of cellular enzymes and increased permeability of cellular membranes. Patients may exhibit irritability, ataxia, delirium, seizures, decorticate posturing, or coma. Treatment is aimed at rapidly reducing core body temperature. Heat edema results in swelling of the hands and feet. This condition occurs during the first week of acclimatization. Treatment consists of cooling, elevation, and support hose for comfort. Heat exhaustion may represent the forerunner of heat stroke and requires early recognition and treatment. Water depletion heat exhaustion occurs when an individual exercises in the heat without adequate fluid replacement. Patients may experience profuse sweating, headaches, nausea or vomiting, muscle weakness, visual disturbances, and cutaneous flushing. Treatment consists of cooling and immediate oral rehydration at a rate of 1L/hr.

Pages: 851–853

179

7: Which of the following statements regarding hypothermia is *not* correct?

    A. Ventricular fibrillation represents the most likely cause of death.
    B. If the patient is not shivering, it can be assumed that his or her core temperature is greater than 90°F.
    C. Affected individuals may appear clumsy, apathetic, or confused.
    D. The diagnosis is confirmed by a core temperature below 95°F.

Answer: B

Critique: Ventricular fibrillation represents the most likely cause of death associated with hypothermia. Care should be taken not to jostle the patient to avoid inducing ventricular fibrillation. If no thermometer is available, core body temperature can be estimated by the presence of shivering. If the victim is shivering, core temperature is usually greater than 90°F. However, core temperature is usually less than 90°F if the patient is obtunded and not shivering. Patients suffering from hypothermia may appear clumsy, apathetic, or confused. The diagnosis of hypothermia is confirmed when the core body temperature measured by a rectal thermometer is less than 95°F (35°C).

Page: 853

8: Which of the following statements regarding hypertrophic obstructive cardiomyopathy (HOCM) is true?

    A. HOCM is the leading cause of nontraumatic death in athletes.
    B. The condition is transmitted in an autosomal recessive pattern.
    C. A thorough history and physical examination should detect all cases.
    D. The pathologic hallmark involves obstruction of the pulmonary outflow tract.

Answer: A

Critique: Hypertrophic obstructive cardiomyopathy is the most common cause of nontraumatic death in athletes. Cardiac causes account for 74% of nontraumatic deaths, and HOCM accounts for 51% of these. HOCM is transmitted in an autosomal dominant pattern with a prevalence of 0.2% in the general population. Ventricular outflow tract obstruction occurs from hypertrophy of the interventricular septum. History and physical examination are the keys to early detection. The two most sensitive screening criteria for cardiovascular disease include a family history of sudden cardiac death in someone younger than 50 or a history of syncope. The symptoms may be vague and require a high index of suspicion and searching for exertional or postexercise symptoms. A systolic ejection murmur may be present in only 25% of patients with outflow tract obstruction. Screening studies for lethal cardiac conditions have not been shown to be effective. Because the condition is relatively rare, the symptoms are vague, and there may be no physical findings, not all cases of HOCM are detected with a thorough history and physical examination.

Page: 863

Match the following clinical descriptions with the correct condition:

    A. Exercise-induced asthma
    B. Exercise-induced anaphylaxis

9: A 14-year-old female was running during gym class and developed shortness of breath. Her symptoms progressed to include headache and nausea as well as a rash on her trunk and neck. She had lunch 1 hour before class.

10: A 17-year-old soccer player complains of chest tightness and coughing while playing. He denies any personal or family history of asthma, but reports that he had eczema as a child. Physical examination is unremarkable.

Answers: 9 - B, 10 - A

Critique: Exercise-induced asthma is a very common pulmonary disorder that affects many athletes. The most frequent symptoms include dyspnea, wheezing, and coughing during or after exercise. Formal diagnosis is made by clinical suspicion and spirometry stress testing. The condition is treated medically by a short-acting beta agonist 15 to 20 minutes before exercise. Exercise-induced anaphylaxis is a rare but life-threatening condition seen in athletes. The most frequent symptoms are flushing, dyspnea, headache, nausea, and an urticarial rash on the neck, trunk, and extremities. Risk factors include food allergies, e.g., some individuals are allergic to celery or nuts eaten before exercise.

Pages: 869, 870

11: Which of the following conditions is an absolute contraindication to strenuous exercise?

    A. Marfan syndrome
    B. Hypertension
    C. Diabetes
    D. Controlled seizure disorder

Answer: A

Critique: Of the conditions listed, only Marfan syndrome is an absolute contraindication to strenuous exercise. The condition is characterized by cystic medial necrosis of connective tissue that may lead to aortic root dilation, aortic regurgitation, or aortic dissection. The diagnosis is made clinically and by ECG and echocardiographic findings. The other conditions mentioned require appropriate medical management but do not limit participation in strenuous exercise.

Pages: 863, 868

12: Which statement about exercise-induced asthma (EIA) is correct?

    A. All patients with general asthma have exercise-induced asthma.
    B. By definition, resting spirometry shows a 15% or greater reduction in FEV_1.

C. Spirometry should be obtained at baseline, immediately postexercise, and every 5 minutes until 30 minutes to confirm the diagnosis.
D. Management includes a short-acting beta agonist 2 to 3 hours before exercise.

Answer: C

Critique: EIA is a very common pulmonary disorder affecting athletes. It is estimated that 10% to 15% of the general population is affected by the disorder. Although common among asthmatics, it is estimated that 80% of patients with general asthma have EIA. Formal diagnosis is made by clinical suspicion and spirometry stress testing. The forced expiratory flow at 1 second (FEV_1) is measured at baseline, immediately postexercise, and every 5 minutes until 30 minutes. A reduction in FEV_1 of 15% or more from baseline is diagnostic. The condition is treated medically by a short-acting beta agonist 15 to 20 minutes before activity.

Pages: 869, 870

13: A high school soccer player runs off the field to the sideline holding his head. He reports that he went up for a header a few minutes earlier and received an elbow to the back of his head. He reports feeling "dazed" and complains of a headache, nausea, and dizziness. His neurological examination is normal, and the back of his head does not reveal any evidence of trauma. He has considerable difficulty performing serial sevens and the months of the year backwards. He knows the score of the game and the name of the opposing team. Medical intervention at this time should include:

A. Immediate transportation to an emergency facility for an MRI examination
B. Immediate transportation to an emergency facility for a CT examination
C. Monitoring the athlete on the sideline with serial examinations
D. Returning the player to the game because he is experiencing only a mild head injury

Answer: C

Critique: An estimated 300,000 cases of sports-related mild traumatic brain injury (MTBI) occur annually. Headache and confusion are the hallmarks of concussions. The quintessential rule for managing athletes with MTBI is to never return an athlete to a game or practice who is experiencing residual neurologic symptoms such as headache or dizziness. Imaging studies (MRI or CT) are used in cases of prolonged headache or persistent postconcussion symptoms. Rapid neurological deterioration determined by serial examinations warrants further evaluation in an emergency medical facility.

Pages: 871–873

14: The female athletic triad includes:

A. Amenorrhea, osteoporosis, and anemia
B. Osteoporosis, eating disorders, and anemia
C. Eating disorders, anemia, and amenorrhea
D. Amenorrhea, osteoporosis, and eating disorders

Answer: D

Critique: The female athletic triad is a disorder of competitive female athletes. The condition includes amenorrhea, osteoporosis, and eating disorders. Regular menstrual periods, sufficient caloric intake, and adequate dietary calcium play critical roles in normal bone metabolism and development and maintenance of adequate bone mineral density.

Page: 873

15: All of the following dermatologic conditions exclude participation from a wrestling tournament, except:

A. Ringworm on the forearm that is easily covered
B. Molluscum contagiosum on the hands
C. Impetigo around the face
D. Herpes gladiatorum on the forehead

Answer: A

Critique: Dermatologic conditions that exclude participation from contact sports (wrestling) include molluscum contagiosum, active herpes gladiatorum, dermatophyte infection that may not be covered, scabies, impetigo, lice, cellulitis, and pediculosis pubis. If an athlete has a small patch of ringworm that is easily covered, he or she may be allowed to participate.

Page: 875

16: Patients with Down syndrome have an increased risk for all of the following conditions, except:

A. Patellar instability
B. Cardiac defects
C. Atlantoaxial instability
D. Exercise-induced asthma

Answer: D

Critique: Exercise-induced asthma is the only condition listed that is not seen more commonly in patients with Down syndrome than in the general population. Atlantoaxial instability is confirmed by lateral radiographs that demonstrate more than 3.5 cm separation between the axis (C1) and atlas (C2).

Page: 884

17: Which of the following statements regarding the pregnant athlete is true?

A. A patient with premature rupture of membranes (PROM) may participate in low-intensity exercise.
B. A low-risk pregnant patient may participate in moderate-intensity exercise.
C. Pregnant athletes should attempt to exercise in hot and humid conditions only.
D. Women who participate in exercise during pregnancy have significantly better outcomes.

Answer: B

Critique: Exercise during pregnancy is safe with appropriate guidelines. A low-risk pregnant patient may participate in moderate-intensity exercise. PROM is a high-risk condition that contraindicates exercise during pregnancy. A recent meta-analysis of 2000 pregnant women found no statistically significant differences in pregnancy outcomes between the patients who exercised regularly and those who did not.

Page: 885

18: Which of the following statements regarding spondylolysis is true?

    A. Spondylolysis most commonly occurs at the L4 level.
    B. Standard AP lumbar radiographs easily detect the defect.
    C. Low back pain is the most common initial complaint.
    D. Single-photon emission computed tomography (SPECT) rarely demonstrates the defect.

Answer: C

Critique: Spondylolysis is a condition among athletes. It results from a unilateral or bilateral fracture through the pars interarticularis without displacement of the vertebrae. The defect is most commonly found at the L5 level. The lesion is usually demonstrated on oblique lumbar radiographs. Low back pain is the most common initial complaint. Bone scan, MRI, and SPECT scanning may be helpful in confirming the diagnosis.

Page: 884

Match the following clinical descriptions with the correct condition:

    A. Ankle sprain
    B. Sever disease
    C. Patellofemoral syndrome
    D. Epiphyseal fracture
    E. Slipped capital femoral epiphysis

19: A 10-year-old male was playing football and rolled his ankle during a tackle and was unable to continue playing. There is significant swelling and ecchymoses on the lateral aspect of the ankle as well as significant tenderness on palpation 4 cm above the lateral malleolus. Routine ankle radiographs are negative for fracture or dislocation.

20: A 12-year-old tennis player complains of pain in her right heel. She is unable to recall an acute injury and reports that the pain developed insidiously. She plays on three different teams but is nearing the end of her season.

21: A 13-year-old male complains of left knee pain. The pain developed over the last 2 weeks and has progressively become more severe. His mother reports that he has grown 3 inches in the last year. Examination of the knee is unremarkable. He walks with an antalgic gait and is noted to have markedly reduced internal rotation of the left hip.

22: A 17-year-old female soccer player complains of bilateral knee pain. She is unable to recall an acute injury. She denies any locking or buckling of the knee. She reports that the knee "pops" a lot and occasionally appears swollen. Climbing stairs and sitting for prolonged periods exacerbate the pain.

Answers: 19 - D, 20 - B, 21 - E, 22 - C

Critique: Epiphyseal fractures require a high index of suspicion because early detection and proper treatment can limit long-term morbidity. Any tenderness on palpation over a growth plate should be treated as an epiphyseal fracture until proved otherwise. It is not uncommon for the initial radiographs to be negative. Sever disease represents a traction apophysitis of the calcaneal apophysis. Believed to be an overuse injury, it results from repetitive loading of the apophysis. Slipped capital femoral epiphysis, the most common hip disorder of adolescence, occurs between the ages of 10 and 15 years. During periods of rapid growth, the epiphysis of the capitellum begins to separate from the metaphysis. It commonly manifests as referred pain from the knee and loss of internal hip rotation. Patellofemoral syndrome, also known as chondromalacia patellae, is a very common cause of knee pain. The syndrome results from a relative imbalance between the vastus medialis obliquus and the vastus lateralis that leads to abnormal tracking of the patella through the trochlea.

Pages: 877–884

Chapter 39

Orthopedics

Sam Sandowski and Nicole Solomos

1: Which part of the gait cycle has the most clinical significance:

  A. Swing phase
  B. Stance phase
  C. Toe clearance
  D. Toe off

Answer: B

Critique: A patient's gait should be observed as part of the physical examination. The gait cycle may be divided into the swing phase and the stance phase. The swing phase includes the movement of the leg, including toe-off and toe clearance. The stance phase starts with the heel strike and includes a foot-flat and heel-off incident. These are critical events in the gait cycle in which there is maximum weight bearing and tends to reproduce the patient's symptoms.

Page: 892

2: A patient who is being evaluated for loss of power of a large muscle group is found to have a grade 3 muscle strength. This indicates that:

  A. The patient can move this muscle group against gravity, but not against any resistance.
  B. The muscle can contract but cannot move the joint at all.
  C. There is normal muscle strength in that muscle.
  D. The muscle can move against gravity but not against a normal amount.
  E. The patient cannot even contract the muscle.

Answer: A

Critique: Muscle strength is graded from 0 to 5. Grade 0 indicates no muscle movement. Grade 1 indicates that the muscle can contract but not move the joint. Grade 2 suggests that the patient can only move the extremity when the forces of gravity are removed. Grade 3 indicates that the patient can move against gravity but not against resistance. Grade 4 indicates that the patient can move against some resistance but not normal strength. Grade 5 is considered normal strength.

Pages: 893–894

3: A 47-year-old runner presents with knee pain. You diagnose a grade 1 anterior cruciate ligament injury. Which of the following statements best describes your findings:

  A. There is increased laxity of the ligament.
  B. There is decreased laxity of the ligament.
  C. There is severe laxity and instability of the ligament.
  D. There is no laxity, and the ligament is intact.
  E. There is a complete tear of the ligament.

Answer: D

Critique: Ligamentous injuries are described in grades. A grade 1 injury reveals an intact ligament without laxity. A grade 2 injury has elongated ligaments and increased laxity. A grade 3 injury denotes instability with total disruption of the ligament.

Page: 896

4: Most office visits for spinal pain and discomfort are generated by the:

  A. Thoracic spine
  B. Cervical spine
  C. Lumbar spine
  D. Sacrum

Answer: C

Critique: The most common reason for office visits for back pain caused by a spinous process is secondary to the lumbar spine. The cervical spine is the second most common reason for spinal pain.

Page: 896

5: A 50-year-old woman presents with a cervical spine injury. Which of the following *cannot* be attributed to the injury:

  A. Decreased motion of the head
  B. Numbness and weakness of the arm
  C. Concern that there is instability of the head
  D. Inability to do alternating rapid movements (diadochokinesis)

Answer: D

Critique: The cervical spine has three major functions. It permits mobility of the head, including turning and bending; it supports and stabilizes the head; and it protects neural elements of the central nervous system, which innervate the arm. It does not protect the cerebellum, where diadochokinesis is determined.

Page: 896

6: The atlas (C1) differs from the other cervical vertebrae because:

A. It has no transverse process.
B. It has no body and no spinous process.
C. It has no body and no transverse process.
D. It is the same as the other cervical vertebrae.

Answer: B

Critique: The atlas is also known as C1. Together with C2, also known as the axis, it forms a unit called the dens. It is this unit that permits most of the rotational movement of the head.

Page: 896

7: The functions of intervertebral disks include all of the following, except:

A. Providing protection for the spinal cord
B. Providing mobility
C. Absorbing shock
D. Distribution of stress over a wide area of vertebrae

Answer: A

Critique: The intervertebral disks have three main functions: providing mobility, acting as a shock absorber for the vertebrae, and distributing stress over a wide area of the vertebrae, thus helping reduce the likelihood of fractures. They do not directly protect the spinal cord. When a disk herniates, it may damage the cord.

Page: 897

8: All of the following tests can elicit symptoms caused by cervical spine pathology, except:

A. Lhermitte's maneuver
B. Spurling's test
C. Distraction test
D. Axial compression test

Answer: C

Critique: The axial compression test is executed by pressing straight down on the patient's head. The Spurling's test also consists of a downward force on the patient's head, with lateral flexion and rotation of the head. Both of these tests elicit symptoms of radiculopathy, with the Spurling's test eliciting pain on the same side as the compressed nerve. The Lhermitte's maneuver, performed by maximally flexing the cervical and thoracic spine, elicits pain from cord compression or spinal stenosis. The distraction test causes relief of radicular pain because traction is placed on the patient's head.

Pages: 897–898

9: A 69-year-old male presents with difficulty holding on to objects. On examination, you notice weakness in flexing the fingers. Which nerve root innervates the extrinsic flexors of the fingers:

A. C3
B. C4
C. C6
D. C7
E. C8

Answer: E

Critique: C3 and C4 innervate the diaphragm. C6 and C7 innervate the wrist and elbow flexors. C8 innervates the extrinsic finger flexors.

Page: 898

10: After examination of a patient with suspected cervical spine instability, you order flexion-extension lateral neck films. Which of the following findings is associated with cervical spine instability:

A. Displacement greater than 5 mm and any angulation greater than 30% between the vertebral bodies.
B. The posterior borders of the cervical spine forming a straight line
C. Anterior displacement of greater than 3.5 mm or angulation between vertebral bodies greater than 11 degrees
D. An avulsion fracture
E. A soft tissue shadow of 3 mm at the level of C4

Answer: C

Critique: The posterior borders of the cervical spine usually form a straight line. The loss of this straight line suggests pathology. While avulsion fractures or facet joint widening may be seen on a lateral film, it is anterior displacement greater than 3.5 mm or angulation between vertebral bodies greater than 11 degrees that suggests cervical spine instability. A soft tissue shadow at the level of C4 is considered abnormal if it is greater than 8 to 10 mm.

Pages: 899, 900

11: All of the following muscles are commonly involved in neck pain, except:

A. Supraspinatus
B. Trapezius
C. Levator scapulae
D. Rhomboids
E. Long cervical muscles

Answer: A

Critique: The trapezius, levator scapulae, rhomboids, and long cervical muscles are commonly the cause of neck pain owing to muscle spasm or injury. Patients often describe a "knot" or "tightness" over a specific area. The injury is usually caused by a repetitive insult, such as carrying a heavy handbag to work every day, and specific insults or trauma to the area is not easily recalled.

Page: 900

12: Treatment of whiplash includes all of the following, except:

A. A soft cervical collar day and night for 1 to 2 weeks
B. Traction in a home traction device after the acute pain has subsided
C. Rest during the first few days after the injury
D. Cold compresses after the initial insult
E. NSAIDs after the injury

Answer: B

Critique: Treatment for whiplash includes wearing a soft cervical collar day and night for 1 to 2 weeks after the injury. Cold compresses and NSAIDs after the insult may be of benefit. Although patients may not have any symptoms for hours to days after the injury, rest during the first few days after the injury may be of benefit as well. Range-of-motion exercises, not traction, should begin after the pain has subsided.

Page: 902

13: (True or False) Regarding congenital torticollis:

    A. It always self-corrects.
    B. Initial treatment includes gentle stretching of the sternocleidomastoid by the parent.
    C. It is not noticeable until 6 months of age.
    D. The head is tilted toward the involved side and rotated in the opposite direction.

Answers: A - False, B - True, C - False, D - True

Critique: Congenital torticollis is noticed at birth and is caused by a unilateral contraction of the sternocleidomastoid muscle. It is more common with breech deliveries and congenital problems, such as hip dysplasia. The child has a shortened, contracted sternocleidomastoid muscle. His or her head is tilted toward the affected side and rotated in the opposite direction. Treatment is usually successful with gentle stretching. However, if unresponsive, surgical correction may be necessary. When untreated, irreversible asymmetry of the face may result.

Pages: 902, 903

14: All of the following statements are true about spasmodic torticollis, except:

    A. It primarily affects adults.
    B. Muscles in the neck other than the sternocleidomastoid may be involved.
    C. Psychologic problems can complicate recovery.
    D. Spasms may be bilateral or unilateral.
    E. Surgical correction is very effective.

Answer: E

Critique: Spasmodic torticollis occurs in adults. It is caused by unilateral or bilateral spasm of several cervical muscles in the neck, not just the sternocleidomastoid. The cause of the spasms is unclear, but stress may exacerbate the problem and delay recovery. Surgery usually results in only minimal relief.

Page: 905

15: The most common cause of cervical radiculopathy is:

    A. Disk disease
    B. Vertebral fracture impinging on cervical nerve roots
    C. Cervical arthritis with foraminal encroachment
    D. Tumors impinging on cervical nerve roots

Answer: C

Critique: The most common cause of cervical radiculopathy is foraminal encroachment with arthritis. Disk disease is the second most common cause of cervical radiculopathy and occurs in younger adults. Vertebral fractures impinging on cervical nerve roots and tumors impinging on cervical nerve roots are rare.

Pages: 903, 904

16: A 33-year-old high diver presents with pain over the scapulae and numbness and weakness in the left hand and arm. What would you *not* expect to find on physical examination:

    A. Improvement by the distraction test
    B. Loss of ability to fully rotate the neck
    C. Limited extension of the neck
    D. A negative Spurling's test
    E. A positive axial compression test

Answer: D

Critique: Diving is a common mechanism of injury causing cervical radiculopathy. Patients with cervical radiculopathy lose the ability to fully extend and rotate the neck. Symptoms of pain or neuropathy may be reproduced with the axial compression test and Spurling's test. The distraction test may alleviate the patient's symptoms.

Pages: 903, 904

17: Cervical disk lesions are most likely to occur at the level of:

    A. C1–C2
    B. C2–C3
    C. C3–C4
    D. C5–C6
    E. C7–T1

Answer: D

Critique: Most (90%) disk lesions occur in the area of greatest mobility. In the neck, this is C5–C6.

Page: 905

18. (True or False) A 44-year-old male is suspected of having cervical disk disease. Which of the following statements are true and which are false:

    A. Plain films are necessary for the diagnosis.
    B. Plain films may be normal.
    C. Imaging such as CT, MRI, or myelography should be done for all patients under age 50.
    D. Myelography is more sensitive than CT scans are.

Answers: A - False, B - True, C - False, D - False

Critique: A good history and physical examination are usually sufficient to diagnose cervical disk disease. If AP and lateral plain films are obtained, a loss of disk space height and/or osteophyte formation with encroachment of the intervertebral foramen may be evident, especially if owing to an arthritic process. Conversely, 35% of asymptomatic patients may have abnormal radiographs. Disk disease secondary to nuclear herniation or disk protrusion often produces normal plain films. Advanced imaging, such as CT and MRI, should be reserved for cases refractory to conservative treatment, when surgery is considered, and when pathology such as a tumor is suspected. Both CT and MRI have a better sensitivity than does myelography alone.

Pages: 906, 907

19: (True or False) Regarding the straight leg–raising test:

    A. The patient will describe back pain in a positive test.
    B. The patient lies supine.
    C. The patient first lifts the unaffected leg and then the affected leg.
    D. Lasegue's test increases symptoms.
    E. The patient may describe pain radiating to the foot in a positive test.

Answers: A - False, B - True, C - False, D - True, E - True

Critique: Low back pain often presents between ages 30 and 60. Physical examination includes a straight leg–raising test, in which the patient's straightened leg is lifted by the examiner while the patient is supine. A positive test produces pain radiating down the posterior or lateral aspect of the thigh, going distal to the knee and often into the foot, without eliciting back pain. The Lasegue's test (dorsiflexion of the foot while performing a straight leg test) amplifies the symptoms.

Pages: 910, 911

20: A 39-year-old male has low back pain and pain down one leg. You perform a crossed straight leg–test. Which of the following statements about the crossed straight leg–raise test is true:

    A. The unaffected leg is raised.
    B. If symptoms occur in the leg that is not raised, the patient is probably malingering.
    C. A positive test indicates posterolateral disk herniation.
    D. It is useful in detecting muscle strains of the leg.

Answer: A

Critique: The crossed straight leg–test is used to detect disk disease. It is performed by passively raising the unaffected leg. If pain or symptoms are reproduced on the affected leg, the test is positive and suggestive of central disk herniation.

Pages: 910, 911

21: In nerve impingement syndromes of the thoracolumbar spine, the test that can localize the problem to three nerve roots (L2, L3, L4) is:

    A. Crossed straight leg raise
    B. Lasegue's test
    C. Femoral nerve traction test
    D. Straight leg raise

Answer: C

Critique: The crossed straight leg–raise test, the straight leg–raised test, and the Lasegue's test can detect disk disease, but only the femoral nerve traction test can detect nerve root compression at L2, L3, and L4.

Page: 911

22: The most common cause of low back pain is:

    A. Nerve impingement
    B. Repetitive use of improperly stretched and toned muscles
    C. Spondylolisthesis
    D. Pathologic fracture
    E. Disk herniation

Answer: B

Critique: Although disk herniation, nerve impingement, spondylolisthesis, and pathologic fractures may cause back pain, the most common reason for back pain is poorly stretched and toned muscles. Obesity, being a "weekend warrior," bad work habits, and even high-heeled shoes may predispose a person to low back pain.

Page: 912

23: (True or False) Low back pain:

    A. Is the most common cause of absenteeism from work
    B. Is a leading cause of work-related disability
    C. Is the most common cause of acute pain
    D. Is the most common cause of chronic pain
    E. Usually leads to chronic pain

Answers: A - False, B - True, C - True, D - True, E - False

Critique: Low back pain is a common complaint, occurring in 60% to 90% of the adult population. Although only in 5% to 10% of the cases does it develop into a chronic pain syndrome, low back pain is still the most common cause of both acute and chronic pain. It is a leading cause of work-related disability and the second most common cause of absenteeism from work.

Pages: 911, 912

24: A 34-year-old male complains of low back pain for 3 days. On physical examination, you notice significant paraspinal muscle spasm. Straight leg–raise test is negative, and the neurologic examination is normal. What is the next step?

    A. Order x-rays of the lumbosacral spine
    B. Order an MRI of the lumbosacral spine
    C. Order a CT myelogram
    D. Treat the patient with rest and pain medication

Answer: D

Critique: This case is suggestive of a lumbosacral strain. Treatment can be started with pain medications and rest. Radiographs are not indicated initially, unless there is suggestion of severe radiculopathy with neurologic findings, tumor, compression fractures, or processes other than a lumbosacral strain. MRI or CT myelograms may be useful for further evaluation of these causes. Even if asymptomatic, most adults over age 40 show some defects on plain films.

Page: 912

25: In the acute phase of lumbosacral strain, which treatment modality may be of *least* benefit:

    A. NSAIDs
    B. Acetaminophen

C. Narcotic analgesics
D. Muscle relaxants
E. Rest

Answer: A

Critique: In the acute phase of lumbosacral strains, rest and pain treatment with acetaminophen, narcotic analgesics, and muscle relaxants are appropriate. NSAIDs may not be of benefit because inflammation is not part of the mechanism causing pain or the strain.

Page: 912

26: A 41-year-old male presents with a new onset of lumbosacral strain. You suggest back-stretching exercises Which of the following is *not* a back-stretching exercise:

A. Modified sit-ups
B. Knee-chest pulls
C. Pelvic rocks
D. Side bending

Answer: A

Critique: Knee-chest pulls, pelvic rocks, and side bending are back-stretching exercises. Modified sit-ups are a back-strengthening exercise and should be performed only after flexibility has been restored with 3 to 6 weeks of back-stretching exercises.

Pages: 915, 916

27: The most common site for lumbar disk herniation is:

A. L1–L2
B. L2–L3
C. L3–L4
D. L4–L5
E. L5–S1

Answer: D

Critique: Most (95%) lumbar disk herniations occur at L4–L5 during the third and fourth decades of life. Almost all the rest occur at L3–L4. Herniation usually occurs at the weakest point: the posterolateral aspect of the disk.

Page: 914

28: In what part of the leg are numbness and tingling most likely to occur in a patient with lumbar disk syndromes:

A. Anterior thigh
B. Posterior thigh
C. Lower leg
D. Buttock and iliac crest
E. Popliteal fossa

Answer: C

Critique: Most lumbar disk syndromes occur at L4–L5. The nerve root of L4 innervates the anterior tibialis, and L5 affects the extensor hallucis longus. Therefore, symptoms of lumbar disk syndromes most commonly present with numbness and tingling over the lower leg.

Pages: 914, 918

29: All of the following are indications for early advanced imaging in lumbar disk syndromes, except:

A. Cauda equina syndrome of the lumbosacral spine
B. Central disk herniation of the lumbosacral spine
C. Tumor of the lumbosacral spine
D. Trauma of the lumbosacral spine
E. Infection of the lumbosacral spine

Answer: B

Critique: Patients with cauda equina syndrome, tumor, infection, or trauma of the lumbosacral spine should all be imaged with CT or MRI. Patients with symptoms of classic central disk herniations should not have CT or MRI done immediately but benefit from empiric therapy. If symptoms do not respond in 4 to 6 weeks, then CT or MRI should be considered. Waiting 4 to 6 weeks permits the herniation to decrease, and earlier readings may prove to be falsely positive.

Page: 918

30: Which of the following statements about the success rate of surgery for lumbar disk syndromes is true:

A. The long-term success rates for patients treated either conservatively or surgically are not statistically different.
B. Success is highest with automated percutaneous diskectomy.
C. Success is highest with chemonucleolysis.
D. Laminotomy (laminectomy) has a 50% success rate.

Answer: A

Critique: Because the success rates for patients treated conservatively or surgically are not statistically different, surgery should not be used as a first-line treatment option. When surgery is done, three techniques can be used. One technique is a laminectomy, in which the disk is removed under direct visualization. It has a success rate that approaches 95% in the properly selected patient. Another technique is automated percutaneous diskectomy, in which a small suction cutter is placed with the use of fluoroscopy. The success rate is about 75%. A third technique is chemonucleolysis, in which an enzyme is injected into the affected disk and dissolves the nucleus pulposus. The success rate is also 75%.

Page: 918

31: A 45-year-old female presents to the office complaining of cramping in both legs, mostly in the thighs but also in the calves; some weakness of her legs; and feeling as if her lower back is flat. Her symptoms are lessened when she squats or lies down in a flexed position. What is the most likely diagnosis:

A. Lumbar disk herniation
B. Scoliosis
C. Spinal stenosis
D. Cauda equina syndrome
E. Vascular claudication

Answer: C

Critique: The listed symptoms are suggestive of spinal stenosis, which usually starts between ages 40 and 50 years. Lumbar disk herniation and scoliosis do not typically cause a cramping pain in both legs. Vascular claudication is sometimes difficult to differentiate from the neurogenic claudication of spinal stenosis. However, vascular claudication more typically starts in the calves, and neurogenic claudication symptoms are often relieved with flexion of the knees and hips.

Pages: 919, 920

32: Which of the following statements about idiopathic scoliosis is true:

    A. It is more common in males.
    B. It is more common in children 6 to 10 years old.
    C. There is no associated rib hump.
    D. It is the most common of all spinal deformities.
    E. Young patients usually have mild to moderate pain.

Answer: D

Critique: Idiopathic scoliosis accounts for 90% of all cases of scoliosis, and it is the most common of all spinal deformities. It is most common in females ages 10 to 13 years. A rib hump, where one side of the back is higher than the other when bending forward, is commonly found on physical examination. Young patients are generally asymptomatic; if there is pain, causes for nonidiopathic scoliosis should be sought.

Page: 921

33: A 12-year-old girl has just been diagnosed with scoliosis. When is surgery most indicated:

    A. In patients with a curvature of less than 20 degrees:
    B. In growing patients with a curvature of greater than 20 degrees
    C. In patients with a curvature of greater than 40 degrees
    D. In patients responding to a Milwaukee brace

Answer: C

Critique: For curvatures of less than 20 degrees, patients who have immature skeletons may be monitored every 4 to 6 months, because 50% of these patients improve spontaneously. When the curvature is greater than 40 degrees, surgery is generally recommended. Surgery may also be recommended for patients who have progressive disease or who have not responded to a Milwaukee brace. Milwaukee braces are generally indicated for patients who are growing and have a curvature of greater than 20 degrees. Most patients with a curvature of greater than 20 degrees will probably benefit from a referral to a scoliosis specialist.

Page: 922

34: Which is the most commonly sprained joint:

    A. Ankle
    B. Knee
    C. Wrist
    D. Elbow
    E. Shoulder

Answer: A

Critique: The incidence of ankle sprains is approximately 1 per day per 10,000 people. It is usually caused by an inversion injury. One quarter of these sprains result in instability of the ankle.

Page: 922

35: While running, a 28-year-old male stepped on a rock and twisted his ankle, causing an inversion injury. Which ligament is most likely to be injured:

    A. Anterior talofibular ligament
    B. Posterior talofibular ligament
    C. Calcaneofibular ligament
    D. Deltoid ligament
    E. Anterior cruciate ligament

Answer: A

Critique: The anterior talofibular ligament, which lies on the lateral aspect of the ankle, is most subject to injury during inversion of the ankle. The posterior talofibular ligament and the calcaneofibular ligament are affected when there is a severe injury with both inversion and dorsiflexion. The deltoid ligament may be injured if the foot is everted and externally rotated.

Page: 923

36: A 14-year-old female presents to the emergency room after twisting her ankle. The ankle is swollen and tender. You do not suspect a fracture, but you do suspect a complete rupture of the anteriorfibular ligament. What grade ligamentous injury does she have:

    A. Grade I
    B. Grade II
    C. Grade III
    D. Grade IV

Answer: C

Critique: Ligamentous injuries are graded from I to III. A grade I injury reveals swelling but an intact ligament. A grade II injury indicates a partial tear of the ligament, and a grade III injury has a complete rupture of the ligament.

Page: 923

37: The Ottawa ankle rules provide guidance for determining which patients who have sustained an ankle injury require x-rays. For a patient who has pain in the malleolar area, all of the following findings indicate the need for x-rays of the ankle, except:

    A. Bony tenderness anywhere along the lower 6 cm of the posterior edge of the fibula
    B. Inability to bear weight immediately or in the emergency department
    C. Bony tenderness over the posterior edge or tip of the medial malleolus
    D. Paresthesias in the toes

Answer: D

Critique: The Ottawa ankle rules provide guidance for selecting patients for whom x-rays should be obtained. If the patient has pain in the malleolar zone, x-rays should be obtained when (1) any bony tenderness exists along the posterior lower 6 cm of the fibula or the tip of the lateral malleolus; (2) any bony tenderness occurs along the posterior edge or tip of the medial malleolus; or (3) the patient is unable to bear weight immediately or in the emergency department. Paresthesias of the toes are not included in the ankle x-ray indicators.

Pages: 923–924

38: Which of the following is *not* appropriate for grades I and II ankle sprains:

    A. Rest
    B. Elevation
    C. Heat
    D. Range-of-motion exercises
    E. Weight bearing as tolerated

Answer: C

Critique: *R*est, *i*ce, *c*ompression with an Ace bandage, and *e*levation (RICE) are all part of the treatment for grades I and II ankle sprains. Range-of-motion exercises and weight bearing as tolerated maintain flexibility and function. Heat should be avoided.

Page: 924

39: A 20-year-old male presents to the emergency room after falling onto his outstretched arm. Physical examination reveals pain on palpation over the radial aspect of the wrist, proximal to the first metacarpophalangeal joint. X-rays show no fracture. The best initial course of action is:

    A. Application of a sugar tong splint
    B. Application of a short arm-thumb spica cast
    C. Application of an Ace (elastic) bandage
    D. Buddy taping the thumb to the index finger
    E. Application of a volar plaster splint

Answer: B

Critique: The scenario is typical for a possible carpal scaphoid fracture. Despite normal x-rays, the injury should be treated as a fracture and reevaluated in 2 weeks. A short arm-thumb spica cast should be applied, and after 2 weeks the patient should be re-examined and x-rays should be repeated. Fractures not apparent on initial examination may now be evident. If a fracture is identified, the cast should be reapplied and maintained for 8 to 10 weeks.

Page: 924

40: (True or False) Determine whether the following statements about carpal instability are true or false:

    A. Patients almost always have a history of pain, clicks, or clunks.
    B. Radiographs help differentiate fractures from dislocations or instability.
    C. The physical examination may help identify carpal instability.

    D. Carpal instability may be acute or chronic.

Answers: A - False, B - True, C - True, D - True

Critique: Not all patients with carpal instability complain of pain, clicks, clunks, and so forth, and many are unaware of any injury. The instability may be acute or chronic. Therefore, a careful physical examination, including stress tests, needs to be performed. AP, lateral, and oblique views of the wrist should be done, because they may have findings consistent with instability. Additionally, certain radiographic findings, such as angling of the lunate dorsally or volarly, may suggest instability.

Page: 924

41: Treatment of ganglion cysts includes all of the following, except:

    A. Steroid injections
    B. Aspiration
    C. Compression bandage
    D. Surgery
    E. Warm compresses

Answer: E

Critique: The initial treatment of a ganglion cyst is aspiration and steroid injection, followed by a compression bandage for 48 to 72 hours. Symptomatic ganglions that are not responsive to initial treatment may require surgical intervention. There is no role for warm compresses in the treatment of ganglion cysts.

Page: 925

42: Which of the following fractures is *not* caused by the corresponding mechanism of injury:

    A. Transverse fracture: direct blow to or bending of bone
    B. Oblique fracture: crush injury to bone
    C. Stress fracture: repeated assault to bone
    D. Avulsion fracture: indirect force to bone, in which a ligament or tendon pulls out bone
    E. Spiral fracture: a twisting of the bone, usually with resultant sharp edges

Answer: B

Critique: The mechanism of injury is important to know, because it may heighten the suspicion for certain types of fractures. All of the listed fractures are caused by the corresponding mechanism of injury except for oblique fractures, which are caused by a twisting or torsion of the bone.

Page: 926

43: Which of the following processes best describes the third stage of fracture healing:

    A. Formation of osteoid matrix around the fracture site
    B. Hematoma formation around the fracture site
    C. Macrophage and inflammatory cell infiltration
    D. Callus remodeling and lamellar bone formation

Answer: D

Critique: Bone healing involves several stages after an acute fracture. The initial response includes inflammatory cell infiltration and hematoma formation. The second stage entails development of an osteoid matrix and callus formation. The final stage involves callus remodeling and lamellar bone formation.

Pages: 927–928

44: Which of the following fractures is best suited for closed reduction:

    A. Fracture of a lower extremity in the elderly
    B. Joint fractures in a weight-bearing joint
    C. Joint fractures in which early mobilization is preferred
    D. Colles' fracture
    E. Epiphyseal fractures

Answer: D

Critique: When reduction of a fracture is necessary, closed reduction is preferable because it decreases chances of infection, causes less soft tissue and periosteal trauma, and decreases chances of devascularization. Although many fractures are easily treated with closed reduction (often under anesthesia), the following fractures will usually be treated with internal fixation: joint fractures in weight-bearing joints or where early mobilization is necessary, fractures of lower extremities in the elderly, epiphyseal fractures, and comminuted fractures.

Page: 928

45: Which of the following statements about the basics of casting is false:

    A. The extremity should not be moved before casting, because doing so may exacerbate the fracture.
    B. One joint above and one joint below the fracture should be immobilized.
    C. Padding should be rolled so that 50% of the prior layer is covered with each turn.
    D. The cast should be applied to the joint in its functional position.

Answer: A

Critique: Casting should be done after reduction is performed. The joint should be placed in its functional (neutral) position. One joint above and one joint below should be immobilized, because this best immobilizes the broken bone. Padding material must be placed below the actual casting material. Padding should be covered by 50% overlap with each turn to provide even and maximal protection.

Page: 928

46: Which of the following requires a referral to an orthopedist:

    A. Nonarticular fracture of the proximal third of the clavicle
    B. Fracture in the middle third of the clavicle
    C. Nondisplaced fracture of the distal third of the clavicle
    D. Displaced fracture of the distal third of the clavicle

Answer: D

Critique: Not all fractures require casting. Immobilization with splinting or slings often may be appropriate. However, it is important to realize that the location as well as any displacement must be considered before a decision to treat non-operatively is made. One such example is that many clavicular fractures can be treated with a figure-of-8 splint or a simple sling, but when the fracture is associated with a rib or in the distal third of the clavicle and associated with a dislocation, orthopedic consultation is warranted.

Pages: 929–930

47: Which of the following can be managed nonsurgically:

    A. Navicular fractures
    B. Distal radius fracture with foreshortening and 30 degrees of angulation
    C. Boxer fracture of the 5th metacarpal (MC) with 30 degrees of angulation
    D. Displaced radial head fractures

Answer: C

Critique: Boxer fractures of the 5th MC with less than 40 degrees of angulation can be managed non-operatively. Only those distal radius fractures without foreshortening and less than 20 degrees of angulation should be managed non-operatively. Displaced radial head fractures are unstable and navicular fractures risk avascular necrosis. These fractures should be referred to an orthopedist.

Pages: 929–930

48: All of the following structures are prone to complications by supracondylar fractures, except:

    A. Axillary artery
    B. Median nerve
    C. Brachial artery
    D. Radial nerve

Answer: A

Critique: The radial nerve is especially prone to entrapment with fractures of the midshaft and upper end of the humerus. The brachial artery and radial nerve may be lacerated or entrapped with fractures at or above the elbow. The axillary artery lies proximal to this area.

Page: 933

49: All of the following clinical findings are associated with pulmonary fat embolism, except:

    A. Mental confusion
    B. Arterial PO_2 greater than 80 mmHg
    C. Tachycardia
    D. Tachypnea
    E. Fever

Answer: B

Critique: Fat embolism is a complication seen within 72 hours of long bone fractures. Clinical findings include mental confusion, tachycardia, tachypnea, and fever. A low arterial PO_2 helps confirm the diagnosis. Fat embolisms may be fatal; prevention includes early mobilization of the patient.

Page: 933

50: Under the Gustillo classification system, an open fracture with a clean laceration greater than 1 cm in length is a:

  A. Class I open fracture
  B. Class II open fracture
  C. Class IIIA open fracture
  D. Class IIIB open fracture

Answer: B

Critique: A clean, open fracture associated with a laceration greater than 1 cm in length represents a class II open fracture. A class I open fracture involves a clean laceration less than 1 cm. Class III injuries are considered "dirty." A class IIIA open fracture connotes a crushing injury associated with the open fracture. A class IIIB open fracture indicates a severe open fracture with loss of tissue overlying the fractured bone. A class IIIC open fracture is a class IIIB open fracture with vascular compromise.

Pages: 933–934

51: After applying a cast, all of the following actions should be recommended, except:

  A. Movement of the joints that are distal to the cast should be limited.
  B. Antihistamines can be helpful in reducing pruritus under the cast.
  C. Cool air blown under the cast may help reduce itching.
  D. Lotion and gentle soap should be used after the cast is removed.
  E. After the cast is removed, moderate activity involving the recently casted joint should begin.

Answer: A

Critique: Movement of joints that are not immobilized helps prevent vasomotor disturbances. Itching under the cast, a common complaint, may be soothed with blowing cool air under the cast or antihistamines. Scratching under the cast should be avoided. After the cast is removed, using gentle soap and lotion is recommended to improve skin care. Moderate activity should be prescribed to overcome any muscle weakness and atrophy that have developed.

52: All of the following treatments are appropriate for an open class III fracture, except:

  A. Copious irrigation
  B. Immobilization
  C. Early would closure
  D. Surgery
  E. Débridement

Answer: C

Critique: Open fractures should be cleaned with débridement and copious irrigation. Immobilization is necessary for all open fractures, and primary closures should be delayed. All class III fractures require open surgical reduction and repair.

Page: 934

53. (True or False) Determine which of the following statements are true or false about reflex sympathetic dystrophy:

  A. It is also known as Sudeck's atrophy.
  B. It occurs in about 20% of fractured limbs.
  C. It is treated easily with nonsteroidal anti-inflammatory drugs (NSAIDs).
  D. It is characterized by a burning pain out of proportion to the injury sustained.

Answers: A - True, B - False, C - False, D - True

Critique: Reflex sympathetic dystrophy is also known as Sudeck's atrophy. It can occur in 3% to 5% of limb fractures. It is characterized by a burning pain during and after the healing process that is disproportionate to the extent of the injury. Treatment may be difficult and often requires consultation with a pain management team.

Page: 936

Chapter 40

Rheumatology and Musculoskeletal Problems

Peter M. Nalin

1: What percentage of all adult medical visits, according to the Centers for Disease Control and Prevention (CDC), is for arthritic conditions?

    A. 1.5%
    B. 5%
    C. 15%
    D. 30%

Answer: C

Critique: In a CDC national ambulatory medical care survey, 15% of all medical adult visits and nearly 30% of office visits by patients age 65 years and older were found to be for arthritic conditions.

Page: 950

2: What percentage of the U.S. gross national product is spent each year on rheumatic disease?

    A. 0.5%
    B. 1.0%
    C. 1.5%
    D. 10%

Answer: B

Critique: The authors indicate that the impact of rheumatic diseases on our health care system is 1% of the U.S. gross national product spent annually on rheumatic diseases.

Page: 950

3: Which of the following usually causes localized rather than diffuse periarticular pain:

    A. Carpal tunnel syndrome
    B. Fibromyalgia
    C. Polymyalgia rheumatica
    D. Polymyositis

Answer: A

Critique: Causes of defuse periarticular pain include fibromyalgia, polymyalgia rheumatica, and polymyositis. Causes of periarticular pain include bursitis, tendinitis, and carpal tunnel syndrome.

Page: 950

4: Symmetric arthritis is characteristic of each of the following, except:

    A. Rheumatoid arthritis
    B. Systemic lupus erythematosus (SLE)
    C. Sjögren syndrome
    D. Reiter disease

Answer: D

Critique: Symmetric arthritis is the term used to describe the same joint on contralateral sides of the body being affected. These joints are not necessarily affected to the same degree. Symmetric arthritis is characteristic of rheumatoid arthritis, SLE, Sjögren syndrome, polymyositis, and scleroderma. Reiter disease in not characterized by symmetric arthritis.

Page: 950

5: The abbreviation IADL means:

    A. Instrumental activities of daily living
    B. Intra-articular diagnostic ligands
    C. Idiopathic anti-DNA lysis
    D. Isolated acute degenerative ligaments

Answer: A

Critique: The abbreviation IADL means instrumental activities of daily living. Examples are buying groceries, cooking, using the telephone, opening jars, and so on. ADL refers to health care activities of daily living, for example, bathing, dressing, and eating.

Pages: 950, 951

6: Serial grip strength measurements can be made using a blood pressure (BP) cuff initially inflated to:

    A. 2 mm Hg
    B. 20 mm Hg
    C. 120 mm Hg
    D. 200 mm Hg

Answer: B

Critique: Serial grip strength measurements can be made by using a BP cuff inflated to 20 mm of mercury and recording the maximal grip force in mm Hg.

Page: 952

7: The name of a useful diagram for recording comprehensive joint examination findings:

A. Audiogram
B. Myelogram
C. Skeleton
D. Matrix

Answer: C

Critique: The simple diagram used for recording comprehensive joint examination findings is a skeleton diagram.

Pages: 952, 953

8: Which of the following antigens is associated with increased incidence and severity of rheumatoid arthritis:

A. HLA-B52
B. HLA-B27
C. HLA-BRht
D. HLA-DR4

Answer: D

Critique: Presence of HLA-DR4 antigen is associated with increased incidence and severity of rheumatoid arthritis. Choices A and C are nonsense. Choice B the HLA-B27 antigen is found in a higher percentage of patients with ankylosing spondylitis and other spondyloarthropathies as compared to the general population.

Page: 952

9: Obesity is an identified factor in osteoarthritis of which joint:

A. Metatarsophalangeal great toe
B. Ankle
C. Knee
D. Sacroiliac

Answer: C

Critique: Obesity is an identified factor in osteoarthritis of the knee. It is possible that this identified risk factor is implicated both mechanically and metabolically.

Page: 953

10: Which infectious agent has not been known to cause arthritis:

A. *Borrelia burgdorferi*
B. Parvovirus B19
C. *Neisseria gonorrhoeae*
D. Human immunodeficiency virus (HIV)
E. Laughter, the best medicine

Answer: E

Critique: All of the infectious agents listed have been known to cause arthritis except choice E.

Page: 953

11: What percentage of patients with rheumatoid arthritis has a positive rheumatoid factor:

A. 18%
B. 50%
C. 80%
D. 98%

Answer: C

Critique: Of patients with rheumatoid arthritis, 80% test positive for rheumatoid factor.

Page: 953

12: Rheumatoid factor is frequently positive in patients with:

A. Viral pancreatitis
B. Exercise-induced asthma
C. Laryngotracheobronchitis
D. Sarcoidosis

Answer: D

Critique: Rheumatoid factor is frequently positive in patients with sarcoidosis. Viral hepatitis and chronic obstructive pulmonary disease (COPD) can lead to a positive rheumatoid factor result.

Page: 953

13: Rheumatoid factor is a serum autoantibody against which immunoglobulin:

A. IgA
B. IgE
C. IgG
D. IgM

Answer: C

Critique: Rheumatoid factor is a serum autoantibody against immunoglobulin (IgG).

Page: 953

14: The percentage of individuals in the normal population with positive antinuclear antibody (ANA) is:

A. 0.1%
B. 0.5%
C. 1.0%
D. 5.0%

Answer: D

Critique: The percentage of positive ANA in the normal population is 5%.

Page: 953

15: Patients with systemic lupus erythematosus (SLE) can have the following associated conditions, except:

A. Hemolytic anemia
B. Thrombocytosis
C. Thrombocytopenia
D. Lymphopenia

Answer: B

Critique: Patients with SLE can have hemolytic anemia, thrombocytopenia, or lymphopenia. Thrombocytosis is the condition of elevated platelet count, which is not characteristic of SLE.

Page: 953

16: Elevated uric acid suggests:

A. Gangrene
B. Gout
C. Grip strength
D. Gross pathology

Answer: B

Critique: Elevated uric acid suggests gout.

Page: 953

17: Select the incorrect pair:

A. Antiphospholipid antibody syndrome—antiphospholipid antibodies
B. Wegner granulomatosis—antineutrophil cytoplasmic antibody
C. Lyme disease—parvovirus serology
D. Spondyloarthropathy—HLA-B27

Answer: C

Critique: Choices A, B, and D correctly identify disease and associated test pairs. For Lyme disease, the IgM and IgG ELISA tests are not related to parvovirus serology.

Page: 953

18: One type of crystal arthropathy is:

A. Pseudotumor
B. Pseudogout
C. Pheochromocytoma
D. Scleroderma

Answer: B

Critique: Pseudogout is a type of crystal arthropathy.

Page: 953

19: In established rheumatoid arthritis on radiographs, one would *not* expect to view:

A. Overhanging edges
B. Marginal erosions
C. Soft tissue swelling
D. Periarticular osteoporosis

Answer: A

Critique: Overhanging edges result from reparative changes associated with gouty erosions. On radiographs in rheumatoid arthritis patients, one often finds marginal erosions, soft tissue swelling, and or periarticular osteoporosis.

Page: 953

20: MRI studies can be particularly useful in each of the following anatomic locations, except:

A. Medial meniscus of right knee
B. Lateral meniscus of left knee
C. Medial meniscus of left knee
D. Lateral malleolus of right knee

Answer: D

Critique: MRI studies can be particularly useful in the medial and lateral meniscus of both knees. The lateral malleolus is an anatomic site of the ankle, not the knee.

Page: 954

21: The iatrogenic infection rate from arthrocentesis is estimated as:

A. 1 in 10
B. 1 in 100
C. 1 in1000
D. 1 in 10,000

Answer: D

Critique: The iatrogenic infection rate for arthrocentesis is estimated at 1 in 10,000.

Page: 955

22: Joint injection using corticosteroids should be limited to no more than how many per joint per year:

A. 0 to 1
B. 1 to2
C. 3 to 4
D. 5 to 6

Answer: C

Critique: Joint injection using corticosteroids should be limited to no more than three to four injections per joint per year.

Page: 956

23: NSAIDs do the following:

A. Prevent tissue injury
B. Prevent joint damage
C. Increase prostaglandin synthesis
D. Reduce inflammation

Answer: D

Critique: NSAIDs reduce inflammation. They have not been proven to consistently prevent tissue injury, prevent joint damage, or increase prostaglandin synthesis.

Page: 956

24: Cyclooxygenase-2 (COX-2) inhibitors are characterized by all of these, except:

A. Reduced gastrointestinal toxicity
B. High cost
C. Lack of COX-1 inhibition
D. Antiplatelet effect

Answer: D

Critique: Cyclooxygenase-2 (COX-2) inhibitors and reduced gastrointestinal toxicity currently are expensive and characteristically lack COX-1 inhibition. The COX-2 inhibitors do not exert an antiplatelet effect.

Page: 956

25: Which drug has not been shown to decrease the incidence of both gastric and duodenal ulcers during concomitant use of COX-1 NSAIDs:

A. Famotidine
B. Omeprazole
C. Ferrous sulfate
D. Misoprostol

Answer: C

Critique: Famotidine, omeprazole, and misoprostol have all been shown to decrease the incidence of both gastric and duodenal ulcers during concomitant use of COX-1 NSAIDs. Ferrous sulfate has not demonstrated this benefit.

Page: 956

26: Lyme arthritis cannot cause:

   A. Migratory monoarthritis
   B. Oligoarthritis
   C. Erythema chronicum migrans
   D. Diabetes mellitus

Answer: D

Critique: Lyme arthritis cannot cause diabetes mellitus. Lyme arthritis can cause migratory monoarthritis, oligoarthritis, and erythema chronicum migrans.

Page: 957

27: Arthritis is associated with:

   A. Atrial fibrillation
   B. Inflammatory bowel disease
   C. Oligohydramnios
   D. Pyridoxine overdosage

Answer: B

Critique: Arthritis has been associated with inflammatory bowel disease. It has not been associated with pyridoxine overdosage, oligohydramnios, or atrial fibrillation specifically.

Page: 957

28: Osteoarthritis can be subclassified into all of the following categories, except:

   A. Idiopathic
   B. Primary
   C. Secondary
   D. Tertiary
   E. Hereditary

Answer: D

Critique: Osteoarthritis can be separated into primary (idiopathic), hereditary, and secondary forms. Tertiary arthritis is not defined.

Page: 957

29: An inflammatory variant of osteoarthritis of the distal interphalangeal (DIP) joints affects which of the following nodes:

   A. Sinoatrial nodes
   B. Bouchard nodes
   C. Cervical nodes
   D. Heberden nodes

Answer: D

Critique: Although osteoarthritis is considered a noninflammatory type of arthritis, one osteoarthritis variant affects primarily the hands. This variant runs in families. Women experience it more commonly than men. At the DIP joints, this inflammatory variant of osteoarthritis causes Heberden nodes. Bouchard nodes occur at the proximal interphalangeal (PIP) joints.

Page: 957

30: Osteoarthritis is more common in women than in men after the age of:

   A. 35 years
   B. 45 years
   C. 55 years
   D. 65 years

Answer: C

Critique: The frequency of osteoarthritis is approximately equal in the two sexes between the ages 45 and 55. After age 55, osteoarthritis is more common in women.

Page: 957

31: The majority of hip osteoarthritis affects which of the following:

   A. Anterior pole
   B. Inferior pole
   C. Superior pole
   D. Posterior pole
   E. North pole

Answer: C

Critique: The majority of hip osteoarthritis affects the superior pole. It is usually unilateral, more common in men than in women, and occurs without other joint involvement.

Page: 958

32: Which of the following drugs is FDA approved for osteoarthritis of the knee:

   A. Glucosamine sulfate
   B. Hyaluronate sodium
   C. Chondroitin sulfate
   D. Doxycycline

Answer: B

Critique: Both hyaluronate sodium and hylan G-F 20 (Synvise) are FDA approved for osteoarthritis of the knee. These substances replace the viscous substance in synovial fluid that lubricates and protects the joints.

Page: 960

33: The hallmark of rheumatoid arthritis is:

   A. Anemia
   B. Asymmetric synovitis
   C. Symmetric synovitis
   D. Obesity

Answer: C

Critique: Symmetric synovitis is the hallmark of rheumatoid arthritis.

Page: 962

34: A palpable, rubbery mass of inflamed synovium is called:

   A. Septic embolus
   B. Pannus
   C. Ganglion cyst
   D. Porous

Answer: B

Critique: Pannus is a palpable, rubbery mass of inflamed synovium.

Page: 962

35: Palindromic rheumatoid arthritis can be easily misdiagnosed as:

- A. Osteoarthritis
- B. Legg-Calvé-Perthes disease
- C. Sickle cell trait
- D. Gout

Answer: D

Critique: Palindromic rheumatoid arthritis is characterized by brief episodes of swelling of a large joint such as a knee, wrist, or ankle and can be easily misdiagnosed as gout.

Page: 962

36: The boutonniere deformity results from:

- A. Carpal tunnel syndrome
- B. Avulsion of the extensor hood of the PIP joint
- C. Flexion of the DIP joint
- D. Ulnar compression syndrome

Answer: B

Critique: The boutonniere deformity results from avulsion of the extensor hood of the PIP because of chronic inflammation. This subsequently causes the PIP to pop up in fluxion while the DIP stays in hyperextension.

Page: 962

37: Posterior herniation of the knee joint capsule into the popliteal area is called:

- A. Indirect hernia
- B. Cystic hygroma
- C. Baker cyst
- D. Inclusion cyst

Answer: C

Critique: A Baker cyst is the posterior herniation of the joint capsule into the popliteal area of the knee. A Baker cyst can be diagnosed by ultrasonography. Rupture of a Baker cyst into the posterior leg may clinically mimic thrombophlebitis.

Page: 962

38: Which of the following do not arise from the synovitis of rheumatoid arthritis:

- A. Ligaments weakened by collagenases
- B. Cartilaginous erosions
- C. Cataracts
- D. Tendon shortening

Answer: C

Critique: Synovitis of rheumatoid arthritis can cause ligaments to be weakened by collagenases, erosion of cartilage, and shortening of tendons. Synovitis of rheumatoid arthritis does not cause cataracts.

Pages: 962, 963

39: Pulmonary manifestations of rheumatoid disease can include all of the following, except:

- A. Oat cell lung cancer
- B. Interstitial fibrosis

- C. Multiple nodular lung disease
- D. Pleural effusions

Answer: A

Critique: Pulmonary manifestations of rheumatoid arthritis include pleural effusions, interstitial fibrosis, solitary or multiple nodular lung disease, and pleurisy. Oat cell lung cancer is not a pulmonary manifestation of rheumatoid disease.

Page: 963

40: Felty syndrome is characterized by each of the following, except:

- A. Lymphadenopathy
- B. Splenomegaly
- C. Thrombocytosis
- D. Leg ulcers

Answer: C

Critique: Felty syndrome includes rheumatoid arthritis, splenomegaly, leukopenia, leg ulcers, lymphadenopathy, thrombocytopenia, and association with the HLA-DR4 haplotype. Thrombocytosis (elevated platelet count) is not associated with Felty syndrome.

Page: 963

41: When extremely rare spontaneous remission of rheumatoid arthritis occurs, it happens within what duration from disease onset:

- A. 2 days
- B. 2 weeks
- C. 2 months
- D. 2 years

Answer: D

Critique: An extremely low rate of spontaneous remission occurs in rheumatoid arthritis. When spontaneous remission does occur, it usually takes place within 2 years of disease onset.

Page: 963

42: Radiographs in late-stage rheumatoid arthritis may often show each of the following, except:

- A. Open growth plates
- B. Marginal bony erosions
- C. Joint space narrowing
- D. Periarticular osteoporosis

Answer: A

Critique: In late-stage rheumatoid arthritis, radiographs may show marginal bony erosions, periarticular osteoporosis, and joint space narrowing, especially in the hands and feet. Open growth plates are not associated with late-stage rheumatoid arthritis.

Page: 963

43: Which substance reduces methotrexate-induced mouth sores:

- A. Thiamine
- B. Ascorbic acid

C. Cyanocobalamin
D. Folic acid

Answer: D

Critique: Methotrexate-induced mouth sores are reduced by folic acid. Folic acid at 1 mg per day reduces mouth sores without decreasing the efficacy of methotrexate.

Page: 964

44: Methotrexate toxicities include all of the following, except:

A. Subcutaneous nodules
B. Blue-gray discoloration of skin
C. Hepatotoxicity
D. Hypersensitivity pneumonitis

Answer: B

Critique: Methotrexate toxicities include subcutaneous nodules, hepatotoxicity, hypersensitivity pneumonitis, bone marrow suppression, rare development of non-Hodgkin's lymphoma, and opportunistic infections. Blue-gray discoloration of skin is a side effect of amiodarone, the antiarrhythmic cardiac medication.

Page: 964

45: An important risk factor in the development of gout is:

A. Alcohol
B. Tobacco smoking
C. Seatbelt avoidance
D. Airplane travel

Answer: A

Critique: Alcohol is an important risk factor in the development of gout. Tobacco smoking is an important risk factor in adenocarcinoma, coronary ethereal sclerosis, and many other diseases, but not gout. Seatbelt avoidance is associated with increased morbidity and mortality associated with automobile accidents. Airplane travel is a contributing risk factor in the development of deep venous thrombosis.

Page: 970

46: Each of the following is a gastrointestinal side effect of colchicine, except:

A. Abdominal cramps
B. Vomiting
C. Diarrhea
D. Duodenal ulcer

Answer: D

Critique: Gastrointestinal side effects of colchicine include nausea, vomiting, abdominal cramps, and diarrhea. Duodenal ulcer is not a side effect of colchicine.

Pages: 970, 971

47: The treatment of choice for calcium pyrophosphate deposition (CPPD) disease is:

A. Allopurinol
B. Methotrexate

C. Inhaled corticosteroids
D. NSAIDs

Answer: D

Critique: Gastrointestinal ulcer is a common side effect of NSAIDs.

Page: 972

48: The spondyloarthropathies include the following, except:

A. Reiter syndrome
B. Juvenile onset arthropathy
C. Psoriatic arthropathy
D. CPPD

Answer: D

Critique: The spondyloarthropathies are a group of multisystem inflammatory disorders that affect predominantly the spine but also other joints and extra-articular tissues. Spondyloarthropathies include Reiter syndrome, juvenile onset arthropathy, psoriatic arthropathy, ankylosing spondylitis, reactive arthritis (Reiter syndrome), and enteropathic arthropathy. CPPD crystals can cause acute gout-like attacks called pseudogout. CPPD crystals can deposit not only on articular cartilage but also in ligaments, tendons, soft tissue, and synovium. CPPD is not a spondyloarthropathy.

Page: 972

49: Extra-articular manifestations of ankylosing spondylitis include all of the following, except:

A. Aortitis
B. Temporal arteritis
C. Acute uveitis (iritis)
D. Diaphragmatic breathing

Answer: B

Critique: Extra-articular manifestations of ankylosing spondylitis include acute uveitis (iritis), aortitis, and neurologic complication from C-spine fractures. Diaphragmatic breathing and limited chest excursion results from costovertebral involvement. Temporal aortitis and giant cell aortitis are two names for the same condition. It usually presents in patients older than 50 years and is not a manifestation of the ankylosing spondylitis.

Pages: 972, 973

50: Which is *not* part of the classic triad of reactive arthritis (Reiter syndrome):

A. Nongonococcal urethritis
B. Arthritis
C. Conjunctivitis
D. Tinnitus

Answer: D

Critique: The classic triad of reactive arthritis (Reiter syndrome) includes nongonococcal urethritis, arthritis, and conjunctivitis. Tinnitus is not part of this classic triad.

Page: 973

Chapter 41

Dermatology

David Vander Straten

1: In describing a dermatological lesion, all of the following terms are appropriate, except:

    A. Vesicle
    B. Papule
    C. Crust
    D. Petechia
    E. Knot

Answer: E

Critique: Larger intradermal lesions should be referred to as cysts, nodules, or tumors, depending on their size and location. The other choices are appropriate terminology.

Pages: 993, 994

2: All of the following are considered primary lesions, except:

    A. Bullae
    B. Macules
    C. Keloids
    D. Wheals
    E. Cysts

Answer: C

Critique: Keloids, otherwise known as hypertrophic scars, are secondary manifestations from a prior trauma to the skin surface. The other lesions listed all arise from the skin de novo.

Pages: 993, 994

3: (True or False) A 10-year-old boy presents in your office complaining of a recent onset of a rash to the bilateral forearms and lower extremities. He reports intense itching and discomfort. There is no history of fever. On examination, you find erythematous linear papulovesicular streaks, which do not extend below the sock line. This condition is:

    A. Caused by an allergic contact dermatitis
    B. Caused by an ingested substance
    C. Responsive to topical compresses
    D. Requires intravenous therapy for complete resolution
    E. May be prevented by oral desensitization therapy

Answers: True - A, C, False - B, D, E

Critique: Poison ivy, poison oak, and poison sumac account for more cases of allergic contact dermatitis in the United States than all other contact irritants combined. The example detailed in the question illustrates the typical streaking pattern of the oleoresin across the skin surface by the plant leaf or stem, whereas other unusual patterns may be seen if the patient is exposed via contaminated clothing or smoke. Washing the affected area with soap and water, application of cold wet compresses, use of oral or intramuscular steroid preparations, cool tub baths with colloidal oatmeal, and calamine lotion all provide palliative effects. No evidence shows that oral desensitization therapy is effective.

Pages: 998, 999

4: (True or False) In the examination of a potential fungal lesion, a slide preparation may prove useful. Slide preparation may be facilitated by the use of:

    A. 10% to 20% potassium hydroxide (KOH) solution
    B. 40 mEq potassium chloride (KCl) solution
    C. Dimethylsulfoxide (DMSO)
    D. Gentle heat
    E. Scrapings from over the top edge of a nail

Answers: True - A, C, D, False - B, E

Critique: The use of KOH, DMSO, or gentle heat accelerates the cellular maceration process, thus revealing the spore, hyphae, or budding yeast forms more quickly. KCl is an electrolyte-replacement medication. Fungal organisms are obtained by scraping under the free edge of the affected nail.

Pages: 994, 995

5: The effective initial management of lichen simplex chronicus includes all of the following, except:

    A. Intralesional steroid injections in the affected area
    B. Occlusive dressings to protect against further injury
    C. Educating the patient as to the necessity to cease scratching
    D. Considering the use of systemic antipruritic medication
    E. Confirming the absence of a superficial fungal infection

Answer: A

Critique: Although intralesional steroid application may be used in the management of lichen simplex chronicus, the initial steps listed can result in a significant decrease in further skin injury. Successful treatment of the lesions at times is hampered by the patient's inability to avoid self-manipulation of the lesions, thus aggravating the overall inflammation rate.

Pages: 999, 1000

6: (True or False) Cetirizine, loratadine, hydroxyzine, and diphenhydramine may:

A. Be useful in the management of pruritus
B. Have no role in the treatment of petechiae
C. Hasten the resolution of hives
D. Cause excessive somnolence

Answers: True - A, C, D, False - B

Critique: The presence of petechiae may indicate a worrisome clinical condition of septicemia, given the correct clinical scenario. One should consider disseminated meningococcal disease and act accordingly, with the prompt initiation of broad-spectrum antibiotic coverage pending the identification of a specific organism.

Page: 996

7: (True or False) Potential etiologies for contact dermatitis include:

A. Nickel
B. Rubber
C. Leather
D. Adhesive tape
E. Neomycin

Answers: True - A, B, C, D, E

Critique: Causes of contact dermatitis are extensive and include both natural and synthetic materials such as dyes, cosmetics, metals, bandage materials, and topical medications (antibiotics, anesthetics, antiseptics, antihistamines, and corticosteroids). Nickel is found in jewelry, watches, and belt buckles. Rubber and leather allergies are sometimes discovered when the patient presents with lesions isolated to the feet. Neomycin is notorious for causing a contact dermatitis, especially when used in a periorbital location.

Pages: 998, 999

8: (True or False) In infants, atopic dermatitis is suspected when which of the following areas are affected:

A. Face
B. Palms
C. Elbows
D. Chest
E. Intertriginous areas

Answers: True - A, C, False - B, D, E

Critique: Atopic dermatitis commonly affects infants on the face, scalp, and extensor surfaces of the extremities. The chest and palms are spared. Intertriginous areas are common sites for *Candida* infections.

Page: 1000

9: (True or False) In contrast, older children with atopic dermatitis may show involvement of which areas:

A. Face
B. Antecubital fossa
C. Trunk
D. Wrists
E. Chest

Answers: False - A, C, E, True - B, D

Critique: Children may manifest papules, erythema, and lichenification on the flexor surfaces, wrists, and the neck.

Page: 1000

10: (True or False) Treatment options for atopic dermatitis include:

A. Use of a mild astringent to clean the skin of oily residue
B. Avoidance of any identified triggers that lead to exacerbation
C. Initiation of immunotherapy to promote desensitization to the offending agents
D. Avoidance of the prolonged use of high-potency topical steroids
E. Identifying allergic rhinitis, asthma, or hay fever as a coexisting condition in the patient

Answers: False - A, C, True - B, D, E

Critique: Patients may make a tremendously positive impact on their condition by using mild bath soap, low-potency topical steroids, and oral antihistamines on an as-needed basis. A conscientious effort to identify and eliminate potential triggers such as certain foods, inhalants, or chemicals, especially for children, is warranted. Reduction in household dust mites is also recommended. Although helpful for lichenoid areas, the chronic use of either high-potency or systemic corticosteroids is not safe. A history of upper respiratory conditions is frequently encountered in the patient's background or in a family member.

Page: 1000

11: (True or False) Treatment options for comedonal acne involve:

A. Reduction of *Propionibacterium acnes* in the skin follicles
B. Use of retinoids to increase adherence of keratinized cells to each other
C. Application of topical benzoyl peroxide four times daily in combination with an astringent
D. Initiation of minocycline along with limiting dietary chocolate intake

Answers: True - A, False - B, C, D

Critique: Acne vulgaris presents in many forms—comedonal, pustular, cystic, and papular—and may include scar formation. *P. acnes*, the main bacterial inhabitant of the follicle, causes a breakdown of the sebaceous gland products into an inflammatory milieu, leading to the typical papules, pustules, cysts, and scars. The keratinized cells sloughed into the follicular channel are quite sticky, and thus a "plug" is created. Topical retinoids serve to decrease comedogenesis by lowering the adherence of the keratinized cells to each other. Overzealous scrubbing or astringent use may actually cause further skin irritation and therefore discourage the patient from compliance with topical therapy. Tetracycline and minocycline are useful adjuncts in the management of cystic acne.

Pages: 1000, 1001

12: The presence of rhinophyma, papules, pustules, or nodules and facial hyperemia leads one to suspect a diagnosis of:

    A. Lupus
    B. Scleroderma
    C. Rosacea
    D. Vancomycin use
    E. Intranasal cocaine use

Answer: C

Critique: Vancomycin, when infused rapidly, is associated with the "red man" or "red neck" syndrome. Frequently patients who use cocaine present to the emergency department with moderate to severe elevations in body temperature and manifest hyperemia. Lupus is characteristically described as having a facial rash in the form of a butterfly. Diffuse scleroderma may involve the skin of the face with thickening and swelling causing a mask-like appearance. The presence of rhinophyma (hyperplasia of the nasal soft tissues associated with enlargement and deformity) should alert the practitioner to the possibility of rosacea.

Pages: 1001, 1002

13: An unmarried 54-year-old business executive presents to your office with a complaint of a scaly rash to his face associated with "dry" irritated eyes. He has tried a cortisone cream without improvement. His social history is notable for extensive travel and unprotected intercourse with multiple partners. A differential diagnosis would include all of the following, except:

    A. Seborrheic dermatitis
    B. Cutaneous tuberculosis
    C. Rosacea
    D. Acne
    E. Mycosis fungoides

Answer: E

Critique: This patient most likely has rosacea with ocular involvement. His topical steroid use deserves further query, because this may actually worsen his condition. Given his extensive travel history, consideration of exposure to tuberculosis is warranted. HIV disease, with facial seborrheic dermatitis as an initial manifestation, should be investigated. Mycosis fungoides, also known as cutaneous T cell lymphoma, presents with either a red, scaly eczematous-like eruption or an atrophic, mottled telangiectatic eruption, usually on the thigh, buttock, or abdomen.

Pages: 1001, 1002

14: (True or False) A 28-year-old Asian male presents with sweaty palms, generalized anxiety symptoms, and a painful bilateral gait. Evaluation and management at this time may include:

    A. Ordering TSH and ESR tests and obtaining a chest x-ray
    B. Placing a PPD
    C. Starting an oral hypoglycemic medication
    D. Applying an aluminum chloride preparation to the hands
    E. Referring semi-urgently for surgical sympathectomy

Answers: True - A, B, D, False - C, E

Critique: The differential diagnoses for this patient who has hyperhidrosis include hyperthyroidism, hypothalamic disorders, lymphomas, hypoglycemia, pheochromocytoma, drug withdrawal, cholinergic substance exposure, and tuberculosis among others. Successful treatment involves reduction of the underlying anxiety and localized therapy to the affected areas. Drysol application to the feet and hands may help reduce perspiration, thus limiting maceration to the skin and reducing discomfort.

Page: 1003

15: (True or False) Common etiologies for folliculitis include:

    A. *Staphylococcus aureus*
    B. Malnutrition
    C. Industrial hydrocarbon exposure
    D. Streptococcal organisms
    E. Halogen ingestion

Answers: True - A, B, C, D, E

Critique: Despite the multitude of potential causes, the treatment for folliculitis generally involves removal of the offending causative factor(s), clothing changes, and initiation of oral antibiotics if needed.

Page: 1004

16: (True or False) Predilection for preschool-aged children, peak incidence during summer, and highly communicable status refer to a condition:

    A. Such as varicella
    B. Incontinentia pigmentosa
    C. Where use of either topical or oral antibiotics is necessary
    D. Due to *Staphylococcus aureus* and group A streptococci

Answers: False - A, B, True - C, D,

Critique: Impetigo contagiosa presents as vesicular eruptions followed by the development of honey-colored crusts sitting on a normal or eroded base of skin. Scratching causes autoinoculation from one part of the body to another, thus propagating the infection to self and others. Topical mupirocin ointment three times daily is the preferred initial therapy, but dicloxacillin or a cephalosporin may be indicated if local therapy fails. Incontinentia pigmentosa is a rare X-linked dominant trait. Varicella, although highly communicable, has a peak incidence in children aged 5 to 9 years and is seen mainly from January to May.

Page: 1005

17: (True or False) Which of the following statements are true regarding erysipelas:

A. The causative agent is group D streptococci.
B. It has a predilection for patients at either end of the age spectrum
C. A rapid onset, presence of bacteremia, and association with glomerulonephritis are found.
D. Differential diagnosis would include herpes zoster, contact/irritant dermatitis, and osteomyelitis of the facial bones.

Answers: False - A, True - B, C, D

Critique: The culprit in erysipelas is group A streptococci. The other statements above all are pertinent to the diagnosis.

Page: 1005

18: (True or False) Molluscum contagiosum:

A. May appear similar to varicella lesions
B. Will resolve spontaneously
C. Requires biopsy for full diagnostic confirmation
D. Is best treated with sharp curettage in children

Answers: True - A, B, False - C, D

Critique: Molluscum contagiosum is a viral disease that may mimic varicella, warts, papillomas, and epitheliomas. The lesions usually regress spontaneously in 2 to 4 months, but autoinoculation may occur as well as spread to sexual partners. Treatment modalities include application of topical cantharidin, liquid nitrogen, or curettage. The trauma and discomfort of curettage, however, precludes this maneuver in children.

Page: 1007

19: A 22-year-old college senior presents to the university health clinic following spring vacation. The student reports malaise, low-grade temperature elevations, dysuria, and painful "bumps" in the groin. Examination reveals the absence of any oral lesions but tender bilateral inguinal adenopathy, a urethral discharge, and genital lesions. Differential diagnosis for this condition includes all of the following, except:

A. Secondary syphilis
B. Herpes simplex
C. Chancroid
D. Gonorrhea and chlamydia
E. Granuloma inguinale

Answer: A

Critique: Secondary syphilis characteristically produces a diffuse generalized papulosquamous rash involving the head, neck, palms, and soles. The astute clinician, however, recalls that syphilis is the great imitator and must be distinguished from pityriasis rosea, drug eruptions, psoriasis, and fungal infections. Genital herpes manifests as a group of clustered vesicles 3 to 14 days following contact. These vesicles may coalesce and then ulcerate. Women may have cervical lesions, but no external genital lesions, which may cause mucopurulent discharge. Tender inguinal lymphadenopathy, malaise, and dysuria are hallmarks of herpes simplex. Both *Neisseria gonorrhoeae* and

Chlamydia trachomatis may be associated with urethritis and cervicitis. Chancroid, due to infection with *Haemophilus ducreyi*, may cause tender lymphadenopathy leading to inguinal abscesses. Granuloma inguinale, caused by *Calymmatobacterium granulomatis*, may manifest as a genital papule, subcutaneous nodule, or ulcer. The nodule may be confused with lymphadenopathy.

Pages: 1007, 1008

20: (True or False) Other physical signs that aid in establishing the diagnosis of the patient in question 19 are:

A. Identifying multinucleated giant cells on a Tzanck smear
B. Visualizing a genital ulcer with a clear base and smooth, sharply defined border
C. Noticing a small inconspicuous, painless genital erosion that subsequently heals without scarring
D. Finding a broad-based painful superficial ulcer that is raised above the skin surface

Answers: True - A, B, C, False - D

Critique: Identification of multinucleated giant cells on a Tzanck preparation is pathognomonic for herpes infection. A genital ulcer with a smooth, well-defined border is consistent with primary syphilis. A small genital ulcer that is followed by purulent-draining inguinal lymphadenopathy is indicative of lymphogranuloma venereum (LGV); the causative agent is *Chlamydia trachomatis*. Granuloma inguinale may be suspected when a superficial ulcer is visualized with rolled borders and friable, beefy red granulation tissue. This lesion, however, is painless and is not associated with regional adenopathy as is the case with both LGV and chancroid.

Pages: 1014, 1015

21: (True or False) Common complications from herpes zoster include:

A. Postherpetic neuralgia
B. Localized hypoesthesia
C. Secondary bacterial infections
D. Ophthalmic zoster
E. Bilateral dermatomal crusting and scar formation

Answers: True - A, B, C, D, False - E

Critique: Herpes zoster (shingles) invariably causes unilateral findings.

Pages: 1008, 1009

22: The disorder caused by this infection appears as diffuse generalized hypo- or hyperpigmented plaques with overlying fine scales. Lesions are primarily located on the upper chest, back, and proximal extremities and may coalesce into large configurations that invariably itch. In the summertime, lesions appear hypopigmented but then darken during the cooler months. This infection is due to:

A. Tinea cruris
B. Tinea corporis
C. *Candida albicans*

D. Tinea manuum
E. *Malassezia furfur*

Answer: E

Critique: Dermatophytic fungi cause tinea corporis (ringworm) and tinea cruris (jock itch). Tinea corporis manifests as round or oval patches with slightly raised erythematous, scaly, or vesicular borders with central clearing. Lesions may be simple or multiple without any specific grouping or pattern. Tinea cruris affects the intertriginous areas of the genital regions and differs from tinea corporis in that small satellite lesions may accompany the pattern. Tinea manuum, tinea unguium, and tinea pedis refer to dermatophytic infections of the hand, nail plate, and foot (athlete's foot), respectively. *C. albicans* flourishes in the setting of poorly controlled diabetes mellitus, oral contraceptive use, and immunosuppressive conditions and following the use of broad-spectrum antibiotics. Typical areas of infection include mucosal membranes or warm moist areas *M. furfur*, the causative agent in tinea versicolor, responds to topical selenium preparations if used regularly. Oral ketoconazole has also been used with varying degrees of success.

Pages: 1010–1013

23: The disease most likely to be associated with painless nodules with central ulcerations, a spreading pattern involving a linear distribution, and recreational gardening activities is:

A. Tularemia
B. Febrile staphylococcal lymphangitis
C. Mycobacteremia
D. Sporotrichosis
E. Leptospirosis

Answer: D

Critique: *Sporothrix schenckii* is a fungal organism found on thorns and splinters, thus serving as an occupational hazard for the rose garden enthusiast. The typical pattern involves inoculation on the hand or distal extremity, followed by linear proximal lymphangitic spread. Treatment may involve oral potassium iodide administration for localized lesions and oral itraconazole for generalized disease.

Page: 1014

24: Acceptable guidelines for elective excision of a nevus include all of the following, except:

A. Irritation
B. Irregular borders
C. Presence of hair within the nevi
D. Involvement with mucosal surfaces
E. Size greater than 5 mm

Answer: C

Critique: Although some dysplastic nevi involve coarse or darkly colored hair, not all hair-containing nevi are malignant. In any case, if a nevus were to demonstrate any malignant potential, excisional biopsy is always prudent.

Pages: 1015, 1016

25: Pyogenic granuloma must be clinically distinguished from all of the following, except:

A. Melanoma
B. Metastatic renal cell cancer
C. Kaposi's sarcoma
D. Keratoacanthoma
E. Fibrosarcoma

Answer: D

Critique: Keratoacanthoma is a common benign growth usually found on the hands or face as a single dome-shaped lesion with a central crust or plug. Its size and growth vary and, like a pyogenic granuloma, may bleed easily with trauma because of the number of blood vessels present. The other lesions listed are malignant neoplasms, which must be appropriately diagnosed as opposed to a benign pyogenic granuloma.

Page: 1017

26: The following are recognized histopathologic types of melanoma, with the exception of:

A. Lentigo maligna melanoma, usually located on the face
B. Superficial spreading melanoma, frequently found on the upper back or legs
C. Nodular melanoma, found anywhere on the body
D. Acral-lentiginous melanoma, which appears on the palms, soles, terminal phalanges, and mucosal membranes
E. Squamous columnar melanoma, found exclusively on the transformation zone of the cervix

Answer: E

Critique: The first four choices are appropriate nomenclature for the clinical spectrum of disease known as melanoma.

Pages: 1018, 1019

27: A 37-year-old migrant farm laborer presents with an "itching rash" involving the inner aspect of the right lower leg and ankle. He wears thin socks and neoprene-lined work boots. The rash has been present for several months, and he reports that it appears to be getting larger. Despite the use of baby powder and over-the-counter hydrocortisone cream, erythematous macules and plaques persist. Management options include:

A. Obtaining an occupational history to elicit any potential repetitive work habits or industrial chemical exposures
B. Suggesting a trial of different footwear or considering "patch" testing to different allergens
C. Starting a short-term trial of a mid- to high-potency topical steroid preparation in an effort to resolve the pruritus
D. Starting a trial of topical antifungal creams, because this may represent an infection caused by tinea
E. Initiating PUVA therapy in an attempt to arrest this psoriatic lesion before it enlarges

Answer: E

Critique: With the exception of starting PUVA therapy, all of the other choices could be effective initial management options. The differential diagnosis for this individual includes atopic dermatitis, contact dermatitis, neurodermatitis, tinea corporis, and psoriasis. Although psoriasis is in the differential diagnosis, most practitioners would consider a trial of topical steroids, coal tar shampoos, and adjunctive therapy with vitamins A and D before starting PUVA therapy.

Pages: 1019, 1020

28: The individual in question 27 has a KOH slide preparation done, which is negative for any evidence of tinea. He is then treated with a mid-potency topical steroid but fails to improve clinically after a 3-week period. The best management option at this point is to offer the patient:

    A. A higher potency topical steroid preparation
    B. Initiation of PUVA therapy
    C. Initiation of oral methotrexate therapy
    D. Biopsy to rule out cutaneous T cell lymphoma
    E. An oral systemic antifungal medication, because KOH slide preparations may have a high false-negative rate

Answer: D

Critique: Because cutaneous T cell lymphoma may appear as macules, plaques, nodules, or tumors, the diligent clinician will obtain a biopsy for tissue diagnosis confirmation before starting any of the other, more complicated regimens listed above. Even if the preliminary biopsy report reveals nonspecific findings, one should continue to entertain a high index of suspicion and offer the patient frequent surveillance biopsies if the lesion persists or increases in size.

Page: 1019

29: (True or False) Benign self-limiting illnesses include:

    A. Pityriasis alba
    B. Pityriasis rosea
    C. Psoriasis
    D. Pseudofollicular barbae (PFB)
    E. Lichen planus

Answers: True - A, B, E, False - C, D

Critique: Pityriasis alba, pityriasis rosea, and lichen planus are all considered self-limiting illnesses. Symptomatic treatments may be offered for control of itching if present. Although pityriasis alba may be considered a chronic condition by some, the degree to which both psoriasis and PFB can negatively affect the self-consciousness and body image of the patient may be substantial. Despite several treatment modalities of varying success, the social isolation and stigmatization experienced by the patient with psoriasis or PFB is not to be understated.

Pages: 1004, 1020

30: Acral iris lesions, a causative association with sulfa-containing medications, coexisting urticarial plaques, and the potential to progress to development of inflammatory bullae or erosions on mucosal membranes in the setting of systemic illness leads one to suspect a diagnosis of:

    A. Erythema nodosum
    B. Erythema infectiosum
    C. Erythema chronicum migrans
    D. Erythema multiforme
    E. Erythema gyratum repens

Answer: D

Critique: Erythema nodosum is a cutaneous manifestation of an active immune response and should lead the clinician to search for an underlying cause. Lesions typically appear as red nodular swellings over the bilateral anterior shins or extensor surfaces of the forearms, thighs, and trunk. Arthralgia commonly precedes the onset of the rash by several weeks. Erythema infectiosum (fifth disease) is caused by parvovirus B19 infection and usually affects children, first as facial erythema (slapped cheek appearance) and followed by a fishnet-like pattern of erythema on the extremities, trunk, and buttocks. Erythema migrans, a hallmark skin finding indicating Lyme disease, starts as a small papule at the bite site of the *Ixodes* tick. Then a slowly enlarging, reddish ring migrates outward, leaving a normal skin surface behind. Unlike the lesions accompanying tinea, the edge of this lesion is flat and does not have scale at its outside margin. Erythema gyratum repens presents as waxy-appearing bands of erythema, snake-like outlines, and wood grain patterns and is commonly associated with cancers of the breast, lung, stomach, bladder, or prostate. It may be difficult to find a precipitating factor when it comes to erythema multiforme, despite the association with the sulfonamides. The differential diagnosis for erythema multiforme includes urticaria, necrotizing vasculitis, secondary syphilis, septicemia, Rocky Mountain spotted fever, viral exanthems, lichen planus, and bullous impetigo.

Page: 1021

31: Androgenetic alopecia affects all of the following, except:

    A. The crown on men
    B. The crown on women
    C. The parietal areas on men
    D. The parietal areas on women

Answer: D

Critique: In women, the parietal areas are usually spared from baldness. If baldness were to occur in a woman before the age of 60, endocrinologic evaluation is warranted.

Page: 1021

32: Nail dystrophies, cataracts, atopy, and pernicious anemia are most likely associated with:

    A. Traumatic alopecia
    B. Febrile alopecia

C. Alopecia areata
D. Traction alopecia
E. Scarring alopecia

Answer: C

Critique: The named findings indicate alopecia areata, which may be seen in conjunction with thyroid disease, pernicious anemia, Addison disease, vitiligo, systemic lupus erythematosus, ulcerative colitis, and Down syndrome.

Page: 1022

33: (True or False) Findings in a patient infected with scabies might include:

A. HIV-positive status
B. Absence of facial involvement
C. Prominent multiple burrows 10 to 15 mm in length
D. Associated intense nocturnal pruritus
E. Tendency for spontaneous resolution

Answers: True - A, B, D, False - C, E

Critique: The mite *Sarcoptes scabiei* forms a 2- to 3-mm burrow, usually on the forearm or the web spaces of the fingers. The burrows are easy to miss clinically as the secondary eruptions of erythematous papules and excoriations in the web spaces, forearms, axillae, abdomen, and genitalia are more clinically apparent. The pruritus may be intense. Treatment is aimed at mite eradication from the skin surface, clothing, bed linens, and any other family members similarly affected.

Pages: 1022, 1023

34: Appropriate treatment options for pediculosis capitis infection include all of the following, except:

A. Kwell
B. Nix
C. Lindane
D. Imiquimod
E. RID

Answer: D

Critique: Imiquimod, a topical immune response modifier, is indicated in the treatment of genital warts. The other agents listed, as well as ivermectin, sulfur, and crotamiton, are indicated for the treatment of head lice.

Page: 1023

35: (True or False) Bacterial paronychia, when compared to fungal paronychia, has:

A. A delayed onset of symptoms
B. More pain and tenderness
C. A tendency to involve multiple fingers
D. An excellent response to topical antibiotic therapy
E. The potential to result in osteomyelitis

Answers: False - A, C, D, True - B, E

Critique: Patients with infection of the nail fold because of bacterial agents invariably present acutely with complaints of associated pain and tenderness. Single-digit involvement is the typical pattern seen and responds well to systemic antibiotic administration as well as incision and drainage. Left untreated, bacterial paronychia may lead to deeper tissue involvement, including osteomyelitis.

Page: 1023

36: (True or False) Correct descriptions pertaining to Kaposi's sarcoma include:

A. A slow-growing plaque-like appearance
B. Characteristic homogeneous tan-brown coloration
C. Propensity to be found on the trunk and face
D. Uniformly painful lesion

Answers: False - A, B, D, True - C

Critique: Kaposi's sarcoma develops from a reddish-pink macule quickly into a nodule or plaque-like tumor that is deep red or purple in color. Numerous lesions may be seen on the face and trunk, and they are generally painless unless irritated by clothing or jewelry.

Pages: 1024, 1025

37: In the patient with AIDS, *Candida* lesions increase in severity as:

A. The number of killer T cells decreases
B. The number of killer T cells increases
C. The number of helper T cells decreases
D. The number of helper T cells increases

Answer: C

Critique: As the population of helper T cells declines, *Candida* infections in the mouth and esophagus become more apparent, manifesting as white plaques on the tongue, and are associated with a sore throat and dysphagia.

Page: 1025

Chapter 42

Endocrinology

Steven A. Crawford, Michael D. Hagen, David R. Rudy, and Edward T. Bope

1: (True or False) Which of the following clinical features are more characteristic of type 1 than of type 2 diabetes mellitus:

    A. Age of onset less than 30 years
    B. Obese body habitus
    C. Presence of islet cell antibodies
    D. Development of ketosis

Answers: A - True, B - False, C - True, D - True

Critique: Type 1 diabetes is more likely to occur at a younger age and is associated with the presence of islet cell antibodies. Type 1 patients are also prone to ketosis. Type 2 diabetes is more likely associated with obesity.

Pages: 1027, 1028, Table 42-3

2: Which of the following ethnic groups has the least expected susceptibility to diabetes type 2:

    A. Northern European
    B. Black African
    C. Polynesian
    D. Pima Indian
    E. Melanesian

Answer: A

Critique: Black Africans, Polynesians, Pima Indians, and Melanesians all are groups who have markedly increased prevalences of diabetes type 2. Ethnic northern Europeans, while far from being immune to diabetes type 2, have lower rates than do the other groups mentioned, as do ethnic Japanese. However, northern Europeans have a significantly higher incidence and prevalence of type 1 diabetes mellitus, which ethnic Japanese do not.

Page: 1033

3: For a type 1 diabetic patient who presents in mild diabetic ketoacidosis, which of the following insulin regimens is the most appropriate initial management:

    A. 20 units insulin lispro subcutaneously hourly
    B. 5 units Ultralente Insulin intravenous push hourly
    C. 15 units NPH insulin intravenous push hourly
    D. 2 units regular insulin hourly continuous intravenous infusion

Answer: D

Critique: The intermediate acting insulins, such as NPH, and long-acting insulins, such as Ultralente, are used for maintenance therapy and not given intravenously. Insulin lispro has a rapid onset and short duration of action and is given before meals in chronic maintenance therapy. Continuous infusion of low-dose regular insulin provides good control with small doses and represents the optimal selection among the choices.

Page: 1029, Table 42–4

4: Assume that you have determined over several days of observation that a diabetic patient appears to require 35 to 40 units of insulin per day to maintain euglycemia. Which of the following represents the most appropriate selection of insulin doses:

    A. 35 units of Ultralente Insulin each morning
    B. 12 units NPH in the morning and 24 units in the evening
    C. 18 units NPH plus 6 units regular in the morning, 8 units NPH plus 4 units regular in the evening
    D. 12 units Ultralente plus 12 units NPH in the morning, 6 units Ultralente plus 6 units NPH in the evening

Answer: C

Critique: NPH insulin action peaks at 6 to 12 hours after administration, while regular insulin action peaks in 2 to 4 hours. By mixing regular and NPH and splitting into morning and evening doses, insulin levels more closely approximate metabolic needs than is seen with the other possible choices. Additionally, splitting the total dose into two thirds of the total in the morning and one third in the evening approximates the normal physiologic pattern for insulin secretion.

Pages: 1029, 1030

5: Which of the following chemical parameters provides the best estimate of long-term blood sugar control in a diabetic patient:

    A. C-reactive protein
    B. Alphafetoprotein
    C. Glycosylated hemoglobin
    D. Hemoglobin electrophoresis

Answer: C

Critique: Glycosylated hemoglobin provides the best estimate of long-term blood glucose control. The other listed tests provide no information about blood glucose levels.

Page: 1030

6: A 25-year-old man with type 1 diabetes mellitus presents to your office with nausea and abdominal pain. You detect rapid deep breathing and an unusual odor on his breath. On a dipstick urine, you detect a large reaction to ketones. Another feature common to this situation would include a:

A. Glucose level greater than 1000 mg/dL
B. Serum osmolality level around 310
C. Serum sodium of 145 mEq/L
D. Tendency toward stupor, coma, and convulsions

Answer: B

Critique: Diabetic ketoacidosis (DKA) commonly occurs when a patient with type 1 diabetes does not get enough insulin, resulting in a variety of profound metabolic changes. It causes marked dehydration, Kussmaul breathing (rapid and deep respirations), glucose levels averaging 475 mg/dL, serum osmolality of approximately 310, ketosis, acidosis, and mild hyponatremia. It uncommonly results in stupor, coma, or convulsions. Hyperosmolar hyperglycemic nonketotic syndrome usually occurs in elderly patients with noninsulin-dependent diabetes mellitus with long-standing uncontrolled hyperglycemia who have a precipitating event (particularly infection) and who cannot keep up with the resultant osmotic diuresis. It causes marked dehydration, normal to mild hypernatremia, marked hyperglycemia (mean levels of 1166 mg/dL), and hyperosmolality with levels greater than 340. It does not result in ketosis, although mild acidosis may occur. It has a profound tendency to result in coma, stupor, and convulsion.

Pages: 1030, 1031, 1079

7: Which of the following represents the typical fluid deficit seen in patients presenting with diabetic ketoacidosis:

A. 0 to 1 liter
B. 1 to 3 liters
C. 2 to 4 liters
D. 3 to 5 liters

Answer: D

Critique: Patients with diabetic ketoacidosis typically have profound fluid deficits. The average fluid deficit is 3 to 5 liters.

Page: 1043

8: The Diabetes Control and Complications Trial (DCCT) demonstrated that tight control of blood sugar leads to lower rates of retinopathy, neuropathy, and nephropathy. Which of the following statements best describes the effect DCCT levels of control had on the incidence of hypoglycemia:

A. The incidence remained the same in the patients whose blood sugar was tightly controlled.
B. The incidence doubled in the patients whose blood sugar was tightly controlled.
C. The incidence tripled in the patients whose blood sugar was tightly controlled.

D. The incidence quadrupled in the patients whose blood sugar was tightly controlled.

Answer: B

Critique: The DCCT demonstrated that approximately 35% of patients treated with conventional insulin regimens experience hypoglycemia, while 65% of patients whose blood sugar was tightly controlled experienced hypoglycemia.

Page: 1032

9: Which of the following statements differentiates complications of diabetes types 1 and 2 (i.e., which point mentioned distinguishes the patterns of complications from type 1 as opposed to type 2 diabetes mellitus):

A. Most cases of end-stage renal disease (ESRD) among diabetics occur in type 1 cases.
B. ESRD is heralded in type 1 disease by microalbuminuria (24-hour urinary albumen in the range of 30 to 300 mg).
C. A type 1 diabetic has a significantly greater risk of developing ESRD and proliferative retinopathy than does a type 2 diabetic.
D. Complications of diabetes, such as retinopathy and nephropathy, are preventable in type 1 diabetics through conscientious ("tight") blood sugar control.
E. Retardation of progression of glomerulopathy and decreasing renal function are effected by protein restriction, blood pressure and blood sugar control, and use of angiotensin-converting enzyme-inhibiting drugs in type 1 disease.

Answer: C

Critique: Type 1 diabetics are at significantly greater risk for nearly all the complications of diabetes related to glycemic control, but type 2 diabetes is twice as prevalent as type 1. For that reason, the majority of ESRD in diabetes is found in type 2 patients. Choices B, D, and E are true statements, but the facts stated do not differentiate types 1 and 2. It is true, for example, that retinopathy and nephropathy are preventable by tight control of type diabetics as shown in the DCCT study, but such control serves as well in type 2 patients as shown in the UKPD study, published in four separate parts. Sixty-seven percent of type 1 diabetics will have proliferative retinal changes after 35 years with disease, and 90% will have discernible signs of retinopathy after 25 to 30 years.

Pages: 1032, 1033

10: Which of the following tests is *least* relevant to order in a 24-hour urine specimen to plan preservation of renal function in diabetes or hypertension:

A. Urine 24-hour and serum creatinine levels
B. 24-hour urinary urea nitrogen
C. 24-hour urinary sodium
D. 24-hour urinary glucose
E. 24-hour urinary total protein, including albumen fraction

Answer: D

Critique: As creatinine clearance falls from its normal 100± mL/min in any renal disease to around 50 mL/min, several measurements should be performed. First, creatinine clearance calculation requires the measurement of serum creatinine and urinary creatinine over a measured time interval. Once creatinine clearance is thus confirmed, preservational measures must be employed. These include control of blood pressure in hypertensive patients, control of blood sugar in diabetics, and other measures for reduction of glomerular filtration rate. The latter utilize angiotensin-converting enzyme inhibitors and reduction in protein intake to a level just above protein needs, so far as will be tolerated by the average patient. Urine urea nitrogen allows calculation of dietary protein through the formula: dietary protein (grams) = UUN g/24 hr + (0.31 × lean body weight kg) × 0.625, where UUN = urine urea nitrogen. Once this is known, the patient can be educated and instructed in how far to reduce dietary protein. Urinary sodium allows estimation of dietary sodium and instruction of the patient in sodium reduction to assist in blood pressure control, increasingly relevant in hypertensive patients as their renal function deteriorates.

Urinary total protein allows assessment for advanced renal disease through diagnosis of nephrotic syndrome, passage of ≥3 grams/24 hour. At a more subtle degree of renal damage, microalbuminuria can be diagnosed, defined as 30 to 300 mg/24 hours in diabetics.

Finally, the least needed measurement in a 24-hour urine collection, whether in a diabetic patient or not, is the amount of glucose spilled. Blood sugar is quickly and more cheaply followed through serum or blood glucose.

Page: 1033

11: To minimize the likelihood of visual loss due to retinopathy, which of the following is the most appropriate preventive strategy:

A. Perform visual field examination by gross confrontation once every 5 years
B. Perform undilated retinal examination with an ophthalmoscope once every 3 years
C. Have ophthalmologic examination performed annually by an ophthalmologist
D. Have extraocular motions tested annually

Answer: C

Critique: In addition to tight blood sugar control, annual retinal examination by an ophthalmologist is the best strategy of the listed options to minimize sight loss due to retinopathy.

Page: 1033

12: In a diabetic patient who has developed microalbuminuria (30 to 300 mg albumin/24 hours), what is the average time to development of end-stage renal disease, assuming no active intervention:

A. 1 year
B. 4 years
C. 8 years
D. 10 years

Answer: D

Critique: Microalbuminuria indicates early nephropathy, and creatinine clearance rates decline by about 11 cc/minute/year once microalbuminuria appears if no active intervention ensues. On average, this leads to end-stage renal disease in about 10 years.

Page: 1033

13: Diabetic nephropathy is characterized by:

A. Higher prevalence in type 2 diabetics
B. Microalbuminuria early in its course
C. Glomerular basement membrane attenuation
D. Increased insulin requirements as the condition worsens

Answer: B

Critique: Type 1 diabetics are at a much higher risk for the development of diabetic nephropathy than are type 2 diabetics. Microalbuminuria, or loss of 30 to 300 mg/day of albumin, is an early sign of diabetic nephropathy. Glomerular basement membrane thickening and increased mesangium are early histologic changes. Insulin requirements decline as renal failure progresses, and it is not unusual to see more frequent hypoglycemic reactions.

Pages: 1033, 1034

14: (True or False) In a patient with early diabetic nephropathy, which of the following interventions have been demonstrated to reduce the rate of decline in renal function:

A. Angiotensin-converting enzyme (ACE) inhibitor therapy
B. Angiotensin receptor blocker therapy
C. Dietary protein restriction to 0.75 g/kg/day
D. Conventional insulin therapy

Answers: A - True, B - True, C - True, D - False

Critique: ACE inhibitors, angiotensin receptor blockers, and dietary protein restriction have all been demonstrated to reduce the rate of renal function decline in patients with diabetic nephropathy. The DCCT demonstrates that tight control of blood sugar, as opposed to conventional therapy, slows the development of complications such as nephropathy.

Page: 1043

15: Which of the following is the most common motor sign of diabetic neuropathy:

A. Gastroparesis seen on gastrointestinal x-rays
B. Retrograde ejaculation in a male
C. Absent ankle reflex
D. Pupillary reflex sluggishness

Answer: C

Critique: Absent ankle reflex is the earliest motor sign of diabetic neuropathy. Gastroparesis and retrograde ejaculation represent manifestations of autonomic neuropathy.

Page: 1031

16: (True or False) Metabolic syndrome X is characterized by which of the following features:

    A. Normal body weight
    B. Hypertension
    C. Hyperinsulinemia
    D. Dyslipidemia

Answers: A - False, B - True, C - True, D - True

Critique: Syndrome X is characterized by hypertension, dyslipidemia, and hyperinsulinemia. Patients with syndrome X are usually obese.

Page: 1036

17: For a newly diagnosed type 2 diabetic with a fasting blood sugar of 175 mg/dL, which of the following is the most appropriate initial therapeutic regimen:

    A. Glyburide 5 mg p.o. twice daily
    B. Weight reduction diet and exercise regimen
    C. NPH insulin 20 units in the morning, 10 units in the evening
    D. Metformin 500 mg p.o. twice daily

Answer: B

Critique: For a patient whose fasting blood sugar is under 200 mg/dL, a trial of diet and exercise is the most appropriate first step. Subsequent addition of pharmacologic agents will be guided by the patient's response to this regimen.

Page: 1037

18: Mr. G., a 46-year-old man seeing you for an uncomplicated viral URI weighs 230 lb at a height of 5 ft 11 in. He has a blood pressure of 150/95. His father died at the age of 55 from his first heart attack. His father smoked 1 pack of cigarettes a day for 30 years. One paternal uncle has type 2 diabetes, and another has hypertension. Mr. G. never has taken any medication nor has he been told, so far as he remembers, that he has any health problems or risks. You decide to educate the patient as to his cardiovascular risk status and advise him. What is his presumed ideal weight:

    A. 150 lb
    B. 172 lb
    C. 184 lb
    D. 194 lb
    E. 230 lb

Answer: B

Critique: The Hamwi rule of thumb for estimating ideal weight is, for women, 100 lb for 60 inches of height plus 5 lb for every inch over 60 inches; for males 106 lb for 60 inches plus 6 lb for every inch over 60 inches of height. By this reckoning, Mr. G.'s ideal weight is 172 lb. This estimate is corrected upward for people with larger than average muscle mass brought about through isometric exercise, such as weightlifting.

Page: 1038

19: How many calories constitute a diet for maintenance of the patient in question 18 at his ideal weight:

    A. 2300
    B. 1720
    C. 1500
    D. 1000
    E. 600

Answer: B

Critique: Having calculated the ideal weight as 172 lb for this individual, the initial choice of number of calories for maintenance of that weight can be estimated as the ideal weight in pounds multiplied by 10 or 1720.

Page: 1038

20: Given the ideal weight of Mr. G., which of the following is a reasonable breakdown of food types to constitute the diet aimed at calories needed to maintain him at ideal weight:

    A. 50% of calories by fat; 30% of calories by carbohydrates; 20% of calories by protein
    B. 50% of calories by protein; 30% of calories by fat; 20% of calories by fat
    C. 55% of calories by fat; 35% of calories by carbohydrates; 10% of calories by protein
    D. 10% of calories by fat; 70% of calories by carbohydrates; 20% of calories by protein
    E. 55% of calories by carbohydrates; 30% of calories by fat; 15% of calories by protein

Answer: E

Critique: Carbohydrates should supply 50% to 60% of this requirement, or 946 calories in the example given. At 4 calories g, this would be supplied by 237 g of carbohydrate.

Protein content of the diet is prescribed at about 15% of daily calories ingested. For this hypothetical patient, the caloric allowance is 258. At 4 calories/g, these calories are supplied by 64.5 g, or roughly 2 ounces of protein. This picture may be changing in that over the past 3 years much attention has been given to the effect of carbohydrates, especially simple carbohydrates, to overstimulate the beta cells of the pancreas, leading more rapidly to exhaustion of pancreatic insulin-producing capacity in type 2 diabetics. No recommendation now exists to change the division of food types, except in certain fringe theories, such as a popular diet that allows high levels of fatty foods.

The recommended fat content of the diet for people in developed countries is less than 30% of calories. This addresses the need to limit endogenous production of cholesterol and overall calorie consumption to address the epidemic of obesity. For the 172 lb patient with caloric needs of 1720, this is 516 cal ÷ 8 kcal/g = 64.5 g.

Page: 1038

21: You advise walking to lose weight. How many excess calories will your patient burn for every mile walked at his present weight:

    A. 230
    B. 172
    C. 115

D. 153
E. 100

Answer: D

Critique: Calories consumed in moving on foot at any speed, for 1 mile, is estimated by multiplying the subject's actual (not ideal) weight in pounds times 2/3. Therefore, 230 lb., the actual weight for Mr. R., × 2/3 = 153. This rule of thumb holds whether the subject is walking or running, though the faster one moves the shorter the time interval in which the set amount of calories is burned. It does not hold true for locomotion in any mode other than by foot. As Mr. G.'s weight drops, the calories burned per mile will fall as well. Thus, the amount of exercise required to lose weight will rise, accounting in part for the often encountered discouragement on the part of weight reduction patients.

Page: 1039

22: After Mr. G. has walked 1 mile every day and followed the prescribed diet for 4 weeks, he weighs 225 pounds. His resting ECG is normal and an ECG stress test was negative. His blood pressure without any pharmacological intervention is 135/85. He has measured his walking pulse and found it to be 90 bpm while walking 1 mile in 20 minutes. He has begun to ride a stationary bike and finds that at a stable rate for 20 minutes his pulse is measured at 120 bpm. He asks advice as to how many excess calories he can expect to consume if he rides his bike at the same pace for 40 minutes three times per week. Your answer is:

A. 808
B. 408
C. 306
D. 153
E. 75

Answer: B

Critique: The estimate of calories burned in pulse-raising exercise is based on the following model: Calories burned in walking a given distance is related to the weight of the subject as shown in question 21. The time taken to walk or run the mile is measured and "standardized" for the individual, and the steady pulse while walking at the pace required to cover that distance in that same time period is also measured in bpm. Calories burned in any other intensity of exercise at a rate in the same proportion as the "exercising" pulse rate relates to the walking pulse rate. Mathematically this relationship can be illustrated as follows:

$$C_x = C_w \times P_x/P_w \times T_x T_w$$

where C_x = calories consumed in pulse-raising exercise; C_w = calories consumed in locomotion 1 mile at any pace (weight in pounds × .67); P_x = average pulse during that exercise; P_w = pulse while walking 1 mile at a steady pace, e.g., 3 mph; T_x = time exercised in minutes; and T_w = time required to walk 1 mile while maintaining pulse P_w. Applying this equation to the problem, given the number of calories exercising for 20 minutes, the time it takes Mr.

G. to walk 1 mile with a steady pulse of 90 is as follows: The calories burned per mile (153 for this person) is multiplied by the number of 20-minute mile time blocks (2 in this case). Thus, such exercise, if generating a pulse of 90 bpm, is the equivalent of walking 2 miles, and the calorie consumption = 153 × 2 = 306. Exercising at rates above or below his walking pace pulse of 90 bpm burns calories at a rate equal to the ratio of the "exercising" pulse to the "walking" pulse. This would be 120/90 times the calories that would have been burned if the exercise were at the same intensity as that used while walking with a pulse of 90; i.e., 306 × 120/90 = 408. Thus, Mr. G. will burn 408 calories for every 40-minute session of exercise at a pace sufficient to raise his pulse to an average of 120 bpm.

The thought involved is much less complicated than the verbiage of the formula. One simply multiplies the number or fraction of the 1 mile walking time by the calories burned per mile (according to the patient's weight) by the ratio of the exercising pulse to the walking pulse at the standard walking pace. This can be easily worked out "in one's head" after a bit of mental practice.

Page: 1039

23: Characteristics of pregnant diabetics include:

A. A decreased risk of sacral agenesis
B. A decline in the rate of progression of retinopathy
C. An increased risk of neonatal macrosomia
D. A decreased incidence of neonatal respiratory distress
E. A lower risk of ketoacidosis for the mother

Answer: C

Critique: Perinatal mortality rates increase with increasing severity of diabetes, but they have decreased dramatically with improved prenatal care and early glucose control. The infant of a diabetic mother has an increased chance of having anomalies, macrosomia, prematurity, respiratory distress syndrome, and death. One of the most characteristic congenital anomalies of diabetes is sacral agenesis or caudal dysplasia. The mother faces an increased risk of ketoacidosis as well as acceleration of retinopathy and nephropathy.

Page: 1041

24: Graves' disease is a type of thyrotoxicosis. It is commonly associated with which of the following manifestations:

A. Excessive TSH excretion
B. Pretibial myxedema
C. Bradycardia
D. Anorexia

Answer: B

Critique: Pretibial myxedema in the pretibial skin or foot areas is pathognomonic of Graves' disease. The combination of suppressed TSH concentration and elevated free thyroxine index confirms the diagnosis of thyrotoxicosis arising from the thyroid gland. Tachycardia, along with a systolic flow murmur, is a common feature of Graves' disease. Loss of weight, despite a good appetite and adequate caloric intake, is an excellent clue.

Pages: 1047–1048

25: A 35-year-old woman enters your office complaining of "jumpiness," irritability, and a 20-pound involuntary weight loss over a period of 4 months, despite an increase in her appetite. She complains also of double vision with certain lateral gazes. Her skin is moist and velvety in texture. Her sclerae are visible above her corneas and she shows an asymmetrical ocular proptosis. Her pretibial areas on both legs manifest a non-pitting swelling that is found nowhere else on her body. What is the approximate ratio of females to males among those afflicted with this disease:

    A. 1:5
    B. 1:3
    C. 1:1
    D. 2:1
    E. 7:1

Answer: E

Critique: The patient has Graves' disease. The patient has symptoms of increased catecholamines and weight loss despite good or even increased appetite. In addition to physical findings of thyrotoxicosis common to all cases of hyperthyroidism (e.g., velvety, moist skin), she manifests changes that are specific for Graves' disease, an autoimmune disorder. These are exophthalmos (as distinguished from the "stare" and lid lag, common to other forms of thyrotoxicosis) and pretibial myxedema. The vast majority of thyroid disorders occur with greater frequency in women than in men. In the case of Graves' disease, the ratio of the incidence in females to males is 7:1. Some sources say this ratio is as high as 10:1.

Page: 1047

26: All of the following are common symptoms or signs of hypothyroidism, except:

    A. Amenorrhea
    B. Facial edema
    C. Lethargy
    D. Coarse skin
    E. Slow movement

Answer: A

Critique: Menorrhagia, not amenorrhea, is a sign/symptom of hypothyroidism, present in 33% of cases (compared to 0% in normal control subjects). This may appear to be ironic and must be remembered by the student. The descending rank order of excess frequency of signs and symptoms of hypothyroidism features as the top five, weakness in 98% (vs. 21% in normal subjects), facial edema in 95% (vs. 27%), lethargy in 85% (vs. 17%), coarse skin in 70% (vs. 10%), and slow movements in 73% (vs. 14%). At the bottom of this list of 33 signs and symptoms is nervousness, present in 51% of cases but also in 41% of "normal" people.

Pages: 1048, 1049

27: Which of the following laboratory studies serve to differentiate Graves' disease from toxic nodular goiter, that is, which tests support the diagnosis of Graves' disease?

    A. Elevated T_3
    B. Elevated T_4
    C. Suppressed TSH
    D. Elevation of serum total calcium, free calcium, and alkaline phosphatase
    E. Presence of anti-Mc or anti-Tg antibodies

Answer: E

Critique: The presence of anti-Mc, or anti-Tg antibodies. especially in high titer, supports the diagnosis of Graves' disease, although this finding could occur in thyroiditis as well. Usually thyroiditides, including Hashimoto's, manifest other symptoms and signs, such as local pain and tenderness, so that presence of anti-Mc or anti-Tg antibodies is seldom a diagnostic linchpin. The other choices are all laboratory findings in thyrotoxicosis owing to any cause. Elevation of serum total calcium, free calcium, and alkaline phosphatase, though not diagnostic, may occur in thyrotoxicosis owing to any cause, because of accelerated bone metabolism and resultant negative calcium balance leading to osteoporosis.

Page: 1050

28: Which of the following ancillary tests assist in differentiating Graves' disease from silent thyroiditis:

    A. Elevated T_3
    B. Elevated T_4
    C. Suppressed TSH
    D. Radioactive iodine uptake (RAIU)
    E. A normocytic, normochromic anemia

Answer: D

Critique: Thyroiditis in the acute phase may cause hyperthyroidism, and when local pain and tenderness are minimal or absent, the symptoms and signs may be difficult to differentiate from those of Graves' disease. Elevated T_3 and T_4 and suppressed TSH are evidence of hyperthyroidism owing to any cause, as is a normocytic, normochromic anemia. The latter, of course, is not specific. In Graves' disease, as in other forms of primary thyrotoxicosis, the 24-hour RAIU shows an increased uptake, well above the normal of 20% and often as high as 60%. In silent thyroiditis, as well as in factitious hyperthyroidism, the RAIU is 5% or less.

Page: 1050

29: Which of the following combinations of laboratory findings is the first abnormality among those mentioned to occur in the evolution of primary hypothyroidism and is hence the most sensitive indicator of the disease:

    A. Low normal T_4, low TSH
    B. Low T_4 and low T_3, normal TSH
    C. Elevated TSH, normal T_3, low T_4
    D. Low T_4 and low T_3, elevated TSH

Answer: C

Critique: Elevation of TSH in isolation is treated as the earliest finding in the development of hypothyroidism. Though a patient with this finding and normal T_3 and normal T_4 is for an indefinite period of time eumetabolic, even if that situation were to remain permanently an isolated TSH elevation should be treated with thyroid hormone for suppression of TSH. This is done to prevent development of euthyroid goiter or multinodular goiter.

Page: 1052

30: Which of the following combinations of laboratory findings is most indicative of secondary hypothyroidism:

    A. Low normal T_4, normal TSH
    B. Low T_4, low T_3, low TSH
    C. Elevated TSH, normal T_3, low T_4
    D. Low T_4 and low T_3, elevated TSH
    E. Elevated T_3, elevated T_4, low TSH

Answer: B

Critique: Secondary hypothyroidism is the result of a decrease in appropriate response or absence of TSH (thyroid-stimulating hormone) response to falling thyroid hormones. Thus, while the physiologic feedback gives rise to elevation of TSH as T_3 and T_4 levels fall, in this condition the insufficient levels of T_3 and T_4 are directly owing to a relative or absolute lack of thyroid-stimulating hormone from the anterior pituitary. Symptoms and signs of deficiencies of other pituitary hormones usually are present. Confirmation of secondary hypothyroidism is established by blunting of the TSH response to the TRH test, wherein a measured dose of thyrotropin-releasing hormone is administered and blood is drawn at standardized intervals for measurement of the TSH response.

Page: 1055

31: Which of the following conditions is associated with hypercalcemia:

    A. Sarcoidosis
    B. Hypothyroidism
    C. Hypomagnesemia
    D. Pancreatitis
    E. Burns

Answer: A

Critique: Sarcoidosis is an uncommon cause of hypercalcemia (0.9% of cases). Malignancy and hyperparathyroidism are the two most common causes. Hypothyroidism causes decreased bone resorption, which results in hypocalcemia. Pancreatitis and burns, along with either hypomagnesemia or hypermagnesemia, may cause hypocalcemia by preventing parathyroid gland function.

Pages: 1061–1063

32: Precocious puberty is defined as the onset of increased testosterone and all its sequelae of secondary sexual development and spermatogenesis before age 9 in boys or estrogen production, breast development, or menarche before age 7 in white girls and 6 in black girls. Its parameters include which of the following:

    A. Occurs more commonly in boys than in girls
    B. About 20% of girls with true isosexual precocity are idiopathic.
    C. Can be caused by epilepsy
    D. Preferred treatment is by administering progestational agents

Answer: C

Critique: True sexual precocity occurs 5 times more frequently in girls than in boys. About 80% of girls and only 50% of boys with true sexual precocity are found to be idiopathic. The remainder can be caused by neurologic phenomena, including head trauma, meningitis, and epilepsy. The favored endocrinologic therapy has changed from FSH suppression to the prevention of developmental and growth-stimulating effects of estrogen by administering progestation agents (which are also antiandrogenic) to luteinizing hormone–releasing hormone (LHRH) agonism in constant or nonpulsed fashion. The latter has the paradoxic effect, through binding with gonadotropic cells of the pituitary, of suppressing the gonadotropins, follicle-stimulating hormone (FSH) and luteinizing hormone (LH).

Pages: 1087–1091

33: A 51-year-old woman presents to your office for evaluation of hot flashes and lack of menses for 14 months. She had a tubal ligation many years ago. Her periods had been decreasing in amount and frequency over the last 2 years until they stopped completely. About which of the following would it be appropriate to inform her regarding her menopausal state?

    A. FSH must be measured to confirm menopause.
    B. Estrogen replacement therapy (ERT) will prevent approximately 20% of the coronary heart disease (CHD) deaths in postmenopausal women.
    C. Consumption of calcium at 1500 mg/day is as effective as ERT in preventing osteoporosis.
    D. There is no danger in waiting more than 3 years to decide whether to be on hormone replacement therapy (HRT) for preventing osteoporosis.
    E. Transdermal estrogen lacks a portion of the lipid-remediating effect of oral estrogens.

Answer: E

Critique: Clinically acceptable definitions of menopause include typical symptoms in the appropriate setting, such as age, associated vasomotor and emotional symptoms, and cessation of menses, even for only a few months, with the corroborating finding of an elevated FSH level (>40 IU/L), 1 year of amenorrhea in the appropriate clinical setting, or an increased FSH level (>40 IU/L) in the atypical setting. Only if amenorrhea exists for less than 6 months should there be confirmation of FSH, and pregnancy must be ruled out before instituting HRT. It is estimated that HRT or ERT can prevent approximately half of the deaths due to CHD in postmenopausal women. Oral calcium is the most conservative regimen that can be used for long-term prevention of osteoporosis, at dosages that ensure a total intake of 1.5 g/day. This regimen alone is not nearly as potent as ERT for prevention of osteoporosis and obviously has no beneficial effect on the risk for CHD. ERT or HRT should be started as soon as menopause is eminent. The first 3 years appears to be crucial. A disadvantage of transdermal estrogen is that it misses the first pass through the liver and consequently lacks a portion of the lipid-remediating effects.

Pages: 1101–1104

34: Other names for type 1 diabetes mellitus include all of the following, except:

    A. Early-onset diabetes mellitus
    B. Juvenile onset diabetes mellitus
    C. Autoimmune diabetes mellitus
    D. Insulin-resistant diabetes mellitus

Answer: D

Critique: Type 1 diabetes, or IDDM, has been called early-onset, juvenile, and autoimmune diabetes. It usually occurs at an early age, during childhood, and has been associated with an autoimmune reaction involving the islet cells. This reaction, which is thought to be triggered by a viral infection in a genetically susceptible individual, leads to progressive loss of insulin-secretory capacity and ultimately to clinical diabetes. Insulin resistance occurs in type 2, or NIDDM, diabetes.

Pages: 1027–1028

35: Common clinical manifestations of hypoglycemia include all of the following, except:

    A. Bradycardia
    B. Perspiration
    C. Irritability
    D. Hunger
    E. Tremors

Answer: A

Critique: The clinical manifestations of hypoglycemia are explained by the responses to counterregulatory hormones or the consequences of neuroglycopenia. When glucose falls to 40 to 50 mg/dL, epinephrine, growth hormone, glucagon, and cortisol are secreted to counter hypoglycemia. Perspiration, tremors, hunger or nausea, tachycardia, pallor, and irritability occur.

Page: 1032

36: Background diabetic retinopathy causes all of the following changes, except:

    A. Hard exudates
    B. Retinal detachment
    C. Microaneurysms
    D. Intraretinal dot hemorrhages
    E. Cottonwool exudates

Answer: B

Critique: Diabetes is the leading cause of blindness in the United States. There are two types of diabetic retinopathy: background and proliferative retinopathy. Background retinopathy occurs after 5 years and consists of microaneurysms, intraretinal dot hemorrhages, and serous fluid that leaks from abnormal retinal vessels (hard exudates). Cottonwool exudates represent infarctions in the inner retinal layers. Proliferative retinopathy refers to new vessel formation in response to ischemia that extends from the retina into the vitreous cavity. These vessels are fragile, bleed easily, and promote retinal detachment.

Pages: 1032–1033

37: Syndrome X is the name given to the constellation of conditions that includes adult-onset non-autoimmune diabetes as the central focus. Other manifestations of this condition include all of the following, except:

    A. Hypertension
    B. Accelerated atherosclerosis
    C. Hypoinsulinemia
    D. Dyslipidemia
    E. Truncal obesity

Answer: C

Critique: In syndrome X, insulin levels rise owing to a compensatory response in the face of insulin resistance. This hyperinsulinemia results in higher levels of hypertension than in the general population. It also contributes to an increase in atherosclerotic conditions, including coronary artery disease and cerebrovascular disease. It also causes increased hepatic production of very low density lipoprotein (VLDL) and therefore triglyceride. Obesity, particularly of the truncal type, is associated with insulin resistance.

Page: 1036

38: Exercise for diabetics has many salutatory effects. Which of the following is *not* considered an effect of exercise:

    A. Potentiation of insulin
    B. Lowering of the blood pressure
    C. Beneficial lipid effect
    D. Accelerates progression of neuropathy

Answer: D

Critique: For most diabetics, exercise should be an integral part of any regimen. Exercise potentiates insulin, has an alleviating effect on hyperinsulinemia, reduces blood pressure, reduces total and LDL cholesterol, and elevates HDL cholesterol. It may mitigate the complications of neuropathy, nephropathy, and retinopathy.

Page: 1039

39: Signs and symptoms found with hypothyroidism can include all of the following, except:

    A. Increased pulse rate
    B. Hyponatremia
    C. Mental agitation
    D. Shortness of breath

Answer: A

Critique: The insufficiency of thyroid hormones affects all tissues. The cardiovascular system findings include a narrowed pulse pressure and bradycardia. Hyponatremia occurs by secondary antidiuretic hormone excess, which results in water retention out of proportion to salt retention. Common psychiatric symptoms include paranoia and depression. The extreme state, myxedema madness, is characterized by agitation. Shortness of breath occurs, especially if there is pleural effusion.

Page: 1053

40: Pharmacologic agents that can cause hypothyroidism or goiter include all of the following, except:

    A. Lithium
    B. Indomethacin
    C. Phenylbutazone
    D. Ethionamide
    E. Amiodarone

Answer: B

Critique: Several drugs in the standard armamentarium are antithyroid and hence goitrous in their effects. Lithium, phenylbutazone, and the antituberculous drug ethionamide can cause goiters. Amiodarone can cause either hyperthyroidism or hypothyroidism. Indomethacin does not affect the thyroid gland.

Page: 1053

41: Clinical manifestations of hypopituitarism include all of the following, except:

    A. Inability to produce breast milk postpartum
    B. Decreased velocity of growth in an infant
    C. Accelerated bone age
    D. Decreased muscle mass

Answer: C

Critique: The clinical features of hypopituitarism are dependent on which hormones are affected, the age of the patient, and the anatomic area of involvement. Inability to produce prolactin will result in a mother being unable to nurse her infant. Growth hormone deficiency presenting at birth results in decreased velocity of growth. Delayed bone age occurs, and the child has a normal extremity-to-body height ratio. If growth hormone deficiency occurs after growth is completed, symptoms are few. There is also a tendency toward decreased muscle mass in some patients.

Page: 1066

42: Common symptoms of diabetes insipidus include all of the following, except:

    A. Dysuria
    B. Polyuria
    C. Nocturia
    D. Thirst

Answer: A

Critique: A deficiency or absence of vasopressin results in polyuria and the inability to adequately concentrate the urine. This problem also results in nocturia and severe thirst. Dysuria is not a symptom of diabetes insipidus.

Page: 1076

43: Signs and symptoms of chronic primary adrenal insufficiency include all of the following, except:

    A. Salt craving
    B. Hypertension
    C. Weight loss
    D. Hyponatremia
    E. Nausea

Answer: B

Critique: Most cases of primary adrenal insufficiency, also called Addison's disease, are insidious in onset and, therefore, become chronic before the diagnosis is made. The manifestations of this disease are protean; however, aside from hyperpigmentation and vitiligo, are all nonspecific. However, almost 100% of patients have decreased energy, anorexia, and weight loss. Along with the skin changes, these findings are essential to the diagnosis. Variable gastrointestinal symptoms, including nausea in 86% of patients, are proportionate to the severity and acuteness of the disease. Hypovolemia due to sodium loss as a result of hypoaldosteronemia is the basis for orthostatic lightheadedness and hypotension and occurs before the onset of persistent hypotension. Salt craving occurs in about 16% of these patients.

Pages: 1079–1080

Questions 44 to 47: Match each of the following statements about adrenal hormone production with the appropriate area of the adrenal responsible for the hormone production. Each lettered option may be used once, more than once, or not at all.

    A. Zona glomerulosa
    B. Zona fasciculata
    C. Zona reticularis
    D. Adrenal medulla

44: Produces the minor adrenal androgens

45: Produces aldosterone

46: Makes up 75% of the cortex

47: Produces a hormone that causes negative feedback on the release of corticotropin-releasing hormone

Answers: 44 - C, 45 - A, 46 - B, 47 - B

Critique: The adrenal gland is at least two functional endocrine organs that happen to exist within the same capsule—the cortex and the medulla. The cortex consists of three functional units that are related intimately by virtue of their overlapping control mechanisms emanating from the pituitary. The zona fasciculata forms 75% of the cortex. The fasciculata produces the main glucocorticoids, and the zona reticularis synthesizes minor adrenal androgenic steroids and minute amounts of estrone and estradiol. The zona glomerulosa produces aldosterone, which is the main mineralocorticoid.

Pages: 1078–1079

Questions 48 to 51: Match each of the following statements with the best choice from the following agents used to treat hyperthyroidism. Each lettered response may be used once, more than once, or not at all.

A. Radioiodine
B. Subtotal thyroidectomy
C. Antithyroid drugs
D. β-adrenergic blockers
E. Iodine

48: Therapeutic effect lost with chronic use

49: Risk of hypoparathyroidism

50: Contraindicated in pregnancy

51: Used primarily to control symptoms

Answers: 48 - E, 49 - B, 50 - A, 51 - D

Critique: Radioiodine, surgery, and antithyroid drugs have been widely used for many years to treat hyperthyroidism. Each therapy has its benefits and risks. Radioiodine is the most commonly used treatment in adults. It should not be used in pregnant women because it crosses the placenta readily and can be concentrated by the fetal thyroid. Surgical removal of the thyroid is another option for the treatment of thyrotoxicosis. There is a 1% chance of iatrogenic hypoparathyroidism because of total removal of all of the parathyroid glands. Antithyroid drugs, such as propylthiouracil, can also be used. They are in general safe and relatively effective. There is a small risk of agranulocytosis. They are the preferred treatment during pregnancy. Beta-blockers, primarily propranolol, produce symptomatic relief in almost all patients with thyrotoxicosis. Iodine can be useful for acute treatment, but its therapeutic effect is lost with chronic use.

Pages: 1050–1052

Questions 52 to 55: Match each of the following statements with one of the following causes of hypoglycemia. Each lettered response may be used once, more than once, or not at all.

A. Postprandial hypoglycemia
B. Postabsorptive hypoglycemia
C. Insulinoma
D. Ketotic hypoglycemia

52: This is an exceedingly rare cause of hypoglycemia associated with low fasting glucose concentrations.

53: Beta-blockers may offer relief of symptoms.

54: A common cause of hypoglycemia associated with acute alcohol intoxication

55: Benign, short-term starvation phenomenon of childhood

Answers: 52 - C, 53 - A, 54 - B, 55 - D

Critique: Postprandial or reactive hypoglycemia occurs within 4 hours after a meal or glucose load. Preceding meals tend to be rich in carbohydrate (particularly simple carbohydrates) and devoid of protein. The most common complaints are symptoms of sympathetic discharge (tremulousness, inability to concentrate, sweating, and mental irritability) and, therefore, beta-blockers may offer symptomatic relief. Postabsorptive hypoglycemia, defined as clinically low plasma glucose levels during the 12-hour postabsorptive period, can be caused by drugs (e.g., alcohol), critical organ failure, hormonal failure, non–β-cell tumors, endogenous hyperinsulinism, sepsis, and disorders peculiar to childhood. Insulinoma is exceedingly rare (1:250,000 patient-years). A low fasting blood glucose associated with an inappropriately high insulin level establishes the diagnosis. Ketotic hypoglycemia of childhood is a usually benign, short-term starvation phenomenon associated with intercurrent illness.

Pages: 1042–1044

Questions 56 to 59: Match each of the following numbered statements with the correct laboratory test. Each lettered option may be used once, more than once, or not at all.

A. Thyroid antibodies
B. Serum thyroglobulin
C. Serum TSH
D. Free T_4 index
E. Thyroid ultrasonography

56: Important technique for establishing whether a thyroid nodule is solid, cystic, or mixed solid-cystic.

57: Yields an estimate of free thyroxine levels

58: Usually rises early in primary hypothyroidism

59: Used to follow well-differentiated thyroid carcinomas

Answers: 56 - E, 57 - D, 58 - C, 59 - B

Critique: Many laboratory tests are available to measure specific aspects of thyroid function. The free T_4 index is an estimate of the free thyroid hormone concentration, which is calculated using the measurement of the total serum T_4 and thyroid-binding proteins. Serum TSH concentration is a highly sensitive test that can determine thyroid dysfunction, either hyperthyroidism or hypothyroidism, early in the course of the disease. Serum thyroglobulin measurements are of value primarily for the follow-up of people treated for well-differentiated thyroid carcinomas. Thyroid antibodies to thyroglobulin or to thyroid microsomes are useful for diagnosing Hashimoto's thyroiditis.

Pages: 1044–1047

Questions 60 to 64: For each of the following numbered statements, select the most appropriate response.

A. Sulfonylureas
B. Biguanides
C. Thiazolidinediones
D. All of the above

60: Stimulates the pancreas to produce & release insulin

61: Increases peripheral glucose uptake

62: Can be used as first-line agent(s) in type 2 diabetes mellitus

63: Decreases intestinal absorption of glucose

64: Can cause lactic acidosis

Answers: 60 - A, 61 - C, 62 - D, 63 - B, 64 - B

Critique: Several classes of oral agents are available to help in treating patients with type 2 diabetes. The sulfonylureas act by stimulating the pancreatic β cells to produce and release insulin. Biguanides are represented by metformin (Glucophage). It functions to reduce intestinal absorption and hepatic glucose output (gluconeogenesis) and to increase use of glucose in the peripheral tissues. The thiazolidinediones, such as rosiglitazone (Avandia) and pioglitizone (Actos), increase peripheral glucose uptake, suppress lipolysis, and reduce hepatic gluconeogenesis. All three classes of drugs can be used as first-line agents in type 2 DM.

Pages: 1037–1038

Questions 65 to 68: (True or False) Features of type 2 diabetes include:

65: Age of onset less than 30 years of age.

66: Rapid rate of onset

67: Ketosis is uncommon.

68: Prevalence is higher than that of type 1 diabetes.

Answers: 65 - False, 66 - False, 67 - True, 68 - True

Critique: The distinction between type 1 and 2 diabetes is sometimes difficult to make. A history of ketoacidosis or the detection of moderate to strong urine ketones in the presence of hyperglycemia is the most useful indicator of type 1 diabetes mellitus. In most cases, the age of onset of type 2 diabetes is over 40 years of age, the rate of onset is slow, and the prevalence is higher than 2% (compared with < 0.5% for type 1 diabetes).

Pages: 1028–1029

Questions 69 to 73: (True or False) Common manifestations of diabetic neuropathy include:

69: Foot ulcers

70: Hypertension

71: Hyperreflexia

72: Paresthesias

73: Bladder flaccidity

Answers: 69 - True, 70 - False, 71 - False, 72 - True, 73 - True

Critique: Diabetic neuropathy is common in both type 1 and type 2 diabetics. Three general types occur: (1) peripheral polyneuropathy, (2) mononeuropathy, and (3) autonomic neuropathy. Peripheral polyneuropathy primarily affects sensory fibers. Paresthesias, expressed as burning feet, tingling, and numbness, are characteristic manifestations. Insensitivity to mild trauma or compressive shoes may result in a foot ulcer, most commonly on the plantar aspect of the distal metatarsal. Autonomic neuropathy can be extensive. Besides causing orthostatic hypotension, it can cause bladder flaccidity and hyporeflexia and even areflexia.

Pages: 1031–1034

Questions 74 to 77: (True or False) In choosing appropriate antihypertensive agents for diabetics, the following factors should be considered:

74: Thiazide diuretics lower triglycerides.

75: β-adrenergic blockers aggravate cholesterol levels.

76: α-adrenergic blockers increase triglycerides.

77: ACE inhibitors have no adverse effect on carbohydrate metabolism.

Answers: 74 - False, 75 - True, 76 - False, 77 - True

Critique: Thiazide diuretics can elevate blood glucose and triglycerides. β-adrenergic blockers aggravate cholesterol dyslipidemia and may cause hyperglycemia. They also blunt the gluconeogenic response to hypoglycemia and may mask the symptoms of hypoglycemia, depriving type 1 diabetics of important protection. α-blockers do not affect carbohydrate metabolism and may have a slight beneficial effect on serum lipids. Angiotensin-converting enzyme (ACE) inhibitors do not affect carbohydrate metabolism and may improve glucose tolerance. They may also have a beneficial effect on the development or progression of diabetic nephropathy.

Page: 1040

Questions 78 to 82: (True or False) Acromegaly owing to growth hormone excess causes striking clinical manifestations. These include:

78: Prognathism

79: Visual field defects

80: Anhidrosis

81: Diabetes insipidus

82: Nerve entrapment syndromes

Answers: 78 - True, 79 - True, 80 - False, 81 - False, 82 - True

Critique: Clinical manifestations of acromegaly appear gradually, and they are striking. Headaches and visual field defects can occur if the pituitary tumor is large. Other features include prognathism, separation of the front teeth, coarse facial features, an increase in glove and foot size, deepening of the voice, nerve entrapment syndromes, and increased sweating, or hyperhidrosis. Growth hormone causes insulin resistance, and about one fourth of acromegalic patients also develop diabetes mellitus. Diabetes insipidus is not related to growth hormone excess.

Page: 1070

Questions 83 to 87: (True or False) Craniopharyngioma, a tumor arising from the cell rests of the craniopharyngeal canal, is characterized by:

83: Accelerated growth

84: Headaches

85: Delayed puberty

86: Visual symptoms

87: Composition of pituitary-type cells

Answers: 83 - False, 84 - True, 85 - False, 86 - True, 87 - False

Critique: Craniopharyngioma is not a tumor arising from pituitary cells. It is an embryonic Rathke's pouch tumor derived from cell rests of the craniopharyngeal canal. In addition to growth failure, symptoms arise from increased intracranial pressure with headaches and visual symptoms. It is an infrequent cause of sexual precocity during childhood.

Pages: 1075–1076

Questions 88 to 92: (True or False) Pheochromocytomas are tumors of chromaffin cells in the adrenal medulla that produce epinephrine or norepinephrine. Parameters of this condition include:

88: Most secrete epinephrine.

89: Orthostatic hypotension can occur.

90: Very few occur outside the adrenal medulla.

91: They can be associated with neurofibromatosis.

92: They should be suspected if hypertension is present with a family history of diabetes.

Answers: 88 - False, 89 - True, 90 - True, 91 - True, 92 - False

Critique: Most pheochromocytomas secrete norepinephrine, despite 85% of the catecholamine of the normal adrenal being epinephrine. Orthostatic hypotension or paradoxic recumbent hypotension occurs as a manifestation of hypovolemia, refractoriness of overstimulated α_1-receptors, or vasodilatation caused by α_2-receptor stimulation. Of pheochromocytomas, 90% occur in the adrenal medulla. Pheochromocytoma can be associated with neurofibromatosis and with retinal cerebellar hemangioblastosis, von Hippel-Lindau disease. Pheochromocytoma should be considered but not necessarily screened for whenever hypertension is first diagnosed. Suspicion is heightened when hypertension is present in a setting atypical for essential hypertension, such as young age of onset, lack of a family or personal history of hypertension, or diabetes.

Pages: 1084–1086

Questions 93 to 96: (True or False) True statements about the evaluation of infertility include:

93: The cause lies in the male partner as frequently as it does in the female partner.

94: Most women who are found to have tubal disease have a history of previous infections.

95: Anovulation is an infrequent cause of infertility. Ovulation can be confirmed by a basal body temperature (BBT) rise of 0.4°F in midcycle.

96: Varicoceles are a rare cause of male infertility.

Answers: 93 - True, 94 - False, 95 - True, 96 - False

Critique: Infertility is the inability to conceive despite attempts to do so for 1 year. The causes in males and females are approximately equal, 40% in men only, 30% to 40% in women only, and in 20% to 30% the causes are in both partners. Before putting a woman through an expensive and potentially uncomfortable evaluation, a semen specimen should be obtained. Failure to ovulate and tubal abnormalities are the major causes of infertility in women. Many women who are found to have tubal disease or adhesion give no history of previous infections. Verification of ovulation can be documented by a BBT rise of 0.4°F in midcycle. Varicoceles account for 38% of all cases of male infertility.

Pages: 1094–1095

Chapter 43

Nutrition and Family Medicine

Wanda Gonsalves

1: A 30-year-old male has recently received health insurance and wants to establish care with your practice. You have a very busy practice, but you believe every patient should have a nutritional assessment as part of his or her evaluation. Given your time restraints, your assessment should include all of the following, except:

 A. His medical history, which includes illnesses and medications taken
 B. An evaluation of his clinical appearance
 C. His psychosocial history
 D. His cultural and religious food practices

Answer: D

Critique: A nutritional assessment can be obtained as part of the patient evaluation even in a busy practice. A 5-minute evaluation should include the medical history with special attention to medical illness and medications that may directly or indirectly affect absorption of nutrients. An observation of the patient's clinical appearance for signs of weight loss gives important information, as does the psychosocial history, which may identify dependency or social isolation affecting nutritional status. Obtaining cultural and religious food practices is important to include in a more complete nutritional assessment.

Page: 1107

2: A 27-year-old male patient was recently diagnosed with inflammatory bowel disease. He currently takes Azulfidine (sulfasalazine). Which of the following nutritional supplements should you recommend:

 A. Ascorbic acid
 B. Folic acid
 C. Vitamin B_6
 D. Riboflavin

Answer: B

Critique: Folic acid (0.4 to 1 mg), which is absorbed in the small intestine, should be considered for patients taking Azulfidine as treatment of inflammatory bowel disease such as Crohn's disease. Ascorbic acid is recommended for patients taking anti-inflammatory drugs such as aspirin. Vitamin B_6 should be provided to patients taking INH for tuberculosis. Riboflavin should be given to patients using tranquilizers.

Page: 1109, Table 43–1

3: A 65-year-old male patient was recently hospitalized after suffering a stroke. He is currently taking Coumadin. Which of the following foods should he avoid:

 A. Eggs
 B. Beef liver
 C. Pork
 D. Legumes

Answer: B

Critique: Foods rich in vitamin K, important in blood clotting, should be avoided when anticoagulants such as Coumadin are taken. Coumadin inhibits conversion of vitamin K to its active form. Administration of Coumadin leads to the depletion of vitamin K–dependent clotting factors. High intake of green leafy vegetables, cabbage family vegetables such as cauliflower, tomatoes, and beef liver, rich in vitamin K, should be avoided.

Page: 1111, Table 43–3

4: A 15-year-old patient comes to your office with her mother. Her mother is concerned that her daughter has poor eating habits. In reviewing the patient's diet for the past 24 hours, you find that she lacks the minimum number of daily servings for dairy products. You would recommend how many dairy product servings per day:

 A. Two
 B. Three
 C. Four
 D. Six

Answer: C

Critique: The recommended minimum number of servings per day for dairy products for the teenage group is four servings. A child should receive at least three and pregnant and lactating women should receive four.

Page: 1109, Table 43–2

5: A shift in the growth channel with a slowed rate of weight gain but a normal rate of height and head growth for children could indicate which of the following:

 A. Mother or father with a small frame
 B. Failure to thrive

C. Short stature (decreased height for age)

D. Hypothyroidism

Answer: B

Critique: A shift in the growth channel toward the 50% level is normal in the first 2 years of life. A small frame in one of the parents, in the absence of other risk factors, is reassuring. Failure to thrive is a slowed rate of weight gain with normal rates of height and head growth. A common cause of failure to thrive is improper feeding. Hypothyroidism is associated with increasing weight and normal height.

Page: 1110

6: Laboratory investigation for nutritional evaluation in the routine office practice should include all of the following, except:

A. Serum albumin

B. Lipid levels

C. RBC indices

D. Fasting blood glucose

Answer: A

Critique: Albumin and transferrin levels are used to rank nutritional status. Albumin and other liver proteins are discrete markers of protein nutrition only in the absence of other clinical factors that influence metabolism and serum levels and therefore lack sensitivity and specificity for nutritional changes. More commonly, lipid levels, red blood cell indices, and fasting blood glucose levels are obtained to assess nutritional status.

Pages: 1110, 1113

7: Groups most at risk for iron deficiency anemia include all of the following, except:

A. Those living below the poverty level

B. African-American children and women

C. Mexican-American children and women

D. Postmenopausal women with osteoporosis

Answer: D

Critique: Of toddlers aged 1 to 3 years, 9% to 11% are iron deficient. Adolescent girls and women of childbearing age are also at risk for iron deficiency. The prevalence of iron deficiency is higher among low-income groups and those living below the poverty level.

Page: 1117

8: Hypervitaminosis is more likely to occur with which of the following vitamins:

A. Vitamin C

B. Riboflavin

C. Folate

D. Vitamin A

E. Vitamin B_{12}

Answer: D

Critique: Hypervitaminosis is most likely to occur with fat-soluble vitamins. Vitamin A is the only fat-soluble vitamin listed. Water-soluble vitamins are rapidly excreted and are least likely, but not unknown, to cause problems when

taken in excessive amounts. For example, vitamin C, when taken in excessive amounts may cause nausea, abdominal cramps, and diarrhea. There have been no reported cases of riboflavin (vitamin B_2), folate, or vitamin B_{12} toxicities.

Page: 1117

9: Glossitis, an inflamed tongue, can signal a vitamin deficiency. Which of the following vitamins has *not* been associated with this condition:

A. Niacin

B. Vitamin B_6

C. Vitamin B_{12}

D. Vitamin C

E. Folate

Answer: D

Critique: Often, more than one deficiency may be the cause of glossitis. Vitamin C deficiency, or scurvy, may cause bleeding gums in children and adults as well as poor wound healing.

Page: 1112

10: Obesity is defined by a body mass index (BMI) of which of the following values:

A. 18.5 or greater

B. 22 or greater

C. 25 or greater

D. 30 or greater

Answer: D

Critique: A BMI of 18.5 is the lower cut point for the healthy weight range. Overweight is defined by a BMI of 25 to 30. Obesity is defined as a BMI of 30 or greater. Of American adults, 54.9% are overweight or obese, and 11% of children and adolescents are overweight. Overweight and obesity substantially increase the risk of hypertension, dyslipidemia, type 2 diabetes, coronary artery disease, stroke, gallbladder disease, osteoarthritis, sleep apnea, respiratory problems, and certain cancers.

Page: 1110

11: High carbohydrate combined with very low fat diets (20% of calories or less) can induce a dyslipidemia characterized by which of the following:

A. Low HDL cholesterol level

B. High triglyceride level

C. Elevated small-dense LDL cholesterol level

D. Low insulin level

Answer: B

Critique: High carbohydrate intake with concomitant low fat intake can raise triglycerides and lower the HDL cholesterol. The resultant increase in postprandial glucose could predispose persons with insulin resistance to type 2 diabetes.

Page: 1119

12: Elevated serum LDL cholesterol levels are most likely to occur with increased intake of which of the following fats:

A. Omega fatty acids

B. Monounsaturated fatty acids

C. Saturated fats
D. Vegetable oils

Answer: C

Critique: Saturated fats increase serum LDL cholesterol levels. Saturated fats are found in foods of animal origin (meat, poultry, dairy products, and eggs). Triglycerides are esters of glycerol and fatty acids. Fatty acids are further categorized as unsaturated and saturated fats. Unsaturated fatty acids are further divided into monounsaturated and polyunsaturated fatty acids. Vegetable oils, such as safflower oil, are omega fatty acids. Monounsaturated fatty acids, vegetable oils, and omega fatty acids are derived from unsaturated fats.

Page: 1119

13: Folic acid deficiency has been associated with all the conditions below, except:

A. Reduced plasma homocysteine levels
B. Coronary artery disease
C. Glossitis
D. Cerebral vascular disease
E. Neural tube defects

Answer: A

Critique: Folic acid reduces homocysteine levels. Elevated serum homocysteine levels have been associated with coronary artery disease, cerebral vascular disease, and neural tube defects. Glossitis, an inflammation of the tongue, may be caused by folic acid deficiency.

Page: 1121

14: Increased consumption of added sugars since 1980 is largely due to the doubling of the intake of sugar-containing soft drinks. Excessive consumption may lead to the development of which of the following conditions:

A. Osteoporosis
B. Diabetes insipidus
C. Hypotriglyceridemia
D. Gingival gum disease

Answer: A

Critique: Research has found that milk in the diet has been replaced by soft drinks, leading to the risk of low calcium intake and subsequent development of osteoporosis. Increased sugar intake does not cause diabetes insipidus, hypotriglyceridemia, or gingival gum disease. Increased consumption of sugar is a factor in the development of dental caries, especially in the newly erupted teeth of young children.

Page: 1121

15: Nursing bottle syndrome is characterized by:

A. A calcium deficiency
B. Tooth decay
C. Decreased weight-to-height ratio on the growth curve
D. Accelerated tooth eruption

Answer: B

Critique: Allowing a child to sleep with a bottle in his or her mouth for extended periods of time predisposes the child's newly erupted teeth to tooth decay.

Page: 1121

16: The average American consumes how much sodium per day:

A. 2 g
B. 3 g
C. 4 g
D. 5 g

Answer: C

Critique: The average American consumes 4 grams of sodium per day. Only 10% of dietary sodium intake occurs in foods naturally. Processed foods, restaurant preparation, and home cooking provide 75% of sodium intake. Removal of the saltshaker reduces sodium intake by only 1 to 2 grams.

Page: 1122

17: Complex carbohydrates and fiber can lower the incidence of heart disease, diabetes, certain types of cancers, and diverticulosis. Foods containing fiber are plant foods that are resistant to digestive enzymes. Which of the following is an example of soluble fiber:

A. Barley
B. Wheat bran
C. Broccoli
D. Cellulose

Answer: A

Critique: Dietary fibers are characterized as soluble or insoluble fibers. Barley is an example of a soluble fiber. Other foods containing soluble fibers are citrus fruits, olive products, and beans. Evidence shows that diets high in soluble fibers decrease blood cholesterol, postprandial glucose, and insulin levels.

Page: 1120

18: Osteoporosis in postmenopausal women can result in bone fractures. Which of the following has *not* been implicated in the development of osteoporosis:

A. Low calcium intake
B. Increased alcohol intake
C. Low sodium intake
D. Cigarette smoking
E. Physical inactivity

Answer: C

Critique: High sodium intake can adversely affect calcium balance in an individual with low calcium intake. The calcium intake of adult women is approximately 600 mg per day. The adequate intake (AI) in adults older than 51 years is 1200 mg per day. Consumption of two to three servings of nonfat milk provides 600 to 900 mg of calcium per day. Calcium supplementation of 800 to 1200 mg/day has been shown to slow bone loss and reduce fracture rates in older women.

Pages: 1122, 1123

19: In pregnancy, the physiological requirement of most nutrients can be met by diet, except for which of the following:

    A. Calcium
    B. Protein
    C. Iron
    D. Carbohydrates

Answer: C

Critique: The increased requirement for iron during pregnancy cannot be met by diet alone. Prenatal vitamins and mineral supplementation are recommended during pregnancy. In addition, the pregnant woman needs 30 mg of elemental iron supplement. Adhering to the recommended servings for the pregnant woman should meet the physiological requirements for most nutrients, including four servings in the dairy food group, three servings of meat, five to nine servings of fruits or vegetables, and six to 11 servings from the grain food group. The pregnant teenager should increase the recommended dairy servings to five per day to provide extra calcium and protein intake.

Page: 1124

20: Supplementation with folic acid 1 month before conception for a woman with a previous history of neural tube defects should include what daily dose of folic acid:

    A. 1 mg
    B. 2 mg
    C. 3 mg
    D. 4 mg

Answer: D

Critique: Periconceptual supplementation with folic acid has been shown to reduce the incidence of spina bifida and other neural tube defects. Supplementation should begin 1 month before conception and continue through the first trimester. The dose recommended for a woman with a previous history of neural tube defects is 4 mg per day. All women of childbearing age should consume at least 0.4 mg of folic acid daily. Sources of folic acid include liver, legumes, green leafy vegetables, peanuts, sunflower seeds, and oranges.

Page: 1124

21: Which of the following vitamins has been associated with teratogenic effects when intake is excessive:

    A. Vitamin C
    B. Thiamine
    C. Vitamin A
    D. Riboflavin

Answer: C

Critique: Excessive intake (over 10,000 IU) of vitamin A has been associated with teratogenic effects. Caution the woman who is planning to become pregnant to avoid high doses of vitamin A. The other vitamins listed are water-soluble and are least likely to have toxic effects.

Page: 1125

22: Which of these statements is false for lactating women:

    A. Lactating women typically lose 0.6 to 0.8 kg body weight per month.
    B. Lactating women require an additional 800 kcal per day.
    C. Successful lactation is not compatible with gradual weight loss.
    D. Lactating women should avoid caffeine-containing products.

Answer: C

Critique: Lactating women typically lose between 0.6 and 0.8 kg per month during the first 6 months. More than 20% of them will not lose or gain weight. Successful lactation is compatible with gradual weight loss. Moderate ingestion of caffeine-containing products (one to two cups of coffee per day) is not prohibited.; however, excessive caffeine intake results in an irritable, wakeful infant.

Page: 1126

23: A 27-year-old lactating mother with a 2-week-old infant is concerned that she is not producing enough breast milk. Which of the following statements represents the most important determinant of milk volume:

    A. Maternal exercise
    B. Maternal rest
    C. Increased nursing frequency and duration of nursing
    D. Increased maternal fluid intake

Answer: C

Critique: Maternal stress and the nursing behavior of both mother and infant are potentially the most important determinants of milk volume. Infant appetite spurts at about 3 and 6 weeks of age and again at 3 and 6 months of age also increase milk volume.

Page: 1127

24: Women who are pregnant and are strict vegetarians should include more of which of the following nutrient supplements:

    A. Vitamin A
    B. Calcium
    C. Vitamin D
    D. Vitamin C
    E. Folic acid

Answer: C

Critique: Strict vegetarians and those with inadequate exposure to sunlight should receive nutrient supplementation of 10 μg/day of vitamin D. Calcium supplementation is indicated for women younger than 25 years whose daily dietary calcium intake is less than 600 mg. The recommended dose is 600 mg/day. Vitamin B_{12} at 2 μg/day for strict vegetarians is also recommended. Excessive intake of vitamin A can be teratogenic.

Page: 1126, Table 43–11

25: Which of the following nutrients is most commonly found to be deficient in adolescents:

    A. Vitamin A

B. Vitamin C
C. Iron
D. Vitamin D

Answer: C

Critique: Iron and calcium are most commonly deficient in the diets of adolescents. Iron-containing foods include red meat, iron-fortified cereals, legumes, nuts, eggs, and dark green, leafy vegetables.

Pages: 1128, 1129

26: A mother is very concerned about her teenage daughter who is a "model child." She has an "A" average in school and is quite the perfectionist. Her daughter recently has lost 10% of her body weight expected for height. She is constantly concerned about her weight, has rapid weight fluctuations, and exercises excessively. The most likely diagnosis in this case is which of the following:

A. Thyroid disorder
B. Diabetes
C. Eating disorder
D. Depression

Answer: C

Critique: Adolescent girls and athletes are particularly susceptible to anorexia nervosa and bulimia. Signs of the development of an eating disorder include weight 15% below that expected for height, other weight fluctuations, excessive exercise, and "feeling too fat" when underweight. A history of binge eating as evidenced by self-induced vomiting and laxative or diuretic use is common in bulimia. Bulimia is more often associated with impulsive behavior and substance abuse.

Pages: 1129, 1130

27: Vitamin supplementation should be recommended in all the following groups, except:

A. Adults over 50
B. Pregnancy
C. Breast-fed infants
D. A person on a diet with a daily intake of less than 1200 calories
E. Poor eating habits

Answer: C

Critique: There is some indication that elderly patients have an increased need for protein; vitamins D, B_6, and B_{12}; and folate. Breast-fed infants do not need a supplement unless anemic or if the mother is a strict vegetarian. Individuals who are on constant diets of less than 1200 calories per day risk nutritionally deficient intake over time. People with poor eating habits, such as adolescents and those on fad diets, may require supplementation. Supplementation of individual vitamins or minerals should be avoided unless multivitamins do not provide a large enough dose of the required nutrient (e.g., calcium).

Page: 1132

28: Vegetarian diets include a variety of eating practices that rely mainly on plant foods. A lacto-ovo-vegetarian consumes all except which of the following foods:

A. Plant products
B. Dairy products
C. Eggs
D. Fish

Answer: D

Critique: A strict vegetarian, or vegan, diet relies solely on plant foods. The lacto-vegetarian diet adds dairy products as well as fruits, vegetables, legumes, grains, nuts, and seeds. The ovo-lacto-vegetarian diet adds eggs, and the lacto-ovo-pesco-vegetarian consumes plant products, dairy products, eggs, and fish.

Page: 1135

29: Endurance athletes and those participating in sports requiring repeated burst efforts benefits most from which of the following foods:

A. Grilled steak
B. Breads and cereals
C. Dairy products
D. Fruits and vegetables

Answer: B

Critique: Athletes who participate in endurance sports such as football, basketball, and soccer benefit from carbohydrate loading and routinely consuming a high-carbohydrate diet. Carbohydrate loading should begin 6 days before the event. The precompetition meal should be eaten at least 2 hours before the event starts. A carbohydrate intake of 1 g/kg body weight may improve performance.

Page: 1136

30: A healthy, active 35-year-old male with a family history of hyperlipidemia and coronary artery disease requests a fasting lipid profile. You learn that his LDL is 160 mg/dL, HDL is 35 mg/dL, triglycerides are 90 mg/dL, and total cholesterol is 210. During his follow-up visit, you recommend which of the following:

A. Give him medication and re-evaluate in 1 year
B. Exercise and weight loss if he is overweight
C. Begin a Step One diet
D. Begin a Step Two diet

Answer: C

Critique: The National Cholesterol Education Program (NCEP) recommendation for borderline high LDL cholesterol level (130 to 160) with two risk factors for coronary artery disease is dietary intervention. However, if risk estimation yields a 10-year risk for coronary artery disease of 10% or higher, drug therapy should also be instituted (a coronary risk calculator, based on Framingham data, is available at the National Heart, Lung and Blood Institute's web site, www.nhlbi.nih.gov). Individuals with LDL cholesterols greater than 160 are considered high risk and treatment would still begin with diet intervention for primary prevention of coronary heart disease but also include drug therapy for those with two risk factors and a 10-year estimated risk of less than 10%. Patients with borderline high cholesterol (200 to 240) or LDL cholesterol levels and fewer than two other risk factors for coronary heart disease should be given instruction in dietary modification and exercise and be re-evaluated in 1 year. Recommended dietary therapy for elevated blood cholesterol comes in two steps: the Step One and the Step Two diets. The Step One diet consists of total fats less than 30% of calories, saturated fats less than 10% of calories, and less than 300 mg of cholesterol per day. If response to Step One is insufficient, Step Two is implemented. Saturated fat intake should be less than 7% of calories, with a total cholesterol of less than 200 mg per day. A minimum of 6 months of intensive dietary therapy and counseling is carried out before beginning drug therapy. Therapy can be initiated sooner if the LDL cholesterol is greater than 220 or the patient has known coronary heart disease. Patients with known coronary heart disease should immediately begin the Step Two diet.

Page: 1137

31: A 45-year-old male with known coronary artery disease comes to your office to establish care. In taking his history, you learn he is a smoker with no history of coronary heart disease. He is not taking any medications. Physical examination reveals that he is overweight and has stage I hypertension. Recommendations for his management could include all of the following, except:

    A. Begin Step Two diet
    B. Obtain fasting lipid profile; initiate drug therapy if necessary
    C. Decrease dietary fiber
    D. Folic acid for elevated homocysteine levels

Answer: C

Critique: Secondary prevention of coronary artery disease includes beginning the Step Two diet. Saturated fat intake is reduced to less than 7% of total calories and cholesterol intake should be less than 200 mg per day. Initiate drug therapy for elevated cholesterol to decrease the LDL cholesterol to less than 100. Other recommendations include weight loss as necessary and exercise. The patient should be counseled about the benefits of exercise, which include a reduction in total cholesterol levels, a reduction in triglycerides, an increase in HDL cholesterol, and a reduction in blood pressure. Addition of soluble fiber to the diet may produce an additional 3% to 10% reduction in serum cholesterol. Foods rich in soluble fiber include oat bran, barley, legumes, root vegetables, apples, pears, figs, and berries. Current evidence is not strong enough to recommend routine screening or supplementation with folic acid except for individuals who have high homocysteine levels (greater than 10.0 mmol/L)

Page: 1137

32: Syndrome X is characterized by all of the following, except:

    A. Elevated triglycerides
    B. Elevated HDL cholesterol
    C. Obesity
    D. Insulin resistance
    E. Hypertension

Answer: B

Critique: Syndrome X, also called metabolic syndrome, is characterized by high triglycerides and low HDL cholesterol levels, obesity, insulin resistance, and hypertension.

Pages: 1138, 1139

33: You see a 45-year-old, obese, type 2 diabetic in your office for follow-up of his diabetes and review of his recent fasting lipid profile. His lipid profile shows elevated triglycerides and cholesterol as well as a low HDL level. Lifestyle recommendations would include all of the following, except:

    A. Begin an exercise program
    B. Increase carbohydrate intake
    C. Decrease total and saturated fat intake
    D. Supplement diet with 300 mg to 500 mg of omega-3 fatty acids

Answer: B

Critique: Obesity, excess calories, dietary fat, and excessive alcohol intake are associated with hypertriglyceridemia. The Step One diet is recommended for all patients with elevated triglycerides, with progression to a Step Two diet if the desired lipid levels are not achieved. The Step One diet consists of a total fat intake of less than 30% of calories, saturated fat less than 10% of calories, and cholesterol less than 300 mg/day. Weight loss alone may normalize triglycerides, and when combined with exercise, the HDL cholesterol levels may increase 10% to 20%. Diets that replace fat with carbohydrates raise triglycerides and lower HDL cholesterol. Reduced fat and saturated fat intake without caloric replacement with carbohydrate result in a low-calorie carbohydrate-controlled diet. Weight loss is most effective in treating hypertriglyceridemia in patients with obesity or type 2 diabetes. Also, consider supplementing with 4 g of omega-3 fatty acids, which is a potent reducer of serum triglycerides by as much as 30%.

Pages: 1138–1140

34: A 38-year-old black female is found to have stage I hypertension on routine physical examination. Her blood pressure is 142/92. She is moderately obese. Which of the following lifestyle modifications would be most effective in lowering her blood pressure:

    A. Decrease alcohol intake to no more than two drinks per day
    B. Weight reduction
    C. Restricting sodium intake to no more than 2.4 g per day
    D. Magnesium supplementation

Answer: B

Critique: The average effect of a 2-pound decrease in body weight is a decrease in systolic blood pressure of 8 mm Hg and a 6 mm Hg decrease in diastolic pressure. Sodium restriction may be additive. Limiting alcohol to no more than two drinks per day for a person who currently drinks more than four per day can lower the systolic blood pressure by 5 to 6 mm Hg and decrease diastolic blood pressure by 2 to 4 mm Hg. Lowering sodium intake in patients who are salt sensitive (e.g., the elderly, African-American patients, diabetics) may lower the average systolic blood pressure by 5 mm Hg and diastolic blood pressure by 2.5 mm Hg. Magnesium deficiency may also develop as a result of increased urinary excretion with use of thiazide and loop diuretics. In such patients, magnesium supplementation may lower blood pressure.

Pages: 1139, 1140

35: The American Diabetes Association (ADA) has made several recommendations for patients with diabetes who have normal weight and lipid levels. Which of the following statements is incorrect regarding ADA dietary recommendations:

A. Dietary guidelines recommend 30% or less of calories from total fat and 50% to 60% of calories from dietary carbohydrates.
B. Cholesterol should be restricted to 300 mg/day or less to reduce cardiovascular risk.
C. Additive sweeteners such as sucrose, saccharin, and NutraSweet are unacceptable in diabetes management.
D. Supplementation with chromium and magnesium is unnecessary when dietary intake is adequate.

Answer: C

Critique: The percentage of calories from carbohydrates should be based on the individual's eating habits, blood glucose level, and lipid goals. Individuals who have a normal blood lipid level and maintain a desirable weight should implement the U.S. Dietary Guidelines of 30% or less of calories from total fat and 50% to 60% of calories from dietary carbohydrates. Alternative sweeteners are acceptable.

Page: 1141, Table 43–21

36: The glycemic index of foods attempts to quantify the blood glucose and insulin response to different types of carbohydrates. Which of the following statements about the glycemic index is true:

A. High-fiber foods have lower glycemic potential.
B. The form of the food, the preparation method, and the influence of food combinations make the glycemic index reliable.
C. The glycemic index may help identify foods that should be avoided.
D. Simple sugars have been shown to have high glycemic responses and should be avoided to prevent hyperglycemia.

Answer: C

Critique: The glycemic index compares the total amount of glucose appearing in the bloodstream after eating a food with the total amount of glucose appearing in the bloodstream after eating the same amount of carbohydrate in the form of white bread. That high-fiber foods have a lower glycemic potential has not been borne out. The glycemic index has proved unreliable because of the variability in glucose response as a result of different forms of foods and preparation methods. The glycemic index has been helpful in identifying high glycemic potential foods, such as bananas and baked potatoes. Simple sugars have not been consistently shown to aggravate hyperglycemia. Simple sugars, such as sucrose, should be limited to 1 to 3 teaspoons/day, or 5% of carbohydrate intake.

Page: 1141

37: A 42-year-old woman, referred to you by one of your patients, weighs 250 pounds. She has no other medical problems. During her initial visit, you decide to counsel the patient about her obesity. According to the National Institutes of Health obesity guidelines, which of the following statements is incorrect:

A. Providers should address the issue of body weight at each office visit.
B. Establish a reasonable weight loss goal.
C. Establish medical goals for weight loss and tie the successive weight loss to these end points.
D. Guide the patient, and design a weight loss program.
E. Recommend increasing physical activity as part of her weight-reduction program.

Answer: A

Critique: Do not address the issue of body weight unless the patient voices a concern and there is a true medical necessity for weight loss. Because this patient has no medical problems besides her obesity, a discussion of weight loss is unnecessary; however, the risk of developing obesity-related disease is high with a body mass index (BMI) greater than 30 and extremely high with a BMI greater than 40. Establishing a reasonable weight loss goal should be individualized, taking into consideration the patient's weight history. If the patient has been overweight since childhood and has tried multiple weight-loss regimens, it may be more reasonable to use weight maintenance as a goal. If the patient has a history of a medical problem, it is also important to tie the success of weight loss to improvement in the medical problem. Increased physical activity will help the patient lose additional weight as well as improve any medical condition such as hypertension or reduction of cardiovascular risk. A successful weight-loss program involves the patient in the design of the program.

Pages: 1143, 1146

38: Bulimia, an eating disorder characterized by grossly disturbed eating behavior, eventually leads to disease or disability. Which of the following statements is true regarding bulimia:

A. Bulimia is less common than anorexia.
B. The bulimic patient might not present for first evaluation until age 30 to 40 years.
C. Bulimic patients demonstrate personality traits similar to those observed in anorexics.
D. Depressive symptoms are uncommon.

Answer: B

Critique: Bulimia has an onset between the ages of 17 and 25 years, but it is not uncommon for a bulimic woman to present for the first evaluation at age 30 or 40. Bulimia is characterized by binge eating followed by purging. Bulimics are difficult to diagnose. They have fluctuating weight and the condition may occur in both normal and overweight individuals. Their personality features differ from those of patients with anorexia nervosa, who restrict their intake. Bulimics often have impulse control problems, manifested as shoplifting or other forms of stealing, and depressive symptoms are common.

Pages: 1147, 1148

39: Which of the following statements is true regarding anorexia nervosa:

A. Patients usually present between the ages of 20 and 25.
B. The diagnosis should be suspected when significant weight loss cannot be explained by physical illness in adolescent girls.
C. Weight loss fluctuates and is associated with complaints of constipation, bloating, and abdominal pain.
D. Patients do not engage in a binge-purge cycle.

Answer: B

Critique: Anorexia nervosa is characterized by self-starvation, usually occurs between the ages of 13 and 20 years and is eight to 12 times more common in females than in males. Low weight is secondary to restrictive caloric intake and is sometimes coupled with excessive exercise and purging behavior similar to that seen in bulimia. Two subtypes of anorexics include restrictors and bulimics, who also engage in the binge-purge cycles.

Pages: 1147, 1148

40: You have received a consultation request to evaluate a 65-year-old man with a history of colon cancer. He is malnourished and has a small bowel obstruction. Your recommendations for nutritional support would include which of the following:

A. Oral and enteral feeding
B. Enteral and parenteral nutritional support
C. Parenteral nutrition alone
D. Megace

Answer: C

Critique: A well-nourished cancer patient fares better with a better sense of well-being. Tube feeding, or enteral support, is useful for patients who can effectively utilize their GI tract. It should be avoided when patients cannot tolerate the use of the GI tract because of nausea, vomiting, obstruction, or malabsorption. Total parenteral nutrition has not consistently proved to augment the response rate or survival of adult patients treated with radiotherapy or chemotherapy. Megace would be considered as an appetite stimulant in the patient with low appetite.

Pages: 1148, 1149

41: The goal of nutritional care for patients with chronic renal insufficiency is to slow the progression of renal disease. Nutrients that should be restricted in these patients include all of the following, except:

A. Protein
B. Phosphorus
C. Calcium
D. Potassium

Answer: C

Critique: Calcium supplementation is necessary to achieve the 1200 mg to 1600 mg recommended calcium intake required to achieve calcium balance. Protein and phosphorus restriction is recommended when the glomerular filtration rate drops below 70 mL per 1.73 m^2/min. If serum potassium is elevated, potassium is restricted to 40 mEq to 70 mEq/day.

Page: 1149

42: (True or False) Which of the following statements regarding nutritional management of gastrointestinal disease are true:

A. A low-fiber diet reduces the recurrence of peptic ulcer disease.
B. Coffee, caffeine, smoking, and alcohol stimulate gastric acid and should be avoided to prevent gastroesophageal reflux disease (GERD).
C. A high-fiber diet is recommended for the treatment of constipation, some phases of irritable bowel syndrome, and nonacute phases of diverticular disease.

Answers: A - False, B - True, C - True

Critique: No evidence supports a causal role of diet in peptic ulcer disease. Some evidence suggests a higher risk for recurrence of peptic ulcer disease in patients on low-fiber diets. Gastroesophageal reflux disease (GERD) may be exacerbated by coffee, caffeine, alcohol, and smoking, all of which stimulate gastric acid. A high-fiber diet is recommended for the treatment of constipation. Insoluble fiber, such as wheat bran, is very helpful for relieving constipation. Soluble and insoluble fiber is recommended for irritable bowel syndrome unless symptoms are severe with bloating, gas, pain, and excessive diarrhea. In such cases, a low-fiber, bland diet may be helpful. In the acute phase of inflammatory bowel disease and diverticulitis, fiber should be restricted.

Pages: 1149, 1150

43: Michael is a 45-year-old male new to your practice who was recently diagnosed with ulcerative colitis. Which of the following findings suggests a need for nutritional support in this patient:

A. Weight loss of 5% of previous weight
B. Persistent diarrhea for less than 1 week
C. Presence of mucosal lesions
D. Low serum albumin found on nutritional assessment

Answer: D

Critique: The decision to initiate nutritional support depends on the nutritional status of the patient and the probable clinical outcome. The low albumin level, although not specific, is a good indicator of poor nutritional status, given the clinical picture. More than a 10% loss of previous weight is considered significant. Gastrointestinal symptoms that last longer than 2 weeks are considered significant for a high-stress disease such as a severe flare of ulcerative colitis with high-volume daily bloody diarrhea. Symptoms present for 7 to 10 days may require total parenteral nutrition or tube feedings.

Page: 1150

44: (True or False) Which of the following statements regarding enteral nutrition are true:

A. Enteral nutrition should be chosen over total parenteral nutrition when a patient is unable to ingest adequate nutrients by mouth and has an intact GI tract.
B. Tube feedings should not continue for more than 8 weeks.
C. Commercial enteral solutions demonstrate a nitrogen-to-calorie ratio of 1:150.

Answers: A - True, B - True, C - True

Critique: Enteral nutrition is the preferred method of nutritional support in the absence of GI tract dysfunction such as gastroparesis, complete intestinal obstruction, paralytic ileus, severe diarrhea, and malnutrition. Enteral nutrition that preserves the function and structure of the GI tract is a more efficient use of nutrients. It should be considered when the nasogastric tube will be used for less than 4 to 8 weeks. After this time, an enterostomy tube should be utilized. The nitrogen-to-calorie ratio of most commercial enteral solutions is 1:150.

Pages: 1152, 1153

45: The complications of total parenteral nutrition may include all of the following, except:

A. Hyperlipidemia
B. Electrolyte abnormalities
C. Nutrient deficiencies
D. Hypoglycemia

Answer: D

Critique: The more common metabolic side effect is hyperglycemia. The components of parenteral alimentation include dextrose, amino acids, lipids, electrolytes, vitamins, and trace minerals. Dextrose monohydrate is primarily available in 30% to 70% concentrations. A healthy adult can clear up to 14 mg/kg/min of dextrose, but higher rates may lead to glucosuria with dehydration and increased production of CO_2 with a resultant poor ventilation. Excess glucose may result in fatty liver. Thiamine is required with high-dose glucose.

Pages: 1153, 1154

Chapter 44

Gastrointestinal Diseases

Alan R. Roth

1: The most common final diagnosis for the presenting symptom of abdominal pain in adults in a family physician's office is which of the following:

    A. Abdominal pain (cause undocumented)
    B. Acute gastroenteritis
    C. Urinary tract infection (UTI)
    D. Irritable bowel syndrome (IBS)
    E. Pelvic inflammatory disease (PID)

Answer: A

Critique: Gastrointestinal illness ranks in the top 10 most common complaints of adults to family physicians' offices. The incidence of gastrointestinal illness increases with age; among people over 65 years of age, more than 50% will suffer from hiatal hernia, constipation, or diverticulosis.

Abdominal pain of undetermined etiology accounts for approximately 50% of the diagnoses in adults presenting to family physicians' offices with abdominal pain. Acute gastroenteritis is the most common known etiology (9.2%), followed by UTI (6.7%), IBS (5.8%), and PID (3.8%).

Page: 1159, Table 44–2

2: The correct diagnosis of acute abdominal pain can be made by the experienced physician based on history and physical examination in what percentage of patients:

    A. 99%
    B. 85%
    C. 50%
    D. 25%
    E. 10%

Answer: B

Critique: In the well-regarded text by Copes, *Early Diagnosis of the Acute Abdomen,* the importance of an accurate history and physical examination is well established in the accurate diagnosis of abdominal pain. Analysis of the symptoms of abdominal pain using the mnemonic PQRST (P=provoking, palliating; Q=quantity, quality; R=region; S=severity; T=temporal issues) is extremely helpful. The diagnosis of acute abdominal pain can often be missed if a careful history is not taken. In addition, a thorough and complete physical examination should be performed and should always include rectal and pelvic examinations. The correct diagnosis can be made in 85% of the cases through history taking and physical examination.

Page: 1160, Table 44–3

3: A 20-year-old male presents with a complaint of anorexia, nausea, and right lower quadrant pain in the periumbilical region that started several hours earlier. He denies vomiting or diarrhea. Which of the following is the most likely diagnosis:

    A. Acute appendicitis
    B. Acute gastroenteritis
    C. Acute diverticulitis
    D. Acute cholecystitis
    E. Acute intestinal obstruction

Answer: A

Critique: Less than 50% of patients present with the above "textbook" presentation of appendicitis. Appendicitis occurs most frequently in patients between the ages of 10 and 30. A careful physical examination to elicit guarding, tenderness, or rebound tenderness at McBurney's point is helpful in the diagnosis. A digital rectal and a pelvic examination are essential to the diagnosis. A rigid abdomen with no bowel sounds indicates that peritonitis is present, and immediate surgical consultation is indicated.

White blood cell (WBC) count is usually moderately elevated, and on urinalysis a few red blood cells and or WBCs may be present. Diagnosis can often be confirmed with CT scan or abdominal ultrasound.

Pages: 1160, 1162, 1164

4: Which of the following is the most appropriate therapy for asymptomatic cholelithiasis in an otherwise healthy patient:

    A. Laparoscopic cholecystectomy
    B. Endoscopic retrograde cholangiopancreatography
    C. Ursodiol (Actigall)
    D. Oral cholecystogram
    E. Low-fat diet and observation

Answer: E

Critique: Between the ages of 55 and 65, 23% of females and 10% of males will have gallstones. The incidence increases with age and is most common in obese females, women with prior pregnancy, individuals with diabetes, and Native Americans. In the National Cooperative Gallstone Study, most patients without a history of pain will remain asymptomatic and therefore surgery is not indicated. However, patients who do present with a history of biliary colic pain will most likely have repeat episodes and should be referred for a cholecystectomy.

The pain of biliary colic is often abrupt in onset, usually severe, and localized to the epigastrium or right upper quadrant. The pain is usually colic in nature and associated with nausea and vomiting.

Page: 1162

5: Which of the following is most diagnostic of acute cholecystitis:

    A. Presence of calculi on ultrasound
    B. A positive oral cholecystogram
    C. Nonvisualization of the gallbladder on technetium 99m (^{99m}Tc) scan
    D. Elevated serum alkaline phosphatase level
    E. Increased white blood cell (WBC) count

Answer: C

Critique: An elevated WBC and alkaline phosphatase are helpful tools in the diagnosis of an acute abdomen. The presence of calculi, wall thickening, and sludge on ultrasound help confirm the diagnosis and should be the first-line test. However, the presence of calculi alone is not diagnostic for acute cholecystitis. With a ^{99m}Tc scan, isotope is injected and images are obtained after 1 hour and after 3 to 6 hours. If the cystic duct is obstructed, the isotope does not fill the gallbladder and the gallbladder therefore is not visualized, indicating acute cholecystitis. The diagnosis of acute cholecystitis is an indication for urgent surgical intervention.

Page: 1163

6: Which of the following is *least* likely to be found in a patient presenting with acute diverticulitis:

    A. Left lower quadrant pain
    B. Fever
    C. Left-sided tenderness on rectal examination
    D. Leukocytosis
    E. Diverticular hemorrhage

Answer: E

Critique: Diverticulitis is an inflammation of one or more diverticula. Diverticulosis is present in up to 60% of patients older than 60 years. Signs and symptoms of diverticulitis resemble those of a left-sided appendicitis and include pain, fever, and elevated white blood count. As the disease progresses, peritoneal signs may be present. Of adults who present with lower GI bleeding, diverticular hemorrhage is the cause in 20% to 40%. It occurs as bleeding in an otherwise asymptomatic patient and is not associated with acute diverticulitis.

Pages: 1163, 1164

7: Which of the following is the most appropriate diagnostic test to evaluate a patient with acute diverticulitis:

    A. Ultrasound
    B. CT scan
    C. Flexible sigmoidoscopy
    D. Colonoscopy
    E. Barium enema

Answer: B

Critique: CT testing is the method of choice in the diagnosis of acute diverticulitis. Abdominal ultrasound does not give as much information as CT scanning. Sigmoidoscopy, colonoscopy and barium enema are all contraindicated and may be associated with an increased risk of perforation. Medical therapy and stabilization of the patient are indicated before performing any invasive procedure. In general, the patient should be managed with intravenous fluids and antibiotics when symptoms are severe. Outpatient management with oral antibiotics is appropriate in less severely ill patients. In either case, the patient should be evaluated several weeks to months later with an endoscopic procedure.

Page: 1164

8: Which of the following diets is most appropriate to recommend to a patient with chronic diverticulosis:

    A. Bland diet
    B. Low-fiber diet
    C. Low-seed diet
    D. Low-residue diet
    E. High-fiber, low-fat diet

Answer: E

Critique: Epidemiologic data suggest that high-fiber diets are associated with fewer symptoms of recurrence than are other diets. Other diets have not shown to have any beneficial effects in the management of diverticulosis. For patients who cannot tolerate a high-fiber diet, bulk agents such as Metamucil, Modane, and others may be used.

Page: 1165

9: Which of the following tests is most useful in the diagnosis of acute pancreatitis:

    A. Serum amylase
    B. Amylase-creatinine clearance ratio
    C. CT scan
    D. Abdominal ultrasound
    E. Abdominal x-ray

Answer: A

Critique: Serum amylase is the most important diagnostic test in the evaluation of a patient with suspected pancreatitis. Other diseases that may cause an elevation in amylase include perforated viscus, intestinal obstruction, tubal pregnancy, and parotiditis. The serum amylase has a sensitivity of 99.9% and a specificity of 98.4%. Serum lipase may occasionally be useful and will remain elevated for 7 to 14 days after testing. Amylase-creatinine clearance ratios are not helpful. Abdominal x-ray, CT scanning, and abdominal ultrasound may be of help when the diagnosis is in doubt or the patient's condition is not improving. In most patients, the cause of acute pancreatitis is either chronic alcoholism or cholelithiasis. Other less common causes include trauma, neoplasm, hypercalcemia, hyperlipidemia, drug use, viral infections, or perforated peptic ulcer.

Page: 1166

10: The most common cause of intestinal obstruction in the pediatric patient is which of the following:

A. Hernia
B. Pyloric stenosis
C. Intussusception
D. Atresias of the bowel
E. Adhesions

Answer: A

Critique: Hernias are by far the most common cause of intestinal obstruction in the pediatric patient, accounting for 38% of cases. Other common causes include pyloric stenosis, intussusception, atresias, and annular pancreas. Adhesions are much less common in children. In adults, hernia is also the most common cause of intestinal obstruction, accounting for 41% of cases. Other common causes include adhesions, intussusception, and cancer.

Patients with intestinal obstruction often present with severe abdominal pain associated with abdominal distention, nausea, vomiting, and constipation. Bowel sounds are usually hyperactive, and plain x-ray films of the abdomen often confirm the diagnosis.

Page: 1168, Table 44–7

11: A 6-month-old infant presents with a history of several days of watery diarrhea without blood, pus, or mucus. The child also had several episodes of vomiting and has a temperature of 101°F. Which of the following is the most likely diagnosis:

A. Rotavirus
B. Enteric adenovirus
C. Norwalk agents
D. *Escherichia coli*
E. Campylobacter

Answer: A

Critique: Rotavirus is the most common cause of gastroenteritis in infants and children. It is a febrile illness that is often associated with vomiting, respiratory distress, and dehydration. Symptoms usually last 7 to 10 days. Adenovirus is the second most common cause of viral gastroenteritis in children, whereas Norwalk agents are the most common cause of gastroenteritis in adults. All bacterial infections account for less than 50% of cases of gastroenteritis in children, and therefore a culture should be performed only if symptoms persist.

Page: 1168

12: Which of the following is the most appropriate initial therapy in a child presenting with gastroenteritis and mild dehydration on physical examination:

A. Diphenoxylate hydrochloride (Lomotil)
B. Cola beverages
C. Kaopectate or Pepto-Bismol
D. Intravenous rehydration therapy
E. Oral rehydration therapy (ORT), Pedialyte, and so forth

Answer: E

Critique: Gastroenteritis with mild dehydration should be treated with oral rehydration therapy with solutions such as Pedialyte, Lytren, or Gatorade. If the child is more severely dehydrated, cannot tolerate oral therapy, or is toxic appearing, admission for intravenous hydration is indicated. Caffeinated beverages such as colas should be avoided. Fruit juices should probably be avoided as well because of their high osmolality and malabsorption potential. Opiates and other anticholinergic agents are not indicated because they have many side effects and can possibly convert gastroenteritis into sepsis or toxic megacolon.

Pages: 1170, 1171

13: Rectal bleeding characterized by the passage of bright red blood after a bowel movement would be seen most commonly with which of the following conditions:

A. Diverticulitis
B. Angiodysplasia
C. Colitis
D. Ischemic colitis
E. Hemorrhoids

Answer: E

Critique: Bleeding from a hemorrhoid follows a bowel movement and is usually associated with blood streaks on the stool, in the bowl, and on the toilet paper. Bleeding from other colon sources usually presents as large amounts of bright red to burgundy-colored stool. Melanotic or black, tarry stools are usually associated with an upper gastrointestinal bleed or a slow bleed from a colon polyp or tumor. The differential diagnosis of hemorrhoids includes anal fissures, proctitis, and rectal tumors and polyps.

Pages: 1171, 1172

14: Which of the following therapies is *not* indicated in the management of a patient with acute thrombosed external hemorrhoids:

A. Sitz baths
B. Stool softeners
C. Analgesics
D. Incision and clot removal
E. Rubber band ligation

Answer: E

Critique: Symptomatic treatment is the cornerstone of management in patients with external hemorrhoids. Sitz baths, analgesics, and stool softeners should be used routinely. An acutely thrombosed hemorrhoid may be opened and the clot removed under local anesthesia, affording some pain relief. Rubber band ligation is indicated only for internal hemorrhoids. Entrapment of the squamous epithelium of an external hemorrhoid by ligation is an extremely painful procedure that should not be used.

Pages: 1173, 1174

15: The most sensitive and specific examination in screening for colon cancer is which of the following:

A. Digital rectal examination
B. Digital rectal examination and stool guaiac
C. Sigmoidoscopy
D. Colonoscopy
E. Sigmoidoscopy and air contrast barium enema

Answer: D

Critique: The AAFP and American Cancer Society guidelines have changed several times in the past few years. Problems with screening include low yield for digital rectal examination (3% to 5%) and poor compliance with fecal occult blood testing (22% to 80%). Routine screening for occult blood yields 5% to 20% of colon polyps and 25% to 70% for cancer of the colon. Sigmoidoscopy is a good screening tool but sensitivity is only 40% to 80%, depending on the depth of insertion. Colonoscopy is the most sensitive and specific tool both for screening asymptomatic individuals and as a diagnostic procedure when symptoms are present.

Pages: 1175, 1176

16: At what bilirubin level should phototherapy be started in a term newborn who is 22 hours old and is icteric:

    A. 2.5 mg/dL
    B. 5.0 mg/dL
    C. 10.0 mg/dL
    D. 14.0 mg/dL
    E. 20.0 mg/dL

Answer: D

Critique: For a full-term newborn, phototherapy should begin at 10 mg/dL before 12 hours, at 12 mg/dL before 18 hours, and at 14 mg/dL before 24 hours.

Exchange transfusion is usually indicated for a bilirubin of greater than 20. Physiologic jaundice rarely increases by more than 5 mg/dL/day. In unusual presentations of neonatal jaundice, one should look for signs of sepsis, hemorrhage, isoimmunization, polycythemia, and congenital liver anomalies. One should also expect higher levels of bilirubin in Asian, Indian, and Hispanic infants.

Benign physiologic jaundice is the most frequent type, but it is usually not associated with bilirubin levels greater than 2 mg/dL. Higher bilirubin levels are expected in breast-fed infants, and overaggressive treatment of breast milk jaundice has led to a decline in breast-feeding.

Page: 1176

17: A 25-year-old male presents with a several-day history of nausea, vomiting, fatigue, and anorexia. On physical examination, the sclera is icteric. The patient is heterosexual with no recent unprotected sex and denies drug abuse. Which of the following is the most likely etiology of these symptoms:

    A. Hepatitis A
    B. Hepatitis B
    C. Toxoplasmosis
    D. Hepatitis C
    E. Mononucleosis

Answer: A

Critique: Hepatitis A is common in industrialized nations and is spread by poor hygiene. The disease is usually self-limited, with no carrier state. Hepatitis B and C are spread by direct contact with blood and body fluids, and both may present as an acute or a chronic disease state. Mono-nucleosis, toxoplasmosis, and cytomegalovirus are rarely associated with hepatitis. Initial diagnosis is made based on the classical history. Physical examination may reveal icterus, fever, and right upper quadrant pain. Bilirubin and hepatic enzymes are elevated, and the diagnosis is confirmed with serologic studies.

Pages: 1177, 1178

18: In a previously unvaccinated patient who is exposed to an unknown source of blood through percutaneous exposure, which of the following treatment protocols is indicated:

    A. Observe only
    B. Test patient for presence of hepatitis B antibodies
    C. Initiate hepatitis B vaccine series
    D. Hepatitis B immune globulin and begin hepatitis series
    E. Hepatitis B immune globulin only

Answer: C

Critique: An unvaccinated patient who has a percutaneous exposure to blood or body fluids should immediately begin vaccination with the hepatitis B vaccine series. If the source is known to be hepatitis B surface antigen positive or is high risk, then hepatitis B immune globulin and the hepatitis B series should be started immediately. If a person who was previously immunized is exposed to a high-risk source, then titers should be tested for hepatitis B surface antibody. If inadequate antibody levels are detected, the patient should receive hepatitis B immune globulin and a hepatitis B booster vaccine.

Page: 1179, Table 44–15

19: The most common cause of dysphagia in an adult patient is which of the following conditions:

    A. Peptic esophagitis
    B. Achalasia
    C. Scleroderma
    D. Pseudobulbar palsy (from stroke)
    E. Extrinsic compression of the esophagus

Answer: A

Critique: Dysphagia, which is difficulty in swallowing, is often secondary to constriction of the lumen of the esophagus. This condition most often results from peptic esophagitis, strictures, esophageal rings, and esophageal neoplasm. The other disorders are rare causes of dysphagia but must be considered when the diagnosis is uncertain. Achalasia is regurgitation of food secondary to the failure of the lower esophageal sphincter to relax and permit passage of food to the stomach. Dysphagia secondary to a stroke is often complicated by cough, aspiration pneumonia, and weight loss. Upper GI endoscopy is the procedure of choice in evaluating a patient with persistent dysphagia.

Page: 1179

20: A 62-year-old male with a history of gastro-esophageal reflux disease (GERD) presents with worsening symptoms of heartburn. An upper endoscopy is performed, which shows columnar epithelium extending up into the esophagus. Which of the following conditions is most likely, based on this description:

A. Hiatal hernia
B. Plummer-Vinson syndrome
C. Barrett's esophagus
D. Schatzki's ring
E. Zenker's diverticulum

Answer: C

Critique: Barrett's esophagus is a condition often seen in patients with severe, persistent gastroesophageal reflux disease. It is frequently associated with stricture, and the metaplastic epithelium may be premalignant. Adenocarcinoma of the esophagus may develop in 1% to 3% of patients, and yearly endoscopy is recommended in following these patients.

Plummer-Vinson syndrome is atrophic gastritis associated with iron deficiency anemia and esophageal webs.

Schatzki's ring is a band surrounding the lower esophageal sphincter that leads to an abrupt onset of esophageal obstruction secondary to food particles.

Zenker's diverticulum is a rare cause of dysphagia and is associated with the regurgitation of undigested food.

Page: 1180

21: A 27-year-old female presents with a complaint of abdominal discomfort following large meals. She notices distention of the abdomen with belching and flatulence. You diagnose non-ulcer dyspepsia. Which of the following is the most appropriate next step:

A. Upper GI series
B. Esophagogastroduodenoscopy (EGD)
C. Trial of an H_2 blocker
D. Trial of a proton pump inhibitor
E. Dietary modification only

Answer: C

Critique: Non-ulcer dyspepsia is one of the most common GI complaints in adults. It is often associated with overeating. Symptoms include abdominal pain, heartburn, nausea, bloating, belching, and flatulence. Approximately 15% to 25% of such patients have organic disease, which is a serious one in less than 1%. Initial management should include dietary modification and an H_2 blocker. If the patient does not respond within 7 to 10 days or if the symptoms recur after 8 weeks of therapy, then EGD is indicated.

Pages: 1181, 1182

22: All of the following factors are associated with an increased risk for the development of gastric malignancy, except:

A. Age greater than 50
B. Females
C. Smoking
D. Previous gastric ulcer
E. Presence of vomiting

Answer: B

Critique: Gastric carcinoma is a condition that often is present in patients with symptoms of dyspepsia, anorexia, and weight loss. Weight loss is the key sign that should lead to an early investigation with endoscopy. The incidence of gastric carcinoma increases with advancing age and is most common in males with a history of smoking and prior peptic ulcer disease. Recurrent vomiting, especially when associated with weight loss, is an uncommon finding with benign disease, and its presence should lead to early intervention and consultation.

Page: 1188, Table 44–17

23: Which of the following medications should the elderly patient with peptic ulcer disease avoid:

A. Sucralfate (Carafate)
B. Ranitidine (Zantac)
C. Famotidine (Pepcid)
D. Nizatidine (Axid)
E. Cimetidine (Tagamet)

Answer: E

Critique: H_2 receptor antagonists are safe and effective first-line therapy in patients with peptic ulcer disease. Due to their ease of use and safety profile they have essentially replaced antacids in medical management.

The H_2 receptor antagonists have a wide margin of safety and have gained over-the-counter status in low doses. Most of the agents are interchangeable; however, cimetidine has increased drug interactions and increased central nervous system side effects when compared with the other agents. Its use should probably therefore be limited in the elderly and patients taking multiple medications.

Pages: 1182, 1183

24: Which of the following combination therapies is *not* indicated in the management of biopsy-proven *Helicobacter pylori* infection:

A. Bismuth + metronidazole + tetracycline + H_2 receptor antagonist
B. Omeprazole + metronidazole + tetracycline + bismuth
C. Omeprazole + clarithromycin + metronidazole
D. Omeprazole + amoxicillin + bismuth
E. Omeprazole + clarithromycin

Answer: D

Critique: Many combination therapies are approved for the eradication of *H. pylori* infection in patients with peptic ulcer disease. With each therapy, one must select an H_2 receptor antagonist or a proton pump inhibitor to be used for 6 to 8 weeks of therapy. This regimen is then combined with antibiotic therapy, usually for 7 to 14 days. Approved antibiotic combinations include bismuth + metronidazole + tetracycline *or* clarithromycin + bismuth + tetracycline *or* clarithromycin + metronidazole or amoxicillin *or* amoxicillin + metronidazole *or* clarithromycin alone.

One should take into account the issue of cost and that dual-drug therapy is slightly less effective than triple-drug therapy. There is also an increasing incidence of the emergence of resistance to antibiotics, including to metronidazole and clarithromycin. This resistance can be diminished by always using two antibiotics.

Page: 1184, Table 46–19

25: All of the following are recommended in the management of a patient with gastroesophageal reflux disease, except:

    A. Avoid greasy, fatty, and spicy foods
    B. Smoking cessation
    C. Avoidance of NSAIDs
    D. Elevation of the head of the bed
    E. Small, frequent meals and a nighttime snack

Answer: E

Critique: Gastroesophageal reflux disease often presents with typical symptoms of heartburn. Up to 44% of the population have monthly symptoms of GERD. Symptoms are made worse by fatty food, spicy food, and large meals. Caffeine and alcohol may also worsen symptoms. Lifestyle modification is extremely helpful in the management of GERD and should include weight reduction, reduction in the size of meals, elevation of the head of the bed, and the patient having nothing to eat for 3 to 4 hours before bedtime.

Pages: 1184, 1185

26: Which of the following medications is associated with numerous drug interactions and has been associated with arrhythmias in patients with underlying cardiac disease:

    A. Cisapride (Propulsid)
    B. Metoclopramide (Reglan)
    C. Omeprazole (Prilosec)
    D. Nizatidine (Axid)
    E. Sucralfate (Carafate)

Answer: A

Critique: Cisapride is a prokinetic drug used as an adjunct in patients with severe GERD. However, cisapride has been shown to have numerous drug interactions, including interactions with the macrolides (clarithromycin) and imidazoles (metronidazole, fluconazole). Severe and fatal cardiac arrhythmias have been reported with the use of this drug. Cisapride is no longer used routinely because of these effects, and it is available only on a limited basis for patients with severe refractory GERD who have not responded to other agents.

Page: 1185

27: A 25-year-old female presents with a 2-week history of bloody diarrhea. The diarrhea is becoming more severe and is awakening her at night. She also admits to low-grade fever, anorexia, and weight loss. A lower endoscopy is performed, which reveals severe proctosigmoiditis spreading proximally and continuously. Which of the following is your most likely diagnosis:

    A. Crohn's disease
    B. Ulcerative colitis
    C. Irritable bowel syndrome
    D. Viral infection
    E. *Giardia lamblia*

Answer: B

Critique: The two major categories of inflammatory bowel disease are Crohn's disease and ulcerative colitis. Both diseases usually produce persistent bloody diarrhea and abdominal pain. Crohn's disease may involve the GI tract from the mouth to anus, but it is much less common in the rectum. The mucosal abnormalities are asymmetrical and discontinuous, involving the entire thickness of the bowel wall. Patients with Crohn's disease are prone to obstruction, abscesses, and fistulas.

Ulcerative colitis is limited to the rectum and colon and involves the rectum in 95% of cases. The spread is proximal and continuous and involves primarily the mucous membrane. Ulcerative colitis increases the risk for development of colon carcinoma.

Both of these diseases may produce systemic symptoms. The presence of diarrhea in the middle of the night suggests an organic pathology. Viral and parasitic infections generally are not associated with severe bloody diarrhea and proctosigmoiditis. A lower endoscopy with biopsy is diagnostic in most patients.

Page: 1186

28: The following are extraintestinal manifestations of inflammatory bowel disease, except:

    A. Iritis
    B. Ankylosing spondylitis
    C. Erosive arthritis
    D. Erythema nodosum
    E. Aphthous ulcerations

Answer: C

Critique: Both Crohn's disease and ulcerative colitis may produce systemic symptoms. Extraintestinal manifestations include iritis, ankylosing spondylitis, erythema nodosum, pyoderma gangrenosum, and aphthous ulceration. Arthritis often manifests in inflammatory bowel disease patients, but it is nondeforming and not associated with erosion of bone.

Page: 1186

29: The most common cause of chronic abdominal pain associated with diarrhea and/or constipation is which of the following:

    A. Irritable bowel syndrome
    B. Inflammatory bowel disease
    C. Infectious colitis
    D. Diverticulosis
    E. Lactose intolerance

Answer: A

Critique: Irritable bowel syndrome is a functional disorder that has no underlying structural abnormality. It affects up to 22% of the population and accounts for 59% of patients seen by gastroenterologists. The syndrome comprises four components: (1) alternating diarrhea and constipation, (2) nervous diarrhea, (3) constipation, and (4) upper GI distress. Lactose intolerance may sometimes mimic irritable bowel syndrome and can be easily diagnosed with a lactose-free diet. Evaluation with barium enema or colonoscopy of the patient with irritable bowel syndrome is normal.

Page: 1188

30: The following agents are useful in the management of patients with irritable bowel syndrome (IBS), except:

A. Psyllium agents
B. Loperamide (Imodium)
C. Donnatal
D. Amitriptyline
E. Milk of magnesia

Answer: E

Critique: The treatment of IBS is empirical and often directed at the prominent symptom (i.e., pain, diarrhea, or constipation). Agents used in treatment include anticholinergics, antispasmodics, sedatives, and bulk-forming agents (psyllium). Other options include simethicone, activated charcoal, and antidepressants (tricyclics or selective serotonin reuptake inhibitors [SSRIs]). Treatment of the patient should include education, diet modification, and multiple therapeutic trials. Routine use of laxatives, including milk of magnesia and senna preparations, should be avoided in patients with irritable bowel syndrome because they may be associated with damage to the myenteric plexus and result in cathartic colon.

Pages: 1188, 1189, Table 44–22

Chapter 45

Oncology

Alex Wilgus

1: One of the primary truisms applicable to the management of patients with cancer is:

- A. Always withhold a grave prognosis from the patient if his or her family requests that you do so.
- B. Telling patients of a poor prognosis will ultimately harm the physician—patient relationship.
- C. Once an oncologic diagnosis is made and the patient is referred to an oncologist, there is little practical need for the involvement of a primary care physician.
- D. Every patient who is capable of understanding his or her diagnosis and prognosis should be given an honest and compassionate assessment.

Answer: D

Critique: When medical care was more paternalistic physicians commonly withheld definitive information from patients about a grave diagnosis; however, as we expect more participation of patients and their families in active decision making and management with respect to their disease, it is generally helpful to give patients an honest assessment of their diagnoses and prognoses. In fact, the most harm comes to the physician–patient relationship when the physician is evasive and dishonest in explaining a patient's condition to him or her, with eventual loss of trust in the physician. Finally, the primary care physician who has long-term, well-developed relationships with patients is in a position to help the patients and their families appropriately interpret medical information and to provide guidance.

Pages: 1193, 1194

2: Among the most common oncologic emergencies that require immediate medical attention is:

- A. Asymptomatic thrombocytopenia
- B. Myocardial infarction
- C. Transient ischemic attack
- D. Severe leukopenia with signs of infection

Answer: D

Critique: Although a myocardial infarction or a transient ischemic attack may be indirectly related to a neoplastic process, neither is strictly considered to be an oncologic emergency. Thrombocytopenia certainly can constitute an oncologic emergency, but some patients may be profoundly thrombocytopenic without any systemic complications. A patient with cancer and thrombocytopenia who is bleeding clearly requires emergent attention. Finally, leukopenia with fever is a common problem encountered in patients with cancer and requires immediate attention.

Page: 1194

3: The Surveillance, Epidemiology, and End Results (SEER) program of the National Cancer Institute relies on a population-based sample of approximately 14% of the U.S. population drawn from:

- A. Specific counties from each state
- B. Portions of the five most populous states
- C. Five specific states and five specific metropolitan areas
- D. Oncology patients from the 10 largest tertiary medical centers in the United States

Answer: C

Critique: The SEER program includes monitoring areas in the states of Connecticut, Utah, New Mexico, Hawaii, and Iowa, as well as the five metropolitan areas of Detroit, Atlanta, Seattle/Puget Sound, San Francisco/Oakland, and Los Angeles. Information is systematically collected on all newly diagnosed cancers in these regions, with the exception of basal cell and squamous cell carcinomas of the skin.

Pages: 1194, 1195

4: The top three *incidence* sites for cancer in males in the United States are, in descending order:

- A. Prostate, lung, colorectal
- B. Lung, prostate, colorectal
- C. Prostate, lung, bladder
- D. Lung, colorectal, bladder

Answer: A

Critique: See Question 7.

Page: 1194

5: The top three *mortality* sites for cancer in males in the United States are, in descending order:

- A. Prostate, lung, colorectal
- B. Lung, prostate, colorectal
- C. Prostate, lung, bladder
- D. Lung, colorectal, bladder

Answer: B

Critique: See Question 7.

Page: 1195

6: The top three *incidence* sites for cancer in females in the United States are, in descending order:

A. Lung, breast, colorectal
B. Breast, lung, colorectal
C. Breast, lung, uterine
D. Lung, breast, uterine

Answer: B

Critique: See Question 7.

Pages: 1194, 1195

7: The top three *mortality* sites for cancer in females in the United States are, in descending order:

A. Breast, lung, uterine
B. Breast, lung, colorectal
C. Lung, breast, colorectal
D. Lung, breast, uterine

Answer: C

Critique: Though the rote memorization of lists is of little value and unlikely to be remembered over the long term, the answers to questions 4 through 7 illustrate some patterns that may be memorable: the highest *incidence* site of cancer subdivided by sex is a sex-specific cancer (prostate or breast). The other two of the top three (lung and colorectal) are independent of sex. The first and third most common sites for cancer *mortality* (lung and colorectal) are likewise independent of sex, and the second most common site for cancer mortality subdivided by sex is sex-specific (prostate or breast). These lists, then, are quite similar, allowing for the common sex-specific cancers, and the most commonly diagnosed cancers (prostate and breast) are less deadly than lung cancer. Also note that the third item of all of these lists is colorectal cancer.

Page: 1195

Questions 8–12: (True or False) The criteria for an optimal cancer screening test include:

8: The condition or risk factor being tested for must be important.

9: The test should be specific but need not be highly sensitive.

10: Preclinical detection of the disease by screening should allow reduction in morbidity and mortality.

11: The screening test should be available only on a limited basis to preselected patients.

12: An acceptable cost-benefit ratio should exist.

Answers: 8 - True, 9 - False, 10 - True, 11 - False, 12 - True

Critique: An appropriate disease screening test should meet several criteria. The condition being tested for should be of some consequence. Additionally, as any good laboratory test should be, a screening test should ideally have both high sensitivity and high specificity to avoid both false-positive and false-negative results. Recall that specificity refers to the proportion of subjects who are disease free and who test negative for the disease, and sensitivity is the percentage of people with the disease who test positive for the disease. As question 9 suggests,

if a test is specific but not sensitive, many people who have the disease will test negative for the presence of the disease. Clearly, early detection of the disease by screening test should make a difference; that is, an early positive test should allow some meaningful treatment to be applied toward the cure of the disease or reduction of associated morbidity. As implied by its very name, a screening test should be widely available to an entire population or to those people considered to be at somewhat higher risk for the disease being tested for. Finally, although it may not be altruistically appealing, an acceptable cost-benefit ratio must exist for widespread application of a practical screening test. A current, somewhat controversial issue focuses on the utility of colonoscopy as a colorectal cancer screening test. Colonoscopy is a relatively expensive test that would provide an uncertain benefit for the expected cost, even though it would certainly detect more cancers than flexible sigmoidoscopy or stool occult blood testing.

Page: 1196

13: The United States Preventive Services Task Force (USPSTF) gives greatest weight in its cancer screening recommendations to:

A. The screening recommendations of other professional medical organizations
B. Evidence from descriptive studies or case reports
C. Evidence from published well-designed case-control or cohort studies
D. Evidence from published randomized controlled trials

Answer: D

Critique: The USPSTF classifies evidence from randomized controlled trials as level I evidence, that is, the best scientific evidence believed to be currently available. Some of the cancer screening recommendations of professional medical organizations are based more on expert opinion and sometimes have limited scientific data to support the recommended screening tests, which is equivalent to USPSTF level III evidence. Descriptive studies, case reports, and well-designed case-control or cohort studies are considered to be different categories of level II evidence.

Page: 1196

14: Based on the 1996 recommendations of the USPSTF, the best scientific evidence supports screening mammography every 1 to 2 years for which age group:

A. 35 to 75 years of age
B. 45 to 80 years of age
C. 50 to 69 years of age
D. 40 to 70 years of age

Answer: C

Critique: Breast cancer screening using mammography every 1 to 2 years, with or without an annual clinical breast examination, is supported by "good" evidence only in the age range of 50 to 69 years. The other age ranges are not actually considered separately; however, mammography in age ranges other than 50 to 69 years is supported only with "insufficient" evidence to recommend for or against the screening. This explains why there is a multitude of varying recommendations on mammography use in breast cancer screening by other organizations.

Page: 1196

15: Based on the 1996 recommendations of the USP-STF, "good evidence" supports which of the following screening tests for preclinical cancer detection:

    A. Annual clinical breast examination
    B. Flexible sigmoidoscopy annually at 50 years of
       age and older
    C. Prostate-specific antigen (PSA) testing
    D. All of the above
    E. None of the above

Answer: E

Critique: The USPSTF recommendations for clinical preventive services are based on a 5-point scale denoting recommendations A to E. When there is "good evidence" to support an intervention, it is given an A recommendation designation. Of all the commonly used cancer screening examinations listed, none is backed by "good evidence" to support the screening test; they are all B or C recommendations.

Pages: 1196, 1197

16: Staging of a neoplastic tumor involves determining:

    A. The degree of differentiation of the cancerous
       cells
    B. The extent of malignant disease spread
    C. The susceptibility of cancerous cells to different
       chemotherapeutic drugs
    D. The physical size of the tumor

Answer: B

Critique: The stage of the neoplastic process identifies the extent of the malignant disease spread when the diagnosis is made. The grade of the tumor has more to do with the degree of differentiation of the cancer cells. The physical size of the tumor itself or the susceptibility of its cells to chemotherapeutic drugs is not considered when determining the stage of a malignant growth.

Page: 1197

17: The TNM tumor-staging acronym letters stand for, respectively:

    A. Tumor type, grade of neoplasia, metastatic
       spread
    B. Tumor type, lymph node involvement, tumor
       maturity
    C. Tumor size, lymph node involvement, metastat-
       ic spread
    D. Tumor size, grade of neoplasia, tumor maturity

Answer: C

Critique: In the commonly used TNM tumor staging system, the *T* stands for tumor size, *N* designates the lymph node involvement (with subscripts noting the loca-

tion and number of nodes), and *M* designates metastatic spread with a subscript of 0 or 1. Other staging classifications have been developed with the collaborative efforts of other professional organizations; indeed, some of these other staging systems are more commonly in use with specific neoplastic processes, such as the International Federation of Obstetricians and Gynecologists (FIGO) system for ovarian or cervical cancer.

Page: 1197

18: The differential diagnosis in a patient with cancer who has lethargy or confusion includes all of the following, except:

    A. Metabolic disturbance
    B. CNS metastases
    C. Hyperviscous blood flow
    D. Hypothyroidism secondary to radiation therapy

Answer: D

Critique: A patient with cancer, and particularly one with cancer that has some potential for metastatic spread, who presents with lethargy or confusion can be suffering from a variety of conditions. Answers A through C are certainly all possibilities in this case. Hyperviscosity of the blood, for instance, is often the result of abnormal protein production in cancers such as multiple myeloma or lymphoma. Hypothyroidism certainly can cause lethargy or confusion but would be uncommonly caused by radiation therapy.

Page: 1198

19: The usual initial symptom in patients suffering the oncologic emergency of spinal cord compression is:

    A. Lower extremity weakness
    B. Lower extremity paresthesias
    C. Bladder dysfunction
    D. Back pain

Answer: D

Critique: Almost all patients who are suffering spinal cord compression present with back pain initially. Certainly, lower extremity weakness or paresthesias could be a consequence of progressive spinal cord compression; however, if symptoms have progressed to that point and are present for more than 24 hours, they are unlikely to regress. These patients typically are examined with diagnostic radiology, and MRI is the first choice. High-dose corticosteroid therapy, surgical decompression, or external beam radiation may all be indicated to decrease the degree of spinal cord compression as rapidly as possible.

Page: 1198

20: In the management of nausea and vomiting in patients undergoing cancer chemotherapy, ondansetron (Zofran) and granisetron (Kytril) are thought to be more effective than other antiemetic agents because:

    A. They are centrally acting
    B. They are peripherally acting
    C. They are specifically designed to counteract the
       emetic properties of chemopharmaceutical agents
    D. They have better quality control because they
       are still proprietary drugs

Answer: A

Critique: The newer antiemetic medications Zofran and Kytril are thought to be more effective in battling the cancer chemotherapy side effects of nausea and vomiting because they are centrally acting. These medications are serotonin receptor antagonists. Metoclopramide (Reglan) has both central and peripheral effects and therefore also may be effective in battling the adverse effects of chemotherapeutic drugs.

Page: 1200

21: (True or False) Electronic medical journals related to oncology available on the Internet are generally trustworthy.

Answer: False

Critique: The World Wide Web has emerged as a powerful tool for access to many types of information; unfortunately, not all of it is good. Many highly reputable medical journals make their text available on line and are subject to the same peer review process as they are on the printed page. The other so-called e-journals are not published on paper and may be part of a reference service provided by a commercial medical company. For these articles, peer review may or may not be part of the Web publishing process. Finally, there is no shortage of disease-specific Web sites, which can be started by any individual with access to a computer and a Web page. These sites can generally be considered the least scientifically reliable.

Page: 1200

22: Common side effects of chemotherapeutic agents include all of the following, except:

    A. Stomatitis
    B. Alopecia
    C. Sexual functioning
    D. Depression

Answer: D

Critique: Chemotherapeutic agents can cause a plethora of side effects, including those listed in answers A to C. Depression certainly can be common among cancer patients, but it is generally not felt to be a direct result of chemotherapeutic agents. Stomatitis is common secondary to the effect of chemotherapy and radiation therapy on rapidly multiplying cells, which includes those lining the gastrointestinal tract and the oropharynx. Alopecia is one of the most visible effects of chemotherapy. Sexual function can be affected in a wide variety of ways, with loss of endogenous estrogens and androgens and a consequent effect on libido. Physical effects of radiation therapy on female cancer patients can include vaginal fibrosis and dyspareunia. Mastectomy can cause psychological distress in female patients as well as in their partners. Erectile dysfunction is a common consequence of surgical procedures such as prostatectomy.

Pages: 1200, 1201

23: Each of the following statements about cancer pain management is true, except:

    A. Cancer pain is multifactorial.
    B. Nonpharmacologic means of pain control have not been shown to be effective.
    C. Opioid pain management should include a bowel regimen to avoid constipation.
    D. The World Health Organization (WHO) guide for cancer pain management advises the initial use of non-opioid medications for mild pain.

Answer: B

Critique: All of these statements are true with the exception of B. Nonpharmacologic forms of pain management can include exercise, massage, biofeedback, guided imagery, thermotherapy, and many other integrative medicine practices. Any pain-control therapy instituted is only as effective as the patient believes it to be; thus, the consideration of any given therapy should take into account the patient's belief system and his or her faith in the therapy's effectiveness.

Pages: 1201, 1202

24: Management strategies for cancer anorexia include:

    A. Regimented weight surveillance to encourage the patient to gain weight
    B. Encouraging the patient to eat protein- and carbohydrate-rich meals
    C. Smaller, more frequent meals
    D. Avoiding certain appetite stimulants that have not been shown to be effective, such as Marinol.

Answer: C

Critique: A primary strategy for the management of cancer anorexia is to offer the patient smaller, more frequent meals and to ensure that food choices include those items that are appealing to the patient, without as much regard for the ideal nutritional value of the choices he or she may make. Although the nutritional needs of the patient with cancer are generally increased because of a normal to elevated basal metabolic rate, it does little good in the long run to harass the patient into eating food that he or she does not care to eat. Appetite stimulants can certainly be part of the treatment; some possibly helpful medications include Reglan, Megace, dexamethasone, and Marinol (which contains an active ingredient of marijuana).

Page: 1203

25: Cancer chemoprevention trials have conclusively proven the effectiveness of which of the following substances:

    A. Vitamin A analogues
    B. Selective estrogen receptor modulators (SERMs) in women at high risk of breast cancer
    C. Betacarotene
    D. Nonsteroidal anti-inflammatory drugs (NSAIDs)

Answer: B

Critique: Cancer chemoprevention concerns the use of natural or pharmacologic agents that may prevent the onset of certain types of cancers or that may reverse premalignant changes. Well-designed studies that prove or disprove the benefit of some of these agents are sometimes difficult to come by and are frequently countered by other equally well-designed studies. Vitamin A analogues have shown activity with respect to epithelial cell differentiation, but they have not been consistently proven to be helpful in chemoprevention. SERMs did demonstrate, in a double-blind randomized trial, a 44% reduction in the incidence of invasive breast cancer in high-risk patients. Several adverse events, however, were noted in the treated population, including an elevated risk of endometrial cancer, pulmonary embolus, deep venous thrombosis, and strokes. Epidemiologic studies have shown a decreased incidence of colon cancer in people who take NSAIDs; however, these have not been supported by randomized blind controlled trials. Betacarotene is a commonly cited supplement thought to have anticancer effects, but it has not been shown conclusively to produce them. It is reasonable in many cases, especially when the possible benefit is opposed by little potential harm (such as in the case of reasonable vitamin supplements), to support patients who wish to supplement their diet with some of these substances, such as selenium or vitamin E.

Pages: 1204, 1205

26: The American Cancer Society (ACS) Advisory Committee on Diet, Nutrition, and Cancer Prevention has identified all of the following as lifestyle objectives to avoid the overall risk of cancer, except:

   A. Alcohol abstinence
   B. Appropriate nutrition (e.g., five servings of fruits and vegetables a day)
   C. Regular aerobic exercise
   D. Avoidance of tobacco products

Answer: A

Critique: The ACS Advisory Committee on Diet, Nutrition, and Cancer Prevention has suggested all of the above objectives to avoid or to reduce the overall risk of cancer except for complete alcohol abstinence. It does recommend, however, a generalized decrease in the amount of alcohol consumed. The campaign promoting five servings of fruits and vegetables a day is fairly well known across the United States. Physical activity or regular aerobic exercise is a part of the recommendation, as is the complete avoidance of any tobacco product use.

Page: 1205

27: The following tumor markers have been proven effective for cancer screening purposes:

   A. Carcinoembryonic antigen (CEA) for ovary and colon cancer
   B. CA-125 for ovarian cancer
   C. PSA for prostate cancer
   D. All of the above
   E. None of the above

Answer: E

Critique: None of these tumor markers has been proven effective for cancer screening purposes. Some of them may be used to follow the tumor load or the

response to therapy of certain cancers, but they generally have not been proven to be helpful for screening because they are all lacking in one or more of the qualities of a good screening test. PSA screening for prostate cancer has not been proven to decrease morbidity or mortality, but it is in wide use as a cancer screening test, most likely because no better test is available.

Pages: 1205, 1206

28: Which of the following chemotherapeutic agents is cell-cycle S-phase dependent?

   A. Alkylating agents that prevent DNA transcription
   B. Antitumor antibiotics with antimicrobial and cytotoxic activity
   C. Antimetabolites such as methotrexate that interfere with DNA synthesis
   D. Mitotic inhibitors such as vinblastine and vincristine

Answer: C

Critique: The cell cycle consists of the G_0, or resting phase; the G_1, or physiological functioning phase; the S, or DNA synthesis phase; the G_2 phase (in which the cell contains duplicated DNA); and the M, or mitosis phase. Alkylating agents that prevent DNA transcription are not, as a class, cell-phase specific. Antitumor antibiotics such as bleomycin and doxorubicin likewise are not phase specific. Antimetabolites, because they do specifically interfere with DNA synthesis, are cell-cycle specific for the S phase. Mitotic inhibitors, as the name suggests, act specifically in the mitosis, or M, phase of the cell cycle.

Pages: 1206, 1207

Questions 29–32: (True or False) Are the following is true or false with regard to radiation therapy for cancer:

29: It should not be used for palliation.

30: Poorly perfused tumor masses are most sensitive to ionizing radiation.

31: Brachytherapy radiation is used most frequently for ovarian cancer.

32: Long-term side effects of radiation therapy occur only up to a few months after treatment is completed.

Answers: 29 - False, 30 - False, 31 - False, 32 - False

Critique: Radiation therapy is a powerful primary and adjunctive treatment for many types of cancer. It can be used for palliation, especially for painful metastatic lesions. Ionizing radiation produces cell death through the production of oxygen-free radicals that affect the cellular DNA. The availability of oxygen is of primary importance in this process; thus, poorly perfused tumors are not as sensitive to ionizing radiation as a well-perfused tumor. Brachytherapy, which involves delivery of seeds of radiation in close proximity to the tumor, is most commonly used in prostate, pharyngeal, and cervical cancers but not in ovarian cancer. Long-term side effects of radiation therapy can occur up to years after completion of the therapy and are often the consequences of damage to the vascular endothelium and stem cells.

Pages: 1207, 1208

33: All of the following cancers include tobacco use as a risk factor, except:

A. Colorectal
B. Ovarian
C. Pancreas
D. Urinary bladder
E. Cervical

Answer: B

Critique: The role of tobacco use as a risk factor for developing cancer is well known; however, there is no known direct correlation between tobacco use and the development of ovarian cancer. Certainly it is widely known that tobacco use plays a role in lung cancer; however, the role of tobacco use and the development of colorectal, pancreatic, bladder, and cervical cancer is not as well known.

Pages: 1209, 1210, 1215

34: The risk of developing colorectal cancer is increased for individuals with each of the following, except:

A. Familial adenomatous polyposis
B. High-fat/low-fiber diets
C. Ulcerative colitis
D. Excessive alcohol consumption
E. Long-term NSAID use

Answer: E

Critique: There are many risk factors for the development of colorectal cancer, some of which may be more intuitive than others. The genetic syndrome of familial adenomatous polyposis is a condition that we normally learn about in medical school but may rarely encounter. Dietary influences such as high-fat, low-fiber nutrition and excessive alcohol consumption also can lead to an increased risk of colorectal cancer. Inflammatory bowel diseases are risk factors in the development of colorectal cancers—ulcerative colitis more so than Crohn's disease. NSAID use epidemiologically decreases the risk of colorectal cancers. This has not yet been proved in randomized trials.

Page: 1209

35: It is estimated that nearly what percentage of all lung cancers are related to tobacco use and exposure to environmental tobacco smoke:

A. 75%
B. 85%
C. 90%
D. 95%

Answer: C

Critique: Roughly 90% of all lung cancers are thought to be related to tobacco use, either directly by the cancer victim or through exposure to environmental tobacco smoke. Patients who are not smokers should be aware of this so that they can take steps to ensure that they are in a smoke-free environment. Tobacco products are disproportionately named as significant risk factors for the development of a wide range of cancers.

Page: 1210

36: The risk of breast cancer is increased in people with first- or second-degree relatives who have had:

A. Colon cancer
B. Cervical cancer
C. Benign breast disease
D. All of the above
E. None of the above

Answer: A

Critique: The risk of developing breast cancer is increased in people who have first- or second-degree relatives who have suffered cancer of the breast, ovary, uterus, or colon. There is no known risk correlation in having relatives who have had cervical cancer or benign breast disease. Epidemiologic studies have also indicated an increased risk associated with a high-fat diet and exposure to endogenous or exogenous estrogens.

Pages: 1211, 1212

37: Definitive diagnosis of bladder cancer is most frequently made with:

A. Urine cytology
B. Cystoscopy
C. Hematuria
D. Urinary obstructive symptoms
E. Elevated CA-125

Answer: B

Critique: A definitive diagnosis of bladder cancer is most frequently made by a cystoscopy, by which the tumor is directly visualized with a cystoscope. Urine cytology may be used as a preliminary study for those in whom you suspect bladder cancer; however, the sensitivity of urine cytology and flow cytometry is approximately 70%, so it should not be the final negative test in the search for a bladder cancer diagnosis. Hematuria or urinary obstructive symptoms could be a presenting symptom; however, the obstructive symptoms would likely appear late in the disease process. CA-125 is a tumor marker used to monitor therapeutic response to the treatment of ovarian cancer.

Pages: 1212, 1213

38: The increased incidence of prostate cancer diagnosis has been attributed to which one of the following factors:

A. More autopsies that indicate subclinical prostate cancer in those who died of other causes
B. An increase in the relative population of African Americans, who themselves suffer an increased incidence of prostate cancer
C. Widespread use of PSA testing
D. An increase in the incidence of tobacco use

Answer: C

Critique: The increased rate of prostate cancer diagnosis is attributed to widespread use of PSA testing, despite the fact that its use as a screening test is controversial at best. Answer A is somewhat true, although the proportion of people who show subclinical prostate cancer at autopsy has probably not increased. It is well known that the more elderly a man is at death, the more likely he is to have evidence of subclinical prostate cancer. Answer B implies truthfully that African Americans suffer an increased incidence of prostate cancer; however, this author is unaware of any particular increase in the relative affected population of African Americans. Finally, there does not appear to be convincing evidence that tobacco use is a risk factor for the development of prostate cancer.

Page: 1213

39: All of the following statements about cervical cancer are true, except:

A. There is increased risk with early age at first intercourse.
B. There is increased risk with human papillomavirus (HPV) infection.
C. Recommended prevention measures include use of spermicidal contraception.
D. More cervical disease is now detected at a premalignant stage as CIN as a result of increased Pap smear screening rates.

Answer: C

Critique: All of the statements with respect to cervical cancer are true with the exception of C. A recommended prevention measure includes use of a barrier contraceptive method, not a spermicidal one. There is an increased risk of contraction of HPV disease in the absence of a barrier contraceptive method. It is certainly true that more cervical disease is now detected in the premalignant stage because of increased Pap smear screening rates.

Page: 1214

40: Malignant melanoma:

A. Is the most common form of skin cancer
B. Has an overall 5-year survival rate of more than 90%
C. Should be screened for by whole-body skin examination
D. Is more common in dark-skinned individuals

Answer: C

Critique: Malignant melanoma is not the most common form of skin cancer; that designation belongs to basal cell carcinoma. The overall 5-year survival rate for malignant melanoma is actually less than 90%, and is worse the more widespread the melanoma has become. The ABCD acronym detailed in the text provides a good reminder of how skin should be examined for possible malignant melanoma lesions. Malignant melanoma is more common in fair-skinned individuals, particularly those who have been exposed to chronic ultraviolet radiation.

Pages: 1216, 1217

41: Non-Hodgkin's lymphoma (NHL):

A. Is the most common form of cancer in persons aged 30 to 50
B. Is diagnosed by the presence of Reed-Sternberg cells on bone marrow biopsy
C. Is commonly staged after a laparotomy and splenectomy
D. Of the subtype Burkitt's lymphoma may have an etiologic relationship to the Epstein-Barr virus.

Answer: D

Critique: NHL is the most common form of cancer in persons aged 20 to 40, rather than 30 to 50. The presence of Reed-Sternberg cells on bone marrow biopsy is a feature of Hodgkin's disease (HD), not NHL. Similarly, staging of NHL is typically achieved with the collection of a tissue specimen, chest x-ray, CT scan of the abdomen and pelvis, and bone marrow biopsy. Laparotomy is infrequently used to stage NHL. HD is typically staged surgically with laparotomy, splenectomy, and lymph node biopsy. Burkitt's lymphoma, a subtype of NHL, does have an apparent etiologic relationship to the Epstein-Barr virus, which is also true of HD in general.

Pages: 1217, 1218

42: Chronic lymphocytic leukemia (CLL):

A. Is the most common type of leukemia in the United States
B. Is more highly correlated with the presence of the Philadelphia chromosome than any other leukemia
C. Uncommonly causes death through comorbid complications
D. Has a median age at diagnosis of about 50 years

Answer: A

Critique: CLL is the most common type of leukemia found in the United States. The relationship to the Philadelphia chromosome is one that is more common with chronic myelogenous leukemia, being found in approximately 95% of patients with that disease. CLL commonly causes death through comorbid complications, such as an infection, because of immunologically less functional lymphocytes. The median age of diagnosis of CLL is closer to 70 years.

Page: 1220

Chapter 46

Hematology

Robert G. Hosey

1: Red blood cell distribution width (RDW) may be falsely elevated by all of the following, except:

   A. Splenectomy
   B. Presence of cold agglutinins
   C. Beta thalassemia
   D. Prosthetic heart valves

Answer: C

Critique: RDW is an indicator of red blood cell (RBC) size distribution. It may be falsely elevated in patients who have had a splenectomy, a blood transfusion, or a prosthetic heart valve or in the presence of cold agglutinins. It is not elevated in thalassemia.

Pages: 1224, 1225

Questions 2 to 4: Match the inclusion body type with the clinical syndrome in which it is found:

   A. Siderotic granules
   B. Heinz bodies
   C. Howell-Jolly bodies
   D. Basophilic stippling

2: Functional asplenia

3: Lead poisoning

4: Megaloblastic anemia

Answers: 2 - C, 3 - D, 4 - A

Critique: In a peripheral blood smear, red blood cell inclusion bodies can be helpful in making a diagnosis. Siderotic granules can be seen in patients with sideroblastic anemia, hemoglobinopathies, or megaloblastic anemia and after splenectomy. Heinz bodies are seen in unstable hemoglobin, hemoglobinopathies, and erythrocyte enzyme deficiencies. Howell-Jolly bodies can be seen in functional asplenia or postsplenectomy. Basophilic stippling is seen in lead poisoning and thalassemia.

Page: 1225

5: Regarding reticulocytes, which of the following statements is *not* true? Reticulocytes:

   A. Spend 24 hours in peripheral blood before maturation
   B. Account for 1% to 2% of total red blood cells in normal states
   C. Have a higher affinity for O_2 than do mature RBCs
   D. Are approximately twice the size of normal RBCs

Answer: C

Critique: Reticulocytes are immature red blood cells. They are produced in the bone marrow, spend 24 hours in the peripheral circulation before maturation, are approximately twice the diameter of mature red cells, and total 1% to 2% of the RBC count in normal situations, but they do not exhibit a higher affinity for oxygen than do mature RBCs.

Page: 1225

6: Bone marrow biopsy may be useful in all of the following, except:

   A. Detecting myelofibrosis
   B. Monitoring osteoporosis
   C. Monitoring leukemia
   D. Assessing iron stores

Answer: B

Critique: Bone marrow examination is commonly used to assess iron stores, detect bone marrow abnormalities such as myelofibrosis, and monitor blood malignancies (leukemia). It is not typically employed to monitor osteoporosis. Positron emission densitometry scanning is a noninvasive test that can be used to assess bone mineral density and monitor osteoporosis.

Page: 1225

7: Which of the following states does not increase erythrocyte 2,3-DPG:

   A. Anemia
   B. Acidosis
   C. High altitude exposure
   D. Alkalosis

Answer: D

Critique: 2,3-DPG is one factor that determines release of oxygen molecules from RBCs. 2,3-DPG binds to hemoglobin to reduce its oxygen affinity and increase delivery of oxygen to the tissues. It is increased in states such as anemia, acidosis, high altitude exposure, hypoxia, and blood loss. It is not increased in the alkalotic state.

Page: 1227

Questions 8 to 13: Match the blood cell with the most appropriate clinical state or characterizing feature:

   A. Neutrophils
   B. Eosinophils
   C. Basophils

D. Monocytes
E. T-lymphocytes
F. B-lymphocytes

8: Allergies

9: Fight infection by phagocytosis

10: Cell surface has high affinity receptors for IGE

11: Granules contain interleukin-1

12: Responsible for humoral immunity

13: Responsible for cell-mediated immunity

Answers: 8 - B, 9 - A, 10 - C, 11 - D, 12 - F, 13 - E

Critique: Neutrophils help the body fight infection by engulfing (or phagocytizing) invading organisms. They also produce bactericidal toxins to help combat infections. Eosinophils have protein-containing granules that bind to parasites and disrupt their membranes. Eosinophils also act as immune modulators in allergic diseases. The surface of basophils has receptors for IgE. Basophils have granules that contain histamines, leukotrienes, serotonin, bradykinin, and heparin that may be released once IgE is bound to the cell surface. Monocytes have granules that contain IL-1, which is an inflammatory agent. T- and B-lymphocytes are responsible for cell-mediated and humoral immunity, respectively.

Page: 1228

Questions 14 to 16: Match the anemia with the correct corresponding red blood cell (RBC) morphology:

A. Iron deficiency anemia
B. B_{12} deficiency anemia
C. Anemia of chronic disease

14: Microcytic hypochromic RBCs

15: Normocytic RBCs

16: Macrocytic RBCs

Answers: 14 - A, 15 - C, 16 - B

Critique: Erythrocyte size and pigmentation can be clues to the underlying problem in anemic patients. Iron deficiency results in failure of the bone marrow to produce adequate numbers of RBCs. The RBCs that are produced are small (microcytic) and hypochromic. B_{12} deficiency results in impaired DNA synthesis and ineffective erythropoiesis. Resultant red blood cells are typically macrocytic. Anemia of chronic disease occurs secondary to a chronic disease such as renal insufficiency. RBCs are usually normocytic in anemia of chronic disease.

Pages: 1229, 1231, 1234

17: Which of the following is not consistent with iron deficiency anemia:

A. Low serum iron
B. Elevated serum ferritin level
C. Elevated total iron binding capacity (TIBC)
D. Low mean corpuscular volume (MCV)

Answer: B

Critique: Iron deficiency anemia is associated with low serum iron, a decreased ferritin level, elevated total iron binding capacity, and a low red blood cell MCV.

Page: 1227

18: All of the following are true about iron, except:

A. Iron is absorbed in the large intestine.
B. Iron serves as a catalyst for cytochrome oxidase.
C. Total iron content in the body is 40 to 50 mg/kg.
D. Gastric acid aids in absorption.

Answer: A

Critique: Iron is an important mineral in hemoglobin synthesis. It also acts as a catalyst for many enzymes, including cytochrome oxidase. Normal iron stores in the body typically range from 40 to 50 mg/kg. Values are somewhat higher for males on the average than for females. Absorption of iron occurs in the duodenum and upper part of the jejunum and is enhanced by an acidic environment.

Page: 1229

19: Which of the following is true regarding iron replacement therapy:

A. Replacement is commonly given as ferrous sulfate 325 mg once weekly.
B. Replacement should be continued for 1 year.
C. Hemoglobin concentration should normalize by 6 weeks after replacement.
D. Reticulocytosis begins after 2 weeks.

Answer: C

Critique: Iron replacement therapy requires management of ongoing iron loss as well as supplementation of iron. Iron therapy is typically in the form of ferrous sulfate 325 mg given between one and three times a day for up to 6 months. With replacement therapy, reticulocytosis begins within a few days and peaks at 8 to 10 days. Hemoglobin concentrations normalize by 6 weeks, although it may take months for RBC indices to normalize.

Pages: 1229, 1231

20: Which of the following is associated with vitamin B_{12} (cobalamin) deficiency:

A. A decrease in serum homocysteine
B. Hyposegmentation of neutrophils
C. Microcytic hypochromic red blood cells
D. Loss of intrinsic factor

Answer: D

Critique: Vitamin B_{12} deficiency affects approximately 1% of the population at some point during life. B_{12} is absorbed in the terminal ileum as cobalamin-intrinsic factor complex. Loss of intrinsic factor is the most common cause of B_{12} deficiency. B_{12} deficiency is also associated with an increase of homocysteine and hypersegmented neutrophils. B_{12} deficiency leads to macrocytic, rather than microcytic, RBCs.

Page: 1231

Questions 21 to 25: (True or False): The neurologic syndrome associated with B$_{12}$ deficiency may be characterized by:

21: Paresthesias

22: Decreased vibratory sensation

23: Dysarthria

24: Ataxia

25: Reversible symptoms with treatment

Answers: 21 - True, 22 - True, 23 - False, 24 - True, 25 - False

Critique: Vitamin B$_{12}$ deficiency can result in a neurologic syndrome. Clinical features of this neurologic syndrome include paresthesias, decreased vibratory sensation, ataxia, clonus, hyperreflexia, and muscle spasticity. Institution of B$_{12}$ therapy will not reverse neurologic symptoms once they are present.

Pages: 1231, 1233

26: Which of the following is true regarding B$_{12}$ therapy:

    A. Treatment should be continued for patient's lifetime.
    B. Oral preparations of B$_{12}$ are most effective.
    C. Treatment should be withheld until Schilling test results are known.
    D. Treatment should not be given unless the patient is anemic.

Answer: A

Critique: B$_{12}$ therapy is most effective when given intramuscularly. It is recommended for patients with a low B$_{12}$ level and in patients with neurologic syndrome with or without anemia. The suggested dose is 1 mg given intramuscularly every week for 8 weeks and then every month for life.

Page: 1234

27: Which of the following would be unlikely to cause an anemia of chronic disease:

    A. Systemic lupus erythematosus
    B. Chronic osteomyelitis
    C. Coronary artery disease
    D. Chronic renal insufficiency

Answer: C

Critique: Anemia of chronic disease may be the result of inadequate iron utilization, inhibitory effects of cytokines (chronic infection, collagen vascular diseases), or decreased response to erythropoietin (chronic renal insufficiency). It is unlikely to result from coronary artery disease.

Page: 1234

28: Anemia of chronic disease is associated with all of the following, except:

    A. Increased total iron binding capacity
    B. Decreased serum iron
    C. Increased ferritin
    D. Normocytic anemia

Answer: A

Critique: In anemia of chronic disease, the red blood cells are usually normocytic and ferritin is increased, which helps distinguish anemia of chronic disease from iron deficiency anemia. Serum iron and total iron binding capacity are decreased.

Page: 1234

29: Which of the following is true regarding erythropoietin (EPO):

    A. It is recommended for patients with anemia of chronic disease.
    B. It is produced in the adrenal gland and pancreas.
    C. It needs to be given with iron supplementation.
    D. It is not useful in treating anemia associated with human immunodeficiency virus (HIV) infection.

Answer: C

Critique: EPO is commonly used in the treatment of anemia of chronic renal failure and for anemia associated with HIV but not for all causes of anemia of chronic disease. It is produced in both the kidney and the liver. Iron supplementation needs to be given with EPO because of increased iron utilization caused by EPO stimulation of erythropoiesis.

Page: 1237

30: Which of the following is *not* a hematologic effect of chronic alcohol use:

    A. Impairment of iron utilization
    B. Decreased body iron stores
    C. Decreased RBC survival
    D. Thrombocytopenia

Answer: B

Critique: Thrombocytopenia, and decreased red blood cell survival are all associated with long-term use of alcohol. Ethanol itself impairs iron utilization. Iron body stores, however, are usually elevated because of increased absorption and ingestion of iron-containing alcoholic beverages.

Page: 1237

Questions 31 to 37: (True or False) Determine which of the following statements are true or false regarding hereditary hemochromatosis:

31: It has an autosomal dominant inheritance pattern.

32: Intestinal iron absorption is increased.

33: Typical onset is in the second and third decades of life.

34: Hepatoma is a rare (<5%) complication.

35: Clinical manifestations include cirrhosis, diabetes, and hyperpigmented skin.

36: Increased ferritin and decreased transferrin saturation occur.

37: Initial treatment consists of weekly phlebotomy.

Answers: 31 - False, 32 - True, 33 - False, 34 - False, 35 - True, 36 - False, 37 - True

Critique: Hereditary hemochromatosis (HH) is an autosomal recessive disorder manifested by accumulation of iron in various organs. The primary defect in HH is increased intestinal absorption of iron. HH affects 2 to 5 per 1000 Caucasians, with a typical onset in the fourth or fifth decade of life. Clinical manifestations include cirrhosis and so-called bronze diabetes. Both ferritin and transferrin saturation are increased in HH, with (fasting) transferrin saturation being the best screening test for HH. Unfortunately for patients with HH, hepatoma is not uncommon, and approximately 29% of HH patients develop it. Initial treatment of HH is weekly phlebotomy to decrease iron stores and prevent organ damage.

Pages: 1238–1240

38: All of the following are associated with risk of venous thrombosis, except:

  A. Protein C deficiency
  B. Protein S elevation
  C. Antithrombin III deficiency
  D. Activated protein C resistance

Answer: B

Critique: An increased risk of venous thrombosis is associated with a deficiency of protein C, protein S, and antithrombin III and also with activated protein C resistance.

Page: 1240

39: Activated protein C resistance results from a mutation in which of the following:

  A. Factor V
  B. Factor VIII
  C. Factor VII
  D. Factor III

Answer: A

Critique: Activated protein C (APC) resistance is the most common inherited tendency to venous thromboembolism. It is produced by a mutation in coagulation factor V and is also known as factor V Leiden. This mutation causes factor V to be resistant to APC. This mutation is found in up to 50% of individuals with unexplained venous thrombosis.

Page: 1240

Questions 41 to 49: (Matching) Match the coagulation abnormality with the appropriate statement. (Each response may be used once, more than once, or not at all.)

  A. Resistance to activated protein C
  B. Protein C deficiency
  C. Protein S deficiency
  D. Antithrombin III deficiency
  E. G20210 prothrombin mutation
  F. Hyperhomocysteinemia
  G. Antiphospholipid syndrome

41: Affects coagulation factors II, IXa, and Xa

42: Affects coagulation factors V and VIII

43: Recurrent fetal loss and cardiac valve abnormalities

44: Results from mutation in coagulation factor V

45: Can be treated with folate and pyridoxine supplementation

46: Associated with increased prothrombin levels

47: Reduces effectiveness of heparin

48: Has propensity to cause arterial thrombosis

49: Homozygous deficiency results in purpura fulminans of neonate

Answers: 41 - D, 42 - B, 43 - G, 44 - A, 45 - F, 46 - E, 47 - D, 48 - G, 49 - B

Critique: Resistance to activated protein C results from a mutation in coagulation factor V and is also known as factor V Leiden. Protein C is a vitamin-dependent protein that acts as an anticoagulant by inactivating coagulation factors V and VIII. Homozygous deficiency of protein C results in purpura fulminans of the neonate and is uniformly fatal. Protein S is a cofactor for protein C, and deficiency has similar effects on the coagulation pathway as those of protein C deficiency. Antithrombin III inactivates thrombin (factor II), factor IXa, and factor Xa. It also serves as a cofactor for heparin and, in the deficient state, reduces the effectiveness of heparin over time. G20210 mutation is a point mutation of the prothrombin gene, which results in elevated levels of prothrombin. The result is an increased risk of venous thromboembolism in these patients. Elevated levels of homocysteine are associated with both arterial and venous occlusive disease. Treatment involves supplementation of folate and pyridoxine on a daily basis. Antiphospholipid syndrome (APS) is an acquired disorder that is associated with the presence of lupus anticoagulant and anticardiolipin antibody. APS has a propensity to cause arterial thrombosis.

Pages: 1240–1242

50: Which of the following statements is true regarding heparin-induced thrombocytopenia:

  A. It may be avoided by using low molecular weight heparin.
  B. It results only in venous thrombosis.
  C. It is managed by gradual withdrawal of heparin therapy.
  D. It occurs in approximately 5% of patients treated with a therapeutic course of heparin.

Answer: D

Critique: Heparin-induced thrombocytopenia (HIT) occurs with the formation of IgG antibodies to the heparin-platelet complex. Platelet counts may fall to <50,000/mm^3 and should be cause for concern. HIT has been associated with low molecular weight heparin and unfractionated heparin. It occurs in approximately 5% of patients treated with a therapeutic course of heparin. Venous and arterial thrombosis (including stroke and myocardial infarction) may occur. HIT is treated by immediate withdrawal of heparin therapy.

Page: 1243

51: Which of the following statements is true regarding warfarin necrosis of the skin and subcutaneous tissue:

    A. It typically occurs 10 to 14 days after institution of oral anticoagulation therapy.
    B. It has a predilection for affecting the penis.
    C. It likely occurs because of a transient hypercoagulation induced by warfarin.
    D. It results in thrombosis of small veins, capillaries, and arteries.

Answer: C

Critique: Warfarin necrosis may occur in up to 0.1% of treated patients, most often in obese women. Symptoms typically start 3 to 5 days after institution of therapy and usually affect areas with abundant subcutaneous tissue (buttocks, thighs, and breasts). The penis is an unusual site of necrosis. Thrombosis of small veins, capillaries, and venules is seen on histology. Arteries are spared. The cause of warfarin necrosis is likely a transient hypercoagulation state that is induced by the warfarin.

Page: 1243

52: Hemolytic anemia resulting from an enzyme defect in the glycolytic pathway is consistent with a diagnosis of which of the following:

    A. Pyruvate kinase deficiency
    B. Glucose 6 phosphate dehydrogenase (G6PD) deficiency
    C. Spherocytosis
    D. Creatine kinase deficiency

Answer: A

Critique: Pyruvate kinase deficiency can cause a hemolytic anemia by means of an enzyme defect in the glycolytic pathway. G6PD deficiency may result in a hemolytic anemia because of a lack of ability to deal with oxidative stresses. G6PD is the enzyme that produces NADPH in the erythrocyte from NADP.

Spherocytosis is a congenital RBC structural abnormality that may lead to hemolytic anemia. Creatine kinase is an enzyme that is responsible for the production of adenosine triphosphate from creatine phosphate and adenosine diphosphate in the mitochondria.

Pages: 1243, 1244

Questions 53 to 58: (Matching) Match the following causes of hemolytic anemic with the appropriate corresponding characteristics:

    A. Glucose 6 phosphate dehydrogenase (G6PD) deficiency
    B. Pyruvate kinase deficiency
    C. Thrombotic thrombocytopenic purpura
    D. Hemolytic uremic syndrome

53: Increased RBC rigidity results from decreased ATP in RBCs

54: Fragmented RBCs and schistocytes

55: Associated with *E. coli* 0157:H7 infection

56: Ingestion of fava beans can lead to massive hemolytic anemia

57: Deposition of platelet microthrombi in kidney and brain

58: Associated with formation of Heinz bodies in affected RBCs

Answers: 53 - B, 54 - C, 55 - D, 56 - A, 57 - C, 58 - A

Critique: G6PD is the enzyme that produces NADPH in the erythrocyte from NADP. G6PD deficiency may result in a hemolytic anemia because of a lack of ability to deal with oxidative stresses. Ingestion of fava beans may increase oxidative stress and lead to massive hemolysis. Heinz bodies (in RBCs) may be seen in individuals with G6PD deficiency and hemolytic anemia. This occurs when oxidized glutathione reacts with hemoglobin and causes precipitation into Heinz bodies. Pyruvate kinase deficiency may lead to hemolysis as a result of increased rigidity of the RBC membrane caused by decreased ATP in the RBC. Thrombotic thrombocytopenic purpura (TTP) is caused by platelet aggregation mediated by large von Willebrand factors that have entered the circulation. It is characterized by platelet microthrombi deposition in the kidneys and brain as well as by fragmented RBCs or schistocytes on peripheral blood analysis. Hemolytic-uremic syndrome typically affects children and is caused by enteric infections with either *E. coli* or *Shigella*.

Pages: 1243–1245

59: The laboratory features of ITP include all of the following, except:

    A. Decreased white blood cell (WBC) count
    B. Normal RBC morphology
    C. Normal hemoglobin (Hb)
    D. Decreased platelets

Answer: A

Critique: Idiopathic thrombocytopenic purpura (ITP) should be suspected in an individual with a decreased platelet count, mucosal bleeding, and petechiae. Although platelets are decreased, RBC morphology, hemoglobin, and WBC counts are usually normal.

Pages: 1245, 1246

60: The treatment of choice in adults with idiopathic thrombocytopenic purpura (ITP) is which of the following:

    A. Intermittent platelet transfusions
    B. Bone marrow transplantation
    C. Splenectomy
    D. Chronic prednisone therapy

Answer: C

Critique: Because ITP is a chronic disease with few spontaneous remissions, splenectomy is the treatment of choice.

Page: 1246

61: Which of the following laboratory tests is not consistent with a diagnosis of disseminated intravascular coagulation (DIC):

A. Elevated aPTT
B. Increased fibrinogen
C. Decreased levels of antithrombin III
D. Decreased levels of plasminogen

Answer: B

Critique: DIC is characterized by simultaneous systemic coagulation and fibrinolysis. Patients with DIC have evidence of coagulopathy in the form of elevated PT and aPTT. In addition, they have decreased levels of fibrinogen, antithrombin III, and plasminogen.

Page: 1247

62: Which of the following should not be considered in the treatment of DIC:

A. Intravenous estrogen therapy
B. Heparin
C. Fresh frozen plasma (FFP)
D. Cryoprecipitate

Answer: A

Critique: Because DIC involves both simultaneous coagulation and fibrinolysis, heparin, FFP, and cryoprecipitate may all be appropriate in management. IV estrogen therapy is not indicated for use in DIC.

Page: 1247

Questions 63 to 64: (True or False) Patients with autoimmune hemolytic anemia (AHA) typically demonstrate:

63: Positive direct Coombs test

64: Negative indirect Coombs test

Answers: 63 - True, 64 - False

Critique: AHA is associated with autoantibodies directed against RBC antigens and loss of immune tolerance. These autoantibodies can fix complement and cause direct lysis of RBCs. Individuals with AHA have a positive direct Coombs test and also generally have a positive indirect Coombs test.

Page: 1249

65: Hapten mediation is a mechanism for which of the following types of hemolytic anemia:

A. Autoimmune
B. Drug induced
C. G6PD deficiency
D. Spherocytosis

Answer: B

Critique: Hapten mediation occurs when a patient makes antibodies against a drug. The resultant antibody-drug complex binds to RBCs. When additional amounts of the drug are given, the resultant antibody response causes hemolysis.

Page: 1249

66: Ineffective erythropoiesis in sideroblastic anemia results in which of the following:

A. Decreased iron values
B. Increased iron values
C. Decreased zinc values
D. Increased zinc values

Answer: B

Critique: Sideroblastic anemia results from ineffective erythropoiesis. As a result, iron stores in the body are increased. Zinc body stores are not affected by sideroblastic anemia.

Pages: 1249, 1250

67: Recommended treatment of hereditary sideroblastic anemia includes which of the following:

A. Vitamin B_{12} therapy
B. Iron supplementation
C. Prednisone therapy
D. Vitamin B_6 (pyridoxine) therapy

Answer: D

Critique: Most patients with hereditary sideroblastic anemia respond to pyridoxine therapy. A dosage of 200 mg/day is recommended over a 3-month treatment period.

Page: 1250

68: Which of the following drugs has been associated with the acquired form of sideroblastic anemia:

A. Trimethoprim
B. Phenytoin
C. Isoniazid
D. Carbamazepine

Answer: C

Critique: Drugs that interfere with pyridoxine metabolism have been implicated in the secondary form of sideroblastic anemia. Of the above choices, only isoniazid interferes with pyridoxine metabolism.

Pages: 1250, 1251

69: Skeletal abnormalities associated with Fanconi's anemia include which of the following:

A. Osteoporosis
B. Osteopetrosis
C. Hypoplasia of the radii
D. Muscular necrosis of the hip

Answer: C

Critique: Fanconi's anemia is an autosomal recessive aplastic anemia. It is associated with multiple skeletal deformities, including microcephaly, short stature, and hypoplasia of the radii and thumbs.

Pages: 1251, 1252

Questions 70 to 81: (True or False) Determine whether the following statements concerning sickle cell anemia are true or false:

70: Sickle cell crisis is common in newborns with sickle cell disease.

71: Pain crisis is the most common presenting symptom in children under the age of 2 years.

72: Vaso-occlusive crisis resulting in abdominal pain is caused by infarcts of the mesentery and viscera.

73: Splenic infarction typically results in a nonfunctional spleen by the age of 2 years.

74: Acute chest syndrome (ACS) is most often caused by pulmonary embolism.

75: The treatment of choice for ACS is exchange transfusion.

76: The normal half-life of sickled red blood cells is 40 to 50 days.

77: The most common cause of bacterial infection in patients with sickle cell disease is *Streptococcus pneumoniae*.

78: Sickle cell patients with a history of cerebrovascular accident (CVA) are unlikely to have a repeat CVA.

79: Penicillin prophylaxis is recommended for children younger than 5 years.

80: Common causative agents of osteomyelitis include salmonella and *Staphylococcus aureus*.

81: Patients with sickle trait may experience systemic sickling of erythrocytes.

Answers: 70 - False, 71 - False, 72 - True, 73 - True, 74 - False, 75 - True, 76 - False, 77 - True, 78 - False, 79 - True, 80 - True, 81 - True

Critique: Sickle cell anemia is an autosomal codominant disorder of hemoglobin configuration. Abnormal hemoglobin (HbS) causes RBCs to undergo sickling in the deoxygenated state. Sickled RBCs have a shorter half-life (10 to 20 days) and can cause vaso-occlusion. Sickle cell anemia is prevalent in the African-American population, with 1 in 12 having sickle cell trait and 1 in 650 having sickle cell disease. Newborns are protected from sickle cell crisis by a high level of fetal hemoglobin and thus do not typically experience sickle cell crisis. The most common manifestations of sickle disease in children under the age of 2 years are dactylitis and splenic sequestration. Pain crisis is the most common symptom after the age of 2. Vaso-occlusive crisis can occur throughout the organs of the body. Crisis with abdominal pain is likely secondary to infarcts of the mesentery and viscera. Repeated splenic infarction is common and results in a nonfunctioning spleen, usually by the age of 2. ACS is usually the result of microvascular thrombotic disease affecting multiple lobes. Less commonly, it can result from infection or pulmonary embolism. Treatment of choice for ACS involves exchange transfusion.

Because of functional asplenia and defects in opsonization, sickle cell patients are prone to bacterial infections. Encapsulated organisms such as *S. pneumoniae* (most common bacterial pathogen in sickle cell patients) pose significant threat. Osteomyelitis is also a potential problem. Salmonella species and *S. aureus* are common causative pathogens in osteomyelitis. Because of the high risk of infection in children with sickle cell disease, penicillin prophylaxis is recommended for patients younger than 5 years. In patients who have suffered a CVA, the risk of recurrence is 60% to 80%.

Although patients with sickle cell trait do not suffer the major complications associated with sickle cell disease, they may experience systemic sickling of erythrocytes under conditions of severe hypoxia.

Pages: 1252–1255

Questions 82 to 84: (Matching) Match the following thalassemias with the appropriate statements:

    A. α-thalassemia minor
    B. β-thalassemia minor
    C. β-thalassemia major
    D. Both choices B and C

82: Increased accumulation of β-globin chains of hemoglobin

83: Has high percentage of fetal hemoglobin

84: Mild asymptomatic hemolytic anemia

Answers: 82 - A, 83 - C, 84 - B

Critique: Thalassemias are a group of disorders caused by the absence (major) or defective synthesis (minor) of one or more of the polypeptide globin chains of hemoglobin. In α-thalassemia, the absence or presence of defective α-globin leads to an increased accumulation of β-globin chains. β-thalassemia minor is associated with a mild asymptomatic hemolytic anemia. β-thalassemia major leads to severe hemolytic anemia with hemoglobin dropping to 3 to 4 g/dL, most of which is fetal hemoglobin.

Page: 1255

85: Thrombocytopenia in pregnancy is most closely associated with which of the following:

    A. Gestational diabetes
    B. Congenital hydrocephalus
    C. Pregnancy-induced hypertension
    D. Aspirin use

Answer: C

Critique: Thrombocytopenia in pregnancy is most closely associated with pregnancy-induced hypertension. It may also be seen in pre-eclampsia. It is not associated with gestational diabetes or congenital hydrocephalus. Although aspirin affects platelet function, its use is not associated with thrombocytopenia in pregnancy.

Page: 1256

86: Secondary thrombocytosis is characterized by which of the following:

    A. Increased production of platelets
    B. Platelet counts greater than 1,000,000
    C. Thrombotic episodes
    D. Treatment with splenectomy

Answer: A

Critique: Secondary or reactive thrombocytosis may have a number of underlying causes that result in increased production of platelets. In affected individuals, platelet counts are usually less than 1,000,000/mm³. Patients are usually asymptomatic, thrombotic occurrences are rare, and specific treatment is not usually necessary because platelet counts tend to return to normal over time.

Pages: 1256, 1258

87: A platelet count of greater than 1,000,000 may be seen in which of the following:

    A. Essential thrombocythemia
    B. Chronic myelogenous leukemia (CML)
    C. Polycythemia vera
    D. All of the above

Answer: D

Critique: Essential thrombocythemia, CML, and polycythemia vera can all result in platelet counts exceeding 1,000,000/mm³. In these situations, thrombosis of both large and small vessels is possible.

Page: 1258

88: Risk of severe bacterial infection is increased with an absolute neutrophil count that is below which of the following:

    A. 500/mm³
    B. 750/mm³
    C. 1000/mm³
    D. 250 mm³

Answer: A

Critique: Absolute neutrophil counts below 500 mm³ are associated with significant risk of severe infection. Gram-negative bacteria and *S. aureus* are common pathogens in patients with severe neutropenia.

Pages: 1259, 1261

89: Which of the following is not associated with Felty's syndrome:

    A. Splenomegaly
    B. Rheumatoid arthritis
    C. Short stature
    D. Neutropenia

Answer: C

Critique: Felty's syndrome is an autoimmune disorder characterized by rheumatoid arthritis, splenomegaly, and neutropenia. Short stature is not a characteristic of Felty's syndrome.

Page: 1261

90: Which of the following disease processes is not associated with eosinophilia:

    A. Adenocarcinoma of the lung
    B. *S. aureus* abscess
    C. *Strongyloides* infection
    D. Systemic lupus erythematosus

Answer: B

Critique: Eosinophilia can be seen in allergic disorders, malignancies, collagen vascular disease, and parasitic infections. It would not be expected with a bacterial abscess.

Pages: 1261, 1262

91: The laboratory finding suggestive of erythrocytosis due to a secondary cause is which of the following:

    A. Decreased thrombopoietin level
    B. Increased erythropoietin level
    C. Increased reticulocyte count
    D. Increased reticulocyte index

Answer: B

Critique: Numerous diseases, including sleep apnea, renal artery stenosis, chronic pulmonary disease, and hypoxia, may cause secondary erythrocytosis. The hallmark of secondary erythrocytosis is an elevated hemoglobin or hematocrit level with an increased erythropoietin level. Decreased erythropoietin levels are seen in polycythemia vera. Reticulocyte count is not helpful in the diagnosis of secondary erythrocytosis. Thrombopoietin affects the platelet series rather than erythrocyte production.

Pages: 1262, 1264

92: The leading cause of death from polycythemia vera is which of the following:

    A. Congestive heart failure
    B. Pulmonary hypertension
    C. Thrombosis
    D. Acute hemorrhage

Answer: C

Critique: Thrombosis accounts for about 30% of deaths from polycythemia vera (PV). Congestive heart failure can occur in PV but is not the leading cause of mortality. Pulmonary hypertension is a cause of secondary erythrocytosis.

Page: 1264

93: Which of the following is *not* true regarding myelodysplastic syndrome (MDS):

    A. Chromosomal abnormalities are common.
    B. The majority of affected patients are older than 60 years.
    C. Thrombocytopenia is usually present.
    D. Progression to leukemia does not occur.

Answer: D

Critique: MDS is a clonal hematopoietic disorder that causes thrombocytopenia and neutropenia and has a tendency to progress to acute myelogenous leukemia. Eighty percent of patients are older than 60 at the time of diagnosis, and 80% have chromosomal aberrations.

Page: 1265

Questions 94 to 97: (Matching) Match the following statements with the appropriate clinical syndrome:

    A. Chronic myelogenous leukemia (CML)
    B. Chronic lymphocytic leukemia
    C. Multiple myeloma
    D. Acute lymphoblastic leukemia

94: Associated with Philadelphia chromosome

95: Standard chemotherapy includes melphalan and prednisone

96: Associated with high risk for hypercalcemia

97: Most common B cell malignancy

Answers: 94 - A, 95 - C, 96 - C, 97 - B

Critique: CML is a malignant clonal disorder characterized by a translocation of chromosome 9 and chromosome 22, the Philadelphia chromosome. CML accounts for 20% of all adult leukemias. Chronic lymphocytic leukemia is the most common B cell malignancy and is caused by the proliferation of long-lived nonfunctional lymphocytes. Multiple myeloma is caused by a proliferation of neoplastic plasma cells. Typical signs and symptoms include bone pain, anemia, renal insufficiency, recurrent infections, and hypercalcemia. Standard chemotherapy for multiple myeloma is melphalan and prednisone. Acute lymphoblastic leukemia is typically seen in children and is not associated with the listed characteristics.

Pages: 1267–1270

98: Waldenström's macroglobulinemia is associated with which of the following:

    A. High serum levels of immunoglobulin G (IgG)
    B. High serum levels of immunoglobulin M (IgM)
    C. Peak onset is in the third decade
    D. High rate of spontaneous remission

Answer: B

Critique: Waldenström's macroglobulinemia is a low-grade lymphoma. It is associated with high serum levels of IgM. The median age at diagnosis is 63, and median survival is 5 years. There is not a high rate of spontaneous remission because two thirds of patients die from complications of macroglobulinemia.

Page: 1269

99: Hodgkin's disease is associated with which of the following:

    A. A low remission rate
    B. Treatment with chemotherapy in early stages
    C. More common in females
    D. The malignant cell is the Reed-Sternberg cell

Answer: D

Critique: Hodgkin's disease is a B cell malignancy whose malignant cell is the Reed-Sternberg cell. Hodgkin's disease is more common in males and often presents with a nontender enlarged lymph node on clinical examination. It is one of the more curable lymphomas, with cure rates of 90% for early-stage disease and 70% to 80% for late-stage disease. Early-stage disease is treated with extended mantle irradiation. Later stages are treated with chemotherapy and irradiation.

Page: 1269

Questions 100 to 103: (Matching) Match the following statements with the appropriate acute leukemia:

    A. Acute lymphocytic leukemia (ALL)
    B. Acute myelogenous leukemia (AML)
    C. Both A and B
    D. Neither A nor B

100: Most common malignancy of childhood

101: WBC counts >50,000 common

102: Associated with Sweet's syndrome (paraneoplastic dermatologic syndrome)

103: Long-term survival rate is approximately 90%

Answers: 100 - A, 101 - C, 102 - B, 103 - D

Critique: ALL is a malignant disorder of lymphoid cells defined by the clonal proliferation of B cells or T cells. It is the most common malignancy of childhood and accounts for less than 20% of adult leukemias. AML is characterized by clonal proliferation of malignant myeloid precursors. It accounts for more than 90% of acute leukemias in adults. Both ALL and AML patients demonstrate significantly elevated WBC counts, commonly above 50,000/mm^3. Sweet's syndrome is a paraneoplastic dermatologic syndrome associated with AML. It is manifested by tender red plaques or nodules caused by an infiltrate of mature neutrophils in the dermis. Although the remission rate for children with ALL approaches 95%, the long-term survival rate is closer to 70%. Adults with ALL fare much worse and have a long-term survival rate of 30%. Long-term survival for AML is less than 20%.

Pages: 1269–1271

Chapter 47

Urinary Tract Disorders

John O'Handley

1: A urinary symptom that is found most frequently with neurogenic bladder is:

    A. Polyuria
    B. Urgency
    C. Hesitancy
    D. Overflow incontinence
    E. Urge incontinence

Answer: E

Critique: True polyuria (meaning frequent, large amounts of urine) is most common with diabetes mellitus and diabetes insipidus. Urgency (the need to void immediately) is commonly a result of bladder inflammation, but when it is associated with incontinence it can be caused by outflow tract obstruction, infection, or neurogenic problems. Hesitancy (waiting for the stream to start) usually indicates bladder outlet obstruction, such as prostatic hyperplasia. Overflow incontinence is seen predominantly in older men and is usually the result of bladder outlet obstruction caused by an enlarged prostate. With continual stretching, the bladder muscles lose their ability to produce a voiding contraction and urine leaks continuously. Urge incontinence is caused by detrusor instability and also affects older adults. It is frequently associated with CNS problems leading to disruption of the normal bladder inhibitory control from the cortex.

Page: 1275

2: Testicular torsion inside the tunica vaginalis occurs primarily:

    A. Before the first birthday
    B. Around 6 years of age
    C. Around puberty
    D. Around 18 years of age

Answer: C

Critique: Testicular torsion must be diagnosed early. The two common types are torsion occurring outside the tunica vaginalis, which tends to occur before age 1 year, and torsion occurring inside the tunica vaginalis, which is more common at puberty. Sudden onset of pain that is not relieved by elevating the testis and is associated with a firm, tender mass palpable in the scrotum is a classic presentation of acute testicular torsion.

Page: 1276

3: An early symptom of epididymitis is:

    A. Dysuria
    B. Scrotal swelling

    C. Testicular swelling
    D. Groin pain

Answer: D

Critique: Although epididymitis may be preceded by a history of urethritis, an early symptom of the condition is groin pain. The pain moves quickly to the epididymis, which becomes swollen and exquisitely tender. As opposed to testicular torsion, elevation of the scrotal contents relieves the pain. Epididymitis is rare in anyone under 20 years of age.

Page: 1276

Questions 4 to 8: Match each numbered entry with the correct lettered entry:

    A. Hernia (indirect inguinal)
    B. Hydrocele
    C. Malignant tumor
    D. Spermatocele
    E. Varicocele

4: The most common soft mass found in the scrotum; transilluminates except in rare instances

5: Nontender retention cyst of the epididymis or rete testis that transilluminates

6: Soft scrotal mass that may transilluminate and extends from the external inguinal ring into the scrotum

7: Usually left-sided, nontender mass that can disappear when the patient is supine

8: Firm to hard mass that does not transilluminate

Answers: 4 - B, 5 - D, 6 - A, 7 - E, 9 - C

Critique: An indirect inguinal hernia may present similarly to a hydrocele. However, a normal testis and epididymis are usually easily palpated, and bowel sounds may be heard in the scrotum. Hydroceles can be either communicating (early in life) or noncommunicating. Except in the rare instance of a thickened tunica vaginalis, hydroceles always transilluminate. Noncommunicating hydroceles may be caused by lymphatic obstruction and may be posttraumatic, postinfectious, infectious, or malignant in origin. Malignant tumors of the scrotum are usually painless, do not transilluminate, and are usually found by the patient during bathing. Spermatoceles can be palpated as distinct from the testis and are found in the upper portion of the junction between the testis and the epididymis. A varicocele occurs more commonly on the left side because of the acute angle the left spermatic vein makes when entering

255

the renal vein. It is typically described as a "bag of worms" in consistency. Surgical correction is indicated only when fertility is in question.

Pages: 1277–1279

9: The differentiation of syphilis from chancroid can be made by all the following, except:

    A. Appearance
    B. Incubation period
    C. Only one is caused by a bacterium
    D. Dark-field examination
    E. Symptoms

Answer: C

Critique: Syphilis typically causes a sharp-bordered, painless ulcer with a clean base. Adenopathy can be present but is also painless. The incubation period for syphilis is 3 to 6 weeks, unlike that for chancroid, which is 2 to 5 days but can be as long as 14 days. The ulcer of chancroid is more irregular and also painful, as are the inguinal lymph nodes. Both are caused by bacteria: *Treponema pallidum* in the case of syphilis and *Hemophilus ducreyi* in the case of chancroid. Dark-field examination can be the most efficient way to distinguish the two diseases.

Page: 1278

10: All of the following are valuable in imaging the genitourinary system, except:

    A. Magnetic resonance imaging (MRI)
    B. Intravenous pyelography (IVP)
    C. Ultrasonography (US)
    D. Computed tomography (CT)
    E. Nuclear scanning

Answer: A

Critique: An IVP not only allows basic imaging of the genitourinary tract but also displays the functional ability of the system. US is also useful in differentiating cysts from solid masses, assessing kidney and prostate size, and determining postvoiding residual urine volume. It offers little in terms of demonstrating functional activity. CT can identify renal tumors, enlarged lymph nodes, and ureteral tumors. Nuclear scanning provides information about function, perfusion, and obstruction and is especially useful in postoperative follow-up of renal transplant patients. Evaluation of vesicoureteral reflux in children can also be accomplished with nuclear scanning. At present, MRI offers no advantage over the more conventional imaging studies.

Pages: 1279, 1280

Questions 11 to 14: Match each numbered entry with the correct lettered entry:

    A. Calcium urate stones
    B. Calcium oxalate stones
    C. Calcium phosphate stones
    D. Struvite stones

11: Most commonly a result of primary hyperparathyroidism

12: Twenty-five percent of patients with gout develop them

13: Formed in an alkaline pH by urease-producing bacteria

14: The most common kidney stone

Answers: 11 - C, 12 - A, 13 - D, 14 - B

Critique: Calcium urate stones are seen in 25% of patients with gout. Alkalinization of the urine and hydration are important treatment steps for these patients. The most frequently seen stones are calcium oxalate. Hydration and avoidance of foods high in oxalate (tea, instant coffee, spinach, beets, berries, and nuts) help to prevent this form of stone. Parathyroid adenomas frequently play a part in the formation of calcium phosphate stones. Surgical excision of the adenoma is the treatment, but calcium phosphate stones are seen in less than 10% of urinary calculi. Struvite stones are formed around a nidus of several substances in an alkaline pH. The bacteria causing these stones are able to split urea into ammonia. Struvite stones must be removed surgically because of their size, when clinically indicated.

Pages: 1285–1287

15: All of the following are true regarding finasteride in the treatment of benign prostatic hyperplasia (BPH), except:

    A. Lowers prostate-specific antigen (PSA) by 50% within 6 months
    B. Decreases prostate volume, as measured by ultrasonography, 30% after 12 months
    C. Directly inhibits 5 α-reductase to block the conversion of testosterone to dihydrotestosterone (DHT)
    D. Side effects include decreased libido, decreased ejaculate volume, and impotence in less than 5% of patients

Answer: B

Critique: BPH can be evaluated by a scoring system developed by the American Urologic Association (AUA). This brings uniformity to the evaluation of BPH symptoms. Successful medical therapy with alpha-blockers and 5 α-reductase has greatly enhanced the medical treatment of BPH. The side effects of finasteride, a 5 α-reductase inhibitor, are seen in less than 5% of patients according to the Finasteride Study Group. At 12 months, one study showed a 19% reduction in prostate volume. Because finasteride blocks only the conversion of testosterone to DHT, it has no systemic androgenic or antiandrogenic effects. By 6 months, there is a 50% reduction in PSA when finasteride is used for BPH. The PSA assay should be checked annually after the first 6-month check when treating BPH with finasteride. Surgical advances in treating BPH include transurethral incision of the prostate (TUIP), visual laser ablation of the prostate (VLAP), and hypothermia. TUIP is equivalent to transurethral resection of the prostate (TURP) when the gland weighs 30 g or less.

Pages: 1293, 1294

16: Antimicrobial prophylaxis for recurrent urinary tract infections that reduces colonization of the vaginal vestibule by fecal flora includes all of the following, except:

A. Nitrofurantoin
B. Trimethoprim-sulfamethoxazole
C. Trimethoprim
D. Cephalexin

Answer: A

Critique: All the antimicrobials mentioned except nitrofurantoin eliminate most Enterobacteriaceae from fecal flora and also are present in vaginal secretions in bactericidal concentrations. This destroys the bacteria before they can contaminate the urine. Nitrofurantoin does not affect the fecal flora, because it is completely absorbed in the upper gastrointestinal tract and excreted solely in the urine, where it is effective only after the organisms enter the bladder.

Pages: 1298, 1299

17: The first step in evaluating patients with acute renal failure is to:

A. Begin intravenous fluids
B. Discontinue nephrotoxic drugs, including NSAIDs and ACE inhibitors
C. Start dialysis
D. Give Kayexalate orally

Answer: B

Critique: The first step in evaluating patients who appear to have acute renal failure is to discontinue nephrotoxic drugs. Any other drug dosages are adjusted for a glomerular filtration rate (GFR) of less than 5 mL/min. In addition, fluids and potassium administration are limited. Hyperkalemia can be a problem with acute renal failure and needs to be treated, but treating it is not the first step in patient evaluation. Once the patient has reached the stage of requiring dialysis, the prognosis is poor, with an average mortality of 70% despite full supportive therapy.

Pages: 1301, 1302

18: The most common cause of chronic renal failure is:

A. Atherosclerotic renovascular occlusion
B. Diabetes mellitus
C. Hypertension
D. Chronic glomerulonephritis
E. Systemic lupus erythematosus

Answer: B

Critique: Diabetes mellitus is the most common cause of chronic renal failure. By delaying the onset of proteinuria in diabetes with the use of an ACE inhibitor, the deterioration of renal function is decreased significantly. Hypertension can lead to progressive renal failure by contributing to atherosclerotic renovascular disease. Chronic glomerulonephritis is a major cause of chronic renal failure but much less common than is diabetes mellitus. This is also true for systemic lupus erythematosus, which can cause chronic renal failure but is even less prevalent.

Pages: 1302, 1303

19: (True or False) The syndrome of inappropriate ADH (SIADH) secretion is characterized by:

A. A urine sodium concentration above 10 mEq/L
B. Lack of symptoms even in the presence of a serum sodium level of 120 mEq/L
C. Edema of the lower extremities
D. Abnormal adrenal function

Answers: A - True, B - True, C - False, D - False

Critique: To diagnose SIADH, other conditions must be ruled out, such as kidney, adrenal, and thyroid disease. Hyponatremia resulting from edematous states such as nephrosis, cirrhosis, and congestive heart failure results in renal sparing of sodium and urinary levels of 10 mEq/L or less of sodium. Higher concentrations of sodium in the urine in the presence of a lower serum sodium level indicate an inappropriate secretion of ADH. SIADH is most often insidious and serum sodium gradually decreases, leading to lack of symptoms even when the serum sodium level is as low as 120 mEq/L.

Pages: 1303, 1304

Questions 20 to 23: Match the following conditions with the findings:

A. Hyperkalemia
B. Hypokalemia
C. Hypercalcemia
D. Hypocalcemia

20: Symptoms include constipation, weakness, and lethargy and a short QT interval on ECG

21: Seen in patients with a high dietary sodium intake in the presence of a renovascular lesion; U waves are seen on ECG

22: Exacerbated by ACE inhibitors; ECG shows peaked T waves, widening of the QRS, and a prolonged PR interval

23: Seen in patients with hypoalbuminemia; ECG shows prolonged ST and QT intervals

Answers: 20 - C, 21 - B, 22 - A, 23 - D

Critique: The ECG can be a sensitive indicator of potassium and calcium abnormalities even before a patient is symptomatic. Hyperkalemia produces peaked T waves, widening of the QRS, and a prolonged PR interval. Administration of ACE inhibitors can lead to hyperkalemia. Hypokalemia is most commonly seen with long-acting thiazide diuretics, but it can also be seen in hypertensive patients with a high dietary sodium intake in the presence of a renovascular lesion. The classic sign of hypokalemia on ECG is prominent U waves. Hypercalcemia can cause symptoms of constipation and weakness and, if left untreated, progress to lethargy, obtundation, coma, and death. ECG shows a shortened QT interval with hypercalcemia. Although uncommon, true hypocalcemia is seen in patients with hypoalbuminemia. A reduction of serum calcium of 0.8 mg/dL can be expected for each 1.0 mg/dL reduction in serum albumin concentration. The ECG shows prolonged ST and QT intervals.

Pages: 1304–1306

24: Causes of an increased anion gap metabolic acidosis include all of the following, except:

    A. Ethylene glycol ingestion
    B. Starvation
    C. Vomiting
    D. Diabetes
    E. Methanol ingestion

Answer: C

Critique: All of the conditions mentioned cause an increased anion gap metabolic acidosis except vomiting. Since the latter results in loss of H^+ from the digestive tract, it results in a metabolic alkalosis. The other conditions add a new acid to the system and consumption of bicarbonate occurs. The normal anion gap is 12 to 16 mEq/L [$(Na^+ + K^+) - (Cl^- + HCO_3^-)$]. The acidic ion is not quickly eliminated and replaced with chloride, so the gap widens. Conditions causing an increased anion gap metabolic acidosis often can be life-threatening, and appropriate therapy is indicated.

Pages: 1308–1309

25: (True or False) The nephrotic syndrome is associated with significant glomerular damage. Which of the following statements are true regarding the nephrotic syndrome:

    A. Focal glomerulosclerosis is often seen in patients with the nephrotic syndrome.
    B. Renal biopsy is the only way a histologic diagnosis can be made with the nephrotic syndrome.
    C. Most adults with idiopathic nephrotic syndrome respond to corticosteroid therapy.
    D. The syndrome consists of edema, hypoalbuminemia, and hypercholesterolemia.

Answers: A - True, B - True, C - False, D - True

Critique: The common conditions that are associated with the nephrotic syndrome are minimal change disease, focal glomerulosclerosis, membranous glomerulonephritis, and membranoproliferative glomerulonephritis. Focal glomerulosclerosis appears in some of the glomeruli and is common in adolescents and young adults. The mean time from diagnosis of focal glomerulosclerosis to dialysis is 5 to 7 years. The only way a histologic lesion can be identified is by renal biopsy, but the lesions mentioned are all treated with corticosteroids and empiric therapy is equal to biopsy-based treatment. Idiopathic nephrotic syndrome responds poorly to corticosteroids, which, if used, can lead to significant morbidity. In the majority of patients with the nephrotic syndrome, the presenting complaint is edema. The laboratory findings reveal hypoalbuminemia and hypercholesterolemia.

Pages: 1309, 1310

Chapter 48

Ophthalmology

Syed S. Azhar

1: A 46-year-old female complains of redness in her right eye. She is most likely to have an acute bacterial conjunctivitis if she has:

- A. Severe pain in the eye
- B. Photophobia
- C. Rapid onset of symptoms
- D. Mucopurulent discharge in the eye, with normal vision

Answer: D

Critique: Most cases of conjunctivitis are painless. Slight ocular pain may be present, but it is usually mild. Serious ocular pain is caused by conditions such as acute glaucoma, iritis, a foreign body in the eye, or corneal abrasions. Photophobia is rare and indicates involvement of the cornea. A foreign body in the eye causes instant pain and redness. Diminished visual acuity is an important sign, because vision is rarely affected with conjunctivitis. Acute bacterial conjunctivitis causes mucopurulent discharge in the eye.

Pages: 1314, 1315

2: A 27-year-old male developed redness and moderate pain in his right eye over the last weekend. There is no discharge in the eye. His vision is diminished in that eye to 20/80. Vision in the other eye is normal. There is circumcorneal ciliary congestion in the affected eye, and the pupil has slight miosis and reacts sluggishly to light. The most likely diagnosis is:

- A. Acute glaucoma
- B. Acute anterior uveitis
- C. Acute conjunctivitis
- D. A foreign body in the eye

Answer: B

Critique: In acute glaucoma, the pupil is dilated and fixed. With acute anterior uveitis, the pupil has miosis and reacts sluggishly to light because of the formation of posterior synechiae, which are adhesions between the pupil and the anterior part of the lens as a result of inflammatory cells in the aqueous. The pupil is normal with conjunctivitis and with a foreign body in the eye.

Pages: 1343, 1344

3: A 3-year-old child is brought to your office with a history of pain, redness, and swelling of right eye for 1 day. He also has had some cough and cold symptoms for the past week. Periorbital swelling and redness are evident. The conjunctiva is red, and the eye appears slightly pro-

truded. The ocular motility seems to be slightly restricted. The following is true about this condition:

- A. This child should be immediately hospitalized for administration of intravenous antibiotics.
- B. You should give him a third-generation cephalosporin by mouth and ask his mother to watch him closely for fever.
- C. The infection has extended from the nasolacrimal sac.
- D. The infection has extended from a boil on the lids.

Answer: A

Critique: Orbital cellulite causes periorbital swelling, conjunctival edema, limited extraocular movements, and proptosis. The infection extends from the ethmoid sinuses. Immediate hospitalization and ophthalmologic consultation are necessary. Cavernous sinus thrombosis, meningitis, and blindness are serious complications of orbital cellulitis.

Page: 1321

4: A mother brought her 3-month-old infant to your office. She noticed slight redness and crusts on both of her child's eyelids. There was also increased tearing in both eyes. You prescribed a course of topical antibiotics, which resolved the symptoms for a short period of time. The infant is back in your office because the symptoms have recurred. You tell the mother all of the following, except:

- A. To massage the lacrimal area with the tip of her little fingers from above downward
- B. The tear ducts are blocked
- C. That 80% of these inflammations require surgical correction by 6 months of age
- D. If symptoms persist, then a referral to an ophthalmologist will be needed for probing of the nasolacrimal duct

Answer: C

Critique: Neonates have tear secretion at birth. A totally patent and functional lacrimal drainage system is present in 96% to 98%. The 2% to 4% whose lacrimal drainage system is not intact have a thin residual membrane at the distal end of nasolacrimal duct. This membrane spontaneously dissolves in 80% to 90% of patients within the first few months of life. Tearing and mattering is a common symptom. Topical antibiotics should be administered and the parents must be instructed in the proper technique for lacrimal sac compression and massage. More than 90% of these cases clear, and the patients become asymptomatic with a conservative regimen.

Pages: 1316–1318

5: In congenital glaucoma, all of the clinical findings are seen, except:

    A. An increase in corneal diameter
    B. Clouding of cornea
    C. Micro cornea
    D. The infants usually present with excessive tearing and photophobia

Answer: C

Critique: Congenital glaucoma, also called buphthalmos, is a potentially blinding condition in infants and should be suspected at an early stage to prevent vision loss. Affected infants usually present with excessive tearing and photophobia. The corneal diameter is increased, and corneal clouding occurs as a result of increased intraocular pressure. Patients should be immediately referred to an ophthalmologist whenever this condition is suspected.

Page: 1318

6: A 20-year-old female came to your office when one of her friends noticed a swelling on her right lower lid about 2 months ago. She had no pain or blurry vision in that eye. The swollen area has gradually increased in size, which prompted her to come back to your office for advice. Her vision is normal in both eyes. There is a nodular swelling 1 × 1 cm in diameter on the outer third of the right lower lid, 5 mm away from the lid margin. There is mild localized conjunctival congestion. The skin over the swelling is normal except for slight erythema. The swollen area is cystic and nontender to palpation. The most likely diagnosis is:

    A. Stye (hordeolum) of the right lower lid
    B. Chalazion (meibomian cyst) of the right lower lid
    C. Basal cell carcinoma
    D. Molluscum contagiosum

Answer: B

Critique: A stye is an acute staphylococcal infection of the hair follicle. It appears as an acutely tender swelling close to the lid margin. Treatment includes warm compresses and topical antibiotics. A stye generally drains spontaneously within a few days. The offending hair can also be pulled out if a localized pustule is seen. A chalazion, on the other hand, is a chronic granulomatous inflammation of the meibomian glands. It is usually nontender and situated a few millimeters from the lid margin. If it persists for more than 3 months, it may require incision and curettage. Basal cell carcinoma accounts for more than 90% of the malignant tumors of the lids. It typically presents with rolled, pearly, telangiectatic edges and a central depression, which may become progressively eroded. It is usually a slowly progressive lesion and is seen mostly in patients older than 50 years. Molluscum contagiosum is a pearly white lesion with umbilication in the center.

Page: 1319

7: Topical steroids in the eye can cause all of the following, except:

    A. Worsening of active herpetic keratitis
    B. Glaucoma, if used for prolonged periods of time
    C. Cataracts, if used for prolonged periods of time
    D. Worsening of inflammation in acute anterior uveitis

Answer: D

Critique: Topical corticosteroids have potentially serious side effects and should be used with extreme caution. Topical steroids should not be given in active herpetic keratitis because of the possibility of making the viral proliferation worse. Prolonged use of topical steroids has shown to increase intraocular pressure and may also cause formation of cataracts. Topical steroids are indicated in the treatment of acute anterior uveitis.

Page: 1320

8: You get a call from a nursing home about your 86-year-old female patient who has had severe pain in her right eye since last night. The nurse tells you that the vision is severely diminished in that eye and that the eye is very red. You arrange for your patient to come to your office immediately. On examination, the patient's visual acuity is limited to counting fingers close to her face in the affected eye. There is significant lid edema and ciliary congestion. The cornea is cloudy. With the use of a penlight, the pupil can barely be visualized and appears semidilated and not reactive to direct light. The most likely diagnosis is:

    A. Acute anterior uveitis
    B. Acute angle closure glaucoma
    C. Chronic open-angle glaucoma
    D. Acute conjunctivitis with corneal ulcer

Answer: B

Critique: Acute anterior uveitis causes pain, redness, and diminished vision. The pupil shows miosis, is irregular, and reacts sluggishly to light. Acute angle closure glaucoma is a condition in which intraocular pressure is acutely increased because of an obstruction of aqueous flow resulting from closure of the angle of anterior chamber.

Pages: 1321, 1322

9: A 68-year-old hypertensive patient with a history of coronary artery disease takes aspirin regularly. She has had a cough for the past few days. She reports a sudden onset of redness in her left eye. She has no history of pain or vision loss or of trauma to or a foreign body in the eye. After examination, you make the diagnosis of subconjunctival hemorrhage. The following is true of this condition:

    A. It usually resolves spontaneously in 2 to 3 weeks.
    B. Spontaneous subconjunctival hemorrhage is a serious ocular condition.
    C. Subconjunctival hemorrhage in a child does not require any further evaluation.

D. A referral to an ophthalmologist is always necessary.

Answer: A

Critique: Spontaneous subconjunctival hemorrhage is a relatively benign condition. There is no therapy, except reassurance that the blood will clear in 2 to 3 weeks. If trauma is suspected, the patient should be referred to an ophthalmologist to rule out more serious injuries, such as perforation of the eye. Suspect child abuse in a child with subconjunctival hemorrhage, and carefully examine the child for any other evidence of trauma.

Pages: 1320, 1321

10: One of your patients had been hammering a nail in the wall, when he had a sudden onset of sharp pain in his right eye followed by tearing and redness. After instilling an ophthalmic local anesthetic in the eye, you examine his eyes with a penlight. There is generalized conjunctival congestion. Cornea stains with fluorescein. You cannot find an obvious foreign body in the eye. The next step should be all of the following, except:

    A. Patch the eye and prescribe a local antibiotic
    B. Evert the upper eyelid and search further for a foreign body
    C. Do a good irrigation of the eye with normal saline
    D. Look for signs of a penetrating foreign body

Answer: A

Critique: High-velocity foreign bodies can easily penetrate the eye. There should be a high index of suspicion for an intraocular foreign body, especially if it is not visualized outside the eye. A subtarsal foreign body should be looked for under the upper lid. The eye should be thoroughly irrigated. Some of the signs of a small perforation of the eye, which may not be obvious, are a subconjunctival hemorrhage, evidence of a dark uveal tissue underneath the conjunctiva, a shallow anterior chamber, and a distorted pupil. The patient should be immediately referred to an ophthalmologist.

Page: 1322

11: Blunt trauma to the eye may cause:

    A. Dilated pupil
    B. Hyphema
    C. Peripheral retinal tear
    D. Vitreous detachment
    E. All of the above

Answer: E

Critique: A blunt trauma to the eye can cause all of these conditions. Hence, in addition to a good anterior segment examination, it is important to do a dilated fundus examination with the use of an indirect ophthalmoscope in all cases of blunt trauma to the eye to look at the posterior segment.

Pages: 1323–1325

12: Hyphema (blood in anterior chamber) secondary to blunt trauma may cause all of the following complications, except:

    A. Corneal bloodstaining
    B. Optic atrophy
    C. Raised intraocular pressure
    D. Blowout fracture of the orbit

Answer: D

Critique: The patient with traumatic hyphema should have a thorough ophthalmologic evaluation. Corneal bloodstaining occurs primarily in patients with a total hyphema. Optic atrophy may result from either acute, transiently elevated intraocular pressure or chronically elevated intraocular pressure. Blowout fracture of the orbit occurs as a result of blunt ocular trauma but is not a complication of hyphema.

Pages: 1324, 1325

13: In traumatic hyphema, the visual prognosis is favorable:

    A. With secondary hemorrhage
    B. With normal intraocular pressure
    C. When optic atrophy occurs
    D. When there is associated damage to other ocular structures.

Answer: B

Critique: It is important to recognize that the prognosis for visual acuity from traumatic hyphema is directly related to the amount of associated ocular damage, secondary hemorrhage, and other complications such as raised intraocular pressure and optic atrophy.

Page: 1325

14: A 36-year-old man sustained a blunt trauma to his left eye when he was involved in a fistfight. His vision is slightly diminished at 20/30. There is some lid edema and ecchymosis. The conjunctiva is congested. The cornea is clear. No hyphema is present. Pupillary reaction to light and accommodation is normal. Fundus examination is normal through an undilated funduscope. This patient may still have all of the following, except:

    A. Peripheral retinal tear
    B. Vitreous detachment
    C. Large macular hemorrhage
    D. Possibility of later developing a retinal detachment

Answer: C

Critique: All cases of blunt trauma to the eye need not only a thorough external eye examination but also a dilated fundus examination. Peripheral retinal tears at the time of injury can be completely asymptomatic but later can develop into a retinal detachment with loss of vision. A large macular hemorrhage is unlikely, because it would cause a significant loss of vision. Vitreous detachment may cause flashing lights and floaters in the eye but can be asymptomatic.

Page: 1325

14: Children's vision should be screened to detect:

    A. Strabismus at an early stage
    B. Ocular disease

C. Amblyopia
D. Refractive errors
E. All of the above

Answer: E

Critique: Appropriate vision screening is one of the most important factors in pediatric eye care. Because visual stimuli are critical to normal development, early detection and correction of problems can prevent serious vision impairment and blindness. In particular, vision screening is necessary to detect four major conditions: strabismus, amblyopia, ocular disease, and refractive errors.

Pages: 1325, 1326

15: The American Academy of Ophthalmology and the American Academy of Pediatric Ophthalmology and Strabismus recommend that children be examined for eye problems in four stages at the following ages:

A. Newborn, 6 months, 3 years, and 5 years and older
B. Newborn, 1 year, 5 years, and 7 years
C. 3 months, 6 months, 1 year, and 5 years
D. Newborn, 6 months, 1 year, and 5 years

Answer: A

Critique: These associations recommend that children be examined for eye problems in four stages: at birth, at 6 months, at 3 years, and at 5 years and older.

Page: 1326

16: The following statements about retinopathy of prematurity (ROP) are true, except:

A. Premature infants with a birth weight lower than 1700 g are at greater risk of developing ROP.
B. In most infants, ROP causes progressive loss of vision.
C. ROP causes some degree of visual loss in approximately 1300 infants in the United States each year.
D. Premature babies should have a detailed eye examination by an ophthalmologist.

Answer: B

Critique: Premature infants with a birth weight of less than 1700 g are at greater risk of developing ROP. Each year, ROP causes some degree of visual loss in approximately 1300 infants in the United States. In most infants, ROP is a transient disease with spontaneous regression.

Page: 1326

17: Leukokoria (white pupil) in infants is seen in all of the following conditions, except:

A. Congenital cataracts
B. Retinoblastoma
C. Retinal detachment
D. Retinitis pigmentosa

Answer: D

Critique: Cataracts are the most common cause of leukokoria at birth. Retinoblastoma is a life-threatening cause of leukokoria that may be detected within the first few weeks of life. Retinal detachment may cause leukokoria. Retinitis pigmentosa is a degenerative condition of the retina and does not cause leukokoria.

Page: 1326

18: You are doing a preschool eye screening of a 3-year-old. The mother is concerned about strabismus because she noticed that the child's eyes are not perfectly aligned. As a primary care physician, you should do which of the following examinations:

A. Check visual acuity to look for amblyopia
B. Cover test
C. Corneal reflex test
D. Extraocular rotations
E. All of the above

Answer: E

Critique: Visual acuity is diminished in the deviated eye owing to suppression of images in that eye, leading to the development of amblyopia. Vision should be checked in the evaluation of strabismus. This can be done in a 3-year-old with the help of the Snellen chart, the tumbling E game, or the Allen picture cards. The corneal reflex test, the cover test, and extraocular rotations are three basic tests for strabismus.

Page: 1327

19: A positive family history of ocular disease should be taken in all children. All of the following eye diseases in children have a positive family history, except:

A. Congenital cataracts
B. Strabismus
C. Refractive errors
D. Congenital ocular toxoplasmosis

Answer: D

Critique: Congenital cataracts, strabismus, and refractive errors all have a positive family history. Congenital ocular toxoplasmosis is caused by maternal *Toxoplasma* infection.

Pages: 1328, 1329

20: Which of the following statements is true regarding amblyopia:

A. Loss of vision or lazy eye occurs in the undeviated eye (fixating eye).
B. Amblyopia occurs in approximately 50% of patients with strabismus.
C. Amblyopia is usually treatable after the age of 7 years.
D. One of the treatments of amblyopia consists of occlusion or patching of the deviated eye.

Answer: B

Critique: Loss of vision in the misaligned eye is called amblyopia, or lazy eye. Unless treatment begins early, loss of vision in the affected eye (i.e., the deviated eye) may be permanent. Amblyopia is usually treatable if detected at 3 to 4 years of age but is generally irreversible after age 7.

Pages: 1329, 1330

21: You are doing a cover test in a 7-year-old child. You ask the child to look straight at a distant object. When the right eye is covered, the left eye moves outward to take up fixation of the distant object. The diagnosis is:

A. Exotropia
B. Esotropia
C. Exophoria
D. Esophoria

Answer: B

Critique: The cover test is important in the diagnosis of strabismus. Have the child look straight ahead at a distant object. Cover the right eye and look for movement of the uncovered left eye. If the eye does not move, there is no apparent misalignment of the eye. If the eye moves outward, the eye is esotropic. If it moves inward, it is exotropic. For latent strabismus (esophoria and exophoria) a cover/uncover test is done. The uncovered eye does not move in both esophoria and exophoria. Repeat the test by covering the left eye.

Page: 1330

22: Which of the following statements is ^not true of retinoblastoma:

A. It is the second most common primary intraocular tumor in all age groups.
B. The tumor occurs bilaterally in about one third of cases.
C. It is usually diagnosed at birth if a careful eye examination is done.
D. Familial cases of retinoblastoma account for 6% of cases.

Answer: C

Critique: Retinoblastoma is the second most common primary intraocular tumor in all age groups. The tumor occurs bilaterally in about one third cases. It is usually diagnosed between 14 and 18 months of age. Familial cases of retinoblastoma account for 6% of patients.

Pages: 1337, 1338

23: All the following conditions can cause ptosis, except:

A. Oculomotor nerve palsy
B. Facial nerve palsy
C. Horner's syndrome
D. Myasthenia gravis

Answer: B

Critique: Facial nerve palsy does not cause ptosis. The patient is unable to close his or her eye, and therefore the cornea should be protected. All of the other listed conditions cause ptosis.

Page: 1340

24: A 42-year-old female with Graves' disease will usually have all the following ocular signs, except:

A. Lid retraction
B. Ptosis
C. Exophthalmos
D. Esotropia

Answer: B

Critique: Retraction of both upper and lower eyelids has been recognized as one of the cardinal signs of Graves' disease. Bilateral exophthalmos is commonly seen. Esotropia is caused by restrictive myopathy and fibrotic contraction of the medial rectus muscle. When this muscle contracts, the eye is deviated nasally (esotropia). The other muscle, which is commonly involved, is the inferior rectus muscle, which causes hypotropia (pulling the eye downward). Ptosis is not commonly seen in Graves' disease.

Pages: 1341, 1342

25: All the following are the risk factors for chronic open-angle glaucoma, except:

A. Older age
B. Family history of glaucoma
C. African-American heritage
D. Narrow anterior chamber angle

Answer: D

Critique: Chronic open-angle glaucoma becomes increasingly prevalent with each decade over the age of 40 years. African Americans develop glaucoma more frequently and become legally blind from glaucoma more often than Caucasians. A family history of glaucoma is generally accepted as a risk factor. The angle of the anterior chamber is open and wide in chronic open-angle glaucoma.

Pages: 1343, 1344

26: Which of the following statements is true regarding age-related macular degeneration:

A. The exudative type of macular degeneration accounts for more than 90% of all macular degeneration cases.
B. There is a 70% chance of the condition occurring in the other eye.
C. Ophthalmic laser surgery has been found to be beneficial in retarding the spread of the exudative form of macular degeneration.
D. If untreated, age-related macular degeneration causes complete blindness.

Answer: C

Critique: Exudative macular degeneration causes severe vision loss and accounts for 10% of all cases of age-related macular degeneration. There is a 10% chance that the opposite eye will be involved with macular degeneration within 1 year. Age-related macular degeneration causes central loss of vision but does not cause complete blindness. Most patients are able to ambulate at home with the peripheral vision they retain. Patients should be reassured that they are not going to go completely blind. There is no cure, but laser surgery will help retard the progress of exudative macular degeneration.

Page: 1345

27: Diabetics are at a much greater risk of becoming blind from diabetic retinopathy. Which of the following statements is true of diabetic retinopathy:

A. Diabetic retinopathy is the most common cause of blindness in Americans aged 45 years to 74 years.

B. Type 2 diabetics should be screened within 3 to 5 years after being diagnosed with diabetes.

C. Type 1 diabetics should be screened for diabetic retinopathy immediately after the diagnosis of diabetes is made.

D. Macular edema causes the most profound vision loss seen in diabetic retinopathy.

Answer: A

Critique: Diabetic retinopathy is the most common cause of blindness in America in the age group 45 years to 74 years. The American Academy of Ophthalmology recommends eye screening in type 2 diabetics immediately after the diagnosis is made. In type 1 diabetics, the recommendation is to perform the eye screening within the first 3 to 5 years after the initial diagnosis. Macular edema is the most common cause of vision impairment in diabetics, but it does not cause severe loss of vision. Severe loss of vision is caused by the complications of proliferative retinopathy.

Pages: 1346, 1347

28: Sudden, painless loss of vision occurs in all of the following, except:

A. Retinal detachment
B. Ischemic optic neuropathy
C. Acute angle closure glaucoma
D. Central retinal artery occlusion

Answer: C

Critique: Acute angle closure glaucoma causes acute loss of vision with severe pain. The other conditions cause painless acute loss of vision.

Pages: 1347, 1348

29: A 65-year-old male complains of right-sided headache, malaise, and tiredness for the past few days. He also gives a history of jaw pains. On examination, his vision is normal with glasses. The right temple area is tender. The temporal artery on the right side is tender and thickened. All of the following statements are true of this condition, except:

A. A sedimentation rate (ESR) should be obtained immediately.

B. The patient should be started on high doses of corticosteroids immediately if the sedimentation rate is high.

C. The visual loss in giant cell arteritis is caused by an ischemic process in the optic nerve.

D. If one eye is involved with giant cell arteritis, the chances of second eye involvement are less than 5% even in untreated patients.

Answer: D

Critique: Temporal arteritis is a systemic immune disorder. Ocular symptoms include profound loss of vision as a result of ischemic optic neuropathy. The work-up of a patient suspected of having giant cell arteritis includes a careful history of nonvisual symptoms, examination, and laboratory studies including a sedimentation rate. Corticosteroids should be started immediately on making the diagnosis. When one eye is involved with giant cell arteritis, the second eye loses vision in 65% of untreated patients.

Pages: 1347, 1348

30: The patient described in question 29 comes to your office with right-sided headache, malaise, and tiredness. He lost his vision in his right eye that morning, before the office visit. His examination reveals a tender right temple with a hardened and tender right temporal artery. He can barely see a hand movement close to his face with his right eye, but the vision in his left eye is normal. His sedimentation rate is 85 mm/hr. You should do all of the following, except:

A. Start the patient on high doses of corticosteroids.

B. Get a temporal artery biopsy to confirm the diagnosis, and then start the patient on high doses of systemic steroids.

C. Use steroids for 6 months.

D. All of the above.

Answer: B

Critique: Temporal arteritis is a systemic immune disorder that generally occurs in individuals over the age of 55 years. Ocular involvement is usually associated with inflammation of the posterior ciliary arteries that causes ischemic optic neuropathy. Once the diagnosis is established, steroid therapy should be instituted immediately with IV prednisone. Do not wait for the results of temporal artery biopsy to start the treatment. When one eye is involved with giant cell arteritis, the second eye loses vision in 65% of untreated patients. Involvement of the second eye generally occurs within 10 days. The treatment may have to be continued for up to 1 year.

Pages: 1347, 1348

Chapter 49

Neurology

Robert G. Hosey

1: Comprehension of speech but a nonfluent speech pattern is consistent with which of the following:

    A. Broca's aphasia
    B. Wernicke's aphasia
    C. Dysarthria
    D. Aphonia

Answer: A

Critique: Aphasia results from injury or damage to the dominant cerebral hemisphere. Broca's aphasia results in comprehension of speech but a nonfluent speech pattern. Wernicke's aphasia refers to poor comprehension of speech with fluent, often meaningless speech. Dysarthria refers to difficulty with the production of speech, whereas aphonia refers to the loss of voice.

Page: 1353

2: An afferent pupillary defect is seen with damage to which of the following cranial nerves:

    A. IV
    B. VI
    C. II
    D. I

Answer: C

Critique: Pupillary function assesses cranial nerves II and III as well as sympathetic activity. The direct and consensual light responses require that both cranial nerves II and III work correctly. Damage to cranial nerve II can result in an afferent pupillary defect. Cranial nerve I (olfactory) is responsible for the sense of smell. Cranial nerves IV and VI are involved in controlling ocular movements.

Pages: 1353, 1354

3: Sensory divisions of the trigeminal nerve include all of the following, except:

    A. Ophthalmic
    B. Mandibular
    C. Maxillary
    D. Cervical

Answer: D

Critique: Cranial nerve V, the trigeminal nerve, has three sensory branches: ophthalmic, mandibular, and maxillary. There is no cervical branch of the trigeminal nerve.

Page: 1354

4: Which of the following cranial nerves is responsible for supplying the sense of taste to the posterior one third of the tongue:

    A. X
    B. IX
    C. VII
    D. VIII

Answer: B

Critique: Cranial nerve IX (glossopharyngeal) supplies sensation to the pharynx and tonsillar fossa and taste to the posterior one third of the tongue. Taste to the anterior two thirds of the tongue is supplied by the facial nerve (VII). Cranial nerve VIII is responsible for hearing and vestibular function. The vagus nerve (X) is responsible for motor control of the pharynx, palate, and larynx and also carries parasympathetic fibers that innervate the thoracic and abdominal viscera.

Page: 1354

5: Upper motor neuron disease is characterized by which of the following:

    A. Fatigable weakness
    B. Fasciculations and muscle wasting
    C. Increased muscle tone
    D. Diminished reflexes

Answer: C

Critique: Increased muscle tone and reflexes characterize upper motor neuron disease. Lower motor neuron disease is characterized by muscle wasting, fasciculations, decreased tone, and absent reflexes. Fatigable weakness is a characteristic of neuromuscular junction disorders.

Page: 1355

6: A patient with a dermatomal loss of pain, temperature, and pressure sensations would most likely have an injury to what part of the spinal cord:

    A. Dorsal column
    B. Spinothalamic tract
    C. Corticospinal tract
    D. Anterior horn

Answer: B

Critique: In the spinal cord, the spinothalamic tract carries nerves responsible for pain, temperature, and pressure sensations. The corticospinal tract carries motor fibers, whereas the dorsal columns are responsible for proprioception, vibration, and light touch.

Page: 1355

Questions 7 to 12: Match the headache type with the appropriate symptomatology. (Each answer may be used once, more than once, or not at all.)

    A. Cluster headache
    B. Basilar migraine
    C. Tension headache
    D. Rebound headache
    E. Migraine (common)
    F. Migraine (classic)

7: Band-like pressure sensation

8: Alterations of consciousness

9: Photophobia and phonophobia

10: Scotomatous defects

11: Symptoms associated with excessive medicine use

12: Rhinorrhea, ptosis

Answers: 7 - C, 8 - B, 9 - E, 10 - F, 11 - D, 12 - A

Critique: Cluster headaches are associated with transient (15 to 180 minutes), severe unilateral orbital or supraorbital pain. Patients also commonly exhibit conjunctival injection, lacrimation, rhinorrhea, miosis, and ptosis. Basilar migraines are associated with dizziness, visual disturbance, diplopia, ataxia, and alterations in consciousness. These symptoms typically precede the onset of headache. Tension headaches are the most common type of headache. They are classically described as causing a band-like pressure sensation in the head and are typically bilateral in origin. Rebound headaches are characterized by diffuse, bilateral, almost daily headache, often aggravated by mild exertion. These can occur when medication doses are excessive or too frequent. Treatment is aimed at discontinuation of the overused medication. Common migraine headaches are often associated with photophobia and phonophobia. These headaches are usually one-sided and have a pulsating quality. They may also be associated with nausea and vomiting and be exacerbated by physical activity. Scotomatous defects are seen in patients with migraine with aura.

Pages: 1356–1359

13: Treatment options for acute migraine headaches include all of the following, except:

    A. Intranasal lidocaine solution
    B. Sumatriptan
    C. Verapamil
    D. Caffeine

Answer: C

Critique: Intranasal lidocaine, sumatriptan, and caffeine have all been used with some success in the treatment of acute migraine headaches. Calcium channel blockers, such as verapamil, are useful in prophylaxis for migraine headaches.

Page: 1357

14: Lithium may be used in the prophylaxis of which of the following types of headache:

    A. Migraine with aura
    B. Basilar migraine
    C. Rebound
    D. Cluster

Answer: D

Critique: Lithium can be used for the prophylaxis and treatment of chronic cluster headaches. Other medications that may be helpful in the treatment of cluster headaches are corticosteroids, methysergide, and verapamil. Rebound headaches are best treated with discontinuation of the overused medicine. Migraines may be treated with a variety of medications, and prophylaxis of migraines commonly can be accomplished with beta-blockers or calcium channel blockers.

Pages: 1357, 1359

15: Which of the following agents represents effective treatment for trigeminal neuralgia:

    A. Valproic acid
    B. Carbamazepine (Tegretol)
    C. Phenobarbital
    D. Methocarbamol

Answer: B

Critique: Treatment options for trigeminal neuralgia include carbamazepine, baclofen, and gabapentin. Carbamazepine is the initial treatment of choice. Valproic acid and phenobarbital are other antiseizure medicines, but they are not indicated for treatment of trigeminal neuralgia. Methocarbamol is used for muscular spasm.

Page: 1359

16: An 81-year-old man presents with a 3-day history of a bilateral throbbing headache that is worse at night. He also notes increased pain with chewing his food. Temporal arteritis is suspected. Which of the following represents the preferred procedure for confirming the diagnosis:

    A. Temporal artery biopsy
    B. Carotid Doppler study
    C. Arteriogram
    D. Slit lamp examination

Answer: A

Critique: The single best test in the diagnosis of temporal arteritis is temporal artery biopsy. An elevated sedimentation rate in a patient with a clinical picture of temporal arteritis also aids in the diagnosis. Carotid Doppler study does not visualize the temporal artery. Slit lamp examination is not helpful in the diagnosis of temporal arteritis. Arteriograms are helpful for visualizing occlusive disease or infarcts of the cerebral circulation but are not indicated in the diagnosis of temporal arteritis.

Pages: 1359, 1360

17: For patients who survive a stroke, the recurrence rate of stroke is approximately which of the following:

    A. 40% per year
    B. 30% per year

C. 20% per year
D. 10% per year
E. 5% per year

Answer: D

Critique: The mortality rate for stroke is approximately 15%. Patients who survive a stroke experience a 10% risk of recurrence per year.

Page: 1360

18: Which of the following is true regarding transient ischemic attacks (TIAs):

A. The subsequent annual risk of stroke is approximately 15%.
B. The risk of stroke after a retinal TIA (amaurosis fugax) is greater than that after a hemispheric TIA.
C. Subsequent myocardial infarction is a greater risk than is a stroke.
D. The patient who experiences a TIA should receive rT-PA (recombinant tissue plasminogen activator).

Answer: C

Critique: For patients who experience a TIA, the risk of subsequent myocardial infarction is higher than that for a stroke. Patients who experience a hemispheric TIA have a higher risk of subsequent stroke than patients with retinal TIA. The annual risk of stroke after a TIA is approximately 4.5% to 6.6%. RT-PA is used in the treatment of demonstrated ischemic infarct.

Page: 1360

19: Which of the following statements is true regarding elderly patients with isolated systolic hypertension (systolic blood pressure >160 mm Hg):

A. They have no increased relative risk of stroke.
B. They have a twofold to fourfold increased relative risk of stroke.
C. They have a fivefold to tenfold increased relative risk of stroke.
D. They have a decreased relative risk of stroke.

Answer: B

Critique: Elderly patients with isolated systolic hypertension have a twofold to fourfold increase in the relative risk of stroke. Treatment of isolated systolic hypertension (>160 mm Hg) in the elderly is therefore recommended.

Page: 1360

20: A 68-year-old female patient presents with a 2-hour history of transient left-sided paresthesias and weakness. All of her symptoms have now resolved and she has no residual clinical findings. Carotid duplex ultrasound reveals bilateral minimal stenosis less than 50%. Which of the following statements is correct regarding management of this patient:

A. She should be referred for carotid endarterectomy.
B. She needs no further treatment.
C. She should be referred for carotid angioplasty.
D. She should begin antiplatelet therapy.

Answer: D

Critique: This patient presents with symptoms consistent with a diagnosis of transient ischemic attack (TIA). In patients with TIAs and minimal carotid artery stenosis (<50%), medical management is indicated. This includes modification of lipids, blood pressure control, smoking cessation, and antiplatelet therapy. Carotid endarterectomy is indicated for patients who are symptomatic and have more than 70% stenosis. The efficacy, safety, and durability of carotid artery angioplasty, at this time, are unclear.

Page: 1360

21: Which of the following is the major side effect of ticlopidine:

A. Leukopenia
B. Thrombocytopenia
C. Anemia
D. Seizures

Answer: A

Critique: Ticlopidine is an antiplatelet medication that has been used for the prevention of stroke. Its use may cause leukopenia, and therefore patients taking ticlopidine need to have their white blood cell counts monitored every 2 weeks for the first 3 months of therapy. Skin rash and diarrhea may also occur with this medication. Thrombocytopenia, anemia, and seizures are not major side effects of ticlopidine.

Page: 1363

22: Warfarin therapy is indicated as a prophylactic medication for prevention of stroke in which of the following circumstances:

A. After a first transient ischemic attack (TIA)
B. High-grade carotid stenosis
C. Dilated cardiomyopathy
D. Calcific aortic stenosis

Answer: C

Critique: Warfarin therapy is indicated in the prevention of stroke in patients with dilated cardiomyopathy because this condition may predispose patients to embolic stroke. After the first TIA, medical management includes antiplatelet therapy but not warfarin. In patients who have symptomatic high-grade carotid artery stenosis, carotid endarterectomy should be performed. Calcific aortic stenosis is not a risk for embolic stroke, and therefore warfarin is not indicated.

Pages: 1363, 1364

23: A 70-year-old male presents with an acute left hemispheric stroke. His symptoms began 6 hours before he arrived in the office. Computed tomography (CT) scan is negative for bleeding. His current blood pressure is 200/100. Which of the following statements regarding treatment is correct regarding further management:

A. He is a candidate for tissue plasminogen activator (t-PA).
B. His blood pressure requires no immediate management.

C. Immediate magnetic resonance imaging (MRI) should be ordered.

D. Corticosteroids should be given to reduce cerebral edema.

Answer: B

Critique: Patients who present with a hemispheric stroke and elevated blood pressure do not require immediate blood pressure control unless systolic blood pressure is consistently above 220 mm Hg or diastolic blood pressure is greater than 120 mm Hg. Sudden drops in blood pressure can convert an ischemic area to a frank infarction. This patient is not a candidate for t-PA because, for this therapy to be effective, patients must be seen within 3 hours from the time of onset of symptoms. Corticosteroids should not be given to patients with thromboembolic stroke, because they may raise blood pressure and exacerbate hyperglycemia. Although MRI may be helpful in visualizing ischemic strokes, immediate MRI does not alter therapy for the patient and can be obtained at a later time. A CT scan can be helpful in the acute setting to rule out hemorrhagic stroke.

Pages: 1364, 1365

24: Which of the following statements is true regarding cerebral edema following a thromboembolic stroke:

A. Cerebral edema peaks at 24 hours.

B. Hyperventilation is effective in lowering intracranial pressure.

C. Corticosteroids are effective in limiting cerebral edema.

D. None of the above

Answer: B

Critique: After a stroke, cerebral edema typically is not a problem in the first 24 hours. Steroids are generally ineffective in limiting edema and may have deleterious side effects, including exacerbation of hypertension and hyperglycemia. Cerebral edema may be reduced effectively by hyperventilation, which lowers the intracranial pressure by 25% to 30% with a corresponding 5 to 10 mm Hg drop in CO_2.

Page: 1365

25: Which of the following medications should be considered in the acute management of delirium:

A. Lorazepam

B. Buspirone

C. Alprazolam

D. Bupropion

Answer: A

Critique: Lorazepam is a commonly used anxiolytic in the management of delirium. It has an intermediate half-life and a rapid onset of action. Both alprazolam and buspirone are anxiolytics but are not indicated in the treatment of management of delirium. Alprazolam is too short acting to be useful in delirium, and buspirone is available only in oral form. Bupropion is indicated in the management of depression.

Pages: 1365, 1366

26: Dementia is characterized by all of the following, except:

A. Lack of judgment

B. Lack of comprehension

C. Acute onset of memory loss

D. Alterations in mood

Answer: C

Critique: Dementia is characterized by lack of judgment, lack of comprehension, alterations in mood, and memory loss. The memory loss, however, is not acute. The rate of intellectual impairment varies from patient to patient and occurs over months to years.

Page: 1366

Match the dementia type with the following statements. (Each may be used once, more than once, or not at all.)

A. Alzheimer's dementia

B. Vascular dementia

C. Neither A nor B

D. Both A and B

27: Accounts for the majority of dementia cases

28: Is associated with hypercalcemia

29: Requires cessation of driving

30: Is accompanied by focal asymmetric neurologic abnormalities

31: May mildly improve function with treatment with cholinesterase inhibitors

Answers: 27 - A, 28 - C, 29 - D, 30 - B, 31 - A

Critique: Two common etiologies of dementia are Alzheimer's type and vascular type. Alzheimer's dementia accounts for approximately 60% of dementia cases. It is associated with histologic findings of amyloid plaques and neurofibrillary tangles. Medical therapy may include cholinesterase inhibitors such as tacrine (Cognex) and donepezil (Aricept). These medications increase acetylcholine levels, which are low in patients with Alzheimer's dementia. Effects of these medications are moderate with a return to level of function noted within 6 to 12 months considered a good response. Vascular dementia may be subdivided into multi-infarct dementia and subcortical vascular dementia (Binswanger's disease). Multi-infarct dementia should be suspected in patients with focal asymmetric neurologic abnormalities. Neither type of dementia is associated with hypercalcemia, although elevated calcium levels can cause confusion. Patients with diagnosed dementia should not drive automobiles, because they may be a hazard to themselves or others.

Pages: 1367, 1368

32: In a comatose patient, pupils that react normally to light generally suggest the area of origin as which of the following:

A. Midbrain

B. Hemispheric

C. Brain stem

D. Cerebellar

Answer: B

Critique: Pupillary size, shape, symmetry, and light reaction are controlled by structures in the midbrain. As a general rule, a normal pupillary response to light in a comatose patient indicates a hemispheric cause for the coma. A brain stem lesion–causing coma produces abnormal pupillary function. The cerebellum is not involved in pupillary response; it is important in coordination.

Page: 1370

33: A 75-year-old comatose male undergoes cold caloric testing to assess oculovestibular response. No response is seen with testing on either side. This result indicates which of the following:

A. Hemispheric cause of coma
B. Presence of nonconvulsive seizures
C. Abducens nerve palsy
D. Brain stem etiology of coma

Answer: D

Critique: Cold caloric testing is useful in determining the level of neurologic injury in comatose patients. A lack of response is indicative of a brain stem etiology. In hemispheric coma, the slow phase in which the eyes look toward the irrigated ear is preserved, but the fast corrective phase-away is absent. A sudden, rapid, spontaneous jerking motion of the eyes indicates nonconvulsive seizures. Abducens nerve palsy is indicated by lack of outward deviation of one eye.

Pages: 1371, 1372

34: The corneal reflex is maintained by innervation from which of the following nerves:

A. Trigeminal
B. Facial
C. Both A and B
D. Neither A nor B

Answer: C

Critique: The corneal reflex is maintained by the afferent limb of the trigeminal nerve and both efferent limbs of the facial nerve.

Page: 1372

35: Apneustic breathing signifies which of the following:

A. Dysfunction in the cerebrum
B. Pontine lesion
C. Metabolic encephalopathy
D. Cerebellar lesion

Answer: B

Critique: Apneustic breathing is characterized by a deep and prolonged inspiration. This type of breathing signifies a lesion in the pons, which usually is the result of a focal stroke. Cerebral dysfunction and metabolic encephalopathy typically result in Cheyne-Stokes respirations. Cerebellar lesions result in movement disorders.

Page: 1372

36: Motor findings seen in encephalopathic patients include all of the following, except:

A. Abnormal deep tendon reflexes
B. Myoclonus
C. Asterixis
D. Tremor

Answer: A

Critique: Motor findings in encephalopathic patients include myoclonus, asterixis, and tremor. Deep tendon reflexes are generally preserved unless the corticospinal tract is involved.

Page: 1372

Match the sleep disorder with the appropriate clinical finding:

A. Obstructive sleep apnea
B. Narcolepsy
C. Central sleep apnea
D. Restless leg syndrome
E. Night terrors

37: Parasomnia that is more common in children

38: Associated with hypnagogic hallucinations

39: Associated with obesity

40: Cessation of respiratory effort

41: Iron deficiency anemia can be an underlying factor.

Answers: 37 - E, 38 - B, 39 - A, 40 - C, 41 - D

Critique: Sleep apnea is characterized by sleep-related respiratory irregularity, sleep disruption, excessive daytime sleepiness, and oxygen desaturation. Sleep apnea may be categorized as central or obstructive. An apnea is obstructive when respiratory effort produces no airflow. In central apnea, however, there is an absence of both airflow and respiratory effort. Obstructive sleep apnea is associated with obesity. Narcolepsy is characterized by excessive daytime hypersomnolence. It is associated with cataplexy, sleep paralysis, and hypnagogic hallucinations. Night terrors are classified as parasomnias and are more common in children. They are characterized by a sudden arousal with intense fear, tachycardia, diaphoresis, and increased muscle tone. Restless leg syndrome (RLS) is characterized by an irresistible urge to move the legs, usually before the onset of sleep. RLS may be associated with disease states, including uremia, iron deficiency anemia, and peripheral neuropathy.

Pages: 1374–1377

42: Seizures that result in focal EEG abnormalities are consistent with which of the following:

A. Partial seizure disorder
B. Generalized seizure disorder
C. Both A and B
D. Neither A nor B

Answer: A

Critique: Partial seizures arise in a portion of one cerebral hemisphere and are associated with focal EEG abnormalities. Generalized seizures typically involve both cerebral hemispheres at the same time from their onset.

Page: 1377

Questions 43 to 46: (True or False) Which of the following statements regarding febrile seizures are true and which ones false:

43: The risk of recurrence after the first episode is approximately 33%.

44: Of children with a febrile seizure, 15% will develop epilepsy.

45: Lumbar puncture should be performed for all cases.

46: Seizures typically last less than 6 minutes.

Answers: 43 - True, 44 - False, 45 - False, 46 - True

Critique: Febrile seizures occur in febrile children, usually from 3 months to 5 years of age, without a definite etiology. Febrile seizures affect approximately 2% to 4% of children. Approximately one third of children who have a febrile seizure will have at least one more. Less than 5% of children who experience a febrile seizure develop epilepsy. Febrile seizures usually last less than 6 minutes and are most commonly tonic-clonic in nature. Lumbar puncture does not need to be performed unless there is a clinical suspicion of intracranial infection.

Pages: 1377, 1378

47: Which of the following is the preferred agent for the medical treatment of absence seizures:

    A. Phenytoin (Dilantin)
    B. Carbamazepine (Tegretol)
    C. Ethosuximide
    D. Phenobarbital

Answer: C

Critique: Although all of these medications are used in the treatment of seizure disorders, ethosuximide is the drug of choice in treating patients with absence seizures. Valproic acid may also be used in treating absence seizures.

Page: 1379

48: A 1-month-old infant is diagnosed clinically with meningitis. The most likely causative bacterial organism is which of the following:

    A. *Escherichia coli*
    B. *Streptococcus pneumoniae*
    C. *Staphylococcus aureus*
    D. Group B streptococci

Answer: D

Critique: For all populations, the three most common pathogens for community-acquired bacterial meningitis are *Haemophilus influenzae, Neisseria meningitidis,* and *S. pneumoniae.* In the first months of life, however, group B streptococci are the most common causative agent.

Page: 1381

49: All of the following laboratory results on cerebral spinal fluid (CSF) examination would be expected in bacterial meningitis, except:

    A. Increased glucose
    B. Increased protein
    C. Increased white blood cell (WBC) count
    D. Bacterial organisms seen on Gram stain

Answer: A

Critique: CSF examination in patients suspected of having bacterial meningitis offers significant diagnostic help. Individuals with bacterial meningitis demonstrate decreased glucose, increased protein, and increased WBC count on CSF examination. The presence of bacterial organisms on Gram stain of the CSF also offers confirmation of bacterial meningitis.

Pages: 1380, 1381

50: In bacterial meningitis, administration of corticosteroids is indicated for which of the following:

    A. In all cases
    B. In infants and children older than 2 months with *Haemophilus influenzae*
    C. In adults with *S. pneumoniae* as a pathogen
    D. In adults with *Mycobacterium tuberculosis* as a pathogen

Answer: B

Critique: The role of corticosteroids in bacterial meningitis is controversial. However, in children over the age of 2 months with *H. influenzae* as a cause of bacterial meningitis, administration of dexamethasone with or before the first dose of antibiotics is indicated. This treatment has been shown to decrease the risk of neurologic and audiologic sequelae. In other cases, steroids are reserved for patients with a positive CSF Gram stain and increased intracranial pressure. Corticosteroids are not indicated in tuberculous meningitis.

Pages: 1381, 1382

51: Rifampin prophylaxis is indicated for close contacts in documented cases of which of the following:

    A. Meningococcal meningitis
    B. *H. influenzae* meningitis
    C. Both A and B
    D. Neither A nor B

Answer: C

Critique: Rifampin prophylaxis is recommended for close contacts in documented cases of both meningococcal meningitis and *H. influenzae* meningitis. Rifampin prophylaxis is not recommended for other causes of meningitis.

Page: 1383

52: Recurrent cases of meningitis are most likely a result of which of the following:

    A. Chronic sinusitis
    B. Chronic otitis media
    C. Chronic CSF leak
    D. Chronic tonsillitis

Answer: C

Critique: Recurrent cases of meningitis may be secondary to infectious or noninfectious sources. A CSF leak is the most common underlying etiology, accounting for approximately 75% of recurrent cases of meningitis.

Page: 1383

53: The initial diagnostic test of choice in a patient with a suspected brain abscess is which of the following:

    A. Computed tomography (CT) scan
    B. Lumbar puncture
    C. Skull radiographs
    D. Cerebral arteriogram

Answer: A

Critique: Cerebral edema is often present with brain abscesses. When a brain abscess is suspected clinically, a CT scan or magnetic resonance imaging (MRI) should be performed before lumbar puncture. Skull radiographs are of limited value in identifying a brain abscess. Cerebral angiography is not indicated as the initial diagnostic maneuver to identify a brain abscess.

Page: 1385

54: Continuous dizziness is likely to be associated with which of the following:

    A. Meniere's disease
    B. Cerebrovascular accident
    C. Benign positional vertigo (BPV)
    D. Transient ischemic attacks (TIAs)

Answer: B

Critique: Continuous dizziness is most likely to be associated with a cerebrovascular accident. In Meniere's disease, dizziness may last hours to days but is not continuous. Dizziness in TIAs and BPV is typically transient.

Pages: 1385, 1386

55: The Hallpike maneuver is useful in the diagnosis of which of the following:

    A. Cerebellar disease
    B. Orthostatic hypotension
    C. Meniere's disease
    D. Benign positional vertigo (BPV)

Answer: D

Critique: A positive Hallpike maneuver confirms the diagnosis of BPV. (See discussion in text for criteria for a positive test.) Orthostatic hypotension is diagnosed by orthostatic changes in blood pressure and pulse. Meniere's disease is associated with a hearing loss, and dizziness is typically not positional. Cerebellar disease is more likely to result in balance disorders and should not be affected by Hallpike maneuver.

Page: 1386

56: Transient ischemic attacks (TIAs) that result in vertigo are secondary to ischemia in the distribution of which of the following:

    A. Internal carotid artery
    B. External carotid artery
    C. Vertebrobasilar arteries
    D. Temporal arteries

Answer: C

Critique: TIAs that result in vertiginous symptoms are secondary to ischemia in the distribution of the vertebrobasilar arteries. TIAs involving the carotid circulation are more likely to result in motor and sensory changes as well as amaurosis fugax.

Page: 1387

57: Worldwide, the most common cause of peripheral neuropathy is which of the following:

    A. Alcoholism
    B. Human immunodeficiency virus (HIV) infection
    C. Diabetes mellitus
    D. Leprosy

Answer: D

Critique: Although alcohol, HIV, and diabetes can all result in peripheral neuropathy and account for the majority of cases in developed countries, leprosy still remains the leading cause worldwide.

Pages: 1387, 1388

58: Wallerian degeneration is characteristic of:

    A. Myelinopathies
    B. Axonal neuropathies
    C. Neuronopathies
    D. Myopathies

Answer: B

Critique: Wallerian degeneration is characterized by degeneration of the axon and myelin sheath distal to the site of injury and is seen in axonal neuropathies. Myelinopathies, as the name suggests, primarily affect the myelin sheath and may result from acute or chronic conditions (e.g., Guillain-Barré syndrome). Neuronopathies result from damage to the dorsal root ganglia or motor neuron cell bodies in the spinal cord. Degeneration with incomplete recovery is common in neuronopathies. Myopathies involve muscle rather than neurons.

Page: 1389

59: Electromyography (EMG) is not typically useful in the diagnosis of which of the following:

    A. Small-fiber peripheral neuropathies
    B. Entrapment neuropathies
    C. Diabetic neuropathy
    D. Large-fiber peripheral neuropathies

Answer: A

Critique: EMG is helpful in the diagnosis of entrapment neuropathies, diabetic neuropathy, and large-fiber peripheral neuropathies. It is not as good a diagnostic tool in small-fiber peripheral neuropathies and often appears normal in these disease states, in which only pinprick and temperature sensation are affected.

Page: 1390

60: A 17-year-old football player suffers a "burner" during a game. The most common brachial plexus nerve roots affected in this type of injury involve which of the following:

    A. C3–C4
    B. C7–C8
    C. C8–T1
    D. C5–C6

Answer: D

Critique: Brachial plexopathies or "burners" are common injuries in football. They typically result from either a compression or a stretch injury of the brachial plexus. Players most commonly present with symptoms related to the C5–C6 nerve roots. These symptoms are usually transient and do not typically cause any long-term problems.

Page: 1390

61: Risk factors for the development of carpal tunnel syndrome include all of the following, except:

    A. Ulnar styloid fracture
    B. Pregnancy
    C. Thyroid disease
    D. Diabetes

Answer: A

Critique: Pregnancy (fluid retention), thyroid disease, and diabetes (enlargement of the median nerve) are all risk factors for the development of carpal tunnel syndrome. The ulnar styloid is not in close proximity to the carpal tunnel, and a fracture at this site would not put the median nerve at risk of impingement.

Page: 1390

62: Inability to adduct the small finger (fifth digit) may be the initial motor sign of which of the following:

    A. Anterior interosseous syndrome
    B. Carpal tunnel syndrome
    C. Cubital tunnel syndrome
    D. Supinator syndrome

Answer: C

Critique: The ulnar nerve innervates the majority of the intrinsic muscles of the hand and is responsible for the adduction of the small finger. The nerve may be compromised as it passes through the cubital tunnel at the elbow (cubital tunnel syndrome). Carpal tunnel syndrome is an entrapment neuropathy of the median nerve. Supinator syndrome is an entrapment neuropathy of the motor branch of the radial nerve. Anterior interosseous syndrome is an entrapment neuropathy of a branch of the median nerve in the forearm.

Pages: 1391,1392

63: Improper use of crutches may result in injury to which of the following nerves:

    A. Axillary
    B. Median
    C. Radial
    D. Ulnar

Answer: C

Critique: In the proximal arm, the radial nerve is vulnerable to injury in the axilla. This may occur by hyperabduction of the arm, which puts traction on the nerve. This is not an uncommon complication of improperly fitted crutches. Injuries to the median and ulnar nerves are not common in the proximal part of the arm. The axillary nerve may be injured in association with shoulder injuries, especially in glenohumeral dislocation, but it is not commonly injured with improperly fitted crutches.

Pages: 1392, 1393

64: A 50-year-old diabetic female presents with symptoms of pain and paresthesias in the anterolateral aspect of the thigh. These symptoms are suggestive of which of the following:

    A. Femoral neuropathy
    B. Sciatic nerve impingement
    C. Peroneal neuropathy
    D. Meralgia paresthetica

Answer: D

Critique: Compression of the lateral femoral cutaneous nerve or meralgia paresthetica is a common peripheral neuropathy. The nerve is typically compressed as it passes over the anterior superior iliac spine. Risk factors include diabetes, obesity, and excessively tight pants. Paresthesias and pain of the anterolateral thigh are usual presenting symptoms. The femoral nerve supplies sensation to the anteromedial thigh. The sciatic nerve supplies sensation to the perineum, posterior thigh, lateral calf, and foot. The peroneal nerve supplies sensation to the lateral aspect of the calf and dorsum of the foot.

Pages: 55, 56

65: Morton's neuroma most commonly occurs between the metatarsal heads at which of the following web spaces:

    A. First and second
    B. Second and third
    C. Third and fourth
    D. Fourth and fifth

Answer: B

Critique: Morton's neuroma is a benign swelling of an interdigital nerve that can cause symptoms of nerve entrapment in the foot. The most common site for a Morton's neuroma to occur is between the metatarsal heads at the second and third web spaces.

Page: 1394

66: Infection with which of the following bacterial organisms is most closely associated with Guillain-Barré syndrome:

    A. *Escherichia coli*
    B. *Streptococcus pneumoniae*
    C. *Klebsiella pneumoniae*
    D. *Campylobacter jejuni*

Answer: D

Critique: Guillain-Barré syndrome (GBS) is an acute inflammatory demyelinating polyradiculoneuropathy. It tends to be a rapidly progressive paralytic syndrome that seems to occur through an immune-mediated response. Most cases follow a viral illness by 1 to 3 weeks. Other risk factors include pregnancy, human immunodeficiency virus (HIV) infection, and bacterial infection with *C. jejuni.*

Pages: 1394, 1395

67: Beriberi is associated with deficiency of which of the following:

    A. Pyridoxine (vitamin B$_6$)
    B. Vitamin B$_{12}$
    C. Thiamine (vitamin B$_1$)
    D. None of the above

Answer: C

Critique: Deficiency of thiamine may be encountered in chronic alcoholics and is known as beriberi disease. These patients may present with a distal polyneuropathy or with Wernicke-Korsakoff encephalopathy. Pyridoxine and vitamin B$_{12}$ deficiencies can also cause a neuropathy.

Page: 1395

68: Wrist drop (radial nerve palsy) is associated with intoxication by which of the following heavy metals:

    A. Copper
    B. Lead
    C. Aluminum
    D. Cobalt

Answer: B

Critique: Lead intoxication results in a motor neuropathy that starts in the upper limbs. It may affect the radial nerve, leading to a wrist drop. Cobalt intoxication may lead to cardiomyopathy. Copper intoxication is associated with Wilson's disease. Aluminum contributes to encephalopathy seen in patients with severe renal disease who undergo dialysis.

Pages: 1395, 1396

69: Bell's palsy is commonly associated with which of the following:

    A. Bilateral involvement
    B. Sensory deficits over the posterior neck
    C. Paresis of cranial nerve V
    D. Spontaneous remission

Answer: D

Critique: Bell's palsy affects the facial nerve (VII) and occurs for unknown reasons, although it may follow a viral illness. It is characterized by unilateral facial droop, involvement of the forehead (inability to wrinkle the forehead), and spontaneous remission.

Page: 1396

70: Which of the following is true regarding trigeminal neuralgia (tic douloureux):

    A. Usually occurs bilaterally
    B. May occur secondary to acoustic neuroma
    C. Treated most effectively with narcotic analgesics
    D. Usually involves the first and second divisions of the trigeminal nerve

Answer: B

Critique: Trigeminal neuralgia usually involves the second and third divisions of the trigeminal nerve and causes pain in the lips, gums, and teeth. Pain may be severe and is typically cyclical. The symptoms are unilateral in 95% of cases. Trigeminal neuralgia may occur as a result of multiple sclerosis, acoustic neuroma, and meningioma. Most patients can be managed with carbamazepine. Other medications, including tricyclic antidepressants and gabapentin, may also be useful.

Pages: 1396, 1397

Match the muscular dystrophy with the appropriate corresponding statement:
    A. Myotonic dystrophy
    B. Becker's muscular dystrophy
    C. Duchenne muscular dystrophy

71: X-linked recessive inheritance

72: Dysarthria and dysphagia common symptoms

73: Dystrophin present in reduced quantities

Answers: 71 - C, 72 - A, 73 - B

Critique: Duchenne muscular dystrophy is an X-linked recessive disorder in which the abnormal gene fails to produce dystrophin, whose absence allows calcium to enter cells, causing muscle necrosis. In Becker's muscular dystrophy, dystrophin is present but in reduced amounts. Myotonic dystrophy is the most common adult muscular dystrophy. It typically involves the palatal and pharyngeal muscles, producing dysphagia and dysarthria.

Pages: 1397, 1398

74: The underlying pathogenesis in myasthenia gravis is which of the following:

    A. Antibodies against serotonin receptors
    B. Antibodies against acetylcholine
    C. Antibodies against acetylcholine receptor
    D. Antibodies against norepinephrine receptors

Answer: C

Critique: Myasthenia gravis is a disease of the neuromuscular junction. In affected patients, weakness occurs because of failure of normal transmission across the neuromuscular junction owing to a decreased amount of acetylcholine receptors. The number of receptors is decreased secondary to an autoimmune process in which antibodies are directed against the acetylcholine receptors.

Page: 1399

75: All of the following are characteristics of myasthenia gravis, except:

    A. Frequent improvement in patients' symptoms throughout the day
    B. Associated with thymoma in approximately 15% of cases
    C. Pure motor syndrome
    D. More common in women

Answer: A

Critique: Myasthenia gravis occurs 50% more often in women than in men. It is associated with thymoma in 15% of adults. Because it affects the neuromuscular junction, it is a pure motor disease. Patients' symptoms usually progress throughout the day and may be better in the morning.

Pages: 1399, 1400

76: Edrophonium (Tensilon) improves symptoms in myasthenia gravis by which of the following mechanisms:

A. Increased release of acetylcholine
B. Inhibition of acetylcholinesterase
C. Up regulation of acetylcholine receptors
D. Increased release of norepinephrine

Answer: B

Critique: The Tensilon test is useful in the diagnosis of myasthenia gravis. Patients' symptoms improve with the administration of edrophonium, because it acts to inhibit the breakdown of acetylcholine by acetylcholinesterase. This allows better binding of acetylcholine to the available receptors, thus improving symptoms. Edrophonium does not affect the release of acetylcholine or norepinephrine.

Page: 1400

Questions 77 to 81: (True or False) Decide whether the following statements regarding Parkinson's disease are true or false:

77: Degeneration of pigmented neurons in the substantia nigra is a characteristic neuropathologic finding.

78: Symmetric tremor is the most common presenting symptom.

79: Selegiline therapy slows dopamine catabolism.

80: The combination of carbidopa-levodopa slows neurologic degeneration.

81: Thalamotomy may be useful in reducing tremor.

Answers: 77 - True, 78 - False, 79 - True, 80 - False, 81 - True

Critique: Parkinson's disease (PD) is a slowly progressive degenerative disorder that is characterized histologically by degeneration of pigmented neurons in the substantia nigra. Degeneration of these neurons results in dopamine deficiency and accounts for the classical clinical features of PD, which include tremor, rigidity, and bradykinesia. The tremor is an asymmetric resting tremor and is the most common presenting symptom. Selegiline is an inhibitor of monoamine oxidase-B and is useful in the treatment of PD because it slows the catabolism of dopamine. Many other medications, including levodopa, anticholinergics, and dopamine agonists, may be useful in treating the symptoms of PD. No medications, however, have been efficacious in slowing neurologic degeneration. Thalamotomy may be useful in patients with severe unilateral disabling tremors that do not respond to medications.

Pages: 1401–1403

82: Magnetic resonance imaging (MRI) findings associated with a diagnosis of multiple sclerosis (MS) include which of the following:

A. Cerebral atrophy
B. Gray matter lesions on T_1 images
C. Gray matter plaques on T_2 images
D. Periventricular white matter plaques

Answer: C

Critique: MRI is a useful tool in the diagnosis of MS. MRI findings associated with a diagnosis of MS include "plaques," which represent areas of demyelination. MS plaques involve white matter and are typically seen in the periventricular areas of the cerebrum, brain stem, and spinal cord.

Page: 1403

83: Typical cerebrospinal fluid (CSF) findings in multiple sclerosis (MS) include all of the following, except:

A. Elevated protein
B. Normal glucose
C. Presence of oligoclonal bands
D. Normal opening pressure

Answer: A

Critique: CSF evaluation in patients with MS is often helpful in making a diagnosis. Typical findings include normal protein and glucose levels, as well as normal cell count and opening pressure. Oligoclonal bands are found in up to 90% of MS patients.

Page: 1403

84: Medications that reduce the number of relapses in multiple sclerosis (MS) include all of the following, except:

A. Interferon β-1a
B. Interferon β-1b
C. Prednisone
D. Glatiramer acetate
E. Intravenous methylprednisolone

Answer: C

Critique: Disease-modifying therapies for patients with MS work mainly by modulation of immune responses. Newer immunomodulating drugs include interferon β-1a and -1b and glatiramer acetate, all of which have been shown to decrease the frequency of relapses and slow disease progression. Although intravenous methylprednisolone has been shown to lessen relapses of MS, oral corticosteroids have not. In fact, oral corticosteroids may increase the risk of attacks.

Pages: 1404, 1405

85: Neurologic impairment in amyotrophic lateral sclerosis (ALS) patients includes which of the following:

A. Sexual dysfunction
B. Cognitive impairment
C. Upper and lower motor neuron dysfunction
D. Bowel and bladder incontinence

Answer: C

Critique: ALS is a progressive, degenerative disorder that affects both upper and lower motor neurons. Although ALS is typically widespread, certain functions are usually spared, including cognitive, sexual, and bowel and bladder.

Page: 1405

Chapter 50

Sexuality in Family Medicine

Sam Sandowski

1: (True or False) Determine which of the following statements about human sexuality are true or false:

   A. The "sex" of a person is determined by society and must be determined by the parents of newborns with ambiguous genitalia.
   B. The "gender" of a person refers to the characteristics associated with a particular sex.
   C. The term *homosexual* is appropriate only if a person has had sexual relations with another person of the same sex.
   D. *Homosexual, bisexual,* and *heterosexual* are terms used to describe one's sexual orientation.

Answers: A - False, B - True, C - False, D - True

Critique: In Western culture, common terms and colloquialisms in everyday conversations are not always synonymous with the medical definition of these terms. The "sex" of an individual is determined by the chromosomal makeup of the individual or by the genital phenotype. The term *gender* refers to the self-perception of characteristics associated with a particular sex. Sexual orientation refers to the attraction to same-sex or opposite-sex partners or both. The term *homosexuality* refers to the exclusive attraction to a same-sex partner, even if sexual relations have not been encountered.

Pages: 1411, 1412

2: All of the following phases have been described in the human sexual response cycle (SRC), except:

   A. Desire
   B. Excitement
   C. Plateau
   D. Stimulation
   E. Orgasm

Answer: D

Critique: The SRC, first described by Masters and Johnson, described four physiologic phases encountered with sexual stimulation: excitement, plateau, orgasm, and resolution. Singer-Kaplan added a psychological phase, desire, combined the excitement and plateau phases, and eliminated the resolution phase. Stimulation is necessary for the SRC to occur, but it is not one of the phases. Sexual dysfunction may occur at any phase.

Page: 1412, Table 50–2

3: All of the following are true, except that orgasms can:

   A. Result in contractions of the testes, epididymis, vas deferens, urethra, and penis in men

   B. Result in vaginal and uterine contractions in women
   C. Cause a decrease in heart rate
   D. Cause vocalization
   E. Cause loss of voluntary motor control in men

Answer: C

Critique: Orgasms may cause contractions of the testes, epididymis, vas deferens, urethra, and penis in men and of the outer vagina and uterus in women. There may also be vocalization and loss of voluntary motor control. During the excitement phase, there is greater parasympathetic activity, but during orgasm there is greater sympathetic activity and the heart rate increases.

Page: 1413, Table 50–2

4: The most common reason elderly persons do not engage in sexual activity is:

   A. Lack of an appropriate partner
   B. Disability from chronic diseases, such as chronic obstructive pulmonary disease (COPD) and arthritis
   C. Physiologic changes associated with aging
   D. the belief that one should not have sexual activity after a certain age
   E. belief that if one has lost a spouse, people should not engage in sexual activity if they are not married

Answer: A

Critique: Physicians have associated many misconceptions with sexual activity in the elderly. Though physiologic changes associated with age or disease processes may be a reason for some elderly not to engage in sexual activity, according to a study by the American Association of Retired Persons (AARP) the most common reason was lack of an appropriate partner. Many elderly are more liberal in their sexual views than physicians may presume: one third of women ages 75 and older did not agree that "people should not have a sexual relationship if they are not married."

Page: 1413

5: When taking a sexual history, all of the following techniques should be used, except:

   A. Inclusion
   B. Normalization
   C. Universalization

D. Using a nonjudgmental approach
E. Providing direction regarding sexual life choices

Answer: E

Critique: When taking a sexual history, a nonjudgmental approach, making no assumptions, is the most effective way to obtain an honest, accurate sexual history. Universalization "assumes that everyone has done everything" and doesn't presume that certain sexual activities are more or less appropriate than other activities. Normalization allows the person to feel that the activity questioned is prevalent and that they are not the only one encountering such an experience (e.g., letting the person know that sexual abuse is not uncommon before questioning them about it). Inclusion allows the person to know that you question all patients about sexuality and that they are not being singled out. Giving direction as to sexual life choices may be viewed as imposing and unwelcome.

Page: 1415

6: When assessing a patient for sexual dysfunction, which of the following organs and systems needs to be examined:

A. Thyroid
B. Cardiovascular
C. Neurologic
D. Skin
E. All

Answer: E

Critique: Although sexual dysfunction may be psychological, physiologic disorders must be ruled out first, including cardiovascular, neurologic, and endocrine disorders. Additionally, a dermatologic problem causing irritation or embarrassment or a musculoskeletal disorder, such as arthritis, may be the reason for sexual dysfunction.

Page: 1417

7: In treating sexual dysfunction, the P-LI-SS-IT model is often used. Which step may be used by family physicians to determine the patient's concerns:

A. P (permission)
B. LI (limited information)
C. SS (specific suggestions)
D. IT (intensive therapy)
E. None of the above

Answer: A

Critique: The steps in the P-LI-SS-IT model are P, permission; LI, limited information; SS, specific suggestions; and IT, intensive therapy. The first step, permission, validates a person's concerns and permits the patient to discuss them further. Identifying a person's concerns helps the physician determine further treatment or appropriate referrals. The other steps, providing limited information, specific suggestions, and intensive therapy, may be best suited for physicians who specialize in sexual dysfunction.

Pages: 1417, 1418, Table 50–3

8: The percentage of women who experience orgasm with vaginal intercourse alone (i.e., without additional clitoral stimulation) is:

A. 100%
B. 90%
C. 80%
D. 65%
E. Less than 50%

Answer: E

Critique: Most women (more than 50%) do not achieve orgasm with vaginal intercourse alone. They require additional clitoral stimulation.

Page: 1418

9: Which of the following is *not* a cause for secondary inhibited orgasm?

A. Lack of personal or partner knowledge of sexual techniques
B. Inability to reach orgasm with vaginal intercourse alone (i.e., no additional clitoral stimulation)
C. Psychologic illness
D. Substance abuse
E. Dyspareunia

Answer: B

Critique: The inability to reach orgasm with only vaginal intercourse and no additional clitoral stimulation occurs in over 50% of women. This condition is so common that it is not included as a cause of orgasmic dysfunction. Causes of secondary dysfunction—the inability to achieve orgasm after previous satisfactory orgasmic functioning—may be organic or psychological factors, including sexual technique, strained relationships, sexual abuse, dyspareunia, or substance abuse.

10: Treatment options for primary orgasmic dysfunction in women include all of the following, except:

A. Receiving information about female sexuality and function
B. Masturbation
C. Partner education
D. Referral for intensive therapy in cases of significant relationship dysfunction
E. Reassurance that this is normal and acceptable in many women

Answer: E

Critique: Some cultures do not encourage women to discuss or explore their sexuality, but in Western cultures primary orgasmic dysfunction should be addressed, particularly if it is of concern to the patient. Primary orgasmic dysfunction may be a result of the woman's inability to identify an orgasm. Learning techniques that increase clitoral and pre-intercourse stimulation are useful and may be achieved with masturbation. Women with a history of abuse and those with significant relationship dysfunction may benefit from intensive psychotherapy.

Page: 1418

11: Vaginismus is:

  A. A discharge from the vagina for any reason
  B. Usually painful
  C. Caused by voluntary pelvic muscle contractions
  D. Almost always idiopathic
  E. Synonymous with vulvar vestibulitis

Answer: B

Critique: "Vaginismus is an involuntary, usually painful spastic contraction of the pelvic musculature, surrounding the outer third of the vagina." Although vaginismus may be idiopathic, many cases are secondary to trauma to the pelvic region (e.g., abuse, gynecologic examination, episiotomy) or subsequent to a vaginal infection or pelvic inflammatory disease. It must be differentiated from vulvar vestibulitis, in which there is tenderness within the vulvar vestibule and vestibular erythema.

Pages: 1418, 1419

12: The postage stamp test to measure erectile dysfunction:

  A. Measures nocturnal penile tumescence
  B. Costs as much to perform as mailing a letter
  C. Uses a double ring of stamps around the penis
  D. Is likely to be positive (i.e., the ring will break) if erectile dysfunction is due to a physiologic cause
  E. Can determine the amount and velocity of blood flow to the penis

Answer: A

Critique: The postage stamp test is a simple test in which a single thickness of stamps is wrapped around a flaccid penis. If an erection occurs overnight (nocturnal penile tumescence), the ring will break. If this happens, a physiologic cause of erectile dysfunction is unlikely.

Page: 1420

13: Which of the following is true in reference to sildenafil (Viagra):

  A. It should be used before a cause of erectile dysfunction is sought.
  B. It may be used even if a cause is not found.
  C. If sildenafil is effective, further evaluation for erectile dysfunction should continue.
  D. It should be given only after a vascular evaluation of the penis.
  E. It is effective only in patients with compromised blood flow to the penis.

Answer: B

Critique: Sildenafil is effective in a high percentage of patients with erectile dysfunction, regardless of the cause. A sexual and medical history and physical examination are the first steps in evaluating erectile dysfunction and must be done before prescribing sildenafil. Even if a cause is not found, however, a trial with sildenafil may be worthwhile. If it is effective, further diagnostic evaluation of the erectile dysfunction is not necessary. Vascular evaluation of the penis should be done if a trial of sildenafil fails or there is a contraindication to prescribing sildenafil.

Page: 1421

14: (True or False) Determine which of the following statements are true and which are false about testosterone:

  A. All men with low testosterone levels have some form of erectile dysfunction.
  B. Testosterone replacement should be considered for men with low testosterone levels and erectile dysfunction.
  C. Testosterone can be given orally, intramuscularly, or transdermally.
  D. The most effective form of testosterone supplementation is oral.

Answers: A - False, B - True, C - False, D - False

Critique: Low levels of testosterone are not always associated with erectile dysfunction, and many men with very low testosterone levels have normal erectile function. However, if low levels are found in a man with erectile dysfunction, a trial with testosterone supplementation may be considered. Testosterone may be given intramuscularly every 10 to 21 days or via a transdermal patch. No oral testosterone preparations for replacement are currently approved.

Page: 1421

15: (True or False) Sildenafil (Viagra):

  A. Works by inhibiting the 5-isoenzyme of the phosphodiesterase, used to degrade cyclic guanosine monophosphate (cGMP)
  B. Is highly effective in erectile dysfunction with either physiologic and psychological causes
  C. May cause color blindness
  D. May cause death if used together with nitrates

Answers: A - True, B - True, C - True, D - True

Critique: Sildenafil inhibits the 5-isoenzyme of the phosphodiesterase, causing cGMP to break down more slowly. An increased cGMP level permits prolonged cavernous smooth muscle relaxation and enhances erectile dysfunction. Sildenafil is effective in 70% to 90% of patients and is effective in erectile dysfunction that results from both physiologic and psychological causes. Side effects of sildenafil are flushing, headache, color blindness, and gastrointestinal discomfort. Concomitant use with nitrates may cause hypotension and death.

Page: 1421

16: All of the following are methods of treatment for erectile dysfunction, except:

  A. Injectable alprostadil
  B. Intraurethral alprostadil (medicated urethral system for erection, or MUSE)
  C. Vacuum pumps
  D. Beta-blockers
  E. Sildenafil

Answer: D

Critique: Several different methods are currently used to treat erectile dysfunction. Vacuum therapy can be used in almost all cases of erectile dysfunction. The vacuum pressure causes the penis to engorge, and then a band is placed at the base of the penis to maintain the erection. Alprostadil is available in an injectable form and an intraurethral form. Sildenafil is one of the most effective oral agents currently available for erectile dysfunction. Beta-blockers may cause erectile dysfunction.

Page: 1421

17: (True or False) Determine which of the following statements are true and which are false about alprostadil:

    A. Alprostadil injections should be given only in the physician's office
    B. Complications with alprostadil are common and include penile necrosis.
    C. Long-term use of alprostadil injections may result in fibrosis.
    D. Up to 10% of patients have painful erections.
    E. Patients should seek medical attention if erections last more than 4 hours.

Answers: A - False, B - False, C - True, D - True, E - True

Critique: Injectable alprostadil, a prostaglandin E_1, is especially useful in erectile dysfunction secondary to vascular disease. The initial injection should be given in the physician's office. However, once titrated to an effective dose, the intracavernous injection can be self-administered. Although complications of alprostadil are rare, long-term use can lead to fibrosis (not necrosis). Ten percent of patients do have painful erections.

Page: 1421

18: Premature ejaculation occurs:

    A. In less than 5 minutes after erection
    B. In less than 10 minutes after erection
    C. In less than 15 minutes after erection
    D. In less than 20 minutes after erection
    E. None of the above

Answer: E

Critique: Premature ejaculation is defined subjectively as ejaculation that occurs sooner than desired by the person or the person's partner. It is not defined by a unit of time, and one partner may feel premature ejaculation is present, while the other does not.

Pages: 1421, 1422

19: Which of the following is not a technique used in the treatment of premature ejaculation?

    A. Squeeze technique
    B. Start-and-stop technique
    C. Masturbation training
    D. Excessive stimulation or overstimulation of the penis
    E. Selective serotonin reuptake inhibitors (SSRIs)

Answer: D

Critique: The squeeze technique is the application of firm pressure on the ventral side of the penis for 3 to 5 seconds. The start-and-stop technique requires stopping sexual stimulation before imminent ejaculation. This can be practiced alone with masturbation training or with a partner. SSRIs prolong the plateau phase of the sexual response cycle (SRC). Excessive stimulation or overstimulation may be a reason that ejaculation takes place earlier than desired.

Page: 1422

20: Dyspareunia:

    A. Does not occur in men
    B. Occurs in men but much less frequently than in women
    C. Occurs approximately equally in men and women but is less discussed with men
    D. Occurs in women but much less frequently than in men
    E. Is always secondary to psychological stress

Answer: B

Critique: Dyspareunia is much less common in men than in women, but it can occur with certain conditions, such as Peyronie's disease, poor technique, or decreased lubrication. Organic genitourinary disorders must be excluded when evaluating dyspareunia, as do psychological issues, such as exploring the relationship stresses or abuse.

Page: 1423

21: (True or False) Determine whether the following statements are true or false:

    A. Human sexual behavior is learned.
    B. Adolescents' engagement in sexual activity is a result of increased hormonal levels.
    C. Adulthood is defined by society and not by sexual activity.
    D. It should be expected that teenagers can and should refrain from sexual activity until age 18.

Answers: A - False, B - False, C - True, D - False

Critique: Sexual techniques may be learned, but human sexual behavior is instinctive. Adolescents may engage in sexual relations to "prove" their adulthood, not just for sexual satisfaction or biological urges.

Page: 1423

22: Masturbation in women:

    A. Is learned about at an earlier age than in males
    B. Is learned about from peers
    C. Stops when one has a partner
    D. Does not occur in the elderly
    E. Can be used to treat primary orgasmic dysfunction

Answer: E

Critique: In males, masturbation is usually learned about from peers at ages 13 to 15. Females usually learn about masturbation at a later age through self-exploration. Masturbation is a normal sexual activity at all ages and may be particularly useful in primary orgasmic dysfunction in women.

Page: 1423

23: (True or False) Determine whether the following statements regarding sexual activity in adolescents are true or false.

A. Approximately 50% of adolescent males report having sexual intercourse.
B. Most sexual adolescent males are monogamous.
C. Drugs and/or alcohol are used by approximately 25% of adolescents before intercourse.
D. Thirty percent of teens who deny sexual intercourse engage in other sexual activities, including mutual masturbation.

Answers: A - True, B - True, C - True, D - True

Critique: Up to 50% of adolescent males have had sexual intercourse. Generally, adolescents tend to stay monogamous while in a relationship. Relationships, however, are usually short lived and therefore they practice serial monogamy. In approximately 25% of cases, alcohol or drugs are used before an adolescent's sexual activity.

Pages: 1423, 1424

24: (True or False) Which of the following are true and which are false regarding suicide:

A. Suicide is more prevalent in homosexual adults than in heterosexual adults.
B. Suicide attempts are more prevalent in homosexual adolescents than in heterosexual adolescents.
C. The risk of suicide is greatest among adolescents and the elderly.
D. Drugs and alcohol are not risk factors in teen suicide.

Answers: A - False, B - True, C - True, D - False

Critique: Suicide is not more likely in homosexual adults than heterosexual adults, but gay adolescents are three times more likely to attempt suicide. Drugs and alcohol use, which increases the risk of adolescent suicide, may be used by some gay youth to alter their mental status and help them engage in heterosexual activities.

Page: 1424

25: Which of the following physiologic changes in the elderly does *not* occur?

A. Decreased scrotal vasoconstriction
B. Delayed erection
C. Less lubrication of the vagina
D. Disappearance of the multiorgasmic nature of orgasms in women

Answer: D

Critique: Changes in the sexual response cycle (SRC) are noted as people age. In men, this includes decreased scrotal vasoconstriction and testicular elevation, delayed erection, less pre-ejaculatory fluid, and less forceful ejaculations. As women age, they may experience less labial engorgement, less lubrication, and weaker uterine contractions. Multiple orgasms in women, however, continue to occur. Although not all people experience the same number of changes, proper education allows the elderly to continue to enjoy sexual activity.

Pages: 1424, 1425

26: Which of the following statements is correct regarding estrogen replacement as a treatment for physiologic changes in aging women?

A. Estrogen has little effect on the elasticity of the vaginal mucosa.
B. Estrogen has little effect on the lubrication of the vaginal mucosa.
C. If estrogen alone does not increase a woman's sexual drive, testosterone may be considered.
D. Estrogen replacement can be given only orally.
E. It often takes 6 months to achieve significant effects of estrogen replacement.

Answer: C

Critique: Estrogen replacement is used to treat some of the physiologic changes of aging affecting sexual activity in women. Estrogen can be replaced orally or topically, but often takes up to 18 months to achieve significant results. It improves elasticity and lubrication of the vaginal mucosa. Although studies are limited, if estrogen therapy alone is unsuccessful in increasing libido, adding testosterone may be considered.

Page: 1425

27: Which of the following should *not* be monitored when replacing testosterone in men?

A. Prostate-specific antigen (PSA)
B. Creatinine
C. Hematocrit
D. Cholesterol
E. Liver enzymes

Answer: B

Critique: Side effects of testosterone replacement include decreased HDL levels (8%), increased cholesterol-HDL ratios (9%), and polycythemia. Testosterone supplementation may also increase prostatic hyperplasia and promote growth of subclinical foci of prostate cancer. Liver enzymes should be monitored, because hepatitis and cholestatic jaundice may occur. Testosterone is metabolized in the liver, and significant first-round metabolism makes oral supplementation less effective. Therefore, intramuscular or transdermal replacement should be prescribed. Testosterone has little effect on renal function, and creatinine levels do not need to be monitored.

Page: 1425

28: The Kinsey Sexual Orientation Scale suggests which of the following:

A. Homosexuality is a psychological illness and therefore is considered an acceptable diagnosis according to the American Psychiatric Association.
B. A homosexual is defined as anyone who has had sexual relations with someone of the same sex more than once.
C. Sexual orientation lies across a spectrum.
D. Sexual orientation is determined before puberty.
E. Homosexuality is dangerous.

Answer: C

Critique: Sexual orientation is not always clearly defined, and many people do not define themselves as exclusively homosexual or heterosexual. Kinsey and colleagues described a seven-station scale that permitted people to place themselves on a spectrum of sexual orientation, from exclusively heterosexual (station 0) to equally homosexual and heterosexual (station 3) to exclusively homosexual (station 6). Only sociosexual contacts and responses that occurred postpubescently should be considered when using this scale. The Kinsey Sexual Orientation Scale does not address acceptability of a particular sexual orientation within a society.

Pages: 1425, 1426

29: Which of the following statements regarding the prevalence of homosexuality is true?

   A. Up to 50% of the male population in the United States reports having had at least one homosexual experience.
   B. The percentage of men who report at least one homosexual experience is greater than the percentage of women who report at least one homosexual experience.
   C. Studies have consistently reported that 7% of men in the United States consider themselves gay.
   D. The prevalence of homosexuality is increasing.
   E. The prevalence of bisexuality has not been studied.

Answer: B

Critique: Many studies have been done to try to determine the percentage of people who engage in homosexual experiences. The results have produced varied results, with anywhere from 10.9% to 37.0% of men report having at least one homosexual experience. The same studies in women consistently report lower percentages in women, ranging from 4.6% to 17.0%. Because results are varied and inconsistent, it is difficult to determine whether or not the prevalence of homosexuality is increasing.

Page: 1426

30: John, a 34-year-old male, presents to your office with a penile discharge. He is married and has two children. When taking his sexual history, which question is most appropriate?

   A. Is your wife here with you?
   B. What symptoms does your wife have?
   C. How often do you and your wife have intercourse?
   D. Are you sexually active with men, women, or both?
   E. Are you bisexual?

Answer: D

Critique: It would be inappropriate to assume that John contracted a sexually transmitted disease from his wife; sexual activity with other persons should be explored. When taking a sexual history, it is prudent to ask about both sexual desires and sexual activities. Not all patients with homosexual feelings have had homosexual experiences. Furthermore, not all patients who have had homosexual experiences identify themselves as gay or bisexual. Therefore, nonjudgmental, neutral questions should be asked.

Page: 1426

31: Which of the following statements is true regarding the "legality" of sexual activities?

   A. All sexual activities are legal when both partners are consenting and over 18.
   B. Sexual activity with minors (under age 18) is legal if the minor consents.
   C. Anal intercourse is legal in all states when both partners are consenting and over 18.
   D. In some states, fellatio is illegal with homosexual couples but legal with heterosexual couples.
   E. In some states, fellatio is illegal with heterosexual married couples.

Answer: E

Critique: It should be noted that laws on sodomy and "crimes against nature" statutes still exist. Activities such as fellatio and anal intercourse are illegal in some states. Though rarely enforced in a consenting married heterosexual couple, the law is true for heterosexual as well as homosexual couples.

Page: 1426

32: (True or False) Determine which of the following statements are true or false about hate crimes:

   A. Hate crimes against gays are decreasing in the United States.
   B. Gay men experience hate crimes at rates similar to or greater than those in other minorities.
   C. Gay women experience hate crimes at rates similar to or greater than those in other minorities.
   D. Gays no longer face discrimination with housing or employment.

Answers: A - False, B - True, C - False, D - False

Critique: Gay men and women continue to encounter social, housing, and employment discrimination, even when such activity is deemed illegal. Additionally, gay men experience hate crimes at rates similar to or greater than those in other minorities. Lesbians, however, are less likely to report crimes of violence.

Pages: 1426, 1427

33: John is a 28-year-old male whom you have been following for the past 3 years. He is physically healthy but is upset because he is gay and wishes he were not. Which of the following is correct regarding changing one's sexual orientation:

   A. Changing one's sexual orientation is easily achieved with appropriate psychotherapy.
   B. Changing one's sexual orientation is supported by the American Medical Association (AMA) if dysphoria is present.
   C. During a "midlife crisis," changing one's sexual orientation is common.
   D. Changing one's sexual orientation may cause psychological sequelae.

E. Changing one's behavior is proof that sexual orientation can be changed.

Answer: D

Critique: Significant same-sex attractions are unlikely to change at any age. No evidence shows that changing one's sexual orientation is successful with psychotherapy or any other therapy. Attempts (and usually failures) at "reorienting" sexuality can lead to distress and psychological sequelae, and therefore the AMA no longer supports this approach.

Page: 1427

34: Lesbian women are:

A. At lower risk for osteoporosis than are heterosexual women
B. At lower risk of breast cancer than are heterosexual women
C. At lower risk of endometrial cancer than are heterosexual women
D. At lower risk of ovarian cancer than are heterosexual women
E. At higher risk of contracting HIV than are heterosexual women

Answer: A

Critique: Lesbian women may receive less health care because many health care maintenance activities (e.g., Pap smears, breast examinations) are associated with reproduction. Additionally, they may not be entitled to health insurance given to a partner, as would the partner of a heterosexual married couple. Many lesbian women are nulliparous and therefore are at lower risk of osteoporosis but at higher risk of cancer of the breast, endometrium, and ovary. Additionally, female-to-female transmission of HIV is less common.

Page: 1427

35: Gay men:

A. Are more likely to exercise regularly than are heterosexual men
B. Are more likely to be obese than are heterosexual men

C. Are at lower risk of HIV than are heterosexual men
D. Are at lower risk of acquiring resistant gonorrhea and chlamydia than are heterosexual men
E. Require safe sexual practices more than heterosexual men

Answer: A

Critique: Gay men tend to exercise more than heterosexual men and therefore tend to be less obese. Although gay men have a higher risk of acquiring HIV and resistant sexually transmitted diseases than do heterosexual men, everyone engaging in sexual activities should be encouraged to practice safe sex.

Page: 1427

36: (True or False) Determine which of the following are true and which are false about cross-dressing:

A. A cross-dresser was previously referred to as a transvestite.
B. Cross-dressing refers to a person who, at times, dresses as the other sex.
C. All cross-dressers have homosexual desires, even if they do not act on them.
D. Cross-dressing is the first step in becoming a transsexual.
E. Cross-dressing is reported in up to 6% of males in the United States.

Answers: A - True, B - True, C - False, D - False, E - True

Critique: Cross-dressers, formerly known as transvestites, are persons who dress up as the other sex. Cross-dressers may view themselves as heterosexual, homosexual, or bisexual, because cross-dressing does not stipulate sexual orientation. Transsexuals are persons who have surgery (and hormonal therapy) to transform them into the opposite biological sex. Cross-dressers do not necessarily wish to undergo surgery and transform their sex.

Page: 1427

Chapter 51

Clinical Genetics

Alvah R. Cass

1: (True or False) Clinical genetics encompasses several areas of study and application. Of the following areas, primary health care providers are most likely to be concerned with:

A. The study of inherited diseases in families
B. The diagnosis and treatment of genetic disorders
C. Provision of information and counseling related to genetic disorders
D. Application of research to map specific disease genes or chromosomes

Answers: A - True, B - True, C - True, D - False

Critique: Clinical genetics includes the study of inherited illnesses in families, the application of research to map specific disease genes or chromosomes, the diagnosis and treatment of genetic disorders, and the provision of information and counseling related to genetic disorders. Primary health care providers will most likely be concerned with the counseling, diagnosis, and treatment aspects of clinical genetics.

Page: 1431

2: (True or False) Family physicians should provide preconception counseling to women contemplating pregnancy. Preconception counseling should include:

A. Referral to a genetic counseling service
B. Identification of presymptomatic maternal conditions that can adversely affect pregnancy outcomes
C. Discussion of folic acid intake
D. Screening for and counseling about potentially harmful medication
E. Recommendations to avoid known teratogens and illicit drug use

Answers: A - False, B - True, C - True, D - True, E - True

Critique: Family physicians should provide preconception counseling for female patients contemplating pregnancy. Counseling can be provided at scheduled health maintenance visits and should be introduced early in the childbearing years. Preconception counseling should include: (1) discussion of folic acid intake, including before conception and during pregnancy to reduce the risk of neural tube defects; (2) screening for and counseling about potentially harmful medications and the use of illicit drugs; (3) recommendations to avoid known teratogens; (4) identification of presymptomatic maternal conditions likely to affect pregnancy, such as glucose intolerance; (5) ethnic-specific screening, such as that for sickle cell disease and Tay-Sachs disease; and (6) answering patients' questions and providing information about referral sources and support groups as indicated.

Page: 1431

3: Nearly 50% of birth defects do not have an identifiable cause. Which of the following mechanisms accounts for the largest proportion of birth defects that can be linked by a causal relationship:

A. Chromosomal abnormalities
B. Maternal factors
C. Multifactorial etiologies
D. Teratogens
E. Single gene defects

Answer: C

Critique: Up to 3% of all newborns have a major birth defect, often with a genetic basis, and up to 7% of the population will exhibit symptoms of a genetic disease during childhood or adolescence. Unfortunately, nearly 50% of birth defects have no known cause. Multifactorial etiologies account for 20% to 30% of birth defects. Less common causes include maternal factors and teratogens, single-gene defects, and chromosomal abnormalities.

Page: 1432 (Table 51–5)

4: A 28-year-old G3P2 woman is 18 weeks pregnant and has had an uncomplicated pregnancy up to this point. She recently felt fetal movement and is excited about the birth of this child. She agrees to have a "triple screen test" done. The results show a lower than expected maternal α-fetoprotein level and a reduced level of maternal estriol. You ask the patient to return to the office to review the results. Her pregnancy is at increased risk for:

A. Trisomy 21 (Down syndrome)
B. Anencephaly
C. Meningomyelocele
D. XXY (Klinefelter's syndrome)
E. Tay-Sachs disease

Answer: A

Critique: Maternal blood sampling and other forms of fetal testing have been incorporated as standard practices in most primary care practices that provide obstetrical care. Implications of positive results of fetal testing and possible therapeutic choices should be discussed before testing. It should be emphasized that pregnancy termination is not the only possible therapeutic option. One of the more commonly used antepartum tests is the so-called triple screen. The triple screen is usually performed between the 16th and 20th weeks of gestation. An elevated level of α-fetoprotein indicates an increased risk of an open neural tube or abdominal wall defect. A reduced level is seen in pregnancies in which the fetus has trisomy 21. Reduced levels of serum estriol are also seen in pregnancies associated with trisomy 21. An elevated level of human chorionic gonadotropin is also indicative of an increased risk for trisomy 21. Anencephaly and meningomyelocele, examples of neural tube defects, are associated with an elevated serum α-fetoprotein. The triple screen does not detect XXY trisomy. Tay-Sachs disease, a single-gene defect disorder, likewise does not cause changes in the triple screen.

Page: 1432

5: Children born with physical features that are substantially different from familial features may have some form of dysmorphism. Dysmorphic features most commonly involve:

    A. Upper extremities, including the hands and fingers
    B. Facial structures
    C. Truncal malformations
    D. Lower extremities, including the feet and toes

Answer: B

Critique: When infants are born with dysmorphic features, the clinician should be alert for possible genetic abnormalities. Up to 50% of all dysmorphic features occur in facial structures. Some dysmorphic features are not appreciated at birth but may become apparent as the child grows and develops.

Pages: 1433, 1434

6: Primary morphologic defects of an organ or body part resulting from an intrinsically abnormal developmental process best describes:

    A. Dysplasias
    B. Deformations
    C. Malformations
    D. Syndromes
    E. Disruptions

Answer: C

Critique: Dysmorphic features may be classified as malformations, dysplasias, deformations, or disruptions. Malformations are primary morphologic defects of an organ or body part resulting from an intrinsically abnormal development process. Dysplasias are primary defects involving abnormal organization of cells into tissue. Deformations are alterations in the form or location of a normally formed body part by mechanical forces. Disruptions are morphologic organ defects caused by an extrinsic breakdown of an organ or system.

Pages: 1433, 1434

7: A new family moves into your community, and a mother brings her 18-month-old daughter in for a routine visit. She expresses some concern about the child's small stature. Further inquiry reveals some mild developmental delays. On examination, you note that the child has a short, broad neck; a broad chest; and a loud systolic murmur. The mother tells you that the murmur was noted at a well-baby clinic where the family lived previously and was described as a flow murmur. You suspect that the child may have a congenital problem. Which of the following would explain your findings:

    A. Trisomy 21 (Down syndrome)
    B. XXX syndrome
    C. XO syndrome (Turner's syndrome)
    D. Trisomy 18 (Edwards' syndrome)
    E. Marfan syndrome

Answer: C

Critique: XO, or Turner's syndrome, is characterized by short stature, webbed neck, broad chest, infertility, and cardiac or renal defects. Mental development may be normal or delayed. Coarctation of the aorta is seen. The features do not fully describe trisomy 21, which has more distinguishing facial features, and the developmental delays are usually more dramatic. Trisomy 18 is associated with severe and multiple defects, and infants usually do not survive the neonatal period. XXX syndrome has more obvious facial abnormalities and demonstrates multiple anomalies. Marfan syndrome is a disorder of connective tissue, and affected individuals usually have tall stature and disproportionately long extremities and digits.

Page: 1432 (Table 51–2)

Chapter 52

Anxiety Disorders

James B. Dunnan

1: Which of the following statements is false:

  A. Primary care patients with mental disorders use approximately twice as much nonpsychiatric medical care as those without mental disorders.

  B. Anxiety and depression are the two most common mental health disorders seen in medical practice.

  C. Psychiatrists care for the majority of patients suffering from anxiety disorders.

  D. Significant anxiety is found in more than half of patients with known cardiologic disease.

Answer: C

Critique: Studies sponsored by the National Institute of Mental Health have revealed that in the United States the primary care doctor treats the majority of mental health disorders. Many cardiac patients suffer from anxiety, underscoring the fact that anxiety is frequently precipitated by medical disease. Patients with serious medical illness should be carefully monitored for the development of anxiety.

Page: 1438

2: The onset of panic disorder usually occurs in people of which age group:

  A. 10 to 16 years

  B. 17 to 30 years

  C. 31 to 50 years

  D. Older than 50 years

Answer: B

Critique: The onset of panic disorder is typically in the 17- to 30-year-old age group, with a mean age of onset of 22.5 years.

Page: 1439

3: Which of the following statements regarding panic disorder is false:

  A. Panic disorder is often precipitated by stressful life events.

  B. Panic disorder is a familial disease.

  C. Panic attacks are not episodic in nature.

  D. Many patients are seen after the first or second panic attack.

Answer: C

Critique: The episodic nature of panic attacks is an important feature to distinguish them from generalized anxiety or transient states of anxiety associated with life stress. Early aggressive treatment of panic attacks can greatly decrease the possible vocational and social disability that can be associated with panic attacks. Many patients with panic disorder present to their primary care physician after the first or second panic attack, giving the physician the opportunity to have a large, positive impact on the disease course.

Page: 1439

4: Approximately what percentage of patients with chest pain and negative angiographic studies suffer from panic disorder:

  A. Less than 10%

  B. 25%

  C. 50%

  D. 75%

Answer: C

Critique: Three studies have shown that nearly 50% of patients with angiographically proven noncardiac chest pain actually are suffering from panic disorder. One fourth to one third of patients with the presenting symptom of palpitations meet the criteria for panic disorder. Patients who present with these types of cardiac symptoms and whose medical work-up is negative should be screened for panic disorder.

Page: 1440

5: The most common initial somatic symptoms of panic disorder are:

  A. Respiratory, musculoskeletal, and neurologic

  B. Gastrointestinal and visual

  C. Musculoskeletal and cardiologic

  D. Cardiologic, neurologic, and gastrointestinal

Answer: D

Critique: Cardiologic symptoms may include chest pain, palpitations, and tachycardia. Neurological symptoms include headache, dizziness, faintness, and paresthesia. Symptoms associated with the gastrointestinal system include irritable bowel and epigastric pain. All of these symptoms are commonly encountered in a primary care office, but when no physical disease process is detected, panic disorder should be considered.

Page: 1440

6: Social phobia usually begins in which age group:

  A. Teenage years

  B. Twenties

C. Forties
D. Sixties

Answer: A

Critique: This subset of phobic disorders usually presents in the teenage years and is often seen in patients with a childhood history of extreme shyness or social inhibition. This disorder can be precipitated by a particularly embarrassing situation. The peak prevalence of this disorder is in the 15- to 24-year-old age group.

Page: 1441

7: Which of the following statements regarding panic disorder and mitral valve prolapse (MVP) is false:

A. Patients with panic disorder have an increased incidence of MVP.
B. MVP in patients with panic disorder is mild and not associated with thickened mitral valve leaflets.
C. MVP found in patients with panic disorder usually necessitates prophylactic antibiotic therapy before major dental procedures.
D. Patients with panic disorder and MVP respond well to imipramine therapy.

Answer: C

Critique: Studies have shown that 18% of patients with panic disorder had definite criteria for MVP, and 27% met probable criteria. This is in contrast to 1% and 12%, respectively, in normal controls. MVP found in the panic disorder patients was usually of a mild variety and not associated with mitral regurgitation or progressive valvular disease. For this reason, the MVP in panic disorder patients usually does not need prophylactic antibiotics. Patients with both MVP and panic disorder usually respond to imipramine therapy just as well as panic disorder patients without MVP.

Page: 1441

8: Which of the following statements regarding generalized anxiety disorder (GAD) is false:

A. Patients with GAD experience excessive anxiety and worry on more days than not for at least 6 months.
B. GAD patients are readily able to control their worry.
C. GAD patients commonly report being easily fatigued.
D. Sleep disorders are a feature of GAD.

Answer: B

Critique: Excessive worry and anxiety on more days than not for at least 6 months, being easily fatigued, and sleep disorders are all common features of GAD. Restlessness, difficulty concentrating, irritability, and muscle tension are other common features. These symptoms cause significant impairment in the patient's social and vocational function and are, by definition, not directly the result of a substance or medical condition. The patients find it difficult to control their worry.

Page: 1442

9: Which of the following is a feature of posttraumatic stress disorder (PTSD):

A. PTSD patients suffer flashback episodes when exposed to stimuli that resemble an aspect of the traumatic event.
B. PTSD patients usually believe they have a long life ahead of them because they have survived the traumatic event.
C. PTSD patients have multiple close relationships and rely on close personal bonds for support.
D. PTSD patients seek out people, activities, and places to remind them of the traumatic event.

Answer: A

Critique: PTSD patients usually display estrangement from others and have a sense of a foreshortened future. These patients avoid thoughts, feelings, or even conversations that remind them of the trauma. Examples of civilian cases of trauma that might precipitate PTSD are severe automobile accidents, industrial accidents, or natural disasters. Refugees from war-torn countries have also been shown to have a high incidence of PTSD. These patients may present to a primary care office with multiple unexplained symptoms.

Page: 1442

10: Which of the following statements regarding anxiety is true:

A. Some anxiety patients have a medical illness that is at least partially responsible for their symptoms.
B. Hypoglycemia may present with symptoms of anxiety.
C. Anxiety can be seen in a patient who has recently had an MI.
D. All of the above

Answer: D

Critique: Patients may present to primary care offices with fairly straightforward symptoms of anxiety, but a medical illness may be to blame. Other medical disorders that can simulate anxiety are arrhythmias, emphysema, occult pulmonary embolism, thyrotoxicosis, thiamine deficiency, iron deficiency anemia, and amphetamine intoxication. Recent MI patients may experience anxiety regarding resuming work and sexual relations.

Page: 1443

11: All of the following statements regarding alcohol are true, except:

A. Improved sleep is usually seen with alcohol consumption.
B. Anxiety frequently accompanies alcohol abuse.
C. Prolonged alcohol usage often leads to increased arousal of sympathetic nervous system tone.
D. Approximately one third of alcoholics have panic disorder or severe phobic behavior, or both.

Answer: A

Critique: Although excessive alcohol use may cause drowsiness or "passing out," it also usually causes a disturbed sleep pattern with nonrestful sleep and early wakening owing to increased sympathetic tone. Anxiety, panic disorder, and phobic behavior are common comorbid conditions of alcohol abuse.

Page: 1444

12: Probably the single best diagnostic tool in the work-up of an anxious patient is:

    A. Patient history
    B. Physical examination
    C. Comprehensive serum metabolic panel
    D. Cardiac stress testing

Answer: A

Critique: Even though physical examination, laboratory tests, and even cardiac stress testing may be needed in the anxious patient, his or her history is probably the single best diagnostic tool in this work-up. The patient's concerns should be elicited and addressed as well as the current life situation, support systems, and any known medical conditions. Physical examination and any testing should be guided by this history in an attempt to make sure the patient's concerns have been addressed.

Page: 1444

13: Which of the following are common symptoms of anxiety and depression:

    A. Difficulty concentrating and poor memory
    B. Patients being preoccupied with their own physical ailments
    C. Difficulties falling asleep or interrupted sleep
    D. Loss of interest in work or hobbies
    E. All of the above

Answer: E

Critique: All of these symptoms can be found in depressed or anxious patients. Other common symptoms are irritability, tension, fatigue, decreased motor activity, and indecision. Somatic complaints may include aches and pains, tachycardia, chest pain, difficulty swallowing, weight loss, headache, and labile hypertension.

Page: 1445

14: Which of the following statements regarding the management of clinical anxiety is true:

    A. The patient should be advised before an expensive medical work-up that most of the symptoms are "in their head."
    B. Involvement of the patient in developing a therapeutic plan is not necessary.
    C. The patient must believe that an adequate evaluation has been performed before any reassurance or counseling will be effective.
    D. Management of anxiety is the same, regardless of the specific organic and psychiatric diagnosis.

Answer: C

Critique: Even though anxiety may be suspected after the physician takes a careful history, care should be taken that all the patient's concerns have been addressed before approaching the possibility of an anxiety disorder. Steps

must also be taken to ensure that the patient understands how his or her symptoms fit into a specific diagnostic category. An explanation of the connection between the anxiety and the physical symptoms is also helpful. Distinguishing between different subtypes of anxiety is important, because patients with different subtypes respond to different therapies.

Page: 1446

15: Selective serotonin reuptake inhibitors (SSRIs) that studies have shown to be effective in the treatment of panic disorder include:

    A. Paroxetine (Paxil)
    B. Sertraline (Zoloft)
    C. Fluvoxamine (Luvox)
    D. All of the above
    E. None of the above

Answer: D

Critique: Zoloft, Paxil, and Luvox have all been shown to be effective in treating panic disorder in randomized controlled trials. Uncontrolled trials suggest that both fluoxetine (Prozac) and citalopram (Celexa) are also effective. Other classes of drugs that have been shown to be more effective than placebo in treating panic disorder are tricyclic antidepressants, benzodiazepines, and monoamine oxidase inhibitors.

Page: 1447

16: All of the following statements regarding SSRI use in panic attacks are true, except:

    A. SSRIs are effective therapeutic agents for both panic attacks and depression.
    B. The maximum dosage should be initiated immediately.
    C. Anorgasmia occurs in 20% to 30% of patients treated with SSRIs.
    D. Three common side effects of SSRIs that tend to go away after 1 to 3 weeks of therapy are jitteriness, nausea, and headache.

Answer: B

Critique: Use of SSRIs for both depression and panic attacks is common in primary care practice. Side effects such as jitteriness, nausea, headache, and anorgasmia should be anticipated and the possibility that they will occur explained to patients. Starting at a low dose may minimize some of these side effects. A possible strategy is to start out at a low dose of the SSRI (10 mg for Paxil or 25 mg of Zoloft) and then increase the dose every 5 days until the panic attacks stop. The use of BuSpar (buspirone) or Wellbutrin (bupropion) in combination with an SSRI has been shown to reverse the side effect of anorgasmia.

Page: 1447

17: All of the following are characteristics of patients that correlate with successful counseling outcome, except:

    A. Young, attractive, intelligent
    B. High motivation to change

C. Ability to maintain close relationships

D. Belief that their problem is of some physical nature

Answer: D

Critique: Counseling has been shown to be effective in treating anxiety disorders, but certain patients are more likely to have a successful outcome. If a patient believes that his or her problem has a physical origin, the success of counseling is less likely. Other characteristics of good counseling candidates are intelligence, a previous positive counseling experience, dependability, and faith that counseling can be helpful.

Page: 1449

18: Benzodiazepines should not be used in patients with a history of:

A. Side effects or allergy to antidepressant medications

B. Alcohol abuse

C. Generalized anxiety disorder

D. Panic attacks

Answer: B

Critique: Almost all abusers of benzodiazepines have a history of drug or alcohol abuse. For this reason, benzodiazepines should be avoided in these patients. On the other hand, this class of drug has shown effectiveness in the treatment of both generalized anxiety disorder and panic attacks. Care should also be taken when patients are taken off these agents, because severe rebound anxiety and withdrawal symptoms can occur when patients stop taking benzodiazepines.

Page: 1449

19: All of the following have been shown to be more effective than placebo in treating generalized anxiety disorder, except:

A. Calcium channel blockers

B. Beta-blockers

C. Buspirone (BuSpar)

D. SSRIs

E. Benzodiazepines

Answer: A

Critique: Beta-blockers inhibit the sympathetic nervous system symptoms that are prominent in anxiety disorder. Care must be taken with their use, because beta-blockers can precipitate depression, which is a common comorbid condition with anxiety. Benzodiazepines can be effectively used in select patients, and several of the SSRIs have been studied for use in GAD. Calcium channel blockers have not been shown to be effective in this arena.

Page: 1449

20: Which of the following are used for treatment of specific phobias, agoraphobia, and social phobias:

A. Behavior modification with the ultimate goal of desensitization

B. Imipramine in combination with exposure therapy

C. Long-acting benzodiazepine therapy.

D. SSRIs

E. All of the above

Answer: E

Critique: Intense therapy with the goal of desensitizing the patient has been shown to be effective in these patients. Two techniques, one with slowly progressive exposure with relaxation and the other with more rapid in vivo exposure, have been used. Imipramine, SSRIs, and benzodiazepines have been used, as have monoamine oxidase inhibitors. It should be kept in mind that most patients with agoraphobia also have panic attacks, so the two conditions should be treated together.

Page: 1450

Questions 21 to 24: (True or False) Decide whether the following statements are true or false:

21: Anxiety and depression are the two most common mental health disorders encountered in a primary care office.

22: Anxiety is never caused by medical illness.

23: Panic disorder, posttraumatic stress disorder, social phobias, and generalized anxiety are all subclasses of anxiety disorder.

24: Anxiety disorders occur only in people who have no social support system.

Answers: 21 - True, 22 - False, 23 - True, 24 - False

Critique: Because they are so common in practice, all primary care physicians must be prepared to treat anxiety and depression. Many medical illnesses can both cause and mimic anxiety, so care must be taken to fully evaluate physical complaints. Obsessive-compulsive disorder and atypical anxiety are also subclasses of anxiety disorder. Anxiety disorders can be present despite strong social support systems.

Page: 1438

Questions 25 to 30: (True or False) Designate the following statements regarding panic disorder as true or false:

25: Panic attacks, by definition, are episodic in nature.

26: It is not imperative to distinguish between generalized anxiety disorder and panic disorders, because the treatments are the same.

27: Panic attacks are usually idiopathic and are not precipitated by stressful life events.

28: First-degree relatives of a patient suffering from panic attacks are at increased risk for developing panic attacks.

29: Men are twice as likely to develop panic attacks as women.

30: Alcohol abuse is a common finding in the male relatives of panic attack patients.

Answers: 25 - True, 26 - False, 27 - False, 28 - True, 29 - False, 30 - True

Critique: A defining characteristic of panic attacks is their episodic nature. Although similar medicines are used in the treatment of GAD and panic disorder, the strategies for treating the two are different. Immediate pharmacological relief of panic attacks is imperative to avoid maladaptive behaviors, whereas counseling can be effective early in the course of GAD. Benzodiazepines, tricyclic antidepressants, and SSRIs are used in both conditions. Beta-blockers, buspirone (BuSpar), and venlafaxine (Effexor) are also used in the treatment of GAD. Panic attacks are commonly precipitated by stressful life events and can have a familial predisposition. Women are twice as likely as men to develop panic attacks. More alcohol abuse is found in male relatives of panic attack patients than in control relatives.

Pages: 1438, 1439

Questions 31 to 37: (True or False) Determine whether the following statements regarding anxiety and panic disorders are true or false:

31: Relaxation techniques and education by the primary care physician are especially effective when used early in the treatment of anxiety.

32: After panic attacks have ceased, it is imperative that the patient continue to avoid situations that have precipitated panic attacks.

33: Benzodiazepines should never be used in the treatment of panic disorders.

34: Tricyclic antidepressant medicines have been used with success in the treatment of panic disorders.

35: Counseling can be effective in the treatment of GAD.

36: It is helpful for the primary care physician to provide psychological support in patients who have concomitant medical problems with GAD.

37: Abuse of benzodiazepines is common in primary care patients.

Answers: 31 - True, 32 - False, 33 - False, 34 - True, 35 - True, 36 - True, 37 - False

Critique: Counseling as well as relaxation techniques and patient education can be effective in the treatment of GAD. The primary care physician can take advantage of office visits regarding medical conditions to provide brief counseling regarding the patient's concomitant GAD. A goal of therapy in panic attacks is to enable the patient to return to activities that previously caused panic attacks, and not to continue to avoid them. Benzodiazepines can be useful in the treatment of panic disorder but should not be considered first-line therapy. The abuse of benzodiazepines is unusual in primary care practice, but it is most common in patients with a history of alcohol or substance abuse.

Pages: 1447–1450

··· # Depression

Navkiran K. Shokar, Gurjeet S. Shokar

1: With regard to selective serotonin re-uptake inhibitors (SSRIs), which of the following statements is true:

    A. They cause a prolonged QT interval.
    B. They rarely cause gastrointestinal upset.
    C. Sexual dysfunction has been reported.
    D. SSRIs can safely be used with St. John's wort in the treatment of depression.
    E. SSRIs are contraindicated in pregnancy.

Answer: C

Critique: SSRIs are tricyclic antidepressants that cause a prolonged QT interval as well as affect the PR interval and QRS complex. They can cause side effects such as nausea, vomiting, and diarrhea. Sexual dysfunction has been reported in patients who take the SSRIs. Patients should not be treated with SSRI and St. John's wort, because there is a risk for developing serotonin syndrome. SSRIs are the safest medications currently available for the treatment of depression in pregnancy.

Pages: 1462, 1467

2: Seasonal affective disorder (SAD):

    A. Is more common in men than in women
    B. Needs to be present for 3 consecutive months to meet the diagnostic criteria
    C. Is treated effectively with bright light therapy in the majority of patients
    D. Is treated effectively by SSRIs alone

Answer: C

Critique: SAD is more common in women than in men, and the pattern needs to be present for at least 2 years to meet the criteria for SAD. For up to 85% of patients bright light therapy is effective, and most patients do best if this therapy is combined with medication.

Page: 1485

3: In postpartum depression, all of the following are true, except:

    A. It is more commonly found in first-time mothers.
    B. It can occur in 5% to 20% of women within 6 months of delivery.
    C. Postpartum blues usually precedes the depression.
    D. SSRIs should be avoided, especially if the mother is breast-feeding.
    E. Inadequate social support may be a contributing factor.

Answer: D

Critique: Postpartum depression is more common in first-time mothers than in multiparous women. It occurs in 5% to 20% of women within 6 months of delivery and often is preceded by the postpartum blues. Inadequate social support and marital difficulty may be a contributing factor. SSRIs are the drugs of choice during breast-feeding and pregnancy.

Pages: 1459, 1460

4: Factors associated with an increased risk of suicide include all of the following, except:

    A. An elderly patient living alone
    B. A family history of suicide
    C. A history of alcoholism
    D. A recent loss of a sibling or other loved one
    E. The absence of a suicide note

Answer: E

Critique: All of the above except choice E are risk factors for suicide. The presence of a specific plan increases the risk for suicide. Patients who are at the highest risk for suicide generally are depressed, white, elderly, unmarried men with a history of substance abuse.

Page: 1461

5: (True or False) When considering treating a patient with a first episode of depression, which of the following statements are true and which are false:

    A. Vigorous aerobic exercise has shown to be of no value.
    B. Treatment with medication should be for 3 months and then quickly tapered over the next 4 weeks.
    C. Psychotherapy is an effective approach to the management of mild depression.
    D. Patients should receive medication for at least 6 months after resolution of symptoms.
    E. Regular follow-up by the physician helps achieve the best therapeutic results.

Answers: A - False, B - False, C - True, D - True, E - True

Critique: Vigorous aerobic exercise has shown to be of value and has been shown to be about as effective as psychotherapy in treating mild depression. A first episode of depression should be treated for at least 6 months after resolution of symptoms. When discontinuing treatment, the dose should be gradually tapered over 2 months while watching for the reemergence of depression. It has been shown that patients who have a regular follow-up with their physicians achieve the best results.

Pages: 1461, 1462

6: Which of the following SSRIs is preferred when a patient is taking several other medications for chronic medical problems and the physician wishes to keep drug interactions to a minimum:

    A. Fluoxetine
    B. Citalopram
    C. Paroxetine
    D. Fluvoxamine

Answer: B

Critique: Citalopram, because of its negligible effect on the cytochrome P450 system, makes interactions with other medications less likely to occur. Therefore, it is particularly beneficial for patients taking multiple medications and for the elderly. However, all the SSRIs have an advantage over the older tricyclic antidepressants in that they do not cause anticholinergic side effects, have no arrhythmic potential, and do cause postural hypotension. Additionally, an overdose is not lethal.

Pages: 1462, 1463

7: Which of the following statements is true regarding monoamine oxidase (MAO) inhibitors in the treatment of depression:

    A. They are safe when used in conjunction with SSRIs.
    B. Patients should be given a list of gluten-containing foods to avoid.
    C. They are safe to use when combined with the tricyclic antidepressants.
    D. They should be the first-line agents for patients who have significant anxiety as well as depression.
    E. They may have a role in the treatment of depression associated with hypersomnia.

Answer: E

Critique: MAO inhibitors have a role in the treatment of depression associated with hypersomnia and are often reserved for patients who fail to respond to other antidepressants. Patients should avoid foods that contain tyramine. MAO inhibitors can have dangerous interactions with SSRIs and meperidine as well as tricyclic antidepressants.

Pages: 1464, 1465

8: In a 45-year-old female patient with depression, which of the following is not an indication for referral to a psychiatrist:

    A. Diagnostic uncertainty
    B. The need for ECT
    C. Auditory hallucinations
    D. Anticholinergic side effects after using amitriptyline
    E. Associated substance abuse

Answer: D

Critique: Indications include all of the above except choice D. Anticholinergic side effects after using amitriptyline are an indication for using a different antidepressant such as an SSRI. Other indications for referral include suicidal ideation, bipolar disorder, and major depression in combination with severe personality disorder.

Page: 1468

9: Discontinuation syndrome:

    A. Refers to patients who regularly do not follow the physician's orders and stop their medications
    B. Most likely occurs within the first 6 weeks after discontinuing therapy
    C. Is more likely in patients who take SSRIs with a longer half-life, such as fluoxetine
    D. Can always easily be differentiated from a recurrence of depression
    E. Symptoms usually last 7 to 10 days and respond to readministration of the antidepressant

Answer: E

Critique: Recurrence of symptoms is most likely to occur within 10 days of abruptly discontinuing an antidepressant. The symptoms usually last 7 to 10 days and respond to restarting the antidepressant medication. It may not always be obvious whether the patient is suffering discontinuation syndrome or a recurrence of the depression, and careful evaluation is needed. Discontinuation syndrome is more common with SSRIs that have a short half-life, such as paroxetine.

Page: 1468

10: Which of the following statements is true regarding St. John's wort:

    A. St. John's wort has been shown to be safe in the third trimester of pregnancy.
    B. The active ingredient is thought to be tyramine, although the extract contains hundreds of compounds.
    C. Most studies of St. John's wort have been well designed, using randomized controlled trials.
    D. It is an herbal extract of the plant *Hypericum perforatum.*
    E. The usual maintenance dose is 0.1 mg twice a day.

Answer: D

Critique: The safety of St. John's wort in pregnancy is not well established. Most studies of St. John's wort have not been well designed, and most have not used placebos or other antidepressants as controls. The active ingredient is thought to be hypericum, which is an herbal extract of the plant *H. perforatum.* The usual maintenance dose is 300 mg 3 times a day.

Page: 1467

11: In patients who attempt suicide:

    A. Most usually have not seen a physician within the last year.

B. Men attempt suicide twice as often with firearms as do women
C. A family history of suicide is not pertinent
D. Most do not communicate their intent to others before their suicide attempt
E. Schizophrenia is not a recognized risk factor

Answer: B

Critique: In patients who attempt suicide, most have usually seen the physician within the previous month. A family history of suicide and a previous history of suicide attempt are important risk factors for suicide. Schizophrenia, a history of bipolar disorder, major depression, and lack of social support increase the likelihood of a suicide attempt.

Page: 1461

12: Which of the following statements is true regarding childhood depression:

A. Its presentation will always be typical.
B. The rate of suicide among adolescents has remained about the same over the last 40 years.
C. School avoidance in these patients is rare.
D. A decline in school performance should alert the physician to consider depression in the child.

Answer: D

Critique: Depression in childhood is often difficult to diagnose because its presentation is not typical. The rate of suicide among adolescents has increased threefold in the last 40 years. School avoidance is common in these patients, and the physician should be alert to a decline in school performance as a possible indicator of depression in the child.

Page: 1460

13: (True or False) Risk-taking behaviors in adolescents that can serve as predictors of suicide include:

A. Carrying a gun
B. Lack of seat belt use
C. Physical fights
D. Substance abuse
E. Regular school attendance

Answers: A - True, B - True, C - True, D - True, E - False

Critique: All of the above except regular school attendance are risk-taking behaviors in adolescents that can serve as predictors of suicide. Truancy also is a risk factor.

Page: 1460

14: (True or False) Which of the following medications can cause depressive symptoms in the elderly:

A. Beta blockers
B. Steroids
C. Thiazide diuretics
D. ACE inhibitors
E. Benzodiazepines

Answers: A - True, B - True, C - False, E - False, E - True

Critique: Beta blockers, steroids, and benzodiazepines as well as barbiturates, reserpine, hormonal preparations, and chemotherapeutic agents have been known to cause depressive symptoms in the elderly.

Page: 1460

15: (True or False) Which of the following statements regarding depression in the elderly are true and which are false:

A. Depression is a risk factor for heart disease.
B. The medication of choice in the elderly should be a tricyclic antidepressant.
C. Underdosing in the elderly can lead to the unsuccessful treatment of depression.
D. Coexisting anxiety with depression is rare in the elderly.

Answers: A - True, B - False, C - True, D - False

Critique: Depression is a major risk factor for coronary heart disease, and depressed men are twice as likely as men who are not depressed to suffer a myocardial infarction. It is preferred to use an SSRI in the elderly, rather than a tricyclic antidepressant, to minimize the side effects. Although one may start with smaller doses in the elderly, one of the reasons that depression is not effectively treated in the elderly years is underdosing. Approximately 60% of patients with depression have anxiety.

Page: 1460

16: (True or False) Which of the following medical conditions are known to be associated with depression:

A. Parkinsonism
B. Hypothyroidism
C. Congestive heart failure
D. Malnutrition
E. Cancer

Answers: A - True, B - True, C - True, D - True, E - True

Critique: All of the above conditions have been associated with depression.

Pages: 1460, 1461

17: Regarding electroconvulsive therapy (ECT):

A. It is now considered unsafe and ineffective.
B. Best results are usually obtained when the patient is mildly to moderately depressed.
C. It results in remission of depression in more than 90% of cases.
D. Treatment sessions should be done weekly for 6 weeks to decrease the incidence of memory loss.

Answer: C

Critique: ECT is safe and very effective, resulting in remission of depression in more than 90% of cases. Treatment is usually given three times a week for 2 or 3 weeks. It is usually reserved for patients who do not respond to medications, those who are acutely suicidal, or for depressed patients with psychotic or catatonic features.

Page: 1467

18: Which of the following clinical features is not associated with the serotonin syndrome, an uncommon and potentially severe medication reaction with SSRIs:

    A. Hyperreflexia
    B. Hypertension
    C. Dizziness
    D. Myoclonic jerks
    E. Shivering

Answer: B

Critique: All of these except choice B are a part of the serotonin syndrome. In addition, hypotension and not hypertension occurs as part of the syndrome. Other features include restlessness, confusion, flushing, and agitation.

Page: 1467

19: (True or False) You are considering starting a 48-year-old African-American female on venlafaxine. Which of the following statements are true and which are false regarding this medication:

    A. It may be useful in patients who are refractory to other agents.
    B. Hypertension is a recognized side effect.
    C. Gastrointestinal and sexual dysfunction side effects have been reported.
    D. It is chemically related to bupropion.
    E. It is an inhibitor of norepinephrine re-uptake only.

Answers: A - True, B - True, C - True, D - True, E - False

Critique: Venlafaxine is a potent inhibitor of both serotonin and norepinephrine uptake. It is useful in patients who are refractory to other agents, and it is chemically related to bupropion. Side effects include gastrointestinal difficulties and sexual dysfunction as well as hypertension.

Pages: 1465, 1466

20: (True or False) Which of the following statements are true and which are false:

    A. The incidence of depression is two to three times higher in a person who has a first-degree relative with the disease.
    B. Dysthymia is a chronic low-grade depression present most days for at least 6 months.
    C. Persistent insomnia is not associated with a higher incidence of depression.
    D. The lethal dose for a tricyclic antidepressant is about five times the daily therapeutic dose.
    E. Meperidine can be used safely for pain relief in patients who are taking MAO inhibitors

Answers: A - True, B - True, C - False, D - True, E - False

Critique: There is a genetic predisposition to depression, with the incidence being two to three times higher in persons who have a first-degree relative with depression. Dysthymia is a chronic low-grade depression present most days for at least 2 years. Persistent insomnia is associated with a higher incidence of depression, and the lethal dose for tricyclic antidepressants is usually about five times the daily dose. Meperidine must not be used in patients who take MAO inhibitors. Other dangerous interactions occur with SSRIs, tricyclic antidepressants, and some antihypertensive agents.

Pages: 1457, 1458, 1462–1469

Chapter 54

Crisis, Trauma, and Disaster Intervention

William Elder

1: Drawing on the experiences of survivors of the Coconut Grove fire in Boston, Massachusetts, Eric Lindemann discovered that disaster survivors typically develop emotional pain, confusion, anxiety, and difficulty in daily functioning. What is the usual duration of these symptoms:

    A. 2 days
    B. 6 weeks
    C. 3 months
    D. Duration varies depending on pre-existing psychopathology

Answer: B

Critique: Most disaster survivors recover spontaneously within 6 weeks. Lindemann examined group reactions of individuals who lost family members in the Coconut Fire in Boston, which claimed 500 lives, and found that most survivors recovered spontaneously within 6 weeks. Complete recovery from symptoms that are sufficient to warrant a diagnosis of crisis state is unlikely within 2 days. Psychopathology has not been shown to be a predictor of recovery time, although it may affect level of self-management of the crisis.

Page: 1470

2: Gerald Caplan integrated previous work into modern crisis theory. Which of the following statements is true regarding the "crisis state" as described by Caplan:

    A. A crisis state cannot be helped with medication.
    B. Individuals are unlikely to have improved functioning after a crisis state.
    C. Crisis states are psychological upheavals precipitated by a stressor.
    D. Crisis states are psychological upheavals that are secondary to personality deficits that prevent adaptation to a stress.

Answer: C

Critique: A crisis state is a psychological upheaval precipitated by a stressor that produces emotional turmoil to the extent that a person is temporarily unable to cope, adapt, and function in daily activities. A crisis implies both the potential for danger and the opportunity for growth. Improved functioning is a possible outcome from a crisis. Medications have proven helpful for symptomatic treatment. All individuals are vulnerable to their environment and capable of experiencing a crisis state, regardless of personality functioning.

Pages: 1470, 1471

3: Erikson identified the concept of the life cycle, including specific life stages and tasks to be completed during those stages. Which of the following statements is correct regarding an individual's progression through these specific developmental stages:

    A. Progression is not affected by progress during previous stages.
    B. Successful progression does not affect interpersonal relationships.
    C. Successful progression affects one's ability to manage life's transitions and losses.
    D. Progression from one stage to the next results in impaired interpersonal relationships.

Answer: C

Critique: Inability to negotiate a stage successfully affects the ability to progress to the next stage. For example, individuals who do not traverse developmental periods, such as identity formation in adolescence, often have difficulty assuming adult roles.

Page: 1470

4: Regarding the percentage of Americans exposed to traumatic events each year, which of the following trends has been demonstrated:

    A. The rate did not change in the twentieth century.
    B. The rate of exposure appears to be decreasing.
    C. The rate of exposure appears to be increasing.
    D. The rate of exposure appears to be unrelated to man-made disasters.

Answer: C

Critique: The percentage of Americans exposed to traumatic events each year is increasing because of various exposures through the media and increases in man-made disasters.

Page: 1471

5: Which of the following statements is true regarding emotional reactions to natural disasters:

    A. These reactions cannot be helped by medications.

    B. These reactions do not depend on the degree of community devastation.

    C. These reactions are less severe than those seen with man-made disasters.

    D. These reactions affect the individual's ability to cope.

Answer: D

Critique: Emotional reactions to any disaster can be helped, at least symptomatically, with medications. Natural and man-made disasters that result in widespread destruction, such as devastation of the community, may be most traumatic, because contacts and resources are lost. Other variables are more important than man-made versus natural source of the disaster, except that natural disasters are often more destructive to community contacts and resources. Adaptive coping requires some cognitive functioning, such as problem solving, and extreme emotions interfere with this cognitive ability.

Page: 1475

6: Which of the following terms best describes the emotional state that a traumatic event disturbs to create a crisis state:

    A. Equistasis

    B. Homeostasis

    C. Equilibrium

    D. Reality functioning

Answer: C

Critique: Equilibrium is described as a balance among an individual's wishes, fears, skills, capacities, values, and ideas. *Environmental equilibrium* refers to a stable balance internally and externally that is disturbed by extreme stress. *Homeostasis* refers to the individual's conscience and unconscious thoughts, behaviors, and physical responses, which have the potential to return the individual to equilibrium.

Pages: 1471,1472

7: All of the following describe stressors that can precipitate a crisis state, except:

    A. Witnessed environmental events

    B. Psychological meaning of events in the patient's life

    C. Intellectual ability

    D. Life cycle developmental phase

Answer: C

Critique: Stressors are internal or external events that produce stress in the individual. Psychological ability, including intellectual functioning, is not a stressor in and of itself but may affect a person's ability to cope with stressors.

Page: 1472

8: Holmes and Rahe reported a scale for measuring social readjustment. The scale includes 43 life stressors that have effects in most people. For an individual who scores over 300 on this scale, which of the following percentages represents the likelihood that this individual will experience a major medical or psychological disorder in the next 2 years:

    A. 20%

    B. 30%

    C. 40%

    D. 50%

    E. 70%

Answer: D

Critique: The social readjustment scale created by Holmes and Rahe includes events such as death of a spouse, divorce, change in work status, change in social activities, and even response to holidays. A patient who scores over 300 has a 50% chance of developing significant medical or psychiatric illness in the next 2 years.

Page: 1472

9: The item with the highest magnitude of stress on the Holmes and Rahe external stressor scale is which of the following:

    A. Divorce

    B. Holidays

    C. Death of a spouse

    D. Buying a home

Answer: C

Critique: Death of a spouse is listed above divorce on the Holmes and Rahe scale. Holidays and home buying appear on the scale as well but have lower magnitudes.

Page: 1472

10: All of the following statements are true about the crisis state, except:

    A. The crisis state is precipitated by an internal or external stressor.

    B. The crisis state is an intense state of inner turmoil or disorganization.

    C. The individual's ability to cope and adapt is overwhelmed.

    D. The individual is aware of what has upset him or her.

Answer: D

Critique: Crisis states can be defined as psychological upheavals that are precipitated by stressors and in which the individual's ability to cope or adapt is overwhelmed. Individuals can have internalized concerns such as fears activated by external events and remain unaware that the external event was a trigger.

Pages: 1472, 1473

11: Which of the following statements is true regarding crisis states and personality disorders:

    A. Response to a stressor has nothing to do with the presence of pre-existing psychiatric or personality disorders.

    B. Individuals with personality or psychiatric disorders may have difficulty with mild stressors.

C. Individuals with antisocial personalities revert to honesty and altruism during times of stress

D. People with borderline personality disorders become more independent when the stressor is external to the individual and doctor.

Answer: B

Critique: The more severe the stressor, the less important are pre-existing psychiatric and personality disorders. The presence of a personality disorder marks the individual as having chronic interpersonal and coping difficulties, rendering them susceptible to emotional reactions to even mild events. The person's dysfunctional attitudes and behavior are persistent. A person with borderline personality disorder tendencies toward dependence or independence in response to events external to the patient-doctor dyad are difficult to predict. It is likely that the person with borderline personality disorder will become more dependent when the relationship with the physician is neutral.

Page: 1475

12: In trying to understand a patient's complaints of extreme emotional distress, the physician should seek all of the following information, except:

A. Financial status
B. Why the stress is occurring now
C. The losses the patient has endured, if any
D. The meaning of the event to the patient

Answer: A

Critique: The approach to evaluating a patient's crisis state involves assessing the precipitating stressor for the event, the meaning of the event to the patient, the crisis situation itself, the patient's ability to cope with the crisis, and the scope of the patient's support system.

Page: 1475

13: Re-experiencing a traumatic event as real, without inappropriate coping, depressed mood, loss of pleasure, or episodic periods of sudden onset anxiety, suggests which of the following diagnoses:

A. Posttraumatic stress disorder
B. Substance use and abuse
C. Panic disorder
D. Major depressive disorder

Answer: A

Critique: Re-experiencing an event as real is a hallmark of posttraumatic stress disorder. Although this could occur during a major depressive disorder, the absence of depressed mood or anhedonia rules out major depressive disorder. The absence of unexplained onsets of anxiety rules out panic disorder. Substance abuse or use could be a primary disorder or an inappropriate means of coping with the trauma.

Page: Table 54–2

14: Which of the following statements is true regarding physician assistance to the patient in crisis:

A. Restoration of resources to meet basic needs has little therapeutic effect.

B. Patients will be unable to describe the nature of the crisis; therefore, trying to obtain this information is unhelpful.
C. Patients are best helped through a crisis by encouraging them to tell the details of their experiences.
D. Patient's understanding of the precipitant of the crisis has little impact on crisis resolution.

Answer: C

Critique: Patients are best helped through a crisis by encouraging them to tell the details of their experience and their individual traumas. By doing this, the patient will not only become aware of what is stressful about the event but also become aware of why the event is stressful and begin a process of problem solving that results in crisis resolution.

Page: 1476

15: In terms of crisis resolution strategies, which of the following strategies has the potential to provide the greatest relief:

A. Have the patient share his or her most painful feelings and emotions
B. Identify the specific areas of the patient's life that are most affected by the crisis
C. Teach the patient to evaluate his or her support system
D. Teach the patient to understand his or her current coping styles

Answer: A

Critique: Although all of these choices can be components of crisis intervention, expressing painful feelings and emotions has been shown to be the most important step in the patient's discovery of meaning and resolution of psychological disturbance.

Page: 1476

16: Which of the following statements is false regarding critical instance stress debriefing:

A. It can be conducted in individual or group format.
B. It typically occurs between 24 and 74 hours following the traumatic event.
C. It should be performed by individuals trained in this specific technique.
D. It is usually accompanied by pharmacologic intervention.

Answer: D

Critique: Although critical instance stress debriefing may be done with individuals, a group format is much more common and can be helpful to a community where these types of debriefings are most often performed. Debriefers receive specific training in the technique. The technique is usually applied soon after the stressing event. Psychopharmacological intervention is rarely needed and could be contraindicated with the use of this technique.

Page: 1480

17: Which of the following statements is true about critical instance stress debriefing:

    A. Feelings should be sealed over as quickly as possible so the person can return to his or her normal condition.

    B. Even in a group setting, confidentiality is unimportant because these groups are not psychotherapy sessions.

    C. Especially in a group setting, detailed descriptions of the event are unimportant because everyone is likely to have seen and viewed the events differently.

    D. Helping the individual to see that he or she is experiencing normal responses to a normal situation is therapeutic.

Answer: D

Critique: Critical instance stress briefing is a brief psychotherapeutic technique. Assurance of confidentiality improves expression of thoughts and feelings. Descriptions of events help the individuals to share their experience. Each individual should have time to express his or her feelings at the time of the incident as well as subsequently. It is therapeutic for group members to find that others have experienced similar feelings and give them a sense of normalcy about the reaction.

Page: 1480

18: Which of the following statements is most correct regarding crisis intervention treatment:

    A. Crisis intervention works best when patients are moved from their natural environment.

    B. Crisis intervention works best when the patient returns to original circumstances as soon as possible.

    C. Crisis intervention works best when the patient is hospitalized.

    D. Crisis intervention works best when treatment is delayed.

Answer: B

Critique: Early formulations of traumatic neurosis reflected increased understanding of the psychological effects of war. Physicians noticed the difference between French and British soldiers in terms of psychological sequelae: French solders did better, and it was noted that they received immediate psychological treatment and were returned to battle as quickly as possible. Except in extreme circumstances, removal from the natural environment is likely to further disequilibrium.

Pages: 1476–1481

19: Which of the following personality disorders is most likely to be related to emotional trauma or crisis:

    A. Borderline personality

    B. Schizotypal personality disorder

    C. Schizoid personality disorder

    D. Antisocial personality disorder

Answer: A

Critique: Borderline personality disorder may result from repeated traumatic separations from a parent. Schizotypal personality disorder involves symptoms of oddness and eccentricities that may reflect a predisposition toward schizophrenia. Schizoid disorder is a pattern of disinterest in relationships with no related anxiety. Antisocial personality is a pattern of disregard for others, manipulation, and violation of rules and laws. Antisocial personality may be related to genetic factors as well as parental behavior.

Pages: 1474–1476

20: Which of the following psychiatric disorders is commonly associated with emotional trauma or crisis:

    A. Schizophreniform disorder

    B. Mental retardation

    C. Seasonal affective disorder

    D. Brief psychosis

Answer: D

Critique: Brief psychosis is a loss of reality testing in the form of hallucinations, delusions, or disorganization in speech and behavior that lasts longer than 1 day but less than 1 month. Schizophreniform disorder involves similar symptoms that last for less than 6 months but more than 1 month. Mental retardation is a genetic or prenatally acquired disorder except in rare cases of extreme deprivation postnatally. Seasonal affective disorder causes a unique constellation of depressive symptoms, has a repeated seasonal onset, and is unlikely to be related to emotional trauma.

Pages: 1474–1476

21: Common symptoms associated with crisis or trauma include all of the following, except:

    A. Returning to places and people associated with the initial traumatic event

    B. Feeling a sense of emptiness or hopelessness about the future

    C. Recurring traumatic dreams or nightmare

    D. Insomnia

Answer: A

Critique: Rather than return to the origin of the trauma, people in crisis or trauma typically avoid anything associated with the traumatic event. The other symptoms are commonly associated with the crisis or trauma.

Page: 1475

22: With regard to crisis resolution, which of the following strategies is appropriate:

    A. Avoid discussing painful feelings and emotions.

    B. Concentrate on the one coping style that has been the most effective in the past.

    C. If the person does not have substance abuse disorder, 1 to 2 ounces of alcohol a night may be helpful.

    D. Identify parties in the social support system who can be helpful.

Answer: D

Critique: The loss of social support is often one of the primary causes of crisis. Even if it is not the precipitant, social support can greatly ameliorate the crisis stage and facilitate return to equilibrium. Victims in crisis may withdraw and need assistance in returning to equilibrium. Patients should be encouraged to express their emotions. They also should be encouraged to try new coping styles; their preferred one may not be appropriate for the current situation. Use of alcohol is a dysfunctional coping style and may exacerbate symptoms.

Pages: 1476, 1477

23: All of the following represent pathologic coping styles, except:

    A. Impulsive
    B. Random chaotic
    C. Action-oriented
    D. Dissociation

Answer: C

Critique: Coping styles are the unique ways in which patients deal with stress. Some styles work better than others, and pathologic coping styles should be countered. The action-oriented person takes an action to immediately rectify a problem. The impulsive person responds in unpredictable ways without anticipating possible outcomes. Random-chaotic coping reflects impulsivity, as well as irrationality, and may be seen in individuals in psychotic states. Dissociation is a change in one's sense of reality associated with extreme trauma.

Page: 1478, Table 54–4

24: Which of the following is an example of symptom-focused treatment for acute stress disorder:

    A. Encouraging help-seeking behavior
    B. Medication in the form of paroxetine at standard doses for depression
    C. Improving access to social support services
    D. Helping the patient to create logical and rational solutions to his or her problems

Answer: C

Critique: Return of social support helps re-establish a state of equilibrium as an aid to resolving the crisis. Help seeking and logical, rational problem solving are adaptive coping styles that also serve as crisis resolution tools. Medications can be helpful with prominent, major symptoms of acute stress disorder, including trauma-related fears and anxiety as well as difficulty in concentrating.

Pages: 1476, 1477, Table 54–3

25: The first-line medication choice for mood lability and anger outbursts associated with posttraumatic stress is:

    A. Diazepam, 0.5 to 4 mg/day
    B. Clonazepam, 0.5 to 2 mg/day
    C. Fluoxetine, starting dose 20 mg/day
    D. Phenelzine, 15 mg three times daily

Answer: C

Critique: Posttraumatic stress disorder is a persisting condition that tranquilizers such as diazepam and clonazepam are unlikely to help except temporarily. The selective serotonin reuptake inhibitors (SSRIs), such as fluoxetine, can be helpful for this indication. Monoamine oxidase inhibitors, such as phenelzine, might be more useful for trauma-related fear and avoidance.

Page: 1479, Table 54–3

26: Which of the following is considered to be the initial preferred medication choice for general anxiety as a symptom of acute stress disorder:

    A. Fluoxetine, starting dose 20 mg/day
    B. Phenelzine, starting dose 15 mg three times a day
    C. Clonazepam, 0.5 to 2 mg/day
    D. Zaleplon, 5 to 10 mg at bedtime

Answer: C

Critique: Acute stress disorder involves symptoms that last no more than 1 month. Clonazepam is the most effective medication of those listed. Phenelzine is a monoamine oxidase inhibitor. Valproic acid is second-line medication for mood lability and generally is not effective in reducing anxiety. Zaleplon is a nonbenzodiazepine hypnotic.

Page: 1474, Table 54–2

27: Which of the following medications should be considered initially in the treatment of insomnia associated with acute stress disorder:

    A. Citalopram, starting dose 20 mg/day
    B. Nortriptyline, starting dose 50 mg/day
    C. Zolpidem, 5 to 10 mg at bedtime
    D. Haloperidol, 10 mg at bedtime

Answer: C

Critique: Citalopram and nortriptyline are antidepressant medications; nortriptyline is one of the more activating of the tricyclic antidepressants. Haloperidol is an antipsychotic medication that, although sedating, is not a good choice in the treatment of insomnia. Zolpidem has been shown to be effective when used as a brief intervention for sleep improvement.

Page: 1479, Table 54–3

Chapter 55

Office Evaluation and Management of Personality Disorders

Michael P. Rowane and William A. Rowane

1: The prevalence rate for personality disorders in the general population is approximately:

   A. 1%
   B. 10%
   C. 50%
   D. 75%
   E. 90%

Answer: B

Critique: The prevalence rate for personality disorders in the general population is approximately 10%.

Page: 1482

2: One significant reason that personality disorders often go unrecognized is that affected individuals:

   A. Rarely have an unexpected or unpleasant interpersonal interaction
   B. Manifest only in a complete psychotic episode
   C. Do not verbalize or manifest typical psychiatric symptoms
   D. Have severe psychiatric symptoms
   E. Do not present with symptoms that are apparent to family and friends

Answer: C

Critique: Personality disorders often go unrecognized because affected individuals do not verbalize or manifest typical psychiatric symptoms or complaints, even though they may suffer with many personality failures. Most commonly, a patient with a personality disorder is recognized after an unexpected or unpleasant interpersonal interaction.

Page: 1482

3: A personality style is:

   A. The lifelong, habitual way one thinks, feels, and behaves
   B. Not often apparent at birth
   C. Genetically conferred
   D. Identical among individuals of the same race and socioeconomic status

Answer: A

Critique: A personality style is the lifelong, habitual way one thinks, feels, and behaves. Styles that are genetically

conferred are termed *temperament*. These styles, such as the ability to filter external stimuli or shyness, are often observable at birth.

Page: 1482

4: A personality disorder:

   A. Strengthens an individual's personality style
   B. Can improve social skills
   C. Rarely leads to impairment
   D. Can be a rigid and extreme personality style
   E. Allows an individual the opportunity to adapt better to his or her environment

Answer: D

Critique: Personality styles that become rigid, extreme, and maladaptively damaging to oneself or others or that lead to social or occupational impairment are termed *personality disorders*.

Page: 1482

5: According to the fourth edition of *Diagnostic and Statistical Manual of Mental Disorders* (DSM-IV), the preliminary diagnosis of a personality disorder includes which of the following clusters:

   A. Typical, excitable
   B. Average, stable
   C. Happy, relaxed
   D. Dramatic, emotional
   E. All of the above

Answer: D

Critique: The three clusters that make up personality disorders as listed in the fourth edition of DSM-IV are cluster A, odd and eccentric; cluster B, dramatic and emotional; and cluster C, anxious or fearful.

Pages: 1482, 1483, Table 55–1

6: An individual who expects exploitation and harm, questions loyalty and fidelity, bears grudges, and is easily slighted is best described as:

   A. Schizoid
   B. Paranoid
   C. Schizotypal

    D. Antisocial
    E. Narcissistic

Answer: B

Critique: An individual with a paranoid personality disorder expects exploitation and harm, questions loyalty and fidelity, bears grudges, and is easily slighted.

Pages: 1483, 1491, Table 55–1

7: A patient has a history of cruelty, problems with authority, unlawful behavior, dishonesty, irresponsibility, and exploitation of others is probably best described as having which personality disorder:

    A. Histrionic
    B. Avoidant
    C. Borderline
    D. Paranoid
    E. Antisocial

Answer: E

Critique: Patients with antisocial personality disorders expect to be exploited, demeaned, or humiliated. They, in turn, treat others in such a manner and may resort to psychopathic manipulations of deception, lying, cheating, or stealing.

Pages: 1483, 1491, 1492, Table 55–1

8: Which of the following personality disorders best describes a patient with core beliefs and thoughts such as "I am special," "I am important," "I come first," and "The world should revolve around me":

    A. Obsessive-compulsive
    B. Schizotypal
    C. Narcissistic
    D. Dependent
    E. Borderline

Answer: C

Critique: Narcissistic patients have a superior, entitled, self-loving, arrogant attitude. They place themselves above others and become the center of their universe.

Pages: 1485, 1493, Table 55–2

9: A physician feels frustrated with a patient who is not able to adequately articulate his or her fears. The physician also feels annoyed when this patient demonstrates weakness. The patient's behavior also may include social timidity and being withdrawn. Which of the following personality disorders reflects these characteristics:

    A. Dependent
    B. Avoidant
    C. Borderline
    D. Schizoid
    E. Histrionic

Answer: B

Critique: Patients who have avoidant personality disorder typically have feelings of inadequacy and fear of criticism. Their low self-esteem fosters their belief that they are inept and inadequate. Such patients may wish to establish relationships and exchange affection, but their fear of being criticized, rejected, embarrassed, or hurt causes them to avoid social situations or meeting new people.

Pages: 1485, 1493, 1494, Table 55–2

10: Individuals with dependent personality disorder are characterized by:

    A. Preoccupation with details, order, and control
    B. Suffering, depression, and self-sacrifice
    C. Feelings of inadequacy and fear of criticism
    D. An exaggerated need for care or a need for direction from someone else
    E. Frequently becoming dependent on their physician in an extremely demanding, clinging, helpless, or self-destructive manner

Answer: D

Critique: A dependent personality disorder is characterized by an exaggerated need for care or a need for direction from someone else. An obsessive-compulsive personality disorder is characterized by being preoccupied with details, order, and control. An individual with an avoidant personality disorder has feelings of inadequacy and a fear of criticism. A patient who frequently becomes dependent on his or her physician in an extremely demanding, clinging, helpless, or self-destructive manner has a borderline personality disorder.

Pages: 1485, 1494, Table 55–2

11: An individual who is driven to ritualistic behavior, such as excessive hand washing, and who is perfectionistic, rigid, and unyielding may be seen as having which of the following personality disorders:

    A. Narcissistic
    B. Borderline
    C. Antisocial
    D. Dependent
    E. Obsessive-compulsive

Answer: E

Critique: Patients with an obsessive-compulsive personality disorder are perfectionistic, driven to orderliness, and logical and have compulsions, such as excessive hand washing. They also are controlling, critical, stubborn, prone to stinginess, frequently seen as workaholics, and overly rational.

Pages: 1485, 1494, Table 55–2

12: Which of the following is consistent with a neurotic personality organization:

    A. Reality testing lost
    B. Defenses are at a higher level
    C. Changing views of self and physician
    D. Defenses are splitting centered
    E. Identity diffusion is prominent

Answer: B

Critique: A patient with a neurotic personality organization has intact reality testing, defenses at a higher level, and repression centered. The neurotic patient has a stable view of self and physician.

Page: 1486, Table 55–3

13: Which of the following statements regarding personality disorders is true:

    A. There is no mixture of different personality disorders in an individual.

    B. Patients typically have the full disorder with no traits of other personality disorders.

    C. Personality disorders are usually uncomplicated.

    D. It is not unusual for a patient to have elements of more than one personality disorder.

    E. A physician rarely is provoked by a patient with a personality disorder.

Answer: D

Critique: Personality disorders are complicated, and it is not unusual for a patient to meet criteria for two cluster diagnoses and more than one personality disorder diagnosis. Primary care physicians often recognize a patient with a personality disorder by their own reactions to the patient.

Page: 1482

14: When dealing with a patient with a paranoid personality disorder, which of the following is an acceptable intervention by the primary care physician:

    A. Acknowledge complaints, even if arguing with or ignoring the patient is necessary

    B. Withhold information from the patient

    C. Correct reality distortions and unreasonable patient expectations

    D. Confront all delusions

    E. Insist that the patient take all required tests, even if they refuse out of mistrust

Answer: C

Critique: The physician who manages the paranoid patient should empathize with the patient's fear of being hurt and acknowledge complaints without arguing or ignoring the patient. It is best to openly and honestly explain medical illnesses as well as correct reality distortions and unrealistic patient expectations. The physician should gently correct the paranoid patient's irrational thoughts and suggest more rational ones. In the event that the patient refuses care out of mistrust, avoid insisting on your management plan and agree to disagree on the necessity of the test.

Pages: 1487–1489, 1491, Table 55–4

15: A common defense mechanism of splitting for patients with personality disorders is expressed as:

    A. Self and others are seen only as all good.

    B. Self and others are seen only as all bad.

    C. Others are seen only as all bad.

    D. Others are seen only as all good.

    E. Self and others are seen as all good or all bad.

Answer: E

Critique: Patients with personality disorders have certain defenses, including splitting, in which self and others are seen as all good or all bad.

Pages: 1487–1489, Table 55–4

16: The management of this personality disorder involves some of the following points: be careful not to tell the patient what to do; ask the patient what it is about independence that is so frightening; do not abandon or threaten termination; gently elicit irrational thoughts and suggest more rational ones. The personality disorder just described is:

    A. Narcissistic

    B. Borderline

    C. Antisocial

    D. Dependent

    E. Obsessive-compulsive

Answer: D

Critique: Dependent personality disorders require the physician to understand and empathize with the patient's need for caregiving and at the same time to encourage and foster independent thinking and action by the patient. The patient will not benefit from being told what to do. The physician must not cater to the patient's unreasonable expectations for being taken care of and help the patient to modify these expectations.

Pages: 1487–1489, 1494, Table 55–4

17: The physician may be used for secondary gain, which requires verifying symptoms and illness progression with others. The physician must not moralize but instead explain to the patient that deception will only result in poor patient care. Which of the following personality disorders does this management approach describe:

    A. Narcissistic

    B. Borderline

    C. Antisocial

    D. Dependent

    E. Obsessive-compulsive

Answer: C

Critique: Patients with antisocial personality disorders often communicate dishonestly, which requires verifying symptoms and illness progression with others.

Pages: 1487–1489, 1491, 1492, Table 55–4

18: These patients do not appear psychotic or idiosyncratic in their behavior. They are disinterested in intimate contacts with others, appear detached and unemotional, and wish to be left alone. The physician should provide neutral or unemotional expressions of medical information, which will most likely be heard and implemented. To which of the following personality disorders do these characteristics and management approach apply:

    A. Schizoid

    B. Borderline

    C. Schizotypal

    D. Dependent

    E. Obsessive-compulsive

Answer: A

Critique: The schizoid patient may give the physician the opinion that the patient is a "loner." These patients do not have psychotic features and do not desire intimate contact with others. Such patients respond best to neutral or unemotional expressions of medical information by the physician.

Pages: 1487–1489, 1491, Table 55–4

19: The patient who the physician feels is both alone and "weird" or "strange," who demonstrates regressive behavior into fantasies, and to a lesser extent, who uses denial as the main defense, is typical of which personality disorder:

- A. Schizoid
- B. Borderline
- C. Schizotypal
- D. Dependent
- E. Obsessive-compulsive

Answer: C

Critique: Although schizoid patients are seen as "loners," the schizotypal patient is both alone and bizarre. The defenses of patients with schizotypal personality disorders involve schizoid fantasy, in which the patient retreats to idiosyncratic fantasy when faced with a painful experience. Denial is a lesser-used defense mechanism of schizoid patients.

Pages: 1487–1489, 1491, Table 55–4

20: When dealing with a patient with a borderline personality disorder, which of the following is an acceptable intervention by the primary care physician:

- A. Be very flexible with the patient.
- B. Avoid punishing the patient for inappropriate behaviors.
- C. Allow the patient to maintain reality distortions.
- D. Immediately interrogate the patient regarding irrational thoughts.
- E. Avoid confrontation, clarification, and interpretation of the problematic situation.

Answer: B

Critique: Office management of patients with borderline personality disorders requires several measures to avoid anger and frustration in the treating physician. Doing so begins with empathetic understanding of the patient's fears. Firm limits must be set and punishment should be avoided. The patient's reality distortions and unreasonable expectations must be corrected. The physician should establish reality testing, then gently correct irrational thoughts and suggest more rational ones. Once reality testing is determined to be intact, the most helpful interventions can be aimed at decreasing pathological splitting defenses by using confrontation, clarification, and interpretation of the problematic situation.

Pages: 1487–1489, 1493, Table 55–4

21: Which of the following are typical physician reactions to the narcissistic patient:

- A. Intimidation
- B. Improved self-value
- C. Feeling superior

- D. Feelings of warmth and happiness
- E. Increased self-confidence

Answer: A

Critique: The care and management of narcissistic patients is often difficult for the physician. They have a superior, entitled, self-loving, arrogant attitude that can be intimidating. The physician may have feelings of being devalued and inferior or fears of the patient's anger and criticism. One aspect of concern is that the physician may have feelings of anger or the desire to dismiss such patients because their lack of empathy and interpersonal exploitation.

Pages: 1487–1489, 1493, Table 55–4

22: A patient who is often depressed and self-sacrificing and repeatedly makes bad choices that lead to failure or pain may be suffering from which of the following disorders:

- A. Avoidant
- B. Self-defeating
- C. Borderline
- D. Antisocial
- E. Dependent

Answer: B

Critique: Patients with self-defeating characteristics are often depressed and self-sacrificing and repeatedly make bad choices that lead to failure or pain. This diagnostic category was eliminated from DSM-IV, but it is commonly seen and is a challenging clinical problem for physicians.

Pages: 1485, 1495, Table 55–2

23: (True or False) Which of the following statements regarding patients with obsessive-compulsive personality disorder are true and which are false:

- A. These patients have recurrent disturbing thoughts or obsessions that create marked subjective distress.
- B. Many traits, such as orderliness and attention to detail, are short-term patterns that many patients use adaptively in their professional life.
- C. Struggle or conflict with the patient over control should be avoided.
- D. Because they believe they come before all others, these patients feel that people are there to be used and exploited.

Answers: A - True, B - False, C - True, D - True

Critique: Patients with an obsessive-compulsive personality disorder are upset because of their recurring disturbing thoughts or obsessions. They have lifelong traits, including core adaptive traits of orderliness, attention to detail, and an emphasis on rational thinking and logic. The physician must empathize with the patient's loss of self-control and assist in his or her regaining control. The physician must avoid struggling or conflict with the patient over control. Patient core beliefs include that people should do better and try harder and that they must be perfect and make no mistakes. Patients with an antisocial personality disorder feel that people are there to be used and exploited, because they think that they come before all others.

Pages: 1485, 1494, Table 55–2

Chapter 56

Somatic Patient

Dorothy B. Trevino

1: The best diagnostic/treatment approach to patients with vague somatic complaints is:

A. Exhaustively rule out all possible organic explanations
B. Address the fact that malingering is a probable cause of most unexplained somatic complaints
C. Consider the most probable underlining psychological and psychiatric conditions
D. Downplay the importance of somatic symptoms, and emphasize the importance of the negative findings

Answer: C

Critique: Exhaustively ruling out organic disease may prolong somatization and lead to iatrogenesis. Patients with psychological disorders are in need of definitive treatment. Psychosocial and psychiatric difficulties have been found to underlie most somatic complaints not explained by organic problems.

Pages: 1496, 1497

2: The somatic complaints of concentration impairment, poor appetite, fatigue, sleep difficulties, increased agitation, anxiety, pain, and nonspecific physical complaints are most descriptive of which disorder:

A. Generalized anxiety disorder
B. Social phobia
C. Major depression
D. Somatoform disorders

Answer: C

Critique: The symptoms of major depression may include those of other diagnostic categories, such as pain and anxiety, but differ from each of the others in specific symptoms, such as the presence of dyspnea, heart palpitation, sweating, and others, present in anxiety disorders.

Pages: 1496, 1497

3: The only somatic disorder in which the patient is consciously involved in producing the symptoms is:

A. Hypochondriasis
B. Conversion disorder
C. Factitious disorder
D. Somatization

Answer: C

Critique: Factitious disorder and malingering involve the patient consciously deciding to use physical symptoms for gain. The other somatoform disorders are involuntarily produced with no insight into the underlying conflict or secondary gain involved.

Page: 1497

4: The easiest somatic disorder to diagnose is:

A. Somatoform pain disorders
B. Depression
C. Situational stress
D. Hypochondriasis

Answer: C

Critique: Stress-related physical symptoms do not meet the full criteria for psychiatric impairments. The relationship between the symptoms and the triggering circumstance is often readily understandable. The other conditions typically have origins greatly removed in time and are difficult to trace.

Page: 1498

5: Patients with personality disorders often present management difficulties. Which personality disorder is characterized by vacillation between intense positive feelings and intense anger at the caregiver, easily feeling rejected, or sabotaging plans:

A. Dependent personality disorder
B. Antisocial personality disorder
C. Obsessive-compulsive personality disorder
D. Borderline personality disorder

Answer: D

Critique: Patients with borderline personality disorder tend to transfer early childhood conflicts onto the present caregiver, unconsciously repeating earlier distress. Although the other personality disorders may involve anger, it is not as central an issue.

Page: 1498

6: (True or False) Examples of behaviors or circumstances that may operantly condition somatic symptoms are:

A. Attention or sympathy from others
B. Financial compensation for symptoms
C. Attention from health care professionals
D. Eliminating previously required distasteful activities

Answer: A - True, B - True, C - True, D - True

Critique: Symptoms can be inadvertently reinforced if the presence of the symptom is followed with positive consequences to the patient or if a negative consequence is removed.

Pages: 1498, 1499

7: (True or False) Determine whether the following statements accurately describe the process of conditioning somatic symptoms:

A. Physical symptoms may be reinforced if a patient is unable to assertively ask that his or her need be met, yet gets attention when ill.
B. Modeling of somatization occurs when parents teach children about health promotion.
C. Operant conditioning can occur when symptoms become associated with a particular person, place, or situation.
D. Conditioning of symptoms occurs only with personality disorders.

Answer: A - True, B - False, C - True, D - False

Critique: Patients who have poor communication skills, such as lack of assertiveness, may unconsciously have their emotional needs met when others are supportive during illnesses. Modeling occurs when someone grows up observing a close family member who somatizes and pays great attention to physical sensations but not when they learn to prevent illness. Receiving attention or care for somatic symptoms may pair the symptoms with a particular time, place, or person. Conditioning of symptoms occurs in all patient groups.

Pages: 1498, 1499

8: Which of the following statements accurately describes sociocultural factors and disorders involving somatic complaints?

A. Hospitalized patients respond to pain in a similar fashion regardless of their culture.
B. Cultures that are less accepting of direct expression of emotions have less somatization.
C. The vegetative signs of depression are the same across cultures.
D. Affective states in depression do not vary by culture.

Answer: C

Critique: The manner in which a culture deals with affective and cognitive states, cultural beliefs, and attitudes influences how symptoms are expressed, including how pain is perceived. Vegetative signs of depression, unlike affective and cognitive states, are diagnostic across cultures.

Page: 1499

9: The best diagnostic approach to patients with non-significant medical findings is:

A. All possible organic causes should be eliminated before exploring nonmedical causes.
B. Assess the psychosocial stress-related aspects of the case early, but postpone discussing them with the patient until after an extensive biomedical work-up is completed.

C. Consideration of a possible psychosocial disorder should be postponed until the physician can rule out any possible dangerous biomedical problem.
D. Comprehensive biopsychosocial assessment produces a diagnosis with the greatest utility for patient management.

Answer: D

Critique: Studies show that most patients accept a multifactorial approach to diagnosis, especially when this strategy is shared early in the assessment, thus establishing a framework for the patient to make sense of all findings.

Pages: 1499, 1500

10: (True or False) The following statements accurately describe the best assessment of somatic complaints:

A. It is best to operationalize the patient's somatic complaints by analyzing the antecedents, symptomatic behavior, and consequences of symptoms.
B. In acute cases, patients can easily make the connection between obvious stressors and physical symptoms; therefore, inquiry by the physician is not necessary.
C. Somatic symptoms occurring for 6 months or less are usually related to specific environmental stressors and have a good prognosis.
D. If the patient denies the presence of depressive affective or cognitive states, it is not important to ask further about vegetative states.

Answer: A - True, B - False, C - True, D - False

Critique: A functional analysis that specifies triggers, behaviors, and consequences leads to a clear picture for intervention. Patients are often unable to make connections between stressors and the presence of symptoms, and the physician must help them with this. Somatic symptoms of short duration have been found to be highly treatable. The patient should always be asked about vegetative states of depression because these states have been found to be stable.

Pages: 1500, 1501

11: Which statement is *not* a benefit of the self-monitoring device of a symptom diary:

A. A symptom diary collects data that help educate patient and physician about contributing factors and causes of complaints.
B. Constant problems, such as fatigue, are useful in symptom diaries because they can be monitored repeatedly.
C. Symptom diaries identify antecedents by recording items such as the time of day, the environment, and events occurring when the symptom is present.
D. Symptom diaries actively involve patients in their medical treatment, rather than relying on the physician to solve the problem.

Answer: B

Critique: Continuous problems, such as chronic fatigue, may actually be reinforced by self-monitoring devices. Such processes do not yield information about patterns, triggers, and so forth, because the symptoms are always present.

Page: 1501

12: The *one* group that requires a multidisciplinary (e.g., physician, psychotherapist, physical therapist) approach to treatment is:

    A. Children who have multiple unexplained physical symptoms related to family dysfunction
    B. Chronic somatizers who clearly had somatization modeled in their family
    C. Patients with somatic problems whose life functioning, such as participation in the workforce, parenting, and daily activities, have become seriously limited
    D. Patients with acute symptoms whose somatic complaints can be directly linked to current stressors

Answer: C

Critique: Most acute somatizers can be helped readily by physician support and patient education. Long-term somatizers often require collaboration with psychotherapists. When life functioning has become limited by somatization, interdisciplinary teams, as well as special programs used over intermediate time periods, are most helpful.

Page: 1501

13: (True or False) Along with behavioral interventions, antidepressants should be considered for which of the following:

    A. Patients who are obsessing over physical symptoms and sensations
    B. Patients with panic disorder and accompanying physical symptoms
    C. Anxious, fearful patients who tend toward generalized anxiety disorder
    D. Patients with chronic pain

Answer: A - True, B - True, C - True, D - True

Critique: Antidepressants, especially SSRIs, have been found to have interactive effects with behavioral and psychological treatment for all of the stated conditions.

Pages: 1501, 1502

Chapter 57

Dementia

Linda Roethel

1: Of the following statements, which is true regarding dementia:

   A. Dementia and delirium are the same condition, and the terms may be used interchangeably.
   B. In dementia, the deficit is isolated to memory alone.
   C. Dementia affects almost 10% of persons 85 years of age, and this prevalence remains consistent as one ages.
   D. People with mild dementia may be difficult to detect, because they often preserve social skills or develop ego-protective techniques to hide their memory loss and cognitive defects from others.
   E. The cause of dementia in the majority of so diagnosed patients is reversible.

Answer: D

Critique: Dementia and delirium are different conditions, although an individual can suffer from both conditions. Dementia is a heterogeneous group of brain disorders resulting in impairment in memory, language, visuospatial perception, praxis, and executive functions to varying degrees. Dementia affects almost 10% of persons 65 years of age, and the prevalence roughly doubles each decade of life thereafter. Mild dementia is difficult to detect and requires an increased awareness of this possibility on the part of the care provider. Only about 20% of patients diagnosed with dementia have treatable causes of dementia.

Page: 1505

2: The initial diagnostic work-up for dementia includes all of the following, except:

   A. An increased awareness of the possibility of dementia in each elderly patient
   B. A thorough history, including a corroborating history from the patient's spouse, significant other, or adult children
   C. Referral of the patient and first-degree family members for genetic screening
   D. Physical examination, including an assessment of comorbid conditions and cognitive function
   E. Laboratory testing to include CBC, chemistry panel, TSH, B_{12} level, syphilis screening, and urinalysis.

Answer: C

Critique: All of the above, except for genetic screening, are part of the initial diagnostic work-up for dementia. If dementia is diagnosed and it is of a type that has a strong genetic component, then a genetic counseling referral may be indicated.

Pages: 1505, 1506

3: All of the following are true regarding Alzheimer's disease and related dementias, except:

   A. Alzheimer's disease and related dementias account for approximately 70% of the irreversible dementias in the United States.
   B. The life expectancy of a patient with Alzheimer's disease is typically 15 to 25 years from onset.
   C. Dementia with Lewy bodies, Parkinson's disease with dementia, and supranuclear palsy are dementias related to Alzheimer's disease.
   D. Women are at greater risk for Alzheimer's disease than men are.
   E. The clinical course of Alzheimer's disease is somewhat variable.

Answer: B

Critique: Alzheimer's disease and related dementias are the most common forms of irreversible dementia in the United States, accounting for approximately 70% of these dementias. The life expectancy of a patient with Alzheimer's disease is typically 10 years from onset. Dementia with Lewy bodies may be the second most common irreversible dementia after Alzheimer's disease and may be correctly diagnosed only after an autopsy. Parkinson's disease with dementia and supranuclear palsy also may present as clinically similar to Alzheimer's disease. In Alzheimer's disease, as well as related dementias, the clinical course is somewhat variable. Women are at greater risk than are men for Alzheimer's disease. The reverse is true for dementia with Lewy bodies.

Pages: 1506–1508

4: (True or False) Patients with dementia with Lewy bodies (DLB):

   A. Are often clinically misdiagnosed as suffering from Alzheimer's disease
   B. Commonly suffer bizarre visual and global hallucinations
   C. Are more likely to be women than men
   D. Respond extremely well to neuroleptic drugs
   E. Are more likely to suffer from depression than are patients with Alzheimer's disease

Answer: A - True, B - True, C - False, D - False, E - True

Critique: Patients with DLB have a very similar presentation as that of patients with Alzheimer's disease. At autopsy, though, one study showed that 36% of patients clinically diagnosed with Alzheimer's disease had pathologic features of DLB. Bizarre visual and global hallucinations are common in DLB even before cognitive deficits become severe. DLB is more common in men than in women. DLB patients respond poorly to typical neuroleptic drugs. Depression is more commonly seen in DLB than in Alzheimer's disease.

Page: 1508

5: Which of the following is true regarding Parkinson's disease with dementia:

   A. Motor signs must precede dementing illness by at least 5 years for a diagnosis of Parkinson's disease with dementia.
   B. The prevalence of dementia in Parkinson's disease is about 2% to 5%.
   C. Parkinson's disease with dementia is more frequently associated with depression when the patient has an earlier onset of Parkinson's disease.
   D. Patients with Parkinson's disease with dementia may exhibit psychoses.

Answer: D

Critique: For a diagnosis of Parkinson's disease with dementia, motor signs must precede dementing illness by at least 1 year. Patients with Parkinson's disease have an increased risk of dementia, with a prevalence of about 10% to 25%. Patients who are of an older age with the onset of Parkinson's disease, as well as having atypical neurological features, are more likely to have depression associated with their illness. Psychoses may occur in patients with Parkinson's disease with dementia and are sometimes difficult to ascribe to the side effects of L-dopa therapy or the dementing disorder itself.

Page: 1508

6: All of the following are true regarding the pharmacologic treatment of Alzheimer's disease and related disorders, except:

   A. It is best to withhold pharmacologic treatment for Alzheimer's for as long as possible, because it has no effect in the early stages of the disease.
   B. At present, curative treatment is not available.
   C. Donepezil (Aricept), a cholinesterase inhibitor, benefits approximately 80% of patients with Alzheimer's disease and related disorders.
   D. Women who are on estrogen replacement therapy benefit more from cholinesterase inhibitor therapy.
   E. Selegiline (Eldepryl), vitamin E, and gingko biloba have all been found somewhat effective in the treatment of Alzheimer's disease.

Answer: A

Critique: Pharmacologic treatment should be initiated as early as possible for maximum disease modification. Pharmacologic agents result in stabilization and slowing of the disease process in most patients. Some patients may show a modest improvement of cognitive function. There currently is no curative treatment for Alzheimer's; all therapies available at present should be considered symptomatic treatment. Approximately 80% of patients with Alzheimer's disease benefit from donepezil (Aricept), a cholinesterase inhibitor. It has less side effects and easier dosing than tacrine (Cognex), the first cholinesterase inhibitor. Women on estrogen therapy benefit more from cholinesterase therapy than women not on estrogen therapy. Selegiline (Eldepryl), vitamin E, and gingko biloba have all been found somewhat effective, but the combination of selegiline and vitamin E caused a more rapid decline than no treatment.

Pages: 1508, 1509

7: All of the following are true regarding vascular dementia, except:

   A. It is a very rare cause of dementia.
   B. It is a heterogeneous group of disorders with multiple causes.
   C. Vascular dementia and Alzheimer's disease may coexist.
   D. Multiple infarcts can result in vascular dementia.
   E. The risk factors for vascular dementia are the same as for atherosclerosis, stroke, and heart attack.

Answer: A

Critique: Vascular dementia is the second most common cause of dementia in the United States after Alzheimer's disease and related dementias. It represents a heterogeneous group of disorders with multiple etiologies, such as multiple infarcts, a single strategically located infarct, or multiple subcortical lacunar infarcts. The risk factors for vascular dementia include the risk factors for atherosclerosis, stroke, and heart attack. Both vascular dementia and Alzheimer's disease are common and may coexist.

Page: 1509

Questions 7 to 10: Match each numbered entry with the correct lettered heading. Each letter may be used only once.

   A. Alzheimer's disease
   B. Frontotemporal dementias
   C. Creutzfeldt-Jakob disease
   D. Huntington's disease

7: This disease is caused by an infectious spongiform encephalopathic agent or prion

8: Individuals homozygous for Apo E allele E4 are at the greatest risk.

9: Pick's disease is a variant.

10: GABA and glutamic acid decarboxylate levels are deficient in this autosomal dominant genetic disorder.

Answers: 7 - C, 8 - A, 9 - B, 10 - D

Critique: Creutzfeldt-Jakob disease is a rare dementia that exists in sporadic, genetic, and new variant types. It is caused by an infectious spongiform encephalopathic agent or prion with a long incubation period. Apo E allele E4 increases an individual's risk of developing Alzheimer's disease. It probably does not cause Alzheimer's but sets conditions for some environmental factor to trigger the disorder. It also confers a risk for dementia with Lewy bodies and vascular dementia. With Pick's disease, a variant of frontotemporal dementias, disturbances in mood, verbal stereotypy, and progressive language dysfunction are common features. Huntington's disease is a genetic disorder with autosomal dominant transmission; peak onset is between ages 35 and 50.

Pages: 1507–1510

11: (True or False) A 78-year-old male is brought in by his 47-year-old daughter. She has been "helping him out" since his wife died 3 years ago. She states her concerns that over the past 6 to 8 months, her father is becoming confused, forgets to pay bills, is restless, and becomes easily angered. He has hypertension, hyperlipidemia, and coronary artery disease and is being treated with multiple medications. You should:

   A. Immediately refer the patient to the emergency department for a stat MRI of the brain
   B. Reassure the daughter that this is a normal part of aging and no work-up needed
   C. Obtain a thorough history from the patient and his daughter, including all medications being used, both over the counter and prescription
   D. Assess, or have the patient assessed for, cognitive and functional ability

Answers: A - False, B - False, C - True, D - True

Critique: At present, a CT or MRI of the brain remains a controversial element of the work-up for dementia. In this patient, because this case is not of acute onset, a stat MRI is not indicated. A screening MRI may be considered after taking a thorough history and physical and laboratory work-ups. Even though age-related memory impairment is seen with aging, the patient presents with symptoms more consistent with dementia and requires further work-up. The work-up includes a thorough history and physical examination, assessment of cognitive and functional ability, and assessment for depression. Laboratory tests for reversible causes of dementia should be ordered.

Pages: 1505, 1506

12: Which of the following is true regarding human immunodeficiency virus (HIV)-related dementia:

   A. Even though HIV patients are living longer, HIV dementia is very rare.
   B. When a patient with acquired immunodeficiency syndrome (AIDS) presents with dementia, the work-up is the same as for a non-AIDS/non-HIV patient.
   C. HIV-related dementia is now the most common dementia appearing before age 50.
   D. Cholinesterase inhibitors are the first choice of treatment in HIV-related dementia.

Answer: C

Critique: HIV-related dementia is now the most common dementia appearing before age 50. When a patient with AIDS presents with dementia, the work-up must include opportunistic infections that can cause dementia, such as toxoplasmosis, as well as the general work-up for dementia. As the treatments for AIDS improve and patients live longer, we can expect an even greater prevalence of HIV-related dementia. The approach for HIV-related dementia is to treat the underlying cause, AIDS, and psychiatric comorbid symptoms.

Pages: 1510, 1511

13: (True or False) Dementia can present with the following symptoms:

   A. Nondysphoric depression
   B. Memory impairment, with remote memory affected more than recent memory
   C. Bizarre visual and global hallucinations
   D. Disordered behavior, labile mood, and social disinhibition

Answer: A - True, B - False, C - True, D - True

Critique: An older patient with nondysphoric depression who presents with apathy, decreased cognitive ability, nervousness, somatization, and/or insomnia should be treated for depression. That individual should also be monitored for dementia, because an irreversible dementia appears in almost 50% of these patients within 5 years. Recent memory is impaired initially more than remote memory. Patients with dementia with Lewy bodies can present with bizarre visual and global hallucinations even before cognitive deficits are severe. Disordered behavior, labile mood, and social disinhibition are common with frontotemporal dementias, even before cognitive testing shows an abnormality.

Pages: 1505, 1508, 1510

14: Which of the following is true regarding dementia:

   A. Treating comorbid conditions in patients with irreversible dementia will never enhance overall function.
   B. There is never a need to obtain additional history from a family member or close friend of a patient suspected of dementia, because there is no need to diagnose dementia early.
   C. Apo E allele E4 confers protection against dementias.
   D. In dementia caused by normal-pressure hydrocephalus, CT or MRI of the head shows the ventricular system to be enlarged out of proportion to the accompanying cerebral atrophy.

Answer: D

Critique: Patients often preserve social skills or develop ego-protective techniques to hide their memory loss and cognitive deficits from others. A corroborating history may assist in early recognition of a dementia. Therapy for dementia may be of greatest value in the early stages. In addition, attention to comorbid conditions often enhances overall function, even in a patient with irreversible dementia. Individuals expressing Apo E allele E4 have an increased risk of Alzheimer's disease, dementia with Lewy bodies, and vascular dementia. In normal-pressure hydrocephalus, the patient usually presents with gait disorder, urinary incontinence, and dementia. This triad also can be seen in other dementia patients with comorbid conditions. The diagnosis is suspected by the findings on the CT or MRI of the brain.

Pages: 1505, 1507–1510

Questions 15 to 18: Match each numbered entry with the correct lettered heading. Each lettered heading may be used only once.

    A. Donepezil (Aricept)
    B. Calcium channel blockers
    C. Cerebrospinal fluid shunting
    D. L-dopa therapy

15: Can cause psychosis in patients with Parkinson's disease with dementia

16: Will benefit about 80% of patients with Alzheimer's disease

17: Has both neuroprotective and blood pressure–lowering effects in patients with vascular dementia

18: May be of benefit in some normal-pressure hydrocephalus patients

Answers: 15 - D, 16 - A, 17 - B, 18 - C

Critique: L-dopa therapy is used to treat Parkinson's disease with dementia. Psychoses can occur, and it is sometimes difficult to determine whether the psychoses are a side effect of the L-dopa therapy or the dementia itself. When treated with donepezil (Aricept), 80% of Alzheimer's disease patients show either moderate improvement in cognitive function or stabilization. Calcium channel blockers are used to treat hypertension, which is a risk factor for vascular dementia. They also have shown neuroprotective effects, especially when the patient has depression associated with vascular dementia. Some patients with normal-pressure hydrocephalus may benefit from cerebrospinal fluid shunting. Those with relatively greater gait disturbance and less severe urinary incontinence and dementia but, paradoxically, with greater degrees of ventricular enlargement and no accompanying white matter disease are most likely to respond.

Pages: 1508–1510

Chapter 58

Alcohol Abuse

Robert W. Brenner

1: All of the following are true about alcoholism, except:

A. Alcoholism is the second leading preventable cause of death after tobacco abuse in the United States.

B. Alcoholic patients use health resources at a disproportionately high rate when compared with other populations.

C. Cirrhosis of the liver is largely attributable to alcoholism.

D. Of motor vehicle accidents in the United States, 50% are alcohol related.

E. Primary care physicians universally screen for alcoholism.

Answer: E

Critique: One hundred thousand deaths per year have been attributed to alcohol abuse, which makes it the second leading preventable cause of death after tobacco abuse in the United States. Relative to the general population, alcohol abusers are high users of emergency services, trauma-related services, acute hospitalization, diagnostic procedures, transfusions, and psychiatric services. Cirrhosis of the liver continues to be largely attributable to alcohol abuse, with estimates of 60% to 90% of cirrhosis deaths. Of motor vehicle accidents in the United States, 50% are alcohol related and result in a significant loss of life, serious trauma-related morbidity, and associated costs of long-term disability. Screening for alcoholism in primary care and emergency medicine is *not* done universally.

Page: 1513

2: In comparing the prevalence of several chronic medical conditions in family practice, it is clear that the early recognition of and intervention in alcohol abuse is of great importance. Which of the following statements is true:

A. Non–insulin-dependent diabetes mellitus has a higher prevalence than alcohol abuse.

B. The lifetime prevalence of alcohol use disorders is 50%.

C. The prevalence of hypertension is three times greater than that of alcohol abuse.

D. The prevalence of alcohol abuse ranks nearly as high as that of hypertension and is much higher than that of diabetes mellitus.

E. Alcohol abuse cannot be characterized as a chronic illness.

Answer: D

Critique: Alcoholism is a chronic and pervasive medical disorder. The lifetime prevalence of alcohol use disorders is 13.5%. If one assumes that binge drinking is equivalent to alcohol abuse, the prevalence is nearly 15% of the population that consumes alcohol (21 million persons). Hypertension is estimated to affect at least 50 million Americans, which is approximately 18.5% of the U.S. population. Non–insulin-dependent diabetes mellitus affects more than 2% of the U.S population, or 5.4 million adults.

Page: 1513

3: An 18-year-old male presents in your office for a routine college entrance physical examination. On completing his family history, you note several paternal relatives, including his father, who have alcohol-related disorders. Your patient asks you whether alcoholism is genetic. The most appropriate response is:

A. If a first-degree relative is an alcoholic, you have a 100% chance of becoming an alcoholic if you drink.

B. The current evidence shows that no single factor is causative for alcoholism, although it is clear that genetics do play a role.

C. Don't worry, because genetics has no role in alcohol abuse.

D. The inheritance of alcoholism has been identified on chromosome number 7, and a laboratory test is available to test for the disorder.

E. Alcohol abuse is mediated by a neurotransmitter named serotonin.

Answer: B

Critique: Although it is true that no single causative factor can be ascribed to alcoholism, it is clear that genetic markers play a significant role. Family studies show that biological sons of alcoholics have a fourfold risk of this disorder. Chromosome hot spots for alcoholism have been located at chromosomes 1, 2, and 7 for alcohol dependency. No laboratory test is available to identify alcoholism. Current research indicates that alcohol dependency is highly mediated by multiple neurotransmitter pathways, whereas illicit drugs bind only to one receptor.

Pages: 1513, 1514

3: Which of the following is *not* an alcohol-related disorder in the *Diagnostic and Statistical Manual of Mental Disorders* (DSM-IV):

A. Alcohol abuse
B. Alcohol addiction
C. Alcohol dependence
D. Alcohol intoxication
E. Alcohol withdrawal

Answer: B

Critique: The DSM-IV (1994) classified alcohol-related disorders into alcohol use disorders including alcohol abuse, alcohol dependence, and alcohol-induced disorders, including alcohol intoxication and alcohol withdrawal. Alcohol addiction is not a disorder listed in the DSM-IV.

Page: 1514

4: Choose the best answer to describe the difference between alcohol *dependence* and alcohol *abuse*:

A. Abuse is the inability to stop drinking alcohol, whereas dependence requires socially dysfunctional use.
B. Dependence is biological, and abuse is psychological.
C. Dependence is distinguished from abuse in that it requires the development of tolerance or a withdrawal syndrome.
D. No distinction is made.
E. Abuse must precede dependence.

Answer: C

Critique: In 1980, the DSM-III introduced the term "substance" to refer to all alcohol and drugs and codified the distinction between abuse and dependence. Dependence is distinguished from abuse by the requirement of the development of tolerance or a withdrawal syndrome. All other choices do not reflect any currently accepted definitions of abuse or dependence.

Page: 1514

5: All of the following are CAGE questions (a brief screening for alcoholism), except:

A. Do you feel guilty about drinking?
B. Have you ever attempted to cut down on drinking?
C. Do you ever take an eye opener?
D. Are you annoyed when others discuss your drinking?
E. Do you accept your drinking as normal?

Answer: E

Critique: The CAGE questions include asking the patient if they have ever attempted to *c*ut down, are *a*nnoyed when others discuss your drinking, do you feel *g*uilty about drinking, and do you ever take an *e*ye opener? Some clinicians add a D to the CAGE questions for *D*UI: have you ever been charged with driving under the influence?

Pages: 1514, 1515

6: A 14-year-old male presents for a routine preparticipation physical examination. The patient is new to your practice, and you decide to update his medical, social, and family history. His response to your question on alcohol use is, "I do not drink alcohol." The most appropriate next question should be which of the following:

A. Did you ever drink alcohol?
B. Are you telling the truth?
C. Do you have a family history of alcoholism?
D. Do you take any illicit drugs?
E. How many drinks do you consume a day?

Answer: A

Critique: When a clinician receives the answer that the patient does not drink at all, the line of questioning should still be pursued with a question such as "Did you ever drink alcohol?" and/or "Why did you stop drinking alcohol?" Family history is one of the major predictive variables in detecting alcohol abuse but such a question is not an appropriate next question. It is important to convey an atmosphere of trust and privacy when interviewing an adolescent patient (parents should be excluded).

Page: 1515

7: A 52-year-old male presents to the emergency room after having had a generalized seizure that was witnessed by several people at a local shopping mall. He is postictal and a history is unobtainable. On your initial physical examination, you find that his vital signs are: P=90/min, BP=170/100, T=98.7, and RR=20/min. His HEENT examination reveals an erythematous face and a dry oral pharynx. You note an enlarged abdomen with hepatomegaly. His extremity examination is significant for palmar erythema and bilateral Dupuytren's contractures. The only laboratory test available to you at this time is blood alcohol level, which was 20 mg/dL. The most likely cause for his seizure is which of the following:

A. Alcohol intoxication
B. Alcohol withdrawal
C. Elevated magnesium
D. Decreased magnesium
E. Isopropyl alcohol ingestion

Answer: B

Critique: Elevated blood pressure, pulse, or respiration can be a clue to the severity of alcohol withdrawal. Some nonspecific physical findings in alcoholics may include the comorbid "dry mouth," rhinophyma; red, swollen facies; porphyria cutanea tarda; Dupuytren's contractures; and palmar erythema. Other findings related to cirrhosis of the liver are hepatosplenomegaly and ascites. A blood alcohol level of 20 mg/dL is a nadir in a chronic alcoholic and is consistent with a withdrawal seizure. Alcohol intoxication in a chronic alcoholic requires very high blood alcohol levels owing to tolerance. The remaining choices, although possible causes for seizures, are less likely.

Pages: 1515, 1516

Questions 8 to 12: Match the following blood alcohol levels with the corresponding most commonly observed clinical symptoms:

A. 20 mg/dL
B. 100 mg/dL

C. 100 to 200 mg/dL
D. 300 mg/dL
E. >400 mg/dL

8: Coma, respiratory depression, hypothermia, hypothermia, death from central nervous system depression, loss of airway integrity, or pulmonary aspiration

9: Mild euphoria, mild impairment of coordination, and mood alterations

10: Marked ataxia, drowsiness, lethargy, and vomiting

11: Slurred speech and delayed reaction times

12: Grossly slurred speech, ataxia, and incoordination

Answers: 8 - E, 9 - A, 10 - D, 11 - B, 12 - C

Critique: The degree of intoxication is determined by the amount of alcohol ingestion, the time period of the ingestion, and the patient's tolerance, if any. Mild euphoria, mild impairment of coordination, and mood alterations occur at 20 mg/dL. Slurred speech and delayed reaction times occur at 100 mg/dL. Between 100 and 200 mg/dL, grossly slurred speech, ataxia, and incoordination are observed. Marked ataxia, drowsiness, lethargy, and vomiting are seen at 300 mg/dL. In the naïve drinker, levels above 400 mg/dL are associated with coma, respiratory depression, hypothermia, and death from central nervous system depression, loss of airway integrity, or pulmonary aspiration.

Page: 1516

13: All of the following medications are appropriate for use with a patient admitted for alcohol detoxification, except:

A. Atenolol
B. Chloridiazepoxide
C. Thiamine
D. Disulfiram
E. Lorazepam

Answer: D

Critique: The preferred central nervous system agents for detoxification are the benzodiazepines. They provide the best side effect profile and have a better risk-benefit profile than other agents do. Benzodiazepines are not likely to be fatal in overdose unless mixed with other central nervous system depressants. Chloridiazepoxide and diazepam are both effective agents. Additionally, beta blockers such as atenolol may decrease tremulousness and sympathomimetic symptoms. Thiamine and glucose should always be administered, because chronic alcoholism is associated with hypoglycemia and thiamine deficiency states. Disulfiram is used for the treatment of alcohol dependency but not for detoxification.

Pages: 1517, 1518

Questions 14 to 19: Part of any substance abuse intervention is the physician's assessment of the patient's readiness to change. Match the following patient stage of change with the descriptions of the physician's interventions:

A. Precontemplative
B. Contemplative
C. Preparation
D. Action
E. Maintenance
F. Relapse

14: The physician tries to motivate the patient to take action by listing the reasons for urgency.

15: The physician is ready to help the patient again with entry into a recovery program and offers nonjudgmental support.

16: The physician plants the seed of how alcohol is harming the patient.

17: The physician performs follow-up on the patient.

18: The physician assists the patient in preparing for reduction or cessation of use.

19: The physician arranges inpatient or outpatient detoxification.

Answers: 14 - B, 15 - F, 16 - A, 17 - E, 18 - C, 19 - D

Critique: First described by Prochaska and DiClimente in 1983 while studying smokers, assessing the stage of change assists the family physician in targeting the intervention approach to the patient. They described six stages of change. *Precontemplative* occurs when the physician plants the seed of how alcohol is harming the patient. *Contemplative* involves the physician trying to motivate the patient to take action by listing the reasons for urgency. *Preparation* occurs when the physician assists the patient in preparing for reduction or cessation of use. *Action* takes place when the physician arranges inpatient or outpatient detoxification. *Maintenance* is the period of time when the physician performs follow-up on the patient. *Relapse* occurs when the physician is ready to help the patient again with entry into a recovery program and offers nonjudgmental support.

Pages: 1518, 1519

20: A 35-year-old female with a known history of alcoholism presents to the emergency room with the complaints of acute onset of flushing, nausea, respiratory difficulty, vomiting, weakness, and feeling anxious. Her medical history is significant for prior admissions for withdrawal seizures and upper gastrointestinal bleeding. She has been in a day treatment program, which has included the use of disulfiram (Antabuse). Her vital signs are: P=110, BP=150/96, RR=24, and T=98.6. On physical examination, she appears flushed, diaphoretic, anxious, and obviously nauseated. The only other pertinent positive on the remainder of her examination is mild, diffuse wheezing on auscultation of her lungs. The most likely diagnosis is which of the following:

A. Alcohol withdrawal
B. Cardiac asthma
C. Antabuse reaction
D. Gastrointestinal bleeding
E. Anaphylaxis

Answer: C

Critique: The patient presented has a known history of alcoholism and is taking disulfiram as an adjunct to her therapy. She has experienced the classic "Antabuse reaction," which occurs after the ingestion of alcohol. Disulfiram inhibits aldehyde dehydrogenase, the second alcohol degradation enzyme. This inhibition causes acetaldehyde to increase to 5 to 10 times the usual levels found after alcohol consumption. If larger volumes of alcohol are ingested, hypotension, syncope, loss of consciousness, and death may follow.

Pages: 1519, 1520

21: The following statements regarding naltrexone use in the treatment of alcoholism are true, except:

A. It is contraindicated in patients who are concomitantly addicted to opiates.
B. It causes an adverse reaction when taken with alcohol.
C. It is an opioid antagonist.
D. It can cause somnolence or anxiety.

Answer: B

Critique: Naltrexone is an opioid antagonist that lessens the pleasurable effects or "high" of alcohol consumption. It does not cause an adverse response when taken with alcohol, as does Antabuse. It should not be used in patients who are currently abusing opiates, because it may precipitate an acute withdrawal. The side effects of naltrexone include nausea, headache, dizziness, anxiety, and somnolence.

Page: 1520

22: Which of the following statements regarding women and alcohol abuse is true:

A. Women enter treatment earlier than men.
B. The CAGE questions are more sensitive in women.

C. Medical complications develop earlier in women than in men.
D. Men have better treatment outcomes than women.

Answer: C

Critique: Women have lower rates of alcohol abuse than do men. They generally enter treatment later than men and have more psychiatric symptoms. Screening tests such as CAGE have less sensitivity in women. Medical complications of alcoholism develop more rapidly in women than in men and at lower levels of alcohol consumption.

Page: 1520

23: All of the following statements regarding physician impairment are true, except:

A. The prevalence of alcohol abuse among physicians is half that of the overall national prevalence.
B. Physicians have a higher incidence of prescription drug abuse.
C. Treatment outcomes for physicians in structured programs are better than 70% to 80%.
D. Impairment usually occurs first in the physician's family and social life before it appears in the workplace.

Answer: A

Critique: The prevalence of alcohol abuse among physicians is comparable to the national lifetime prevalence of 13.5%. The pattern of physician abuse differs from that of the general population by increased use of alcohol, benzodiazepines, and prescription opiates. Much of the prescription drug use is self-prescribed. Impairment is generally first noted in the physician's social and family life, with eventual progression into the workplace. Treatment outcomes for physicians in structured programs are excellent, with sustained recovery rates of 70% to 80% or better.

Page: 1521

Chapter 59

Nicotine Addiction

Ann M. Aring

1: (True or False) In the United States, tobacco smoking:

- A. Is the leading cause of preventable death
- B. Causes the majority of cancer deaths
- C. Caused more deaths than have occurred in wars in the twentieth century
- D. Causes more cancer death in women than does breast cancer
- E. Decreases a smoker's life expectancy by about 7 years

Answers: A - True, B - False, C - True, D - True, E - True

Critique: Smoking is currently the leading preventable cause of death in the United States, contributing to an estimated 400,000 deaths per year. Smoking has caused far more deaths of United States citizens than have wars in this century. For average 32-year-old men, smoking-related deaths occur about 7 years earlier than do non-smokers' deaths, making smoking the leading preventable cause of cancer deaths but not the cause of most cancer deaths.

Page: 1523

2: Passive smoking has been shown to affect all of the following conditions, except:

- A. Cervical cancer
- B. Lung cancer
- C. Laryngeal cancer
- D. Heart disease

Answer: C

Critique: Sidestream smoke is diluted by ambient air before reaching nonsmokers, but the cooler temperature and lack of filtering by the cigarette and its tip leave high levels of carcinogens in sidestream smoke. Of the problems listed, only laryngeal cancer is not currently thought to be an important concern for those exposed to passive smoke.

Pages: 1528, 1529

3: (True or False) An effective office-based smoking cessation strategy is likely to include which of the following:

- A. Weekly or biweekly office visits during the cessation effort
- B. Behavior modification information
- C. Tapering transdermal nicotine prescription
- D. Setting a quit date within 2 months
- E. Focusing efforts on motivated smokers

Answers: A - True, B - True, C - True, D - True, E - False

Critique: All of these strategies are recommended except the last one. Setting a distant quit date could reinforce excuses to continue smoking. If office interventions are limited to motivated smokers, physicians shirk their responsibility to help unmotivated smokers and might reinforce the notion that it would be too difficult for them to become nonsmokers. Nicotine replacement is an adjunct to other smoking cessation strategies. Nicotine should be started at 80% to 100% intake of the smoker's daily intake to maintain comfort. Daily intake can be estimated at 1 mg nicotine per cigarette when the patient is smoking at will. Nicotine reductions should be done slowly.

Page: 1534

4: Obstacles to office-based smoking cessation include all of the following, except:

- A. Lack of time for counseling
- B. Lack of cost-effective behavioral interventions
- C. Lack of insurance reimbursement
- D. Magazines in the waiting room that contain tobacco advertisements

Answer: B

Critique: Behavioral interventions are extremely cost effective when compared with other medical technologies. Direct insurance coverage for smoking cessation is rare. However, the reduced health care visits and medical costs for ex-smokers are a benefit to providers in health maintenance organizations. Magazines with cigarette advertisements should not be in the waiting room without prominent stickers or rubber-stamped messages warning patients of the health risks associated with smoking.

Page: 1534

5: (True or False) A 25-year-old woman has recently given birth to a small-for-gestational-age female infant. The patient smoked cigarettes throughout the pregnancy. Which of the following criteria must be met to use "fetal tobacco syndrome" to explain the baby's low birth weight:

- A. The infant must demonstrate asymmetric growth retardation.
- B. The mother smoked at least one pack of cigarettes per day.

C. The mother was normotensive throughout the pregnancy.
D. No other cause of intrauterine growth retardation can be found.

Answers: A - False, B - False, C - True, D - True

Critique: A dose-response relationship exists between tobacco use during pregnancy and fetal birth weight. The more a pregnant women smokes, the lower will be the infant's birth weight. On average, the weight of babies born to women who smoke is 200 grams less than that of babies born to comparable nonsmokers. However, a woman who stops smoking by her fourth month of gestation has the same risk as a nonsmoker. The term *fetal tobacco syndrome* provides a label for fetal growth retardation when (1) the mother smoked five or more cigarettes per day throughout the pregnancy, (2) the mother was normotensive throughout the pregnancy, (3) the newborn demonstrates symmetric growth retardation, and (4) no other cause of intrauterine growth retardation is obvious.

Pages: 1529, 1530

6: All of the following are common myths about smoking tobacco, except:

A. Smoking relieves stress.
B. Smoking keeps weight off.
C. The patient needs to be "ready to quit."
D. Menthol found in certain brands of cigarettes causes tobacco smoke to feel less irritating.

Answer: D

Critique: The most important myth surrounding smoking is that it relieves stress. This myth can be debunked by pointing out that the stress that is relieved resulted from being dependent on cigarettes in the first place. In addition, deep breathing in itself has a relaxing effect. Smoking damages the taste buds and other digestive tract cells and inhibits appetite. When a patient stops smoking, the average weight gain is only 5 pounds. Menthol is an anesthetic that deadens the throat to create the illusion of less irritating smoke. The physician should not advise "cutting down," switching to a low-tar cigarette, or changing to a pipe or cigar.

Pages: 1535, 1536

7: All of the following statements about the demographics of smoking in the United States are correct, except:

A. The majority of adult smokers state that they would like to stop smoking.
B. More young women than young men smoke cigarettes.
C. Half of high school seniors who smoke start by age 18.
D. Approximately 40% of all deaths from cancer and 21% of deaths from cardiovascular disease are caused by smoking.

Answer: C

Critique: Half of high school seniors who smoke start by age 14. More young women than young men smoke

cigarettes. In 1986, lung cancer surpassed breast cancer as the leading cause of cancer death in women. Although 80% of adults who smoke say they would like to quit, only 20% of those who try actually succeed in stopping for good.

Page: 1523

8: Compared with nonsmokers, smokers are more likely to develop the following diseases, except:

A. Leukemia
B. Coronary artery disease
C. Macular degeneration
D. Cerebrovascular accidents
E. Bladder cancer

Answer: A

Critique: Cigarette smoking does not increase the risk of developing leukemia. However, a greater than 50% mortality from leukemia occurs in cigarette smokers, and the response is dose related. The risk is greatest for myeloid leukemia and acute nonlymphocytic leukemia. The risk of myocardial infection is proportional to the number of cigarettes smoked. Macular degeneration is the leading cause of blindness after the age of 65. Smoking 20 or more cigarettes a day increases the risk of macular degeneration twofold to threefold. As with the other smoking-related disorders, macular degeneration appears to be dose related. The incidence of stroke in smokers is 50% higher than that in nonsmokers (40% higher in men and 60% higher in women). Forty percent of bladder cancers are smoking related. Smokers have a three to four times higher risk of bladder cancer than people who never smoked.

Pages: 1524–1527

9: (True or False) Parental smoking is associated with the following childhood disorders:

A. Otitis media
B. Asthma
C. Sudden infant death syndrome
D. Teenage smoking
E. Behavioral disorders, such as hyperactivity

Answers: A - True, B - True, C - True, D - True, E - True

Critique: Of patients who smoke cigarettes, 75% have at least one parent who smoked. The risk of a child starting to use tobacco doubles with each additional adult family member who smokes. Numerous studies have shown that otitis media and asthma are more prevalent in children whose mothers smoke. Passive smoking has been linked to children who have died of sudden infant death syndrome. Deficits in growth and emotional development as well as behavioral disorders are also found at an increased rate in children exposed to cigarette smoke.

Page: 1529

Questions 10 to 13: This group of questions explores the similarities and differences between smokeless tobacco and cigarettes. Match the numbered items to the appropriate lettered items.

A. Smokeless tobacco
B. Cigarettes
C. Both
D. Neither

10: Long-term users have a 50-fold increased risk for cancer of the cheek and gum.

11: Contains harmful carcinogens including nitrosamines

12: An upward trend in use among adolescent males

13: Nicotine levels in the blood are similar to those with cigar use.

Answers: 10 - A, 11 - C, 12 - A, 13 - C

Critique: Smokeless tobacco increases the frequency of oropharyngeal cancer and gum recession. Both smokeless tobacco and cigarettes contain harmful carcinogens. Smokeless tobacco, however, contains higher levels of nitrosamines. Even though the National Cancer Institute and Major League Baseball have launched educational programs about the risk of using smokeless tobacco, there is a growing trend among adolescent males to use smokeless tobacco. Nicotine blood levels are similar for cigarette smokers, pipe smokers, and users of smokeless tobacco, despite the different methods of absorption.

Pages: 1527, 1528

Questions 14 to 17: This series of brief clinical scenarios focuses on nicotine replacement systems for use as a part of a comprehensive behavioral smoking cessation program. Select the *best* answer by matching the lettered items to the numbered ones:

A. Nicotine polacrilex (Nicorette gum)
B. Transdermal nicotine patch
C. Nicotine inhaler (Nicotrol)
D. Bupropion hydrochloride SR (Zyban)

14: A 56-year-old automobile mechanic with a seizure disorder who smokes one and one-half packs a day

15: A 31-year-old secretary with labile mood, insomnia, and decreased concentration who smokes one pack a day

16: A 48-year-old alcoholic currently on disability for chronic back pain who smokes two to three packs per day

17: A 19-year-old student who was recently diagnosed with asthmatic bronchitis who smokes one pack a day

Answers: 14 - B, 15 - D, 16 - C, 17 - A

Critique: The best choice for nicotine replacement for the automobile mechanic with the seizure disorder would be the transdermal patch. This patient could not use bupropion SR because it is implied that the patient is also taking an antiepileptic for a seizure disorder. Because this patient is working with greasy hands, the gum or inhaler would not be an optimal choice. The patient described in item 15 also has underlying depression. In this case, bupropion SR would be the best choice to treat both conditions. The best choice for a nicotine replacement system in the 48-year-old alcoholic patient who smokes two to three packs a day is the nicotine inhaler. This patient would benefit from the behavioral aspects of the inhaled delivery system. The final patient, described in item 17, would be a good candidate for nicotine gum. The Nicotrol inhaler has not been studied in asthma or chronic pulmonary disease and might cause bronchospasm.

Pages: 1531–1533

Questions 18 to 20: Cigarette advertising campaigns have long tried to calm the consumer's concern about smoking. In the following set of questions, two types of cigarettes are listed followed by four numbered statements. Match each lettered item with its corresponding numbered item.

A. Filtered cigarettes
B. Low-tar and low-nicotine filtered cigarettes
C. Both
D. Neither

18: People who smoke these cigarettes inhale more frequently and deeply.

19: This type of cigarette accounts for more than 97% of cigarettes sold in the United States.

20: Risk of myocardial infarction is decreased.

Answers: 18 - B, 19 - A, 20 - D

Critique: In the 1950s, tobacco companies began producing filtered cigarettes that they claimed removed harmful components. Today, filtered cigarettes account for more than 97% of cigarettes sold in the United States. People who smoke low-nicotine cigarettes undergo compensatory smoking in which they inhale more frequently and more deeply to maintain their blood nicotine levels. In addition, some brands of cigarettes include perforations in the filter to dilute the smoke. Many smokers block these perforations with their lips or their fingers to obtain a higher concentration of nicotine. Cigarettes with reduced yields of nicotine and carbon monoxide are not safer for people to smoke. The risk of myocardial infarction does not change according to the nicotine content of the cigarette.

Page: 1527

Chapter 60

Abuse of Controlled Substances

George W. Miller, JR.

1: In most cases, the pathophysiologic mechanism of drug addiction primarily involves:

   A. Adaptation of inhibitory neurons in the hypothalamus
   B. Down-regulation of GABA receptors in the ventral tegmentum
   C. Adaptation of noradrenergic neurons in the locus coeruleus
   D. Up-regulation of the mesolimbic dopamine system
   E. None of the above

Answer: D

Critique: Drug addiction is a brain disease that involves permanent changes in the mesolimbic dopamine system in most cases. This system mediates reward and appetite behavior. Most psychoactive substances activate the mesolimbic system and cause structural and functional adaptations in individual neurons and their associated neural circuits. These adaptations form the basis for complex behaviors that are associated with addiction, such as dependence, tolerance, craving, and sensitization.

Page: 1539

2: All of the following are characteristic of substance use disorders, except:

   A. Early onset of symptoms
   B. Behaviorally oriented treatment that results in a favorable prognosis for recovery
   C. The need for routine screening to identify cases early
   D. Complex interplay between genetic predisposition and environmental influences
   E. Unpredictable course

Answer: A

Critique: Substance use disorders are chronic medical conditions that are characterized by late onset of symptoms, unpredictable course, complex etiologies, behaviorally oriented treatment with a favorable prognosis for recovery, and the need for early identification of cases through routine screening. Clinical problems associated with substance use disorders may develop slowly and remain undetected for long periods. The complex interplay between genetic familial predisposition and lifestyle influences the development of these disorders.

Page: 1540

3: All of the following are true regarding cocaine addiction, except:

   A. Rate of cocaine use is highest in 18- to 25-year-olds.
   B. SSRIs are an effective pharmacologic intervention for cocaine addiction.
   C. Withdrawal symptoms of cocaine may be less intense than withdrawal symptoms of methamphetamine.
   D. Metabolites of cocaine, such as benzoyl-methylecgonine, may be detected in the urine for 12 to 72 hours after cessation of cocaine use.
   E. Drug craving after cocaine withdrawal may be treated with bromocriptine and amantadine.

Answer: B

Critique: Cocaine is the second most commonly used illicit drug. Two million Americans use it, with the preponderance occurring among young adults. Withdrawal symptoms such as drug craving, anxiety, depression, hyperphagia, hypersomnolence, anhedonia, and anergy may manifest after cessation of cocaine use. Postwithdrawal drug craving may be treated with dopamine agonists. Although there is no specific cocaine detoxification regimen, SSRIs and other antidepressants may be selected for the treatment of associated depression.

Pages: 1539, 1541, 1546

4: The parents of a 15-year-old boy want to know if their son is abusing drugs. When screening the boy for substance abuse, you should:

   A. Elicit general psychosocial information in a natural order of progression
   B. Avoid increasingly sensitive questions about substance use
   C. Routinely use urine toxicology as part of the screening process
   D. Obtain the parent's consent for urine toxicology
   E. Arrange for ongoing monitoring with an addiction medicine specialist

Answer: A

Critique: Health care of the adolescent requires more time when there is a suspicion of substance abuse. The clinician is in a unique position to be able to determine whether an adolescent is using drugs and whether that use is casual or problematic. The adolescent interview should begin with a general discussion about lifestyle and progress to increasingly sensitive questions about substance abuse. Urine toxicology screening is not routinely indicated but may be reasonable when specific evidence makes substance abuse more likely. Adolescents should be tested with their knowledge and consent, except in a medical emergency.

Page: 1541

5: A patient will test positive on a urine drug screen when the drug has been used within how many hours prior to the test:

    A. The period is variable and depends on the type of drug used.
    B. 12 hours
    C. 24 hours
    D. 48 hours
    E. 72 hours

Answer: E

Critique: The test will be positive when the drug has been used within 72 hours before the test, regardless of whether the patient is dependent on the drug or using it for the first time.

Page: 1541

6: All of the following are signs of a substance abuse problem in a health care professional, except:

    A. Feeling of immunity to the problem
    B. History of frequent illnesses
    C. Numerous visits to the dentist
    D. Curriculum vita that shows unexplained time lapses between jobs, frequent geographic relocations without clear explanations, and vague references
    E. Repeatedly making rounds extra early in the day

Answer: E

Critique: Health care providers who have substance abuse problems may show a predictable collection of signs and symptoms in various life areas. These professionals tend to deny their problem, and peers, family, friends, and patients may form a "conspiracy of silence" around them. Signs and symptoms may become evident in life areas such as family, community, physical status, office, hospital, and professional history. Specific examples of signs and symptoms include (1) frequent illnesses and trips to the doctor or dentist, (2) a feeling of immunity to the problem, (3) the presence of three or more "clues" on an application for employment or staff privileges, and (4) making hospital rounds late.

Page: 1541

7: (True or False) When making a diagnosis of drug addiction:

    A. Criteria for diagnosis vary by drug class.
    B. Symptoms of tolerance and physiologic dependence are essential.

    C. The patient must experience loss of control over use of a substance that results in negative consequences.
    D. A careful history must be obtained from the patient or other reliable source.

Answers: A - False, B - False, C - True, D - True

Critique: The DSM-IV classification system for substance dependence (see Table 60–4) essentially requires loss of control of substance use that results in clinically significant impairment or distress. The diagnosis of substance dependence is established by obtaining a careful history from the patient or other reliable source. Criteria for diagnosis are the same for each drug class and do not require the presence of tolerance and physiologic dependence.

Page: 1542

8: Acceptable psychosocial interventions in the treatment of substance dependence include:

    A. Application of psychodynamic principles to help patients develop alternate modes of behavior
    B. Expression of feelings in a group setting that concern personal experiences
    C. Chemically inducing immediate and consistent discomfort when using a drug
    D. Relapse prevention education
    E. All of the above

Answer: E

Critique: Acceptable psychosocial interventions in the treatment of substance dependence include individual therapy, group therapy, marital therapy, family therapy, relapse prevention, and chemical aversion therapy. Chemical aversion therapy involves counterconditioning of the substance abuser, such as occurs with the use of emetine in marijuana dependence or disulfiram with alcohol dependence. It reduces or eliminates craving for a drug and simultaneously develops in the patient distaste and an avoidance response to the drug. Varieties of aversion therapies exist for treatment of heroin addiction, marijuana dependence, cocaine and amphetamine dependence, alcohol addiction, and tobacco dependence.

Pages: 1542, 1543

9: All of the following are true regarding self-help addiction recovery groups, except:

    A. Data show that self-help groups can help prevent relapse.
    B. Group fellowship, service work, and meeting attendance are important to maintaining abstinence.
    C. Self-help group programs are successful because of their religious basis.
    D. Self-help groups help persons at any point in the recovery process.
    E. Alcoholics Anonymous, Narcotics Anonymous, and Cocaine Anonymous are examples of 12-step self-help groups.

Answer: C

Critique: Bill W., a stockbroker, and Dr. Bob, a physician, founded Alcoholics Anonymous (AA) in 1935. AA is not allied with any religious sect or denomination and includes atheists and agnostics. The principles of AA were published in the "Big Book," entitled *Alcoholics Anonymous*, which includes The Twelve Steps of recovery for AA members. Narcotics Anonymous (NA) was established in 1947 at the U.S. Public Health Service Hospital in Lexington, Kentucky. Cocaine Anonymous (CA) began more recently with the surfacing of the national cocaine epidemic. NA and CA operate under the same guiding principles as AA.

Page: 1543

10: (True or False) With regard to patient confidentiality in substance abuse treatment:

    A. It is permissible to disclose medical information when a patient has signed a valid consent form that has not expired or been revoked by the patient.

    B. Law and regulations contained in 42 Code of Federal Regulations (CFR), Part 2 were instituted to encourage patients to enter treatment without fear of discrimination.

    C. Requirements contained in 42 CFR, Part 2 directly apply to patient records that are generated in general medical settings and hospitals.

    D. Physician-patient privilege is more restrictive of medical information disclosure than the law and regulations contained in 42 CFR, Part 2.

Answers: A - True, B - True, C - False, D - False

Critique: Federal law and regulations ensure strict confidentiality of information concerning persons receiving drug abuse assessment or treatment services. In the early 1970s, Congress passed the law and regulations that are contained in 42 CFR, Part 2. Congress issued a complex set of regulations, entitled "Confidentiality of Alcohol and Drug Abuse Patient Records," in 1975 and amended them in 1987 and again in 1995. Regulations provide for disclosure of medical information when a patient signs a valid, operative consent. They are more restrictive of communication than physician-patient privilege and constitute the universe of legal requirements in this area of law. Amendments to the regulations clarified the requirements for general medical settings and hospitals.

Page: 1543

11: Many withdrawal symptoms mimic those of psychiatric disorders. Psychiatrists therefore recommend that diagnoses for comorbid psychiatric conditions be made after patients have been detoxified from abused substances and observed in a drug-free condition for:

    A. 1 week
    B. 4 weeks
    C. 3 months
    D. 6 months
    E. 1 year

Answer: B

Critique: Psychiatrists recommend observation of the patient for 3 to 4 weeks in a drug-free condition and confirmation of comorbid psychiatric diagnoses before initiating pharmacotherapy for anxiety, depression, or insomnia.

Page: 1543

12: Which of the following identifies a significant difference between alcohol withdrawal and sedative withdrawal:

    A. The presence of pathognomonic symptoms in sedative withdrawal but not in alcohol withdrawal

    B. The presence of hyperpyrexia in alcohol withdrawal but not in sedative withdrawal

    C. A greater risk of orthostatic changes in blood pressure and pulse in alcohol withdrawal than in sedative withdrawal

    D. A greater risk of status withdrawal seizures in sedative withdrawal than in alcohol withdrawal

Answer: D

Critique: Sedative withdrawal is characterized by a variety of adrenergic-autonomic, musculoskeletal, neuropsychiatric, and other symptoms. None of the symptoms and signs of sedative withdrawal is pathognomonic. However, many of the symptoms and signs of sedative withdrawal are similar to the symptoms and signs of alcohol withdrawal, such as autonomic hyperactivity, fever, anxiety, tremor, dizziness, fatigue, and loss of appetite, among others. Potentially life-threatening orthostatic changes in blood pressure and pulse are associated with withdrawal from barbiturates, carbamates, and chloral hydrate. The risk of withdrawal seizures, including repeated and status withdrawal seizures, is higher in sedative withdrawal than in alcohol withdrawal.

Page: 1544

13: A 17-year-old high school athlete presents with new-onset symptoms of asthma. His history includes treatment for allergic rhinitis. He smokes cigarettes and guiltily admits that he recently started smoking marijuana. Which of the following is the most likely cause of his symptoms:

    A. Pollen
    B. Cigarette smoke
    C. Exercise
    D. Marijuana smoke
    E. Fungi

Answer: E

Critique: Marijuana is the most commonly used illicit drug. The respiratory effects of marijuana and tobacco smoke are very similar. Chronic marijuana smoking results in mild obstructive airway disease that may not be reversible with abstinence. In addition, aspergillus and other fungi may contaminate marijuana weed. When contaminated weed is smoked, susceptible individuals may experience asthma symptoms.

Page: 1544

14: Chronic use of which of the following drugs is not associated with a withdrawal syndrome when the drug is stopped:

    A. Marijuana
    B. Flurazepam
    C. Meprobamate
    D. Methamphetamine
    E. Propoxyphene

Answer: A

Critique: Chronic use of cannabis, PCP, hallucinogens, inhalants, and caffeine is not associated with a withdrawal syndrome when the drug is stopped.

Pages: 1544–1546

15: (True or False) Important aspects of the care of hospitalized, medically ill, methadone-maintained patients include:

    A. Verification of the patient's methadone maintenance dose by contacting maintenance program staff
    B. Administration of non-opiate analgesic medications for control of severe pain
    C. Reduction in analgesic dosage because of the additive analgesic effect of methadone
    D. Incremental administration of opiate analgesics until pain is relieved

Answers: A - True, B - False, C - False, D - True

Critique: Methadone-maintained patients who are admitted to the hospital with medical illness should continue to receive their maintenance dose of methadone as usual. Because patients may not reliably report the correct methadone maintenance dose, a medical care provider should verify the patient's maintenance dose by directly contacting maintenance program staff. Opiate medications should be administered in incremental doses until the patient experiences relief of pain. Such doses may be higher than normal owing to opiate tolerance.

Pages: 1545, 1546

16: Pharmacotherapy is an important adjunct in the treatment of drug dependence. Which of the following pharmacologic agents is incorrectly matched with its mechanism of action:

    A. Levomethadyl acetate—ability to saturate opiate receptors, block euphoria, and prevent withdrawal syndrome
    B. Naltrexone—binding receptors to block the effect of an opiate and reduce its reinforcing effects
    C. Clonidine—stimulation of alpha-2 adrenergic receptors, thereby decreasing the intoxicating effects of opiates
    D. Buprenorphine—mixed agonist/antagonist that reduces illicit opiate use with long-term therapy
    E. Disulfiram—sensitizing the body's response to the presence of a drug

Answer: C

Critique: Pharmacologic therapies for addiction assume an ever-increasing role in mainstream medical care. As our understanding of the neurobiology of addiction has improved, new medications with unique mechanisms of action have been introduced. They assist in the treatment of drug intoxication, drug withdrawal, postwithdrawal disturbances, and relapse prevention. Examples of such mechanisms include drug sensitization, saturating receptor sites with agonists, blocking drug receptors, and reducing the reinforcing effects of a drug. Clonidine decreases the withdrawal effects of opiates.

Page: 1545

17: A 33-year-old female suffers from moderate symptoms of opioid withdrawal syndrome. You decide to treat her symptoms with clonidine. All of the following are true concerning its use in this setting, except:

    A. Clonidine patch wearers have fewer drug cravings than those who take the drug orally.
    B. The patient should be monitored for orthostatic hypotension and fatigue.
    C. Oral clonidine is initiated at doses of 0.1 to 0.2 mg every 4 to 6 hours.
    D. Adjunctive medications may be needed because clonidine does not treat all withdrawal symptoms.
    E. Clonidine may be used in both inpatient and outpatient settings.

Answer: C

Critique: Clonidine is an alpha-2 agonist medication that is helpful in the treatment of opioid withdrawal in both inpatient and outpatient settings. Patients should be observed for evidence of hypotension and fatigue that may result from the medication. Clonidine may be administered orally or by wearing a patch. Patch wearers experience fewer drug cravings than those who take the oral form. When clonidine is given in the oral form, an initial test dose should be administered followed by a 45-minute observation period before the start of subsequent therapy.

Page: 1545

18: (True or False) A 21-year-old male smokes marijuana that is laced with PCP. Which of the following statements concerning PCP abuse in this patient are true and which are false:

    A. PCP acts primarily as a dissociative anesthetic.
    B. Low doses of PCP can precipitate psychosis.
    C. Symptoms of PCP withdrawal are treated with benzodiazepines.
    D. Administration of ammonium chloride promotes excretion of PCP.

Answer: A - True, B - True, C - False, D - True

Critique: PCP intoxication results in behavioral toxicity that involves bizarre and violent behavior. Physical findings include elevated temperature, elevated blood pressure, nystagmus, hyperacusis, muscle rigidity, and ataxia. Although there are limited reports of withdrawal effects in humans, no PCP withdrawal syndrome is recognized.

Page: 1546

19: Prevention of relapse in highly motivated heroin abusers involves which of the following:

    A. Administration of a maintenance dose of naltrexone 25 mg daily

    B. Administration of an increased dose of naltrexone before the weekend

    C. Administration of naltrexone immediately on cessation of heroin use

    D. Administration of naltrexone for a beneficial mood-altering effect

    E. Administration of naltrexone for relief of opiate craving

Answer: B

Critique: Antagonist maintenance with naltrexone is started following acute withdrawal from opioids. At least a 5- to 7- and a 7- to 10-day period should exist between the start of naltrexone and the last short-acting and last long-acting dose of opioid, respectively. The initial dose of naltrexone is 25 mg on the first day, followed by 50 mg daily thereafter. The total dose of naltrexone is 350 mg weekly, which is usually divided into three doses (100 mg Monday, 100 mg Wednesday, and 150 mg Friday). Naltrexone does not have a mood-altering effect and does not relieve opiate craving.

Page: 1546

20: A 34-year-old recovering heroin addict works in a saw blade manufacturing company. He sustains multiple lacerations and soft tissue crush injuries to his left hand in an accident that involves a machine press at his workstation. His medical history includes current antagonist maintenance therapy with naltrexone. On presentation to the emergency department, he needs pain relief and repair of the injuries to his hand. Which of the following is the most reasonable next step:

    A. Override opiate blockade with extra therapeutic doses of opiates

    B. Administer opiates 24 to 72 hours after the last dose of naltrexone

    C. Perform a peripheral nerve block and repair the injuries

    D. Consult an anesthesiologist and administer a sedative

Answer: C

Critique: Naltrexone blocks the analgesic effects of opiates for 24 to 72 hours following its last dose. In this case, performing a peripheral nerve block is the most reasonable next step. Peripheral nerve block is the preferred method of relieving pain from peripheral injuries in recovering heroin addicts who receive antagonist therapy with naltrexone.

Page: 1546

21: Abuse of 3,4-methylenedioxymethamphetamine (MDMA) leads to depletion of brain:

    A. Norepinephrine

    B. Serotonin

    C. Dopamine

    D. γ-aminobutyric acid (GABA)

Answer: B

Critique: MDMA is a schedule I controlled drug that produces amphetamine-like stimulant and mescaline-like hallucinogenic effects. It causes depression via depletion of brain serotonin and degeneration of serotonin nerve terminals. SSRIs are indicated as treatment.

Page: 1546

22: Which agent can cause methemoglobinemia when abused as an inhalant:

    A. Nitrous oxide

    B. Aliphatic nitrites

    C. Chloroform

    D. Glue solvents

    E. Halothane

Answer: B

Critique: Inhalants consist of a heterogeneous group of addictive agents that are volatile. Most commonly, agents are sniffed directly from the container ("sniffing"), inhaled from a rag soaked in the substance and held to the face ("huffing"), inhaled from a bag into which the substance is placed and vaporized ("bagging"), or sprayed directly into the mouth. Rarely, inhalation of aliphatic nitrites causes methemoglobinemia, which is treated with methylene blue.

Page: 1547

Chapter 61

Interpreting Laboratory Tests

Michael D. Hagen

1: The accuracy of a clinical test is best described as which of the following:

A. The reproducibility of the test on repeated determinations
B. The sensitivity of the test
C. The ability of the test to reflect the true value of the measured parameter
D. The standard deviation of the test result

Answer: C

Critique: The accuracy of a test represents its ability to reflect the true value of the measured characteristic. Sensitivity represents a test's ability to correctly identify affected individuals as abnormal. Reproducibility is the precision of the test on repeated applications. The standard deviation describes the dispersion of results around a measure of central tendency, such as the mean.

Page: 1548

2: In a population that demonstrates a normal distribution for results on a certain test, what percentage of the individuals will have a normal test result:

A. 5%
B. 10%
C. 90%
D. 95%

Answer: D

Critique: For a normally distributed test result, 95% of the tested normal individuals will demonstrate a normal result. Five percent will have an abnormal, or false-positive, result.

Page: 1548

3: A blood chemistry panel contains 10 biochemical measurements. Assume that the laboratory has defined *normal* as the population mean plus or minus two standard deviations (±2 SD) from the mean. What is the likelihood that the report on a given patient will obtain at least one falsely abnormal result:

A. 15%
B. 30%
C. 40%
D. 55%

Answer: C

Critique: If *normal* for each test is defined as the mean ±2 SD from the mean, each test has a 5% likelihood of a falsely abnormal result. The likelihood of at least one false positive out of a panel of 10 determinations can be calculated as follows: probability of false positive = $1 - (0.95)^n$, where n is the number of tests in the panel. For a single test, this probability is simply $1 - 0.95$, or 5%. For a panel containing 10 results, the probability is $1 - (0.95)^{10}$, or 40%.

Pages: 1548, 1549

4: Assume that a clinical test is performed on two populations: one group is known by other means to represent normal individuals, and the other group represents individuals known to have the disorder in question. After testing a large number of patients from both populations, the distribution of results appears as shown. The laboratory establishes an upper limit for normal as shown. Which one of the areas (labeled "a," "b," "c," and "d") in Figure 61–A

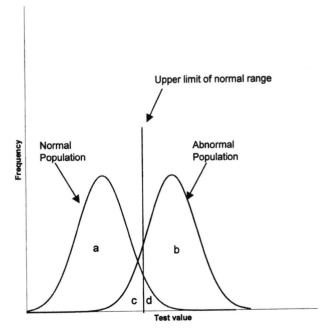

Figure 61-A

represents the "true positive" results (i.e., abnormal individuals who have an abnormal result):

A. Area "a"
B. Area "b"
C. Area "c"
D. Area "d"

Answer: B

Critique: The figure displays two normally distributed populations. The members of the abnormal population who demonstrate a test value above the normal cutoff represent the "true positive" results.

Pages: 1550, 1551

5: Referring again to the figure, which of the labeled areas represents the "false-positive" test results:

A. Area "a"
B. Area "b"
C. Area "c"
D. Area "d"

Answer: D

Critique: The left-most curve in the figure displays the test performance in normal individuals. Because nearly all clinical tests separate normal from abnormal imperfectly, some normal individuals will have abnormal results, and vice versa. In the figure, the normal individuals who demonstrate test results above the normal cutoff represent the "false-positive" results for the test. These results correspond to area "d."

Pages: 1550, 1551

6: Assume that you are embarking on a program to screen for a serious disease for which effective and safe treatment exists and that false-positive results can be identified with safe and inexpensive confirmatory tests. You wish to minimize the chances for missing cases in the population. Referring to Figure 61–A, moving the threshold for normal/abnormal to the left will accomplish which of the following:

A. Increase the false-negative results
B. Increase the true negative results
C. Increase the false-positive results
D. Decrease the true positive results

Answer: C

Critique: Changing the normal/abnormal threshold value to a less stringent cutoff criterion increases sensitivity at the cost of lower specificity, or more false-positive results. The false-negative rate will decrease, the true negative rate will decrease, and the number of true positives will increase.

Page: 1550, Table 61–4

7: On the basis of your clinical examination, you determine that a patient has a 10% probability of having a particular disorder. You perform a test that exhibits a sensitivity of 80% and 75% specificity for the disorder, and the test result is positive for the disorder. On the basis of this result, what can you tell the patient regarding her likelihood of having the disorder in question:

A. It is less than 10%.
B. It is approximately 30%.
C. It is approximately 50%.
D. It is greater than 90%.

Answer: B

Critique: Test results must be interpreted in light of the test characteristics (sensitivity and specificity) as well as the "prior" likelihood that the patient has the disorder in question. In this example, the prior likelihood is 10%. Several techniques can be used to revise the probability of disease on the basis of the new test information. The clinician can use published nomograms or can perform the calculations easily with a pocket calculator using Bayes' theorem:

$$\frac{\text{Prior likelihood} \times \text{Sensitivity}}{(\text{Prior likelihood} \times \text{Sensitivity}) + ((1 - \text{specificity}) \times (1 - \text{Prior likelihood}))}$$

In this case, this reduces to: $(0.10 \times 0.80)/((0.10 \times 0.80) + (0.25 \times 0.90)) \sim 0.26$ or 26%. The odds–likelihood ratio form of Bayes' theorem is somewhat easier to manipulate. First, convert the prior likelihood to odds (0.1/0.9), and multiply the result, 0.11, by the likelihood ratio associated with the test. The likelihood ratio is the true positive rate (sensitivity) divided by the false-positive rate (1-specificity), or 0.80/0.25 in this example. Multiplying $0.11 \times 3.2 \sim 0.36$, which represents the post-test odds that the patient has the disorder. This can be converted back to probability using the formula probability = odds/(1 + odds), or $0.36/1.36 \sim 26\%$.

Pages: 1551, 1552

8: Assume that you have performed a test that has a sensitivity of 80% and specificity of 80%. The prior probability that the patient has the disorder in question is 5%. On the basis of information about costs, benefits, and risks of treatment, you establish a "test-treat" threshold of 50% and a "no test–test threshold" of 10%. If the patient's test result is positive, which of the following is the best next step in the patient's management:

A. Do no further testing or treatment
B. Begin treatment without further testing
C. Perform an additional test
D. Repeat the initial test

Answer: C

Critique: The threshold approach to decision making provides a framework for systematic application of sequential or multiple testing. In this approach, information about test performance, risks and benefits of testing, and risks and benefits of treatment are combined mathematically to establish two thresholds: a testing threshold and a treatment threshold. On the basis of the initial prior probability and the test result, Bayes' theorem is used to calculate the revised probability of disease. If this probability exceeds the treatment threshold, the patient should be treated without further testing. If the revised probability falls below the test threshold, the patient should receive no further testing or treatment. For values in between, further testing should be performed. In this example, the revised probability is about 17%, which falls between the two thresholds. The specifics about these calculations appear in the original work by Pauker and Kassirer.

Pages: 1550, 1551

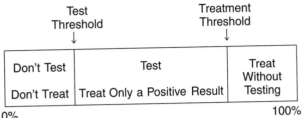

Figure 61-B

9: Assume that two tests are available for diagnosing a clinical disorder (Figure 61-B). You have the option of performing the tests simultaneously or serially (if the first test is abnormal, perform the second test). You elect to perform both tests simultaneously and decide that you will initiate treatment if either test is positive for the disorder. Which of the following statements best describes the effect this approach will have on the operating characteristics of your testing strategy:

    A. Sensitivity and specificity will be higher than for either test used alone.
    B. Sensitivity and specificity will be lower than for either test used alone.
    C. Specificity will be higher and sensitivity lower than for either test used alone.
    D. Sensitivity will be higher and specificity lower than for either test used alone.

Answer: D

Critique: When several tests exist for diagnosing a disorder, the decision maker has several options for designing a testing strategy. He or she can perform both tests simultaneously and make the diagnosis if either test is positive for the disorder (a *disjunctive* positively criterion). He or she can also perform both tests and make the diagnosis only if both tests are positive for the disorder (a *conjunctive* positivity criterion). Alternatively, he or she can perform one test and then a second test if the first is positive for the disorder. The disjunctive approach heightens sensitivity at the price of lower specificity (more false positives). The conjunctive approach increases specificity and lowers sensitivity. The serial testing approach increases sensitivity and specificity, but at the cost of extended time to make the diagnosis. Testing for human immunodeficiency virus (HIV) using ELISA as the first test and Western blot as the second, confirmatory test represents a good example of a serial testing strategy.

Pages: 1551, 1552

10: All of the following options typically lead to lowered albumin levels, except:

    A. Severe infection
    B. Chronic liver disease
    C. Dehydration
    D. Chronic renal disease with proteinuria

Answer: C

Critique: Severe infection and associated catabolism, chronic liver disease, and chronic renal disease with proteinuria can all be associated with hypoalbuminemia. Dehydration can cause elevated albumin levels.

Page: 1553

11: A healthy 14-year-old boy had a screening blood chemistry panel performed at a local health fair and was told that his results were abnormal. Your review of his laboratory report shows all values to be normal except for an alkaline phosphatase of 150 U/L (normal 25 to 100 U/L). On the basis of this result, you should proceed with which of the following courses of action:

    A. Order a computed tomographic scan of the abdomen
    B. Perform diagnostic liver ultrasound
    C. Reassure the patient that this is a normal result for an adolescent
    D. Order an isotope bone scan
    E. Refer the patient for consideration for liver biopsy

Answer: C

Critique: Alkaline phosphatase is present in liver, bone, placental tissue, and intestine. Values can normally be elevated in children and adolescents. The options listed are not warranted in an otherwise healthy adolescent.

Pages: 1553, 1554

12: As part of an annual physical examination of a 48-year-old man, you perform a blood chemistry panel that includes aspartate aminotransferase (AST) and alanine aminotransferase (ALT) levels. The patient's AST is 85 U/L (normal 15–45), and his ALT is 45 U/L (normal 15–40). Which of the following represents the most likely source for these values:

    A. Acute viral hepatitis
    B. Drug-induced hepatitis
    C. Ethanol-induced hepatitis
    D. Gilbert's syndrome

Answer: C

Critique: AST and ALT elevations together indicate probable hepatocellular liver disease. In most of these disorders, AST and ALT demonstrate similar elevations. In ethanol-induced hepatitis, AST levels are typically higher than those for ALT. Gilbert's syndrome presents with indirect hyperbilirubinemia rather than transaminase abnormalities.

Page: 1554

13: A 50-year-old woman has experienced painful interphalangeal joints in both hands for several years. You perform an antinuclear antibody test that demonstrates a speckled pattern at a titer of 1:160. Further testing reveals antibody to nuclear ribonucleoprotein (RNP). On the basis of these results, which of the following is the most likely cause for her joint discomfort:

A. Rheumatoid arthritis
B. Systemic lupus erythematosus
C. Scleroderma
D. Mixed connective tissue disease

Answer: D

Critique: A high titer antinuclear antibody (ANA) with speckled pattern and antibody to nuclear ribonucleoprotein (anti-RNP) is most likely associated with mixed connective tissue disease (MCTD). Although high titer ANA can be seen with systemic lupus erythematosus and scleroderma, the anti-RNP result more strongly suggests MCTD.

Page: 1555, Table 61–10

14: A 25-year-old man is concerned that occasionally, but particularly when he is tired or ill, his sclerae appear yellow. His total bilirubin is 1.7 mg/dL (normal <1.5) and the unconjugated fraction is elevated. Which of the following is the most likely cause of this finding:

A. Gilbert's syndrome
B. Crigler-Najjar syndrome
C. Acute viral hepatitis
D. Common bile duct stone

Answer: A

Critique: Mild unconjugated hyperbilirubinemia in an otherwise healthy individual characterizes Gilbert's syndrome. Crigler-Najjar syndrome and obstructive processes such as a common duct stone are associated with conjugated hyperbilirubinemia. The recurrent history mitigates against acute viral hepatitis.

Pages: 1555, 1557

15: (True or False) Blood urea nitrogen (BUN) is reduced in which of the following circumstances:

A. Dehydration
B. Severe chronic liver disease
C. Third trimester of pregnancy
D. Intrinsic renal disease
E. Syndrome of inappropriate antidiuretic hormone (SIADH)

Answers: A - False, B - True, C - True, D - False, E - True

Critique: The liver produces BUN as a byproduct of protein metabolism. BUN can be reduced in severe chronic liver disease, during the third trimester of pregnancy, and in circumstances associated with SIADH. Dehydration and intrinsic renal disease typically elevate BUN.

Page: 1557

16: A 62-year-old woman presents with a 1-week history of mental confusion. Her history is significant for a mastectomy for intraductal carcinoma 5 years ago. Her examination reveals only the mastectomy scar and confused mental status. Laboratory evaluation reveals a total calcium of 14.7 mg/dL (normal 8.5–10.5 mg/dL) and an albumin of 3.1 g/dL. The remainder of her routine blood chemistry results are normal. Which of the following represents the most likely explanation for these findings:

A. Hyperparathyroidism
B. Hypoalbuminemia
C. Metastatic breast carcinoma
D. Chronic renal insufficiency

Answer: C

Critique: Extremely elevated calcium levels usually suggest malignancy. Hyperparathyroidism is associated with mild calcium elevations, and hypoalbuminemia leads to lower measured total calcium. Chronic renal insufficiency is unlikely in a patient with otherwise normal blood chemistry levels.

Page: 1557

17: A 48-year-old man with known chronic alcohol abuse presents with epistaxis that has persisted for several hours. His physical examination reveals a firm, somewhat irregular liver border and spider angiomata. Coagulation studies reveal an International Normalized Ratio (INR) of 2.1 (normal 0.99–1.1) and an activated partial thromboplastin time (aPTT) of 41 seconds (normal 20–35 seconds). Which of the following is the most likely explanation for these findings:

A. Excessive dietary intake of vitamin K
B. Hyperfibrinogenemia
C. von Willebrand's disease
D. Clotting factor deficiency secondary to liver disease

Answer: D

Critique: A prolonged INR indicates a disorder of the extrinsic coagulation pathway and is associated with defects or deficiencies of clotting factors I, II, V, VII, and X. Liver disease is associated with deficiencies of these factors. Excessive vitamin K intake and hyperfibrinogenemia would not be expected to prolong the INR. von Willebrand's disease is usually associated with a normal aPTT.

Pages: 1558, 1559

18: A 65-year-old woman has experienced weakness for 3 to 4 months. She relates no other complaints. Her physical examination reveals pale oral mucosa and conjunctivae but is otherwise normal for her age. The stool tests negative for occult blood. Her CBC shows hematocrit 28%, hemoglobin 8.5, red cell distribution width (RDW) 19%, and mean corpuscular volume (MCV) 103 fL (normal 76–100 fL). The peripheral blood smear demonstrates hypersegmented neutrophils. Which of the following is the most likely explanation for these findings:

A. Iron deficiency anemia
B. Folic acid and/or vitamin B_{12} deficiency
C. Hereditary spherocytosis
D. Anemia of chronic disease
E. Heterozygous beta-thalassemia

Answer: B

Critique: The scenario describes results consistent with macrocytic anemia such as that seen with vitamin B_{12} or folic acid deficiency. The other listed processes are normal or microcytic red blood cell indices.

Pages: 1559, 1560

19: A 28-year-old man with known type 1 diabetes mellitus has had a flu-like illness for the past 48 hours. Over the past 12 hours, he has become nauseated and experienced several episodes of vomiting. He has not taken his insulin for the past 24 hours because he was afraid he might become hypoglycemic. His blood sugar is 550, and his urine is strongly positive for ketones. Serum electrolytes reveal sodium 130 mmol/L (normal 135–145 mmol/L), potassium 3.2 (normal 3.5–5.1 mmol/L), chloride 94 mmol/L (normal 95–105 mmol/L), and bicarbonate 18 mmol/L (normal 22–29 mmol/L). Which of the following is the most likely cause of these findings:

A. Diabetic ketoacidosis
B. Hypochloremic metabolic alkalosis
C. Renal tubular acidosis
D. Respiratory acidosis

Answer: A

Critique: The increased anion gap (130 - (94 + 18)), or 18 (normal 10 to 12) in this case, suggests the presence of unmeasured ions such as ketone bodies seen in diabetic ketoacidosis. Hypochloremic metabolic alkalosis demonstrates an increased bicarbonate, as does respiratory acidosis. Renal tubular acidosis more likely would be associated with normal anion gap.

Pages: 1560, 1561

20: A 53-year-old man presents for an annual physical examination. His history is normal except that he reports having seen blood mixed with his stools on several occasions. He denies any other gastrointestinal symptoms. His physical examination reveals no abdominal tenderness or masses. Which of the following is the most appropriate next step in his evaluation:

A. Have the patient collect six Hemoccult slide stool specimens over the next week to test for occult blood.
B. Have the patient continue to observe his stools for blood for the next 3 months.
C. Have the patient see an endoscopist for colonoscopy.
D. Have the patient abstain from red meat for 3 days and return for a digital rectal examination and fecal occult blood test on the examination specimen.

Answer: C

Critique: The fecal occult blood test can be used for screening purposes and to confirm the presence of blood in the stool. However, a patient who reports frank blood in the stool needs definitive evaluation, such as colonoscopy, to rule out colon cancer.

Pages: 1563, 1564

21: The American Diabetes Association defines "impaired fasting glucose" as which of the following ranges for fasting plasma glucose:

A. 80 to 109 mg/dL
B. 110 to 125 mg/dL
C. 126 to 140 mg/dL
D. 140 to 200 mg/dL

Answer: B

Critique: The American Diabetes Association criterion for impaired fasting glucose is a fasting plasma glucose between 100 and 125 mg/dL.

Page: 1565, Table 61–20

22: A 48-year-old woman presents for her annual Pap smear and pelvic examination. She relates that she has not had a menstrual period for 10 months, and a urine pregnancy test is negative. Which of the following gonadotropin results is most consistent with menopause as the source for her amenorrhea:

A. Follicle-stimulating hormone (FSH) 45 IU/L (normal 5 to 20 IU/L), luteinizing hormone (LH) 50 IU/L (normal 2 to 20 IU/L)
B. FSH 15 IU/L, LH 25 IU/L
C. FSH 15 IU/L, LH 18 IU/L
D. FSH 1 IU/L, LH 2 IU/L

Answer: A

Critique: In the primary ovarian failure of menopause, the gonadotropins LH and FSH increase to high levels. Choice B describes findings consistent with polycystic ovaries, choice C is in the normal range, and choice D describes levels that suggest a central origin for the amenorrhea.

Page: 1565

23: A 25-year-old heterosexual male has been involved in a monogamous relationship with a woman for over a year. He desires to be tested for human immunodeficiency virus (HIV), and an ELISA test is performed. The result is positive, but a subsequent Western blot test is negative. Which of the following represents the most likely explanation for these findings:

A. The patient has very early HIV infection.
B. The HIV ELISA result represents a false positive.
C. The patient has developed acquired immunodeficiency syndrome (AIDS).
D. The test results indicate incipient connective tissue disease.

Answer: B

Critique: Although the ELISA test for HIV performs with better than 99% sensitivity and specificity, false-positive results can occur. Positive results require confirmation with a Western blot or other, similar test. A positive ELISA result followed by a negative Western blot result should be considered a false-positive test result.

Page: 1566

24: A 25-year-old woman presents for an annual examination. During the examination, you note pale mucous membranes and conjunctivae. A CBC reveals hemoglobin 8.5 g/dL (normal 12–16 g/dL), hematocrit 27% (normal 35–45%), mean corpuscular volume (MCV) 78 fL (normal 80–100 fL), mean corpuscular hemoglobin 24 pg/cell (normal 26–34 pg/cell), and mean corpuscular hemoglobin concentration 29 Hb/cell (normal 31–37% Hb/cell). The red cell distribution width (RDW) is 19 (normal 11.5–14.5). Serum iron saturation is 10% (normal 15–50%). Which of the following represents the most likely explanation for these findings:

A. Beta-thalassemia
B. Anemia of chronic disease
C. Hemochromatosis
D. Iron deficiency anemia

Answer: D

Critique: Iron deficiency anemia is characterized by microcytic indices (low MCH, MCV, and MCHC), an increased RDW, and low iron saturation. Anemia of chronic disease typically presents as normocytic or microcytic but with normal RDW. Beta thalassemia similarly demonstrates normal RDW and normal or high iron saturation. Hemochromatosis is an iron overload disorder and is not associated with iron deficiency.

Page: 1567, Tables 61–16, 61–22, 61–23

25: The National Cholesterol Education Program recommends lipid screening every 5 years over age 20. Which of the following represents the recommended screening lipid assay:

A. Total cholesterol (TC)
B. TC, high-density lipoprotein (HDL), and triglycerides
C. Low-density lipoprotein (LDL) and triglycerides
D. HDL plus triglycerides

Answer: B

Critique: The third report of the National Cholesterol Education Program recommended that lipid screening, using a complete lipid profile, be performed every 5 years beginning at age 20. The lipoprotein profile includes TC, LDL cholesterol, HDL cholesterol, and triglycerides. In screening practice, the LDL value is usually calculated from the TC, HDL, and triglyceride values. This represents a change from earlier statements that recommended TC alone as the screening procedure.

Pages: 1568, 1569

26: (True or False) Which of the following represent the major mechanisms for hypophosphatemia:

A. Decreased intestinal absorption of phosphate
B. Increased renal loss of phosphate
C. Sequela of hypoparathyroidism
D. Chronic systemic corticosteroid use
E. Chronic metabolic acidosis

Answers: A - True, B - True, C - False, D - True, E - True

Critique: Hypophosphatemia can occur through several mechanisms. Decreased intestinal absorption, increased renal losses, chronic corticosteroid use, and chronic acidosis can all lower phosphate levels. Hypophosphatemia is seen in hyperparathyroidism.

Page: 1572

27: Which of the following represents the platelet count level at which clinical evidence of bleeding might be expected:

A. 500,000/μL
B. 250,000/μL
C. 150,000/μL
D. 100,000/μL
E. 50,000/μL

Answer: E

Critique: Clinical evidence of bleeding as a result of thrombocytopenia appears at levels of 50,000 to 70,000/μL, at which point bleeding times become prolonged. At levels below 10,000 to 20,000/μL, spontaneous hemorrhage can occur.

Page: 1573

28: Which of the following clinical circumstances is the most likely cause of an elevated serum potassium level:

A. Profuse and prolonged diarrhea
B. Treatment with loop diuretics such as furosemide
C. Acute metabolic alkalosis
D. Angiotensin-converting enzyme (ACE) inhibitor therapy
E. Prolonged vomiting

Answer: D

Critique: Potassium represents the most abundant cation in the body. Diarrhea, vomiting, alkalemia, and loop diuretics can deplete potassium and result in hypokalemia. ACE inhibitor therapy can raise serum potassium levels.

Page: 1573

29: (True or False) Which of the following might be expected to elevate serum prostate specific antigen (PSA) levels:

A. Sexual intercourse
B. Finasteride therapy
C. Bed rest
D. Acute prostatitis
E. Benign prostatic hypertrophy

Answers: A - True, B - False, C - False, D - True, E - True

Critique: Various organizations have promoted conflicting clinical recommendations regarding the use of PSA for prostate cancer screening. These conflicts arise because of the relatively poor specificity of PSA. Sexual intercourse, acute prostatitis, and benign prostatic hypertrophy can all elevate the serum PSA level. Finasteride and bed rest might be expected to lower measured values.

Pages: 1574, 1575, Table 61–32

30: Serum proteins, as identified on serum protein electrophoresis, include albumin, α_1-globulin, α_2-globulin, β-globulin, and γ-globulin. Which of the following protein responses is most consistent with chronic inflammatory states, such as chronic infection or collagen vascular disease:

A. Increased albumin concentration
B. Decreased α_2-globulin

C. Elevated γ-globulin
D. Polyclonal gammopathy

Answer: C

Critique: Chronic inflammation lowers albumin and elevates γ-globulin and α_2-globulin. Polyclonal gammopathy can be found with cirrhosis.

Pages: 1575, 1576

31: The reticulocyte count serves as a measure of erythropoiesis. In anemia states, reticulocytes are released into the blood earlier in their lifespan, which artifactually elevates the reticulocyte count. The reticulocyte production index (RPI) corrects for this phenomenon. Which of the following represents the RPI associated with a hematocrit of 25% and a reticulocyte count of 4%:

A. 5.5
B. 2.75
C. 1.25
D. 0.5

Answer: C

Critique: The RPI can be calculated with the formula:

(% reticulocytes × measured hematocrit) / (maturation time × normal hematocrit)

The maturation time is inversely related to the measured hematocrit. The maturation times are approximately 1, 1.5, 2.0, and 2.5 days for hematocrits of 45%, 35%, 25%, and 15%, respectively. For a measured hematocrit of 25%, the RPI is approximately 1.25, assuming a normal hematocrit of 40%. An RPI of not greater than 1 in an anemic patient indicates at least some degree of ineffective erythropoiesis.

Page: 1576

32: (True or False) Determine whether the following statements regarding rheumatoid factor are true or false:

A. Rheumatoid factors are usually IgM antibodies directed against IgG.
B. Rheumatoid factors demonstrate 90% sensitivity in identifying rheumatoid arthritis.
C. Rheumatoid factors provide an accurate means for monitoring response to therapy.
D. Rheumatoid factors can be detected in persons with chronic infections and connective tissue disorders other than rheumatoid arthritis.

Answers: A - True, B - False, C - False, D - True

Critique: Rheumatoid factors consist of autoantibodies against the Fc segment of IgG. They demonstrate only 50% to 75% sensitivity for rheumatoid arthritis. Rheumatoid factor frequently fails to decrease with successful therapy and can be detected in persons with chronic infections (such as syphilis or tuberculosis) and other connective tissue disorders.

Page: 1576

33: In a patient who presents with hyponatremia in the context of congestive heart failure, which of the following combinations of findings is most likely:

A. Low urine osmolality and urine sodium greater than 20 mmol/L
B. Low urine osmolality and urine sodium less than 20 mmol/L
C. High urine osmolality and urine sodium greater than 20 mmol/L
D. High urine osmolality and urine sodium less than 20 mmol/L

Answer: D

Critique: In congestive heart failure, diminished effective renal blood flow leads to increased salt and water reabsorption, but water is absorbed proportionally more than sodium. This leads to hyponatremia despite increased total body sodium stores. The increased reabsorption results in high urine osmolality and low urine sodium levels.

Page: 1557, Table 61–35

34: (True or False) Which of the following statements regarding rapid streptococcal antigen tests are true and which are false:

A. A negative test reliably excludes the presence of streptococcal disease.
B. A positive test represents good evidence for the presence of streptococcal disease.
C. Recent antibiotic therapy can cause false-negative results.
D. The sensitivity of the test is affected by swab technique.

Answers: A - False, B - True, C - True, D - True

Critique: The rapid streptococcal antigen tests provide useful clinical information but do have limitations. Their sensitivity of 75% to 80% means that a negative test does not exclude disease. On the other hand, a positive test, particularly in a patient with exudative pharyngitis, represents good evidence for streptococcal infection. Recent antibiotic therapy can cause false-negative results, and the result does depend on rigorous swabbing technique.

Pages: 1578, 1579

35: Which of the following statements is correct regarding clinical tests for syphilis:

A. The fluorescent treponemal antibody (FTA) test returns to negative after successful treatment for syphilis.
B. The Venereal Disease Research Laboratory (VDRL) test returns to negative usually within a year after successful therapy for syphilis.
C. The VDRL test performs with high specificity (>95%) for syphilis.
D. A positive VDRL test result in a newborn infant of a mother infected with syphilis represents a reliable indicator of congenital infection.

Answer: B

Critique: The FTA remains positive in nearly all patients after successful therapy for syphilis. The VDRL and rapid plasma reagin (RPR) tests usually return to negative within a year of successful therapy for primary and secondary syphilis. The nontreponemal syphilis tests perform with only fair specificity, demonstrating about 20% false-positive results. Antibodies responsible for a positive VDRL test result cross the placenta through passive transfer, and their presence in the newborn does not necessarily indicate congenital infection.

Page: 1579

36: Which of the following combinations of thyroid assays is most consistent with hypothyroidism secondary to Hashimoto's thyroiditis:

    A. Decreased T_3 resin uptake (T_3RU) and increased total T_4
    B. Increased T_3RU and increased total T_4
    C. Increased T_3RU and decreased total T_4
    D. Decreased T_3RU and decreased total T_4

Answer: D

Critique: The T_3RU provides a measure of thyroid binding globulin saturation with thyroid hormone. The T_3RU varies inversely with the number of free binding sites on thyroid-binding globulin (TBG). Therefore, clinical circumstances associated with increased TBG levels (e.g., estrogen therapy) lower T_3RU and vice versa. Decreased thyroid hormone production leaves a larger than normal number of binding sites available on TBG, and thereby lowers the T_3RU; thus, hypothyroidism owing to decreased hormone production in the thyroid is associated with both decreased T_3RU and decreased total T_4.

Page: 1580

37: (True or False) Hematologic findings that suggest a leukemoid reaction, rather than leukemia, include which of the following:

    A. A total white blood cell count (WBC) of 40,000
    B. Presence of nucleated red blood cells on the peripheral blood smear
    C. Presence of myelocytes on the peripheral blood smear
    D. Increased leukocyte alkaline phosphatase
    E. Platelet count of 500,000

Answers: A - True, B - False, C - False, D - True, E - True

Critique: Leukemoid reactions can result from toxic conditions, neoplasms, infections, and myeloproliferative disorders. The total WBC is usually less than 50,000 cells/mm^3, and platelet counts rarely exceed 600,000. The leukocyte alkaline phosphatase is increased. Nucleated red cells and myelocytes on the peripheral blood smear suggest a leukemic process.

Pages: 1582, 1583

PART V

MANAGEMENT OF THE PRACTICE

Chapter 62

Problem-Oriented Medical Record

William F. Miser

1: You are starting a new practice with a group of family physicians and have been given the task of developing your office's record system. All of the following statements regarding an office record system are correct, except:

- A. The charting system should be designed so that everyone uses the same format and the same forms in the group.
- B. The ideal record should be kept simple.
- C. A system should be avoided that requires unnecessary paperwork.
- D. Acute illnesses should be viewed in the total perspective of a person's long-term care.
- E. Orderly recording of data is vital to efficient patient care.

Answer: A

Critique: One of the most useful tools available for a family physician is a well-prepared medical record. However, "one size" does *not* "fit all." An office record system should be adapted to the individual preferences and personalities of the physicians using the system. Therefore, the system should be flexible enough to meet the individual needs of all the physicians involved in a group practice. The record should be kept as simple as possible to avoid unnecessary paperwork and organized so that data are readily retrievable for efficient patient care. Acute illnesses are not isolated events but should be viewed in the total context of the patient's longitudinal care.

Page: 1587

2: Which of the following statements is incorrect regarding the problem-oriented medical record (POMR):

- A. The system was developed more than 30 years ago because office records of the past were poorly organized and illegible.
- B. The POMR is also known as the patient-oriented medical record.
- C. The POMR achieves maximum potential in the hands of a subspecialist.
- D. The POMR is best suited for patients who have chronic illnesses or those with complex cases involving multiple problems.
- E. The basic concepts of the POMR serve as a foundation for an efficient office medical record.

Answer: C

Critique: The problem-oriented medical record, also known as the patient-oriented medical record because it emphasizes the individuality of the patient, addresses the many concerns of the past. Developed in 1969, the POMR's concepts serve as an excellent foundation for an efficient office medical record and is best suited for patients who have complex cases involving multiple problems or who have chronic illnesses that are followed over a period of time. The POMR achieves its maximum potential with family physicians, who through continuity provide care over time to patients with complex cases involving multiple problems.

Page: 1587

3: A patient in your practice for the past 10 years is leaving the area and is requesting to take her medical records from your office. Which of the following statements is true regarding patient access to medical records (select only one answer):

- A. Because you have established good rapport over the years, you can give her the original copy of her medical records to take with her.
- B. Because she will no longer be in the area, it is not important for you to keep her medical records on file.
- C. Your patient has no right to see her medical records because they are the property of your practice.
- D. The patient may have a copy of her medical records, unless there is a valid medical reason for refusing to do so.
- E. Sharing medical records with patients is not harmful.

Answer: D

Critique: The medical record today is becoming the joint responsibility and common property of the physician, other health care providers, and the patient. As such, the patient may have access to read and obtain a copy of her medical records, but the original should not be given to her to keep. Although sharing this information with patients could be beneficial, it also may be harmful by causing excessive worry about language and conditions that patients may not understand. Each office should have a well-defined policy concerning how it will handle its medical records. In this case, a good policy involves either mailing a copy of this patient's records to her new physician or providing a copy for her to take with her, unless you have a valid medical reason to believe that providing this information would harm her care.

Page: 1588

4: Which of the following statements is correct regarding medical records:

    A. When referring a patient for consultation, a problem list should accompany the request to the subspecialist only if the problem is pertinent to the consultation.
    B. You should attempt to incorporate the patient's entire medical background into the record as soon as possible.
    C. If you perform a detailed history and physical examination on a new patient, it is not important to obtain all medical information from other physicians and hospitals.
    D. The use of personalized abbreviations and shorthand is all right to use in the medical record so long as the physician has a well-established system in place.
    E. Because the medical record is for the personal use of the physician, it is not important for the writing to be legible to others.

Answer: B

Critique: Because the information found in the medical record is becoming shared property among the physician, other health care providers, and the patient, it must be legible, clear, and concise. Personal shorthand or abbreviations that can be understood only by the physician may prove confusing to other providers. When seeing a new patient, it is important to obtain his or her entire medical background as quickly as possible and obtain all medical information from other physicians and hospitals to confirm the history. Incorporating the problem list with a consultation permits the subspecialist to see the "whole" patient in the context of his or her other problems.

Pages: 1588, 1589

5: Which of the following is the greatest barrier to effective communication and good records:

    A. Numerous physicians involved in the care of one patient
    B. Use of dictation and transcription services for the medical records
    C. Pressure to see more patients at a faster pace
    D. Finances available to purchase an integrated computer system with other providers
    E. Illegible handwriting of the physician

Answer: E

Critique: Illegible handwriting of physicians is the greatest barrier to effective communication and good records. A sloppy, illegible record calls into question the physician's ability to provide quality care and is a liability

in malpractice suits. To correct this problem, many offices are now turning to transcription services for dictation of the medical record. Although the other items mentioned might contribute to ineffective communication, they are not the major barrier.

Page: 1589

6: You are asked to develop a filing system for your office. Which of the following statements is incorrect:

    A. Misfiling is common in those systems that file alphabetically according to the surname.
    B. Terminal digit filing is the least efficient system in retrieving medical records.
    C. Color-coded terminal digit filing virtually eliminates the possibility of misfiling.
    D. Open shelves are better than drawers for filing medical records.
    E. Family filing is difficult with the alphabetical system.

Answer: B

Critique: Various methods exist for filing systems in family practice. Filing alphabetically by surname potentially leads to misfiling and, because of mixed families with different last names, family filing is difficult. Terminal digit filing is an efficient system for family practice and allows for more rapid and accurate placement of records. Misfiling is extremely uncommon in the color-coded terminal digit filing system. Filing using open shelving is better than using file drawers.

Pages: 1589, 1590

7: How long should inactive medical records be kept in the office before being purged to a storage area?

    A. 1 year
    B. 2 to 3 years
    C. 4 to 5 years
    D. 6 years or longer
    E. Medical records should never be purged, regardless of how long they have been active.

Answer: B

Critique: Purging inactive records from the system annually helps keep the medical record area from overflowing with unused charts. It is recommended that records of patients who have not been seen for 2 to 3 years should be considered inactive, removed from the active file, and placed in storage; they should never be destroyed, however. Various methods exist to identify these charts, including color-coding, but require attention to detail by the receptionist or nurse to ensure that the system works.

Page: 1590

8: Which of the following statements is incorrect regarding family charts:

    A. Family charting focuses on the entire family's health, which may subsequently have an impact on the health of the individuals within the family.
    B. Family genogram is an important part of family charting.

C. Recording events such as a wedding anniversary potentially can improve the physician-patient relationship.

D. Primary purpose of family charting is to allow for better billing practices within the office.

E. Family charting assists the family physician in identifying problems that potentially could improve the quality of care to the family.

Answer: D

Critique: Filing charts based on the family structure offers several advantages to the family physician. It can improve the quality of care to the family, as well as have a positive impact on the health of the individuals within that family. A family registration form containing family demographic data, along with a family genogram, are key parts of the family folder. The primary purpose of the family chart system is to provide the family physician with as much information as possible on the family and has nothing to do with billing practices.

Pages: 1590, 1591

9: Which of the following is *not* a basic component of the problem-oriented medical record:

A. A complete medical database
B. A photograph of the patient
C. A problem list
D. An initial plan
E. Progress notes

Answer: B

Critique: The four major elements that form the foundation of the problem-oriented medical record include a database, a list containing the major problems to be addressed, an initial plan for addressing these major problems, and progress notes documenting incremental care.

Pages: 1592, 1593

10: (True or False) Which of the following statements are true regarding the problem list and which are false:

A. It is the most important ingredient of the patient-oriented medical record.
B. It should include only specific diagnoses and chronic problems.
C. It should be kept in a prominent position in the medical record.
D. It provides a dynamic picture of the patient's health problems.
E. Symptoms and risk factors do not belong on the problem list.

Answers: A - True, B - False, C - True, D - True, E - False

Critique: The problem list is the single most important ingredient of the POMR and should have a prominent place in the medical record. It serves as a "snapshot" of the patient's health and reminds the physician to provide care to the whole person. Types of problems listed can include anything that requires diagnosis or management or that interferes with the patient's quality of life. The list can include signs, symptoms, abnormal laboratory results, and risk factors as well as specific diagnoses and chronic problems.

Pages: 1592, 1593

11: Which of the following statements is incorrect regarding the problem list:

A. Recurring acute problems should be placed on the major problem list.
B. Legibility is an important component of the problem list.
C. The problem list should include problems that are temporary in nature.
D. Problems of family members should be included.
E. "Incomplete database" should be listed as the first problem.

Answer: C

Critique: The major problem list should include recurring acute problems, such as bronchitis or otitis media, but not problems that are temporary in nature and that do not recur (e.g., a first-degree ankle sprain). The value of the problem list is that it provides any provider with an overview of the person's health. Hence, it should be legible and problems should be printed for ease of reading. Including problems of family members reminds the physician to look at the family as a whole and that problems of one family member can affect the other family members. "Incomplete database" as the first problem reminds the physician to continually accumulate data.

Pages: 1592–1594

12: Which of the following should be included in the database of the patient-oriented medical record:

A. A detailed history and physical examination results
B. Baseline laboratory studies
C. A list of allergies and immunizations
D. Hospitalizations and consultations
E. All of the above

Answer: E

Critique: The database provides the foundation for developing the problem list. Each physician should identify the minimal information that will be collected on all patients in the practice and should include as a minimum all these listed items.

Page: 1595

13: You are seeing a new patient in your practice. Which of the following statements is incorrect regarding the history that should be obtained:

A. The patient can complete a detailed health history questionnaire in the office waiting room or at home before the visit.
B. Detailed preprinted questionnaires are available commercially for specific systems (e.g., cardiovascular or respiratory).
C. It is not important to have the patient's previous medical records when obtaining a detailed history.

D. The initial history is an essential part of the data-base.

E. A health history questionnaire can be either self-designed or purchased commercially.

Answer: C

Critique: The initial history is an integral part of the data-base. Health history questionnaires, as well as detailed system-oriented questionnaires, completed by the patient are a valuable timesaving tool and can be developed or purchased commercially. However, information obtained should be confirmed by reviewing the medical records from the patient's previous physicians.

Pages: 1595, 1596

14: (True or False) Determine which of the following statements are true and which are false regarding the comprehensive physical examination portion of the data-base:

A. A printed physical examination sheet is advantageous.

B. A nonstructured, open-ended, preprinted format is better than a highly structured "check-off" format.

C. Illustrations of body parts identifying abnormalities should be included.

D. Some practices insist on a comprehensive physical examination before providing treatment beyond the second visit.

E. The patient should be sent a summary of the findings from the physical examination, including the problem list.

Answers: A - True, B - False, C - True, D - True, E - True

Critique: A comprehensive physical examination is an important part of the database and should be completed as soon as possible when caring for a new patient. A highly structured "check-off" format is preferable to one that is nonstructured, because it identifies areas of the examination that still need to be completed. Illustrations identifying abnormalities provide a quick visual reference for other providers. Sending the patient a summary of the findings and the problem list allows him or her to review the material for accuracy.

Page: 1596

15: Which of the following statements is correct regarding placing laboratory and other data into the medical record:

A. Original laboratory slips should always be kept in the chart.

B. The major problem with transferring data from laboratory slips to a standard laboratory data sheet is the probability of incorrectly recording data.

C. Laboratory results, Pap smear results, and radiographs should be kept in chronologic order in the chart.

D. Laboratory slips should be placed at the front of a chart preceding the problem list.

E. Transferring information from laboratory report slips to a standard data sheet is too time-consuming to be worthwhile.

Answer: C

Critique: Family physicians care for patients over time, and laboratory data, radiograph reports, and other information should be easy to access and chronologically placed. Transferring the information from a laboratory slip to a standard laboratory data sheet is a timesaving practice. The fear of incorrectly recording data is largely unfounded. Once recorded, the original laboratory sheets can be discarded. Use of the data sheet allows the family physician to observe subtle changes that occur over time. Actual report forms that indicate patient abnormalities should be filed in the back of the chart.

Page: 1596

Questions 16 to 19: Regarding progress notes, match each numbered entry with the correct lettered entry:

A. Subjective
B. Objective
C. Assessment
D. Plan

16: Furosemide 20 mg orally once a day

17: She complains of increasing shortness of breath over the past 2 weeks.

18: Congestive heart failure

19: BP 160/88, HR 80 irregular, 2+ edema

Answers: 16 - D, 17 - A, 18 - C, 19 - B

Critique: The SOAP format in a progress note provides an organized way to document the clinic visit. Subjective information includes history, symptoms, and feelings. Objective data include examination and all measurements of factual information. The assessment refers to the diagnosis, and the plan includes the diagnostic and therapeutic modalities used in the management of the problem.

Pages: 1596, 1597

20: Which of the following statements is incorrect regarding the SOAP format of a progress note:

A. Only problems pertinent to the visit should be described in the note.

B. The term "doing well" provides a valuable piece of information in the subjective portion of the note.

C. The plan section is the most important portion of the progress note.

D. The three major subdivisions of a plan should include diagnostic tests, therapeutic modalities, and patient education.

E. If one is uncertain of a diagnosis, it is better to list the symptoms rather than guess at a diagnosis.

Answer: B

Critique: The SOAP format is an organized way for family physicians to document the information obtained during the clinic visit. For patients with multiple problems, only those problems pertinent to the clinic visit need be mentioned in the note. Terms such as "doing well" or "status quo" are meaningless and should be avoided. For uncertain diagnoses, it is better to list the symptoms in the assessment (with perhaps a differential diagnosis) than to prematurely label the patient with a diagnosis. The plan is the most important part of the entire note because it outlines the next steps toward resolution or treating the problem. Every plan should include the diagnostic studies to be done, the therapy to be applied, and patient education.

Pages: 1597, 1598

21: You are trying to maintain a complete and accurate medical record that would "stand up" in a court of law in case a malpractice suit were filed against you. All of the following are important ways to avoid legal pitfalls, except:

A. Every page of the medical record should have the patient's name, and every progress note should be signed, dated, and arranged chronologically.
B. The progress note should avoid derogatory comments about the patient.
C. Every telephone call received in the office regarding the patient should be documented in the chart.
D. To change an error, one should completely erase or obliterate the error so that it cannot be read.
E. You should document in the chart when a patient refuses a certain recommended test or treatment.

Answer: D

Critique: One of the best defenses in a malpractice case is a legible and well-maintained record that is accurate and complete. It is not uncommon for one to periodically make an error in the progress notes. When an error is detected, use only a single line to cross out the error (so that it is still legible) and initial and date this line. Never alter medical records after a suit has been filed. All of the other choices mentioned are good record-keeping practices.

Page: 1598

22: All of the following are true regarding the medical record, except:

A. Flow sheets are especially important in monitoring a chronic disease such as diabetes mellitus.
B. If done properly, a flow sheet may substitute for the "O" and "P" portions of the SOAP progress note.
C. Keeping a direct copy of all prescriptions by using pressure-sensitive paper is a good way to maintain the patient's medication list.
D. Patients feel that using computerized patient records interferes with the physician-patient relationship and interferes with their perception of their care.
E. A patient on Coumadin for atrial fibrillation would benefit by having a flow sheet in the chart.

Answer: D

Critique: The use of flow sheets is an excellent way to assist physicians in managing patients with a chronic disease such as diabetes mellitus. Flow sheets serve as a reminder for necessary tests and evaluations and also serve as an appropriate way to document the care that is provided during that visit. If done properly, it is permissible to write "see flow sheet" in lieu of entries in the objective and plan portions of the SOAP note. Flow sheets are also a good way to document problems that require frequent laboratory monitoring, as in the case of a patient who is on Coumadin. Keeping copies of written prescriptions in the patient's chart allows for maintenance of his or her medication list. Studies have shown that patients look favorably on the use of computerized patient records, and they feel that their physicians are practicing up-to-date medicine.

Pages: 1598–1602

Chapter 63

Managed Health Care: Practicing Effectively in the 21st Century

William A. Verhoff

1: All of the following are true regarding managed care, except:

    A. Managed care is a system by which the physician operates within a financial system such as capitation or fee for service.

    B. Managed care delivers a specific set of health care services to a defined population of patients.

    C. Managed care operates within a set network of providers and facilities.

    D. Managed care performs all needed services without regard for quality or patient satisfaction.

Answer: D

Critique: The provider in the manage care system must be and will be held accountable for delivering quality, accessible, and affordable health care with the highest patient and provider satisfaction possible.

Page: 1603

2: Managed care covers a continuum of services from which patients can choose. The plan that allows patients to have complete freedom of choice of physicians and services is:

    A. Group model HMO

    B. Traditional fee for service

    C. Managed PPO

    D. Workers' Compensation

    E. Medicare

Answer: B

Critique: In the typical fee-for-service system, patients typically have complete freedom of choice of physician and services. The health care network consists of any and all physicians and facilities, and most, if not all, services are reimbursed, regardless of necessity. The group model HMO represents the other end of the spectrum. The HMO operates with strict controls, capitation, and a limited, defined network of physicians and facilities. This strict environment allows for monitoring of cost, quality, and utilization.

Page: 1603

3: Managed care can be traced back to 1877. It wasn't until nearly 100 years later that legislation standardized and distinguished health maintenance organizations from traditional fee-for-service plans. This legislation was the:

    A. HCFA Act

    B. CLIA Act

    C. HMO Act

    D. AMA Act

Answer: C

Critique: The Health Maintenance Organization Act of 1972 set the standards for HMOs.

Pages: 1603, 1604

4: What were the two main factors that fueled a dramatic increase in employer-supported enrollment in the alternative managed care arrangements in the 1980s (i.e., PPOs, HMOs, IPAs):

    A. The HMO Act of 1972

    B. The patients' desire to have higher quality service

    C. The failure of the traditional fee-for-services system to control cost and demonstrate value

    D. The need to control physician salaries

    E. The requirement to limit the number of specialists in practice

Answers: A and C

Critique: The HMO Act of 1972 opened the door for a variety of alternative health care financing and delivery systems. They all offered varying degrees of price discounts, a defined provider network, and management of the use of health care services. This approach became attractive to employees seeking to add quality and value with cost savings, which the fee-for-service plans could not offer.

Page: 1604

5: The *primary* organization that started the accreditation process of health plans (e.g., HMOs) in 1991 was the:

    A. JCAHO

    B. AMA

C. VHA
D. NCQA
E. AFL-CIO

Answer: D

Critique: The NCQA (National Committee for Quality Assurance) is a private, not-for-profit organization that is governed by a board of directors and includes employer, consumer and labor representatives, health plans, quality experts, policy makers, and representatives from organized medicine. The NCQA began accrediting health plans in 1991 in response to a need for standardized, objective information about their quality.

Page: 1605

6: (True or False) Health plans and provider networks are being pressured to demonstrate their value on the basis of health outcomes and performance standards. The current standardized health plan performance measures that are issued by NCQA are called HEDIS.

Answer: True

Critique: HEDIS (Health Plan Employer Data and Information Set) resulted from a 4-year effort by employers, health plans, and consumers to define a set of standardized performance measures.

Page: 1605

7: Which of the following HEDIS 2000 performance standards is being required by many commercial, Medicare, and Medicaid payers:

A. Effectiveness of care measures
B. Access to and availability of care
C. Patient satisfaction with care
D. Cost of care
E. All of the above

Answer: E

Critique: The above four performance measures, along with utilization of common ambulatory and hospital services and the overall stability of the health plan, are all being measured as HEDIS indicators. This information is being used by over 250 health plans and submitted to NCQA for accreditation.

Page: 1605

8: (True or False) The measuring and reporting of the various performance data has climaxed and reached a point of maximum usage among consumers.

Answer: False

Critique: Measuring and reporting these data is just in its infancy. Barriers that remain are inadequate information systems, lack of standardized measures, and cost.

Pages: 1606, 1607

9: As managed care systems evolve, innovative reimbursement strategies are applied. Review the list below and match the reimbursement system with the unique problem that exists as a result of each payment system.

1. Fee for service
2. Capitation
3. Salary
4. Risk sharing

A. Ethical issues
B. Decreased productivity
C. Increasing utilization and cost
D. Underutilization of services

Answers: 1 - C, 2 - D, 3 - B, 4 - A

10: (True or False) Discharge planning and case managers are examples of supply-side care management. These supply-side management strategies have not been successful in reducing hospital admissions and lengths of stay, pharmacy costs, and referral rates.

Answer: False

Critique: Posthospital discharge planning begins on the first day of admission, and case managers help to arrange and coordinate posthospital care. These efforts do impact length of stay, referrals, cost, and readmission rates.

Page: 1608

11: Twenty-four-hour nurse health counseling lines, health risk appraisals, wellness programs, and self-care programs are all examples of:

A. Risk management
B. Utilization management
C. Practice management
D. Demand management

Answer: D

Critique: Demand management is the use of self-management and decision support systems to enable, educate, and encourage people to improve their health and make appropriate use of medical care.

Page: 1609

12: Which of the following arrangements is not considered an example of health system integration:

A. Multispecialty group practice
B. IPA (Independent Practice Association)
C. PMO (Physician Hospital Organization)
D. Hospital system mergers
E. Solo family physician performing multiple procedures

Answer: E

Critique: The solo physician is not an example of "integration" and is being replaced by primary care specialty and multispecialty group practices and by larger IPAs, medical groups, and networks.

Page: 1609

13: (True or False) With the advent of managed care, patient, public, and physician subspecialty pressures continue to allow patients to bypass primary care physicians and go directly to specialists, thus minimizing the role of the primary care doctor.

Answer: False

Critique: As managed care continues to evolve, the broadly trained personal physician, who can diagnose and treat people's common problems and help them obtain the care they need to keep them healthy, can be expected to play a central role in health care.

Page: 1610

14: Continuous quality improvement (CQI) is a fundamental competency in today's businesses. Review the CQI process steps below and put them in the proper order.

    A. Measuring and providing feedback
    B. Identifying desired outcome and indicator
    C. Using feedback to identify new ways to achieve desired outcome
    D. Defining the guidelines to obtaining the desired outcome

Answers: B, D, A, C

Page: 1610

15: Which of the following practice management techniques can prove to be the most important first step for the physician to take to improve the overall function of the practice:

    A. Get the most and best from the office staff
    B. Find ways to improve office efficiencies
    C. Hire out as many functions as possible to subcontractors
    D. Use patient satisfaction questionnaires to gather information

Answer: B

Critique: By looking at our own office efficiencies and inefficiencies, we can then look at ways to improve our own practice management techniques. This must be the first thing the provider does before looking at the other factors that may be influencing the practice.

Page: 1611

16: The use of the computer in the physician's office will be in the early 2000s as was the:

    A. Office phone in the 1970s
    B. Fax machine in the 1980s
    C. Stethoscope in the 1960s
    D. Cell phone in the 1990s
    E. All of the above

Answer: E

Critique: As each one of the items above was revolutionary in its time, the computer and information services are evolving at an alarming rate. With each of these items, implementation was relatively immediate. The computer, however, poses many new challenges based on the vast number of potential applications. This can make getting started very difficult. Also, the complete computer system, capable of performing, scheduling, billing, medical records, and Internet access, is somewhat cost prohibitive for many family physicians, but the pressure to become computerized will have to be met.

Page: 1611

17: Which of the following is not required for physicians to become knowledgeable in the area of reimbursements:

    A. Accurate use of coding and documentation
    B. Maximizing revenue with no regard to expenses
    C. Being comfortable with monitoring the practice's financial status
    D. Being able to negotiate good contracts with insurers

Answer: B

Critique: Today's physician must have an understanding of the overall financial status of the practice. He or she must have enough fiscal knowledge to establish a budget as well as have a handle on the costs versus revenues and what factors affect each area.

Pages: 1611, 1612

18: (True or False) Federal and state regulations, recredentialing, accreditation rules for in-office laboratories, liability insurance, risk contracts, and investment restrictions are but a few factors that have made practicing legally and ethically much more difficult for today's physician.

Answer: True

Critique: Unlike the days when having only a medical license was sufficient to open an office, it is now a requirement to have numerous licenses and certificates. Physicians must also be aware of investment regulations, which prohibit them from referring patients for diagnostic tests or treatment services in which they have an ownership interest. All of these factors influence the physician's ethical and legal approach to running a practice.

Page: 1612

19: (True or False) To fulfill the professional responsibilities required in medicine, we need to make sure that the other aspects of our lives take on less importance so we can be devoted to improving our clinical skills, knowledge base, and overall practice management skills.

Answer: False

Critique: This can be a sure way to burn out. As physicians, we need to evaluate and determine our core values associated with being a doctor, a spouse, a parent, and a member of the community and strike a balance between our personal and professional lives.

Page: 1613

20: In a recent survey of 7500 patients, the percentage who valued the role of their primary care physician as a source of first contact for their health care needs was:

    A. 94%
    B. 90%
    C. 89%
    D. 75%

Answer: A

Critique: According to a study by Selby Grunbach, 94% of the more than 7500 patients surveyed said they valued the role of their primary care physician as a source of first contact.

Page: 1613

Chapter 64

Clinical Guidelines

Michael D. Hagen

1: Different organizations use different methodologies to create clinical guidelines. Major organizations, such as the American Medical Association, the Institute of Medicine, and the Canadian Medical Association, have developed standards for such efforts. A recent review of 279 guidelines found that what percentage had adhered to these standards:

    A. 25%
    B. 43%
    C. 67%
    D. 88%
    E. 95%

Answer: B

Critique: Many organizations, such as specialty societies, professional societies, and government agencies have created clinical guidelines over the past decade. Unfortunately, many of these efforts have not been conducted according to standard methodologies and thus must be embraced cautiously.

Page: 1615

2: In 1990, the Institute of Medicine (IOM) created a definition of *practice guidelines* as a means to promote standard approaches to guideline development. Which of the following best represents the IOM definition of *practice guidelines:*

    A. A consensus statement created by experts in a clinical area
    B. A meta-analysis of case-control studies related to the guideline's clinical context
    C. A narrative review of pertinent literature related to the guideline's clinical context.
    D. A systematically developed statement to assist practitioners' and patients' decisions about appropriate health care

Answer: D

Critique: The IOM defined *practice guidelines* as "systematically developed statements to assist practitioners' and patients' decisions about appropriate health care for specific clinical circumstances."

Pages: 1615, 1616

3: A number of terms have been developed to describe various components of clinical guidelines. Which of the following best describes a "Performance Measure":

    A. Systematically developed statements that can be used to assess specific health care decisions
    B. A rule or set of instructions containing conditional logic for accomplishing a task
    C. A documented plan of expected clinical management in which critical treatments are optimally sequenced along a timeline
    D. A method or instrument to monitor conformance to practice guidelines

Answer: D

Critique: A "performance measure" is defined as a method or instrument to monitor the extent to which providers' actions conform to established practice guidelines or standards. Choice A describes medical review criteria, choice B defines an algorithm, and choice C refers to a critical pathway.

Page: 1616

4: (True or False) Potential benefits of clinical guidelines include which of the following:

    A. They can potentially reduce unexplained clinical practice variation.
    B. They can identify gaps in clinical knowledge as a stimulus for research.
    C. They can generally be developed at little cost in time and money.
    D. They encourage innovation in clinical practice.
    E. They provide a means for assessing and promoting quality practice.

Answers: A - True, B - True, C - False, D - False, E - True

Critique: Clinical guidelines can provide the stimulus to reduce unexplained regional variation in clinical practice. Well-crafted guidelines also serve to identify gaps in clinical knowledge and can thus guide research. Well-done guidelines are generally fairly costly to develop. Additionally, they can serve to limit innovative clinical practice. Guidelines can serve as the focus for assessing quality and quality improvement activities.

Page: 1616

5: The Institute of Medicine (IOM) has developed a series of attributes that characterize well-developed clinical practice guidelines. Which of the following best describes "validity" as an attribute of a good clinical practice guideline:

A. The guideline includes statements about how often the guidelines should be reviewed for potential revision.
B. The guideline identifies generally expected exceptions to the guideline recommendations.
C. The guideline uses unambiguous, precise language and terminology.
D. The methodology used in creating the guideline is described explicitly.
E. The guideline leads to the health and cost outcomes projected in the guideline.

Answer: E

Critique: The IOM attributes include descriptions of validity, reliability/reproducibility, clinical applicability, clinical flexibility, multidisciplinary involvement in development, scheduled review for revisions, and explicit documentation. Of the choices provided in this question, choice E describes validity of a guideline.

Pages: 1616, 1617

6: The American Medical Association (AMA) also has described attributes that developers should follow in creating guidelines. The AMA attributes include all but which of the following:

A. Practice guidelines should not be developed in conjunction with physician organizations.
B. Practice guidelines should be based on current professional knowledge.
C. Practice guidelines should assist in decisions about appropriate health care applicable to specific circumstances.
D. Practice guidelines should explicitly describe the methodology used in creating them.

Answer: A

Critique: According to the AMA's recommendations, practice guidelines should be developed by or in cooperation with physician organizations.

Page: 1617

7: The Agency for Healthcare Research and Quality (AHRQ) has developed a model for assessing quality of health care interventions. In this model, clinical care consists of inputs, processes of care, and outcomes. Which of the following represents an input to clinical care, as defined by AHRQ:

A. Preventive measures offered during clinical care
B. Mortality and morbidity associated with a clinical intervention
C. Quality of life associated with a clinical intervention
D. Risk factors that the patient demonstrates
E. Therapeutic procedures conducted in the clinical intervention

Answer: D.

Critique: The AHRQ model of care includes inputs, process of care, and outcomes. Inputs include demographic factors, risk factors, and functional status before the intervention. Process attributes include preventive

measures, diagnostic testing, procedures, and therapies offered to the patient during clinical care. Outcomes include mortality, morbidity, health status, quality of life, and functional status after the intervention.

Page: 1619

8: (True or False) A number of organizations, such as the Agency for Healthcare Research and Quality, have invested substantial time and resources in developing clinical guidelines. Additionally, processes have been suggested for adapting existing guidelines for local use. Which of the following represent appropriate steps in adapting recognized guidelines for local use:

A. Identify and recruit clinical leaders to the adaptation effort.
B. Review critically the guideline proposed for adaptation.
C. Conduct a concurrent data review for feedback to clinicians.
D. Collaborate with appropriate professionals in developing critical pathways.

Answers: A - True, B - True, C - True, D - True

Critique: Because of the time and expense involved in creating guidelines de novo, many organizations prefer to adapt existing guidelines for their local use. Wise and Billi developed a suggested set of steps for such adaptation efforts. Their suggested process includes all of the options listed. Additionally, the process includes selecting the practice area, identifying and recruiting team members, collecting appropriate nationally endorsed guidelines, identifying data elements for review of guideline performance, and evaluating and developing implementation methods.

Page: 1619

9: (True or False) The Shewart cycle describes the process used in quality improvement activities. This model includes which of the following steps:

A. Planning a new or improved process of care
B. Doing or implementing the process
C. Checking or measuring the process outcomes
D. Acting on the information to revise the care process as necessary

Answers: A - True, B - True, C - True, D - True

Critique: Quality efforts have moved from the punitive quality assessment efforts of the 1980s to an emphasis on continuous improvement in clinical care quality. The Shewart cycle describes the quality improvement process in simple form and consists of four components: planning, doing, checking, and acting. This model emphasizes continuous improvement rather than retrospective assessment of historical performance.

Pages: 1619, 1620

10: Good outcomes represent the goal of health care services, but outcomes are difficult to measure. Both direct and indirect measures are available for health outcomes. Which of the following represents a direct health outcome measure:

A. Hospital infection rates
B. Rates of unexpected transfer to a critical care unit
C. Prevention of avoidable death
D. Readmission rates within a specified time of hospital discharge

Answer: C

Critique: Health outcome measures have historically focused on indirect assays of quality, such as hospital infection rates, rates of unexpected events such as transfers to critical care units, and early readmission rates. These measures do not necessarily relate to outcomes that are important to patients. Outcomes such as prevention of avoidable death, cure rates, and functional status represent issues of importance to patients, but they can be more difficult to measure than can indirect measures.

Page: 1620

11: A number of factors can affect practitioners' performance in achieving good clinical outcomes. Patient-related factors, clinician-related factors, organization-related factors, and community-related factors all can influence the delivery of quality health care services. Which of the following represents an organizational factor that can affect outcomes:

A. Clinician level of knowledge
B. Severity of patient illness
C. Community health risk factors
D. Processes for management in the provider's group
E. Allocation of community health resources

Answer: D

Critique: Provider organizational factors that can affect health outcomes include management structures, group resources, and support systems for clinical care. Patient-related factors include normal biologic variation, severity of illness, and comorbidities. Clinician factors include knowledge, technical and interpersonal skills, and clinical judgment. Community factors include risk factors, health care resources, and structure of the health care system.

Page: 1620

Chapter 65

Accounting Systems

Daniel Knight

1: (True or False) When posting transactions from a journal to account ledgers using the accrual method of accounting, all money that is actually spent or received during an accounting period is included in that period.

Answer: False

Critique: Expenses and revenue are charged to the period in which they are incurred or earned, even if the money is actually spent or received at a different time. In the cash method, all money that is actually spent or received during an accounting period is included in that period.

Page: 1625

2: An employee may be exempt from the record-keeping and overtime pay requirements of the Fair Labor Standards Act and may be paid a fixed salary if her or his position includes all of the following, except:

    A. Position requires independent judgment.
    B. Employee earns more than a certain amount.
    C. Employee is an office manager, head nurse, or laboratory technician.
    D. Employee works more than 50 hours per week on a continuing basis.

Answer: D

Critique: An employee is exempt from record keeping if the position meets certain criteria, such as "requires exercise of independent judgment" and earns above a certain amount. "Hours worked per week" is not a criterion for exempt workers.

Pages: 1625, 1626

3: An individual may be declared an "independent contractor" by the IRS if:

    A. The individual spends all employment time working for one employer.
    B. All work must be done on the premises.
    C. The employer provides the training required and tools and pays all expenses of doing the work
    D. Individual provides services to more than one business.

Answer: D

Critique: Several tests are used to evaluate whether an employee is an independent contractor. The tests include whether the employer specifies when, where, and how the work is to be done; whether the work must be done on the premises; whether the employer provides training and tools and pays expenses; and whether the individual spends all employment time working for one employer.

Pages: 1625, 1626

4: The American Medical Association's *Physicians' Current Procedural Terminology* (CPT) codes are used for all of the following, except:

    A. Coding for evaluation and management services
    B. Determining higher levels of reimbursement for more complex medical decision making
    C. Documenting the level of care for office visits, hospital visits, and consultations
    D. Documenting the patient diagnosis
    E. Whether professional fees reflect the time, effort, training, skill, and resources required to render the service

Answer: D

Critique: Diagnosis is documented by *International Classification of Diseases* (ICD-9-CM) to health insurance plans.

Pages: 1627, 1628

5: (True or False) Recording the net value of the charge minus adjustments on the payment and adjustment register gives a true picture of the practice that the family physician can use when deciding whether to participate in a particular health insurance plan.

Answer: False

Critique: Such documentation distorts the statistics of practice operations and obscures information that the family practitioner may use to decide whether to participate in certain insurance plans.

Page: 1629

6: In a traditional indemnity health insurance plan, the following does *not* occur:

    A. The plan typically requires pre-authorization of services, such as referral to other physicians, outpatient procedures, and hospital admissions.
    B. The agreement involves the insurance carrier and the patient only.
    C. The patient is liable for the physician's entire fee for a medical procedure, whatever the amount approved or reimbursed by the insurance plan.

D. Payment is made directly to the insured.

E. The patient may *assign* benefits to the physician.

Answer: A

Critique: Traditional indemnity insurance plans typically do not require pre-authorization for services. Generally, this is required by managed care organizations. All other answers are features of an indemnity plan.

Page: 1629

7: Under capitation for services with insurance plans:

A. The physician is usually paid quarterly.

B. The plan does not ever cover services outside the practice.

C. The patient may be required to pay a deductible amount each year.

D. The patient does not have to pay a co-pay for each visit.

E. Negotiated fees are usually more than a physician's usual fees.

Answer: C

Critique: The physician is usually paid monthly. Capitation sometimes includes a multitude of services, including referrals to specialists and outpatient and in-hospital care. The patient often has a co-pay and may be required to pay a deductible each year. The fees paid are usually less than a physician's usual fees.

Page: 1629

8: (True or False) If a physician participates in an indemnity insurance plan, she or he may bill the patient for and collect charges above the approved amount.

Answer: False

Critique: If a physician participates in a plan, she or he may not bill for charges above the approved amount, a practice called *balance billing*. Therefore, the physician cannot be compensated for the difference between the approved amount and the full fee.

Pages: 1629, 1630

9: *Gross charges* refers to:

A. Full value of the physician's professional services minus expenses

B. Full value of the physician's services despite any adjustments to charges, such as professional courtesies, discounts, or contractual adjustments

C. Full value of the physician's professional services minus professional courtesies, discounts, or contractual adjustments

D. Total charges with deductions for Medicare discounts

E. Total charges excluding co-pays for HMO patients

Answer: B

Critique: *Gross charges* refers to the full value of a family physician's professional services, despite any adjustments such as professional courtesies, discounts, or contractual adjustments that might reduce the amount billed.

Page: 1631

10: Which of the following ratios refers to how much the family physician is discounting fees:

A. Gross charges

B. Collection ratio

C. Contractual adjustments ratio

D. Courtesies and discounts ratio

E. Bad debts ratio

Answer: D

Critique: The courtesies and discounts ratio is determined by dividing the total of the courtesies and discounts by the gross charges.

Page: 1631

11: (True or False) The accounts receivable ratio = total accounts receivable/average monthly gross charges is acceptable if it is as high as 2.5.

Answer: True

Critique: Although the accounts receivable ratio is acceptable up to as high as 2.5, below 2.0 is preferred.

Page: 1631

12: The following service produces patient bills and insurance claims and identifies and produces collection tools for delinquent accounts:

A. Batch processing service bureau

B. Time-sharing service bureau

C. Billing service

D. In-house computing system

E. All of the above

Answer: E

Critique: All of the billing services mentioned produce patient bills and insurance claims and identify and produce collection tools for delinquent accounts. Each differs in the services provided to a practice, with differing benefits and disadvantages.

Pages: 1632, 1633

13: Pegboard accounting systems:

A. Are expensive, difficult to operate, and inefficient

B. Are well-suited to large practices with many accounts

C. Require a computer system to operate

D. Have many transcription errors

E. Are well-suited to small practices with few unpaid accounts

Answer: E

Critique: Pegboard systems are manual systems that have good controls and virtually eliminate transcription errors. These systems may be used successfully in small practices with few unpaid balances.

Page: 1632

Chapter 66

Clinical Informatics in Office Practice

Michael D. Hagen

1: Ways in which electronic medical records (EMRs) can potentially improve clinical productivity include all of the following, except:

    A. They facilitate simultaneous access for multiple users.

    B. They provide means to search for and display information in multiple formats.

    C. They can provide ready access to laboratory and test results.

    D. They can eliminate the need for staff training in record maintenance.

Answer: D

Critique: Electronic medical records have the potential to address many of the shortcomings inherent in paper records. They can provide simultaneous access for multiple users who might need to use the record during a patient's visit. Searching for and displaying information are greatly enhanced compared with the hand-searching methods necessary for paper records. Through links to other databases, the EMR can provide immediate access to laboratory and test results. Although the EMR can improve productivity, systematic prospective training for all users is necessary to limit inevitable productivity losses during an EMR's introduction.

Pages: 1635, 1640

2: Compared with paper records, which of the following statements best describes the impact of an EMR:

    A. The cost for paper supplies is increased.

    B. The initial costs can be high compared to those for paper records.

    C. Storage space costs increase.

    D. Costs for personnel increase.

Answer: B

Critique: A properly chosen and implemented EMR system should decrease total paper, storage space, and personnel costs. However, initial outlays can be high compared with those for paper records; ongoing maintenance costs are relatively modest. Computer hard drive storage typically costs $0.02 per megabyte, which is less than the cost for storing similar information in paper format.

Pages: 1635, 1636

3: (True or False) Which of the following represent ways in which EMRs can facilitate clinical quality improvement:

    A. EMRs can incorporate context-appropriate reminders for preventive services.

    B. EMRs can facilitate the maintenance of accurate problem lists.

    C. EMRs can incorporate practice guideline and decision-support information.

    D. EMRs can provide access to drug-interaction and prescribing information.

Answers: A - True, B - True, C - True, D - True

Critique: EMRs can potentially foster quality improvement in multiple ways. They can provide service reminders for preventive services keyed to diagnosis, age, gender, or whatever parameters are appropriate to the context. They also provide easy access to problem lists for single-entry maintenance and can provide information from practice guidelines and decision-support algorithms. They also can limit prescribing errors by providing information regarding drug interactions and patient-specific drug allergies.

Pages: 1635, 1636

4: Selecting an EMR system involves several steps. Which of the following represents the first step in selecting an EMR:

    A. Contact vendors and request written information and system demonstration disks.

    B. Arrange with a vendor for a system demonstration.

    C. Define the goals the practice hopes to achieve with an EMR.

    D. Request proposals from several vendors.

Answer: C

Critique: The first step in selecting an EMR should entail defining the goals the practice would like to achieve with such a system. These goals and objectives should be identified before seeking out and contacting vendors.

Page: 1636

5: (True or False) Typical motivations for moving to an EMR system include which of the following:

  A. Reduction of required chart storage space
  B. Improvement in chart documentation and legibility
  C. Improved access to records from multiple sites
  D. Limiting misplacement of physical patient records

Answers: A - True, B - True, C - True, D - True

Critique: EMRs can potentially reduce physical space required for record storage and limit physically lost records. They also can provide chart access from multiple practice sites and certainly improve legibility and documentation compared to a handwritten paper record.

Pages: 1636, 1637

6: (True or False) Data elements that should be included in an acceptable EMR include which of the following:

  A. Problem lists
  B. Visit notes
  C. Medication lists
  D. Medical history
  E. Laboratory data

Answers: A - True, B - True, C - True, D - True, E -True

Critique: In assessing the suitability of a particular vendor's EMR software, the clinician should look for several general features. The EMR should have data elements that include patient identifiers, activity status in the practice, medical history, social and family history, risk factors, problem lists, visit notes, medication lists, correspondence, and laboratory data. The EMR also should include the ability to import reports such as hospital discharge summaries and consultants' letters.

Page: 1637

7: (True or False) An acceptable EMR system should include a summary screen that includes which of the following elements:

  A. Copies of correspondence from consultants
  B. An up-to-date problem list
  C. An up-to-date medication list
  D. A list of the patient's known allergies
  E. A list of needed preventive services

Answers: A - False, B - True, C - True, D - True, E - True

Critique: The EMR should provide a summary screen that includes a problem list, medications, known allergies, and preventive services the patient should undergo. Although the EMR should provide access to reports from consultants, these are not included in a summary screen.

Page: 1637

8: (True or False) EMR should provide links to other data sources that might not be available in the provider's office. These data sources should include which of the following:

  A. Laboratory data
  B. Radiology reports
  C. Pathology and other diagnostic test results
  D. Hospital discharge summaries

Answers: A - True, B - True, C - True, D - True

Critique: The EMR should provide links to other information sources so that the provider can access needed reports without necessarily maintaining redundant copies. Examples of such information include laboratory results, radiology reports, diagnostic test and pathology reports, and hospital discharge summaries.

Page: 1637

9: Security measures for EMR systems should include all of the following, except:

  A. Automatic log-outs should occur when an individual station remains unused for a specified period.
  B. The record system should include an audit trail of all access to patient records.
  C. The EMR should have a permanent password for each user.
  D. The EMR should restrict entry of data elements to authorized users only.

Answer: C

Critique: EMRs require multiple levels of security to ensure confidentiality of patient information. The system should log-out individual terminals that remain unused for a specified period. Additionally, the EMR system should maintain a record of all instances of access to patient-specific information and should restrict data entry to only authorized individuals. The system should allow regular, periodic changes of passwords.

Page: 1637

10: An EMR system should provide analytical functions to facilitate patient care. Examples of such functions include all of the following, except:

  A. Patient visit progress notes
  B. Diagnostic decision-support algorithms
  C. Reminder systems for prospective preventive services
  D. Statistical algorithms for defining abnormal clinical variables

Answer: A

Critique: EMR systems provide the potential for functionality beyond simple recording of progress notes and correspondence. These systems should include support systems for therapeutic and diagnostic decision making. They also should include functions to provide timely reminders for ongoing preventive health services. The EMR also should provide facilities for generating graphical reports, such as time-series graphs and statistical process control charts.

Page: 1637

11: (True or False) An EMR system should provide analytical tools, such as statistical process control charts, to facilitate interpretation of data that vary over time. Figure 66-A displays a typical statistical process control chart for a series of blood glucose measurements obtained over time. True statements regarding this process include which of the following:

A. The process appears to be in statistical control.
B. The average blood glucose is approximately 200 mg/%.
C. The upper control limit is approximately 270 mg/%.
D. The lower control limit is approximately 66 mg/%.

Answers: A - True, B - False, C - True, D - True

Critique: Statistical process control charts can provide a visual overview of whether or not a process appears to be operating within acceptable limits. Typically, the upper and lower control limits are established at the average + or − 3σ, or 3 standard deviations. In this case, the average is approximately 166, the upper control limit is about 270, and the lower control limit is about 63 mg/%. The 3σ value is used in industry and may not be appropriate for medical processes. The upper and lower control limits can be established as appropriate for the context. For example, blood sugar value limits clearly need to be more restrictive.

Page: 1637

12: (True or False) An acceptable EMR system should include order-entry capabilities for which of the following options:

A. Therapeutic interventions appropriate for the practice
B. Standard order sets for specific conditions
C. Access to information regarding test cost and insurance coverage
D. Linkage to electronic versions of appropriate practice guidelines to facilitate order selection

Answers: A - True, B - True, C - True, D - True

Critique: The EMR system selected for a practice should include order-entry capabilities appropriate for the providers and their practice style. These features should include order entry for therapeutic interventions appropriate to the practice and standard order sets for specific conditions (e.g., a metabolic panel for hypertensive patients). The system also should provide access to test cost information and whether or not a particular intervention is covered by the patient's insurance carrier. The EMR also should provide links to appropriate practice guidelines.

Page: 1638

13: EMR systems should facilitate rather than complicate data entry. Capabilities that can optimize data entry include all of the following, except:

A. Typing of free-form text directly into the record
B. Preformatted progress note templates
C. "Pick lists" for common responses encountered in creating a progress note
D. Merging of appropriate pre-existing data from other parts of the record into the progress note

Answer: A

Critique: An EMR system should possess a number of options for data entry. Preformatted progress note templates can greatly streamline documentation of patient visits. Pick lists of common responses also facilitate creating the progress note. If relevant data (e.g., interventions entered in the order-entry module of the system) reside in other parts of the record, the system should automatically incorporate this information into the progress note. Free-form typing should be minimized as a data-entry option.

Pages: 1638, 1639

14: Considerations in the final selection process for an EMR system should include all of the following, except:

A. Site visits to offices that already have installed and use the system

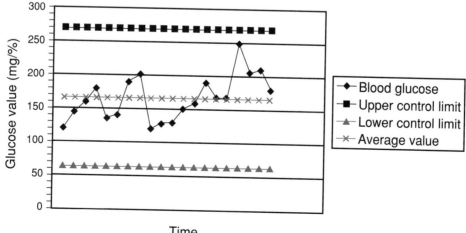

Run Chart for Blood Glucose

Figure 66–A

B. Assessment of ongoing user support
C. Hardware and software requirements for running the system
D. The decision for purchase should rely on the physicians' opinions alone
E. The financial stability of the system vendor

Answer: D

Critique: In making the final decision regarding purchase of an EMR system, the potential purchaser should make site visits to offices and institutions that have already installed and use the proposed systems. The purchaser also should assess ongoing user support by the vendor, the essential hardware and supporting software (e.g., operating systems such as Windows NT or Linux) necessary to run the system, and the financial stability of the vendor. Representatives of all the major users, not just physicians, should be involved in the final selection process.

Pages: 1639, 1640

15: To prevent data loss, an EMR system should have several levels of backup capability, including redundant hard drives and tape backup systems. Which of the following statements is correct regarding the required storage capacity of a tape backup system:

A. The tape system should possess storage capacity greater than that of the hard drive to be backed up.
B. The tape system should possess storage capacity equal to that of the hard drive to be backed up.
C. The tape system can possess storage capacity less than that of the hard drive to be backed up.
D. The tape system's capacity bears no relation to that of the hard drive to be backed up.

Answer: A

Critique: Any EMR system requires redundant backup systems to protect against loss of data. The hardware should include redundant hard drives to guard against data loss from hard drive crashes. Additionally, the system should include a tape backup system that possesses storage capacity greater than that of the hard drives to be backed up.

Page: 1640

16: (True or False) Additional electronic resources can enhance the usefulness of an EMR system. Electronic references, continuing and patient education systems, and diagnostic support packages represent examples of such applications. Which of the following are diagnostic support systems:

A. Iliad
B. Genrx
C. Diagnosis Pro
D. QMR

Answers: A - True, B - False, C - True, D - True

Critique: Several electronic diagnostic support systems are available. Iliad (A.D.A.M. Software, Atlanta, GA: www.adam.com), Diagnosis Pro (Medtech USA, Los Angeles, CA; www.medtech.com), and QMR (First Data Bank, San Bruno, CA; www.firstdatabank.com) are all diagnostic decision support systems. Genrx (Mosby, Inc., St. Louis, MO; www.mosby.com) is a drug-drug interaction system.

Page: 1641

17: (True or False) Electronic mail (e-mail) can enhance the physician-patient interaction but should be conducted according to established procedures. Appropriate subjects for e-mail correspondence with patients include which of the following:

A. Scheduling appointments
B. Sharing of patient education materials
C. Possible emergency situations
D. Discussion of human immunodeficiency virus (HIV) test results
E. Requests for prescription refills

Answers: A - True, B - True, C - False, D - False, E - True

Critique: E-mail can enhance the efficiency of mundane tasks such as refilling prescriptions, forwarding patient education materials, and scheduling appointments. However, e-mail should not be used for conveying sensitive, confidential patient information such as HIV test results. Additionally, possible emergency situations should not be handled via e-mail. The American Medical Informatics Association (www.amia.org) has published guidelines for the clinical use of e-mail. Family physicians who intend to communicate with their patients via e-mail should consider acquiring and reading this useful document.

Page: 1642

18: An EMR system must provide facilities for free-form text entry. Options for entry include dictation and transcription, voice recognition, and typing. Currently available voice-recognition systems demonstrate insufficient accuracy to support clinical use. What level of accuracy will voice-recognition systems need to achieve to become widely adopted in clinical practice:

A. 90%
B. 93%
C. 95%
D. 99%

Answer: D

Critique: Currently available voice-recognition systems have improved markedly but still demonstrate 4% to 10% error rates. These systems must achieve 99% or greater accuracy before they will be widely adopted in medical contexts.

Pages: 1639, 1645

Chapter 67

Risk Management

Dennis LaRavia

1: The physician has the duty to exercise reasonable care when providing advice and treatment to a patient. That duty exists only when a physician-patient relationship has been established. Physicians have the right to decide for whom they will provide professional services. Limits of appropriate physician-patient relationships may include several scenarios as determined by the courts. All of the following statements are true, except:

A. A physician is expected to provide continuity of care to his or her existing patients.
B. A physician is obligated to treat all comers in an emergency room setting for which the local general hospital has advertised its emergency room services.
C. A physician may be legally liable for "curbside advice" he or she gives another physician when the information appears in the medical record after their discussion.
D. A physician acting in the capacity of medical director for a managed care organization will not be held liable in his or her medical treatment determinations because he or she has no direct care relationship with patients.

Answer: D

Critique: A physician may not abandon an existing patient. The physician may terminate care if he or she provides alternative and equivalent coverage until the patient can arrange to have another physician-patient relationship (usually 30 days is reasonable). Even though a patient has not been seen before by a physician, when that physician is working in an emergency department for which services are advertised, that physician is obligated to treat the patient. When a physician offers advice over the telephone or in person to a colleague, a physician-patient relationship may be in effect when this advice finds its way into the medical record. Certain jurisdictions have concluded that a physician-patient relationship does exist for a medical director of a managed care organization, because he or she is making determinations that directly affect management of the patient.

Page: 1646

2: Breach of duty is another element of negligence with which physicians must be familiar. This is commonly referred to as "standard of care." Which of the following statements about "standard of care" is incorrect:

A. The adequacy of the physician's performance is determined by a lay jury composed of people without medical expertise or by a judge.
B. A plaintiff attorney usually will not proceed in a malpractice suit without having an expert witness to testify on behalf of the patient.
C. Standard of care is usually accepted in today's courts as medical practice "quality of care" in the physician's particular locale and specialty.
D. A physician is expected to perform at a level similar to that of an average, not necessarily the best, physician.
E. A physician may be measured by the standard, "Would a reasonable physician have referred this particular patient?"

Answer: C

Critique: The adequacy of a physician's performance is not determined by a group of peers, but by a judge or laypeople with no medical expertise. Expert witnesses are usually a prerequisite for both the defense and plaintiff sides of the issue, but they are not difficult to obtain as a rule because of the wide range of opinions of physicians. "Standard of care" is defined as the degree of skill, care, and the average physician would exercise in the same or a similar circumstance and on the basis of the state of medical knowledge at the time. A growing number of jurisdictions hold physicians to a national standard of care that is not related to locale or specialty. Currently, a physician defendant usually is measured against whether a reasonable physician would have managed the patient problem in a similar manner and whether he or she would have referred the patient with the problem in question.

Page: 1647

3: In a malpractice suit, the plaintiff must prove that damages (an injury or loss) resulted from the physician's negligence. Which of the following statements best describes damages as an element in proving negligence in a malpractice suit:

A. Most plaintiffs do not have obvious injuries.
B. Obtaining adequate informed consent is not an important consideration.
C. An emerging trend by plaintiff lawyers is the allegation that the plaintiff has suffered a "loss of chance" because of the lack of a timely diagnosis.
D. A physician has the sole responsibility for making the right decisions about treatment options.
E. Frivolous claims by plaintiffs for trivial injuries very commonly result in malpractice suits.

Answer: C

Critique: Most plaintiffs do have obvious injuries, and frivolous claims for trivial injuries are uncommon. Some cases award damages where no medical negligence is found but the physician failed to obtain adequate informed consent from the patient or guardian. A physician must determine how much information to give a patient and ensure that treatment decisions are made jointly with the patient throughout treatment and that the medical record clearly shows that shared decision making occurred. Legal trends have supported the concept that even if a diagnosis is made eventually that this "loss of chance" by not having an earlier diagnosis often produces a lesser likelihood of survival and thereby constitutes an injury.

Page: 1647

4: The fourth element that a plaintiff must prove is that the negligent performance of the physician was the proximate cause of the patient's injury. Select the single best answer in regard to proximate cause as an element in proving negligence against a physician:

    A. Even if the injury to the patient would not have occurred except for the negligence of the physician, this is not conclusive evidence to prove proximate cause.
    B. Even if several causes resulted in the injury to the patient, if the physician's error was a substantial factor in the injury, then his or her negligence may be deemed as the "cause in fact," thereby implicating the physician as negligent.
    C. Some acts, such as a hemostat left in the abdomen, are called *res ipsa loquitur* (the thing speaks for itself) and still require an expert witness to affirm negligence on the part of the defendant.
    D. When a physician defendant fails to make an early diagnosis, even in a patient with a poor prognosis, then it is generally conceded that proximate cause has been satisfied and the physician is deemed negligent.
    E. The burden of proof always falls on the plaintiff to confirm guilt of the defendant, even in a *res ipsa loquitur* case such as operating on the wrong leg.

Answer: B

Critique: The plaintiff must first show that the physician's negligence was the "cause in fact" of the alleged injury. Two formulas can be used to demonstrate cause in fact: (1) "but for"—the injury would not have occurred but for the negligence, and (2) "substantial factor"—when several possible causes exist and the physician's error was a substantial factor in the resultant injury. Once cause in fact has been proved, the plaintiff must prove that the defendant's mistake was so closely connected in time and space and of such significance that legal liability should be imposed (proximate cause). With certain acts, the negligence and causation are so obvious that a lay jury is deemed able to make that determination. The doctrine of *res ipsa loquitur* is invoked, and no expert testimony is required. The burden of proof in this case shifts to the defendant to show mitigating circumstances to avoid liability. Proximate cause becomes a more elusive concept, however, when the patient's original prognosis was poor. Traditionally, the patient could not prevail on the causation question unless the prenegligence odds for survival were more likely than not. More recently, some courts have found that a delay of weeks or months in diagnosis may have caused a "loss of chance," which may be compensable. The concept of delay in diagnosis in a patient with a poor prognosis, therefore, is still unsettled regarding predictable outcome on the question of negligence.

Pages: 1647, 1648

5: Education of our public, the patients we take care of, is a challenging goal for us in this age of technology. Which of the following statements is most correct regarding public education by physicians:

    A. Unrealistic patient expectations may lead to patient dissatisfaction, but they are not commonly seen as a causative agent in medical malpractice lawsuits.
    B. Information technology (e.g., from the Internet) affords the public easy, almost always accurate access to sources of information that may affect the physician in his or her choice of treatments.
    C. The modern physician does not have the opportunity or obligation to give an appropriate interpretation and perspective on the information a patient obtains from the Internet before he or she advises the patient on an exact course of treatment.
    D. In the final analysis, the patient expects his or her physician to decide on the correct treatment without the patient's involvement in the discussion or decision-making process.
    E. Unrealistic expectations of patients may often result from hospital advertising that extols state-of-the-art medical care, emergency equipment, birthing suites, and so on to obtain more patient attraction to the facility.

Answer: E

Critique: Unrealistic patient expectations not only lead to patient dissatisfaction, but also are a common thread in all medical malpractice lawsuits. Information technology affords often easy access to sources of information for patients, but the information is often inaccurate and inappropriately interpreted. A physician cannot control the sources of information a patient heeds outside his or her office, but the physician does have the obligation and opportunity to put this information into perspective for the patient. Most patients expect to take part in the discussions and decision making about their own care. Hospitals, in their effort to maintain a strong financial position, frequently help to produce unrealistic expectations among patients by promoting their emergency equipment, cardiovascular suites, birthing suites, and so forth as the best available in medicine.

Page: 1648

6: (True or False) Professional education continues to play an important part in keeping physicians at their best. Determine whether the following statements regarding professional education are true or false:

    A. Reading medical literature is a primary means of staying current in today's fast paced field of medicine.

    B. Risk reduction methods, such as helping patients to set reasonable treatment goals, are usually not effective in reducing unfavorable outcomes.

    C. In the event of a malpractice suit, it is the responsibility of the defendant's lawyer to guide the defense case and make sure that the physician is ready to testify in his behalf.

    D. Continuing to hone medical skills is not extremely important for an already accomplished and experienced physician.

    E. The defendant physician should leave nothing to chance in a malpractice case but should make every effort to educate himself or herself and counsel on appropriate medical knowledge and changing theories of medical negligence.

Answers: A - True, B - False, C - False, D - False, E - True

Critique: Keeping up-to-date with current medical literature, maintaining clinical skills, and staying current on practice risk-reduction techniques are all helpful elements in the maintenance of top-notch professional education. The education of patients is an important tool to help them set reasonable treatment goals. In the event of malpractice claims, it is the physician's responsibility, not the defense counsel's alone, to actively participate in his or her own defense, including efforts to help defense counsel stay current with recent advances in medical knowledge and evolving theories of medical negligence.

Page: 1648

7: (True or False) Enterprise liability has been proposed as an alternative to the current accountability process in professional malpractice. Determine whether the following statements about enterprise liability are true or false:

    A. In this philosophy, the emphasis shifts from the individual physician to all those involved in the delivery of care.

    B. Enterprise liability does not undermine professional autonomy.

    C. Enterprise liability diffuses accountability on an individual basis.

    D. It is likely that this concept would decrease medical costs if it becomes a reality.

    E. Enterprise liability may significantly undermine professional judgment.

Answers: A - True, B - False, C - True, D - False, D - True

Critique: Enterprise liability holds the entire organization, or enterprise, responsible for the care received by a patient, rather than focusing on an individual caregiver. The criticism of this concept is that it undermines professional autonomy and judgment, diffuses accountability, and could ultimately increase medical costs.

Page: 1648

8: (True or False) A "no-fault" system has also been proposed as a replacement for our current professional malpractice system. A modification of the no-fault system would establish accelerated compensation events (ACEs). Decide whether the following statements about ACEs are true or false:

    A. ACEs represent predefined classes of medical injuries that do not normally occur when patients receive good care.

    B. A benefit of an ACE system is that widespread and fair compensation of injured patients would be the rule, rather than the exception.

    C. A problem of the ACE system would be less effective deterrence of poor quality by the system of care.

    D. An ACE system would encourage a reduction in defensive medicine.

    E. An ACE system would likely deteriorate the framework of outcomes-based research.

Answers: A - True, B - True, C - False, D - True, E - False

Critique: ACEs do represent predefined classes of medical injuries that do not normally occur when patients receive good care. The putative benefits of an ACE system would be more widespread and fair compensation of injured patients, more effective deterrence of poor quality by the system of care, a reduction in defensive medicine, standardization of medical expertise about injuries, an opportunity to strengthen the physician-patient relationship, establishment of a framework for outcomes research, and greater confidence in the accuracy and fairness of malpractice determinations.

Page: 1648

9: (True or False) A malpractice lawsuit is a dreaded event in the life of most physicians. Determine whether the following statements about the measures that can be taken to avoid malpractice suits are true or false:

    A. Malpractice suits are less common among physicians who stay focused on individual patient needs.

    B. Risk prevention practices have seldom been helpful in reducing malpractice suits.

    C. Outcomes-based research with appropriate changes in clinical practice may be one of the most reliable methods to reduce malpractice claims

    D. Maintaining a sense of partnership and good communication is usually not helpful in reducing malpractice claims.

    E. Historically, practicing defensively is more reliable than practicing quality of care in diminishing the likelihood of malpractice suits.

Answers: A - True, B - False, C - True, D - False, E - False

Critique: The avoidance of a malpractice suit is best accomplished by a physician who stays focused on individual patient needs; keeps current with changing medical science, including risk prevention practices; continually applies scientifically validated standards of care; and maintains a sense of partnership and communication with the patient. Keeping the focus on quality care is ultimately more effective than practicing defensively to avoid a lawsuit.

Page: 1649

10: Many variables have to be considered when choosing methods for the evaluation and improvement of process and outcome of medical care. Which of the following statements reflects a reliable approach in promoting quality medical care in our society:

    A. The reporting of all incidents or unexpected outcomes, with or without injury, involving a patient is the single most important element in producing quality medical care.

    B. Routine generic outcome screens are unreliable as an indicator of unfavorable patient outcomes.

    C. More watchdog agencies, including the federal government, managed care organizations, and other third-party payers, would definitely improve the quality of care provided by physicians.

    D. Regardless of the approach used, physicians should view the process of ongoing review of the quality of their care and appropriate adjustments in their practice techniques as the key features of good medical practice.

    E. The essential elements for evaluating quality of care are the process the physician used, the outcome achieved, the quality of the medical record, and the opinions of other physicians in the community.

Answer: D

Critique: Several methods for evaluating and improving the process and outcome of medical care have been developed, including incident reporting systems, generic outcome screens, and clinical indicators. In addition to health care organizations, other entities such as third-party payers, the federal government, and managed care organizations are increasingly interested in quality-of-care information. Several elements must be considered when evaluating quality of care: the process the physician used, the quality of the medical record, the use of a consistent and logical approach with each patient, and the patient's satisfaction with the care provided. Regardless of the approach used, physicians should view the process of ongoing review of the quality of their care as a necessary part of good medical practice.

Page: 1649

11: Risk management, loss prevention, and quality improvement are interrelated in the reduction of malpractice lawsuits and of patient injuries in the medical system. Which of the following statements regarding this area of discussion in medical malpractice is correct:

    A. The main purpose of risk management is to improve care while monitoring or reducing costs.

    B. It is important to remember that most malpractice suits begin with a poor result, and not necessarily an unhappy patient.

    C. It is difficult, but not impossible, for patients to sue physicians they like.

    D. Quality improvement focuses on the protection of the financial assets of an organization through strategies to prevent and control patient injuries.

    E. Physicians who spend more time with their patients per visit and display genuine interest in their patients derive more enjoyment from their practice but have no significant reduction in the number of malpractice claims as compared with physicians who spend shorter times with their patients.

Answer: C

Critique: Risk management and loss prevention are efforts to protect the financial assets of an organization through strategies to prevent and control patient injuries, malpractice claims, and malpractice claim losses. On the other hand, quality improvement activities are not created for the purpose of asset protection; they are usually intended to improve care while monitoring or reducing costs. The common ground between risk management and quality improvement is the use of credible data to analyze outcomes and improve practice patterns. It is important to keep in mind that a malpractice suit begins with an unhappy patient. It is difficult, but not impossible, for patients to sue physicians they like. Physicians who spend more time with their patients per visit and display genuine interest in their patients have fewer claims filed against them.

Page: 1649

12: Over the last 15 years, several trends have remained fairly constant in allegations in the field of family medicine. Which of the following statements is correct:

    A. Diabetes and pregnancy are among the top three patient conditions producing claims over the last 15 years in general and family practice.

    B. Family physicians who provide maternity care services have a lower risk of a lawsuit and higher practice satisfaction than do family physicians who do not deliver babies.

    C. Family physicians are least often sued for failure to diagnose common and serious conditions that may initially have nonspecific signs and symptoms.

    D. Educating patients about the significance of important signs and symptoms has promoted earlier detection of medical problems but has not reduced the number of malpractice claims.

    E. More women die of breast cancer than of lung cancer, and more women fear breast cancer than lung cancer.

Answer: B

Critique: According to Table 67-2, diabetes and pregnancy are among the top 10 conditions resulting in claims over the last 15 years, but rank as numbers 7 and 9 and are not among the top three patient conditions. There is evidence that family physicians who provide maternity care services have a lower risk of a lawsuit and higher practice satisfaction than do family physicians who do not deliver babies. Family physicians are most often sued for failure to diagnose common and serious conditions that initially may have nonspecific signs and symptoms and, as a result, may be difficult to diagnose early. Educating patients regarding the significance of important signs and symptoms can promote earlier detection, better treatment, and fewer poor outcomes. Although more women die of lung cancer than of breast cancer, breast cancer is more feared by women and more likely to result in suit for delay in diagnosis.

Pages: 1650–1651

13: (True or False) There are some common pitfalls in the practice of family and general medicine. Determine whether the following statements are true or false:

A. Negative physical examination and negative mammography in a 45-year-old female are adequate more than 95% of the time to assure the patient that there is no cancer or underlying pathology.
B. Negative electrocardiograms coupled with negative cardiac enzyme test results are more than 98% reliable in ruling out a myocardial infarction.
C. Attributing rectal bleeding to hemorrhoids in a patient older than 40 years without doing a proper colon examination is considered poor clinical judgment.
D. Failure to obtain an arterial blood gas study in a suspected pulmonary embolus may be considered a judgment error.
E. Failure to take a chest radiograph in an "at-risk" patient, such as a cigarette smoker or someone with "persistent pneumonia," is deemed a clinical judgment error.

Answers: A - False, B - False, C - True, D -True, E - True

Critique: Overreliance on negative mammography, which has a false-negative rate as high as 20%, can pose substantial liability risks. It is important to establish a follow-up plan to ensure that persisting symptoms are further pursued, that a second opinion is considered, or that another diagnostic test is considered. Other common pitfalls include excessive reliance on falsely negative electrocardiograms or cardiac enzyme test results in the evaluation of chest pain; failure to recognize pulmonary emboli by neglecting to obtain an arterial blood gas study; delayed surgical response for appendicitis; attributing rectal bleeding to hemorrhoids in a patient older than 40 years, when bowel cancer must first be ruled out; and failure to document chest radiograph clearing in an at-risk patient, such as a smoker or a patient with "persistent pneumonia."

Pages: 1650, 1651

14: Medication errors are a common issue in malpractice claims. Off the following statements, which best addresses medications and issues surrounding the use of medications:

A. It is not considered inappropriate in an office practice to have a penicillin allergic reaction in a patient when the physician did not know that the patient was allergic to penicillin.
B. Monitoring prothrombin times and INR values is not necessary in a stable patient with no bleeding problems and no recent changes in medications.
C. Documentation of over-the-counter (OTC) preparations, vitamins, and herbal medicines is equally important as tight maintenance of continuing prescription medications.
D. The use and management of psychoactive medications is relatively straightforward and requires no special management tools to prevent user injury.
E. Using new medications in a patient with no prior history of usage of the specific drug does not raise particular concern in the patient or the physician.

Answer: C

Critique: The continuing release of new medications; the similarity of names and packaging of many medications; the interactions that may occur with other medications, including OTC preparations; and the increasing popularity of alternative or vitamin therapy all pose risks of medication-related adverse events. Anticoagulant, psychoactive, and cardiovascular drugs top the list of medicines that create a risk of injury and liability. Monitoring, as appropriate, of prothrombin times, medication checks, and electrolyte values, respectively, can reduce these risks. Asking about and documenting the current medicines being used by the patient, including OTC preparations and herbal or vitamin products, can reduce the risk of adverse drug interactions. Patient allergies to medications should be noted before each instance of prescribing.

Page: 1651

15: (True or False) Fracture management has its own set of peculiarities. Determine whether the following statements are true of false:

A. A "sprained wrist" may require immobilization for 1 to 2 weeks to ensure that there is no fracture of the navicular bone.
B. Cervical spine radiographs can always be definitively read acutely in the emergency department to confirm a fracture, with appropriate consultation.
C. Femoral head injuries can be difficult to interpret acutely in an elderly female post–acute injury.
D. Soft-tissue injuries seldom require exploration or radiographs before suturing and treating definitively.
E. Evaluation of popliteal injuries requires only distal circulation documentation at the time of the injury.

Answers: A - True, B - False, C - True, D - False, E - False

Critique: Fracture management can prove vexing; this is especially true of fractures involving the carpal navicular, cervical spine, and femoral head. For example, a "sprained wrist" may require continued immobilization in a thumb spica cast, along with follow-up radiographs in 1 to 2 weeks, until a navicular fracture can be definitely ruled out. Other imaging studies, such as computed tomography, may be needed to resolve the question of a cervical spine or femoral head fracture. Soft-tissue injuries should be evaluated for possible foreign bodies, infection, or compartment syndrome. Evaluation of popliteal fossa injuries should include documentation of intact distal circulation and neurologic function.

Page: 1651

16: Scope of practice and practice environment have continued to be in a state of change over the last few years. Which of the following statements is correct:

- A. When a physician chooses to be an employee of a hospital or other organization, he or she does not have the same responsibility as a self-employed physician to provide professional guidance and advocacy for the patient.
- B. No matter what agreements a physician may sign, he or she continues to have an obligation to advocate for patients and good patient care.
- C. Training, experience, and demonstrated competence are no longer legal determinants for deciding who performs certain specialized services in today's practice environment.
- D. Contractual requirements remove the physician from the responsibilities of the past to advocate for the patient in the event that a health plan declines coverage for the care needed.
- E. Employed physicians do not have to adhere to practice guidelines, specific processes for admitting patients to a hospital, or use of specific facilities simply because they are hired physicians and have signed compliance contracts.

Answer: B

Critique: Physicians increasingly are choosing employment status, which does not relieve them of their independent professional duty to their patients. Physicians may be required to sign contracts with third-party payers that specify adherence to referral guidelines, specific processes for admitting patients to a hospital, use of specific facilities and specific practitioners, and procedures for emergency department use. The physician has a continued obligation to advocate for patients and good patient care. Training, experience, and demonstrated competence are the legal criteria against which requests to perform certain services should be measured. Regardless of contractual requirements, physicians retain the responsibility to provide patients with their recommendations for most appropriate care and to advocate for the patient in the event that a health plan declines coverage for that care.

Pages: 1651, 1652

17: The federal government and its array of regulatory agencies and legislation have produced another arena of concern for many physicians. Which of the following statements about agencies and federal legislation is correct:

- A. JCAHO, AAAHC, NCQA, OSHA, and HCFA are all federal agencies dedicated to the support and affirmation of the physician community.
- B. COBRA, or Consolidated Omnibus Budget Reconciliation Act, was primarily enacted to provide fluid transfer of commercially insured patients from private hospitals to public hospitals without complaint from the receiving hospital.
- C. OBRA, or Omnibus Reconciliation Act, was enacted to bolster COBRA and specifically requires that hospitals notify their patients of their rights to care and imposes stricter penalties for violations by physicians.
- D. EMTALA, the most recent federal legislation regarding patient dumping, states that a patient coming to an emergency department is entitled to a medical screening examination and appropriate treatment for stabilization, regardless of ability to pay, but specifically excludes women in the first stage of labor.
- E. HIPAA, or Healthcare Insurance Portability and Accountability Act, passed in 1998, was designed to provide (1) assurance that patients could move from one job to another and still have access to health insurance, and (2) assurance that private physicians would not be pursued for criminal penalties in Medicare miscoding.

Answer: C

Critique: Hospitals seek accreditation through the Joint Commission on Accreditation of Healthcare Organizations (JCAHO). Accrediting Association of Ambulatory Healthcare Centers (AAAHC) is an accrediting body for ambulatory care centers. A body that accredits health plans, especially managed care organizations, and conducts physician office reviews is the National Committee for Quality Assurance (NCQA). COBRA was signed into law in 1985 to prevent private hospitals from routinely diverting patients to public hospitals because of their inability to pay for services, a practice known as "dumping." OBRA requires that hospitals notify patients of their rights to care and imposes stricter penalties for violations. Physicians who violate the OBRA requirements can be fined up to $50,000 per violation. EMTALA requires that a patient coming to an emergency department be entitled to a medical screening examination and appropriate treatment for stabilization, regardless of the ability to pay and before any decision is made regarding discharge, transfer, or treatment. This requirement includes a woman in any stage of labor. HIPAA was designed to ensure that people moving from one job to another or from employment to unemployment are not denied access to health insurance because of an existing medical condition. The legislation also provides government agencies with more investigative funds and enforcement tools so that fraudulent activities are be identified and offenders are punished.

Page: 1652

18: Medicare coding for reimbursement is an area of great concern for the government and most practicing physicians. Which of the following statements is correct:

A. Coding for reimbursement is one of the areas that is most significantly affected by the government's aggressive efforts to ferret out crime.
B. Physicians are expected to code office visits and procedures accurately and have adequate documentation in the patient's chart to authenticate the code as submitted for reimbursement.
C. The rules for governing coding for reimbursement are complex and subject to interpretation.
D. In addition to civil penalties for fraudulent activities, a physician can be found guilty of criminal penalties, which can produce a loss of licensing but not incarceration.
E. When a medical practice is not large enough to have a compliance oversight individual, it is prudent to hire a consultant to assist in setting up a compliance program for coding.

Answer: D

Critique: Coding for reimbursement is one of the areas most significantly affected by the government's aggressive efforts to ferret out crime. It is the information submitted for reimbursement from the Medicare program that may pose the greatest liability risk. The rules governing coding for reimbursement are complex and subject to interpretation, so the potential for error is high. As a result, coding is one of the activities most targeted by governmental agencies. In addition to civil (money) penalties for fraudulent activities, a physician can also be found guilty of criminal fraud and be incarcerated. When a practice is not large enough to hire a dedicated compliance oversight individual, it would be wise to hire an outside consultant to assist in setting up this important system within the practice.

Pages: 1652, 1653

19: Patient expectations, office staff members, and perceptions about a physician's practice are very important in the overall management of communications and staff interchange with patients. Which of the following statements regarding this area of medical risk assessment is correct:

A. Patient brochures usually are not helpful in regard to the patient's perception of what to expect in the physician's practice.
B. The choice of reading material in the waiting room is usually not significant, because most patients do not have high expectations on the dating and variety of reading material in a physician's office.
C. Take-home materials for patients, when used as a reminder of instructions, have not been validated as very effective in improving physician-patient relationships.
D. Documentation of which patient information materials were given and retention of copies of those materials can be helpful years later should litigation result.
E. The patient's perception of a practice primarily includes the physician and the receptionist but not other staff members, such as laboratory technicians or billing clerks.

Answer: D

Critique: A patient's perception of the practice is important. A physician can influence perceptions by making information about the practice available, such as office hours, directions when an emergency occurs, and how on-call situations are handled. Many physicians provide this information to new patients through brochures, which can be a good way to manage patient expectations from the beginning of the physician-patient relationship. The choice of reading material in the waiting room can be significant; current periodicals suggest an up-to-date practice. Take-home materials for patients can remind patients of instructions that the physician has given for medications, when to call back, and similar issues. Documentation of which patient information materials were given and retention of copies of those materials can be helpful years later if litigation results. The patient's perception of a practice includes everyone, not just the physician: the receptionist, laboratory technicians, medical assistants, nurses, and billing clerks. If the physician or any of these people within the practice creates a negative impression with a patient, it may be difficult to overcome. Annual or semiannual competency testing for staff is helpful.

Page: 1653

20: (True or False) Other areas of potential medical malpractice include follow-up on tests, patient behavior, and medical records/documentation problems. Determine which of the following statements are true and which are false:

A. Systematic processing of laboratory results in an office practice is important, but not necessary to maintain proper control of interpretation of laboratory data before filing in a patient's chart.
B. When a patient misses an appointment, it is prudent to arrange a follow-up plan to determine the cause of the missed appointment and then to document the reason in the medical record.
C. It is important to remember that the patient does not own the medical record; the physician owns the physical record and the information it contains.
D. A patient's right to privacy is not likely to be compromised by facsimile transfers, photocopiers, and routine use of electronic records in the average medical office.
E. Written protocols for medical record documentation, including all forms of communication, are not necessary if the office has good personnel.

Answers: A - False, B - True, C - False, D - False, E - False

Critique: A systematic process can include instructing office staff that no follow-up information will be filed in a patient's record until it is seen and signed or initialed by the treating physician. Many malpractice allegations originate from abnormal test results that were not read or acted on by the treating physician. Regardless of the reason for a patient's missed appointment, the physician is best protected against legal liability by initiating a follow-up call to determine why the visit was missed. Documenting attempts at arranging follow-up in the record serves as evidence that a good-faith effort was made on the part of the physician, regardless of the patient's actions. It is important to remember that the physician owns the physical record but the patient owns the information. A patient's right to privacy can be compromised by the use of any of these communication methods (facsimile, photocopiers, and electronic records), particularly if little thought is given to protecting the information. An office should have written protocols for medical record documentation that include all forms of communication, and these protocols should address confidentiality and access.

Pages: 1653, 1654

21: Telephone communications and telemedicine breakthroughs have been blessings and challenges at the same time. Which of the following statements is correct:

    A. Documentation is important, of course, but the use of telephones and cell phones for callbacks and access to the physician by the patient precludes the need to document telephone calls with patients, particularly when using cell phones.

    B. Telemedicine, including (1) real-time use between physicians and between physician and patient and (2) store-and-forward consultations, is a useful tool in rural and remote areas and requires no particular consent of the patient in their use.

    C. The quality of this new state-of-the-art telemedicine equipment is exceptional and is so well rounded in value that no particular concern has to be paid to ensure satisfactory quality.

    D. Specific, written agreements may be constructed between sender and recipient that indicate how confidential patient information will be stored and secured.

    E. Telephone pads and dictation devices available at all telephone locations are relatively inexpensive but have not been of any particular benefit in improving documentation of patient calls.

Answer: D

Critique: Telephone conversations can be troublesome for a practice, especially conversations that do not become part of the documented medical record. Continuity of care can be compromised when these communications are lost. Telephone pads are inexpensive and should be available at any phone that a physician is likely to use in the care of patients. A small recorder for dictating notes can serve the same purpose. Telemedicine refers to providing health care consultation and education over telecommunication networks. Two

forms of telemedicine are acknowledged, including (1) real-time consultations between physician and patient or between two physicians, and (2) store-and-forward consultations, where the information is viewed at a later time. Telemedicine techniques can be a useful new tool, but clinicians must exercise reasonable caution to ensure appropriate use, including attention to informed consent and security issues. Certain liability issues are inherent in the use of telemedicine. The protection of patients' rights to privacy and confidentiality should be a particular concern. In addition to creating documented policies governing forms of electronic communication, a physician has the responsibility to verify the credentials and reliability of other parties involved. Specific, written agreements should be constructed between sender and recipient that indicate how confidential patient information will be stored and secured and under what circumstances it will be disclosed. Another concern is the quality of the equipment being used. When using store-and-forward communications for teleradiology, for example, it is important that the recipient's equipment provide a high-quality image so that decisions regarding care are made with the best information available.

Pages: 1654, 1655

22: (True or False) Liability issues may arise in the use of the Internet through e-mail, chat rooms, and Web sites. Determine whether the following statements are true or false:

    A. A physician should at least be familiar with the types of offerings on the Internet so that adequate assistance can be given to patients as they seek guidance about their medical problems and to help them recognize reputable sources.

    B. Web sites are fairly easy to set up and may be very helpful as a source of medical information to patients, with little or no medical liability.

    C. Chat rooms have become increasingly popular and provide an easy interchange with minimal likelihood of resulting in medical liability.

    D. Chat rooms are an excellent way to develop new patients and are recommended for new physicians who need to build up a patient clientele.

    E. In this modern technological era, electronic or telephone communication still cannot substitute for an office visit when a personal evaluation is needed.

Answers: A - True, B - False, C - False, D - False, E - True

Critique: A physician should be familiar with what is available to consumers over the Internet and assist patients in sorting out information that applies to their health care. Web sites are easy to set up but can be a source of liability. A physician who chooses to establish a Web site should be very clear at the outset regarding the purpose of that site. If medical advice is offered or if it appears that medical advice has been offered, the interaction could be characterized as one that occurs between a physician and patient and thereby establishes a physician-patient relationship, regardless of the intent of the physician. A physician approaching a chat room and considering communicating through this forum should think twice before doing so. The presence of two-way communication immediately raises the issue of a potential physician-patient relationship. It would be difficult, if not impossible, for a physician to participate in a chat group without giving advice, regardless of his or her intent. Although a new and enticing communication format, chat rooms are not recommended for inclusion in the practice of medicine. Electronic or telephone communication should not substitute for an office visit when an in-person assessment is needed.

Page: 1655

23: Informed consent is an everyday event in office and hospital practice for many physicians. Which of the following statements is correct:

A. Informed consent is a form to be signed and must be present to protect the physician, regardless of the verbal communication between the physician and patient.
B. All risks in regard to the procedure covered by the informed consent must be listed, including the uncommon and rare side effects of the procedure to be performed.
C. The physician should educate, inform, and assist the patient in making a correct decision regarding the proposed procedure and document the process as evidence that an informed decision occurred.
D. More serious procedures, such as allergy injections, antibiotic injections, steroid injections, minor surgical procedures, and the use of prescriptive medications, require not only a written informed consent but also a notary to witness the signature.
E. Billing complaints and personnel disagreements can usually be ignored in an office setting and do not necessarily need to be reported to the physician manager in a medical practice.

Answer: C

Critique: Informed consent is not a form to be signed—it is a process of communicating vital information between the patient and physician. Informed consent and refusal require that the patient's options and their outcomes be reviewed, concerns be addressed, and questions be answered. Not all risks must be listed, only those that are most common and significant. The process and results of the discussion must be documented. Ultimately, the physician has a twofold responsibility: to educate, inform, and assist the patient in making a decision regarding diagnosis or treatment and to document

that process as evidence that an informed decision occurred. A more formal process to obtain and document an informed decision should be considered for any recommended treatment or procedure that is more than minimally invasive or carries a risk of infection, anaphylaxis, excessive bleeding, or serious reaction. This definition includes allergy injections, antibiotic or steroid injections, minor surgical procedures, and a variety of prescriptive medications. A complaint of any type, whether a billing issue, personnel problem, or undesirable outcome, is an indication of patient dissatisfaction and can become a much larger problem if not handled effectively.

Page: 1656

24: The only guarantee for avoiding a medical malpractice suit is to avoid medical practice. A diligent physician can do only so much to avoid or diminish the likelihood of a malpractice allegation. Which of the following statements is correct:

A. Disagreements over patient care can be discussed appropriately verbally and documented in the patient record, generally without damaging your physician colleagues.
B. Nurse's notes are important and should be read regularly by the physician, but the physician should not discuss areas of disagreement in regard to a patient with the nurse in question.
C. Competence is determined by training, experience, and expertise, coupled with the physician's ability to perform at specific point in time.
D. The medical record is important, but malpractice cases are seldom lost by the defendant because of an inadequate record.
E. Practicing thoughtful, reflective medicine is helpful to the patient, but it is unlikely to reduce patient injury, dissatisfaction, and malpractice litigation.

Answer: C

Critique: Disagreements over patient care, or "jousting," should not be aired gratuitously in the medical record. Nurses' notes should be read, and when disagreements arise, they should be addressed. Physicians should perform only those services that they can provide competently. Competence is determined by training and expertise, as well as by the physician's ability to perform at that moment. Approximately one third of malpractice cases are lost because of an inadequate record. Practicing reflective medicine can reduce patient injury and dissatisfaction, and it can represent the best prophylaxis against malpractice litigation.

Page: 1656